SECOND EDITION

Geropsychiatric and Mental Health Nursing

Edited by

Karen Devereaux Melillo, PhD, GNP, ANP-BC, FAANP, FGSA
Professor, Chair
Department of Nursing
School of Health and Environment
University of Massachusetts Lowell
Lowell, Massachusetts

Susan Crocker Houde, PhD, ANP-BC
Professor, Associate Dean
School of Health and Environment
University of Massachusetts Lowell
Lowell, Massachusetts

JONES & BARTLETT
LEARNING

World Headquarters

Jones & Bartlett Learning
40 Tall Pine Drive
Sudbury, MA 01776
978-443-5000
info@jblearning.com
www.jblearning.com

Jones & Bartlett Learning Canada
6339 Ormindale Way
Mississauga, Ontario L5V 1J2
Canada

Jones & Bartlett Learning International
Barb House, Barb Mews
London W6 7PA
United Kingdom

Jones & Bartlett Learning books and products are available through most bookstores and online booksellers. To contact Jones & Bartlett Learning directly, call 800-832-0034, fax 978-443-8000, or visit our website, www.jblearning.com.

Substantial discounts on bulk quantities of Jones & Bartlett Learning publications are available to corporations, professional associations, and other qualified organizations. For details and specific discount information, contact the special sales department at Jones & Bartlett Learning via the above contact information or send an email to specialsales@jblearning.com.

The authors, editor, and publisher have made every effort to provide accurate information. However, they are not responsible for errors, omissions, or for any outcomes related to the use of the contents of this book and take no responsibility for the use of the products and procedures described. Treatments and side effects described in this book may not be applicable to all people; likewise, some people may require a dose or experience a side effect that is not described herein. Drugs and medical devices are discussed that may have limited availability controlled by the Food and Drug Administration (FDA) for use only in a research study or clinical trial. Research, clinical practice, and government regulations often change the accepted standard in this field. When consideration is being given to use of any drug in the clinical setting, the health care provider or reader is responsible for determining FDA status of the drug, reading the package insert, and reviewing prescribing information for the most up-to-date recommendations on dose, precautions, and contraindications, and determining the appropriate usage for the product. This is especially important in the case of drugs that are new or seldom used.

Production Credits

Publisher: Kevin Sullivan
Acquisitions Editor: Amy Sibley
Associate Editor: Patricia Donnelly
Editorial Assistant: Rachel Shuster
Associate Production Editor: Lisa Cerrone
Associate Marketing Manager: Katie Hennessy
V.P., Manufacturing and Inventory Control: Therese Connell
Composition: Arlene Apone
Cover Design: Kristin E. Parker
Cover Image: © Pavalache Stelian/Dreamstime.com
Printing and Binding: Malloy, Inc.
Cover Printing: Malloy, Inc.

Library of Congress Cataloging-in-Publication Data
Geropsychiatric and mental health nursing / [edited by] Karen Devereaux Melillo, Susan Crocker Houde. — 2nd ed.
   p. ; cm.
 Includes bibliographical references and index.
 ISBN 978-0-7637-7359-5 (pbk.)
 1. Geriatric psychiatry. 2. Geriatric nursing. 3. Psychiatric nursing. I. Melillo, Karen Devereaux. II. Houde, Susan Crocker.
 [DNLM: 1. Geriatric Nursing—methods. 2. Psychiatric Nursing—methods. 3. Aged. 4. Geriatric Psychiatry—methods. 5. Mental Disorders—nursing. WY 152]
 RC451.4.A5G479 2011
 618.97'689—dc22
                                                                                                2010026999
6048
Printed in the United States of America
14 13 12 11 10   10 9 8 7 6 5 4 3 2 1

Contents

Contributors   *ix*

Contributors to the First Edition   *xi*

Acknowledgments   *xiii*

Part I   Overview of Aging and Mental Health Issues   **1**

1   Introduction and Overview of Aging and Older Adulthood   **3**

Karen Devereaux Melillo

Mental Health and Older Adults   3

Introduction to Mental Health Issues and Disorders   5

Introduction to Gerontology   14

Summary   25

Acknowledgment   25

References   26

2   Geropsychiatric Nursing as a Subspecialty   **31**

Karen Devereaux Melillo
Lee Ann Hoff

Review of Standards   35

Theoretical Foundations for Geropsychiatric and Mental Health Nursing   37

The Nursing Paradigm Applied to Geropsychiatric Nursing   44

Acknowledgments   48

References   48

3   Comprehensive Mental Health Assessment: An Integrated Approach   **53**

Lisa A. Brown
Lee Ann Hoff

Overview of Assessment Methods   54

Cognitive Assessment Tools   57

Comprehensive Mental Health Assessment Tool   57

CMHA and McHugh's "Essentials": Description and Commonalities   60

Data-Based Service Planning   69

References   71

4   Ethnic Elders   **73**

Jane Cloutterbuck

Demographic Change   73

Who Are Ethnic Elders?   74

Prevalence Rate for Mental Disorders of Ethnic Elders   75

Disparities in Mental Health Care   75

Key Terminology: Race, Culture, Ethnicity, and Minority Group   76

The Sociocultural Context of
Mental Illness — 77

Access to Care — 83

Quality of Care — 84

Cultural Competence — 87

Summary — 88

References — 92

5 Mental Health Promotion — 101
Charles Blair

Stressors Impacting Mental Health — 102

Comprehensive Mental
Health Assessment in
Clinical Practice — 105

Assertiveness and Problem-Solving
Skills Training as Part of Social
Skills Training — 107

Late Life Challenges That Can
Contribute to Mental
Health Problems — 108

Therapeutic Interventions to
Address Mental Health
Promotion and Wellness — 110

Family and Community
Resources to Enhance
Mental Wellness — 114

Clinical Research Pertaining to
Mental Health Promotion in
Older Adults — 114

References — 117

6 Psychopharmacology — 121
Geoffry Phillips McEnany

Challenges in Prescribing for
Older Adults — 122

Factors Influencing Pharmacotherapy in Older Adults — 123

Psychotropic Drugs — 128

Summary — 141

References — 141

**Part II Psychopathology of
Late Life — 145**

**7 Nursing Assessment and Treatment
of Depressive Disorders of Late Life — 147**
Eva Heemann Byrd
Nancie A. Vito

Consequences of Depression — 147

Global and National Initiatives for
Mental Health — 148

Etiology — 150

Assessment and Screening of
Late-Life Depression — 151

Diagnosis of Mood Disorders — 156

Suicide — 157

Treatment Options — 160

Pharmacological Treatment Options — 161

Psychotherapy — 164

Electroconvulsive Therapy — 166

Nursing Interventions — 166

Evidence-Based Models of
Care Delivery — 168

References — 170

**8 Nursing Assessment and
Treatment of Anxiety in Late Life — 175**
Marianne Smith

Anxiety Disorders in Late Life — 176

Comorbid Conditions — 177

Assessment of Anxiety in Later Life — 183

Treatment of Anxiety in Late Life — 185

Summary and Conclusions — 195

References — 197

9 Psychosis in Older Adults — 203
Janet C. Mentes
Julia K. Bail

Background — 203

Assessment — 209

Treatment 212

Ethical and Legal Issues 218

Summary 222

References 223

10 Substance Abuse in Older Adults 227

Betty D. Morgan
Donna M. White
Ann X. Wallace

Prevalence of Substance Abuse
in Older Adults 227

Definitions 228

Comorbid Conditions 229

Drugs of Abuse 229

Review of the Literature 231

Screening Tools for Identification
of Substance Abuse in the
Older Adult 231

Alcohol Abuse and the
Older Adult 235

Gender Issues, Alcohol, and
the Older Adult 236

Health Assessment 237

Medication Assessment 238

Medical Consequences of
Substance Abuse 238

Review of Systems 239

Treatment Issues 242

Treatment Philosophies 242

Medications Used in Treating
Addictive Disorders 245

Nursing Interventions to Address
Substance Abuse in the
Older Adult 247

References 249

**Part III   Issues in Geropsychiatric
and Mental Health of
Older Adults 253**

11 Delirium 255

Karen Dick
Catherine R. Morency

Introduction 256

Terminology 257

Definition 257

Pathophysiology 258

Risk Factors 258

Subtypes and Patterns 259

Relationship Between Dementia
and Delirium 260

Clinical Course 260

The Problem of Recognition 260

Assessment and Evaluation 261

Supporting Safety and Recovery 265

Documentation 267

Ethical Issues 269

Summary 269

References 270

**12 Nursing Assessment of Clients
with Dementias of Late Life:
Screening, Diagnosis, and
Communication 273**

Kathleen Sherrell
Madelyn Iris
Tracy Ann Ramos

Alzheimer's Disease and
Other Dementias 274

The Neurobiology of Dementia 275

Behavioral and Psychological
Symptoms of Dementia 276

The Role of Nurses in the
Dementia Assessment Process 277

The Process of Diagnosis Seeking
in Dementia ... 283

Communicating the Diagnosis ... 284

Summary ... 287

References ... 287

13 Nursing Management of Clients Experiencing Dementias of Late Life: Care Environments, Clients, and Caregivers ... 291

Ruth Remington
Linda A. Gerdner
Kathleen C. Buckwalter

Care Environments ... 291

Frameworks for Intervention ... 294

Interventions Directed Toward
the Person ... 295

Interventions Directed Toward
the Environment ... 301

Interventions Directed Toward
the Caregiver ... 303

Dementia Care Resources ... 306

Summary ... 307

References ... 307

14 Addressing Problem Behaviors Common to Late-Life Dementias ... 313

Ruth Remington
May Futrell

Agitation ... 313

Pain ... 317

Other Problem Behaviors ... 324

Summary ... 329

References ... 330

15 Family Caregiving ... 335

Susan Crocker Houde

Emotional Responses to Caregiving ... 336

Caregiver Assessment and the
Geropsychiatric Nurse ... 351

Interventions to Support Caregivers ... 354

Summary ... 361

References ... 361

16 Normal and Disordered Sleep in Late Life ... 367

Geoffry Phillips McEnany

Physiology of Sleep ... 368

Common Sleep Disturbances
in Older Adults ... 370

Assessment of Sleep Disorders
in Late Life ... 374

Therapeutic Nursing Interventions
to Address Sleep Disorders ... 375

Indications for Pharmacological
Therapies ... 382

Environmental Approaches in
Institutional Settings ... 388

Patient Education and Counseling ... 389

Referral and Consultation ... 389

Evaluation of Treatment
Effectiveness with Follow-Up ... 389

References ... 392

17 Pathological Gambling Among Older Adults ... 395

Cindy Sullivan Kerber

Prevalence of Pathological Gambling ... 395

Pathological Gambling Among
Older Adults ... 396

Assessment and Diagnosis of
Pathological Gambling in the
General Population ... 397

Assessment and Diagnosis of
Pathological Gambling Among
Older Adults ... 397

Therapeutic Nursing Interventions
for Problem and Pathological
Gambling 404

Evaluation of Treatment
Effectiveness with Follow-Up 406

Related Issues Pertaining to
Problem and Pathological
Gambling in Older Adults 406

Summary 407

References 408

18 Elder Mistreatment 411

Terry Fulmer
Jamie Blankenship
Angela Chandracomar
Nina Ng

Types of EM 411

Incidence and Prevalence 412

Population at Risk 413

Theories of EM 413

Institutional Mistreatment 413

Clinical Presentations 414

Evaluation and Referral 418

Legal Considerations 418

Prevention 418

Summary 420

Acknowledgments 420

References 420

19 End of Life 423

Michelle Doran
Karyn Geary

Gold Standard for End-of-Life
Care: Hospice and
Palliative Care 424

Advance-Care Planning 427

Determining Prognosis 429

Patient–Family Assessment 431

Pain 432

The Dying Process 432

Grief and Bereavement 433

Future End-of-Life Care 436

References 436

**20 Social, Health, and Long-Term
Care Programs and Policies
Affecting Mental Health in
Older Adults 439**

Kathy J. Fabiszewski

Role of the Professional Nurse 441

Federal Programs Supporting
and Financing Mental
Health Care 443

Reimbursement Issues for the
Geropsychiatric Nurse 454

Creating a Mental Health Policy
Agenda for Older Adults 457

References 461

**21 Envisioning the Future of
Geropsychiatric Nursing 465**

Kathleen C. Buckwalter
Cornelia Beck
Lois K. Evans

New Service Delivery Models
and Settings for Care 466

Expanded Roles 468

Needed Research 469

Emphasis on Translation of
Research into Practice 470

Need to Prepare More
Geropsychiatric Nurses 471

Health Promotion and
Disease Prevention 472

Conclusion 472

References 473

Appendices 477

A Recommended Geropsychiatric Competency Enhancements for Entry Level Professional Nurses 479

B Recommended Geropsychiatric Enhancements for Gerontological Clinical Nurse Specialists 483

C Recommended Geropsychiatric Competency Enhancements for Gerontological Nurse Practitioners 487

D Recommended Geropsychiatric Enhancements for Clinical Nurse Specialists Who Provide Care to Older Adults But Are Not Geriatric Specialists 494

E Recommended Geropsychiatric Competency Enhancements for Nurse Practitioners Who Provide Care to Older Adults But Are Not Geriatric Specialists 498

F Recommended Geropsychiatric Competency Enhancements for Psychiatric Mental Health Clinical Nurse Specialists 506

G Recommended Geropsychiatric Competency Enhancements for Psychiatric Nurse Practitioners 510

Index 519

Contributors

Julia K. Bail, MS, APRN, BC
Geriatric Nurse Practitioner,
    Clinical Nurse Specialist
West Los Angeles Veterans Administration
Los Angeles, California

Cornelia Beck, PhD, RN, FAAN
Louise Hearne Chair in Dementia and
    Long-Term Care
University of Arkansas for Medical Sciences
Little Rock, Arkansas

Charles E. Blair, PhD, RN, CS
Nurse Practitioner
Tyler VA Mental Health Clinic
VA North Texas Health Care System
Tyler, Texas

Jamie Blankenship, BA
Elder Mistreatment Research Assistant
College of Nursing
New York University
New York, New York

Lisa A. Brown, MS, APRN, BC
Psychiatric Nurse Practitioner
Pelham, New Hampshire

Kathleen C. Buckwalter, PhD, RN, FAAN
Sally Mathis Hartwig Professor of
    Gerontological Nursing Research
College of Nursing
University of Iowa
Iowa City, Iowa

Eve Heemann Byrd, MSN, MPH, FNP-BC
Executive Director, Fuqua Center for
    Late-Life Depression
Emory University
Atlanta, Georgia

Angela Chandracomar, BS, RN
Clinical Nurse I
Head and Neck Medical/Surgical Oncology
    Department
Memorial Sloan-Kettering Cancer Center
New York, New York

Jane Cloutterbuck, PhD, RN
Associate Professor
College of Nursing and Health Sciences
University of Massachusetts Boston
Boston, Massachusetts

Karen Dick, PhD, GNP-BC, FAANP
Hartford Scholar
Clinical Associate Professor
University of Massachusetts Boston
Boston, Massachusetts

Michelle Doran, APRN, BC, ACHPN
Palliative Care Service
North Shore Medical Center
Salem, Massachusetts

Lois K. Evans, PhD, RN, FAAN
Van Ameringen Professor in
    Nursing Excellence
School of Nursing
University of Pennsylvania
Philadelphia, Pennsylvania

Kathy J. Fabiszewski, PhD, APRN, BC
Gerontological Nurse Practitioner
Lynnfield Medical Associates
Peabody, Massachusetts

Terry Fulmer, PhD, RN, FAAN
Dean, Erline Perkins McGriff Professor
College of Nursing
New York University
New York, New York

May Futrell, PhD, RN, FAAN, FGSA
Professor Emerita
University of Massachusetts Lowell
Lowell, Massachusetts

Karyn Geary, MS, APRN, ANP, GNP, ACHPN
Nurse Practitioner
Hospice of the North Shore
Danvers, Massachusetts

Linda Gerdner, PhD, RN
School of Nursing
University of Minnesota
Minneapolis, Minnesota

Lee Ann Hoff, PhD, MSN, MA
International Consultant: Violence, Crisis,
    and Gender Issues
Boston, Massachusetts

Susan Crocker Houde, PhD, ANP-BC
Professor, Associate Dean
School of Health and Environment
University of Massachusetts Lowell
Lowell, Massachusetts

Madelyn Iris, PhD
Director
Leonard Schanfield Research Institute
CJE SeniorLife
Chicago, Illinois

Cindy Sullivan Kerber, PhD, APRN, BC
Assistant Professor
Mennonite College of Nursing
Illinois State University
Normal, Illinois

Geoffry Phillips McEnany, PhD, APRN, BC
Professor
Department of Nursing
University of Massachusetts Lowell
Lowell, Massachusetts

**Karen Devereaux Melillo, PhD, GNP, ANP-BC,
    FAANP, FGSA**
Professor, Chair
Department of Nursing
School of Health and Environment
University of Massachusetts Lowell
Lowell, Massachusetts

Janet C. Mentes, PhD, APRN, BC
School of Nursing
University of California Los Angeles
Los Angeles, California

Catherine R. Morency, MS, GNP-BC
Health Care Coordinator
Society of Jesus of New England
Watertown, Massachusetts

Betty D. Morgan, PhD, PMHCNS, BC
Associate Professor
Department of Nursing
University of Massachusetts Lowell
Lowell, Massachusetts

Nina Ng, RN
Emergency Department
New York-Presbyterian Hospital/
    The Allen Hospital
New York, New York

Tracy Ann Ramos, RN, MS, GNP-BC
Gerontological Nurse Practitioner
Geriatric Outreach
Mount Auburn Professional Services
Waltham, Massachusetts

Ruth Remington, PhD, ANP, GNP-BC
Department of Nursing
University of Massachusetts Lowell
Lowell, Massachusetts

Kathleen Sherrell, RN, PsyD
Associate Professor Emeritus
Northwestern University
Oak Park, Illinois

Marianne Smith, PhD, ARNP, BC
Assistant Professor
College of Nursing
University of Iowa
Iowa City, Iowa

Nancie A. Vito, MPH
Program Coordinator
Fuqua Center for Late-Life Depression
Emory University
Atlanta, Georgia

Ann X. Wallace, NP-C, GNP-BC
Geriatric Nurse Practitioner
Newton-Wellesley Hospital
Newton, Massachusetts

Donna McCarten White, RN, PhD, CS, CADAC
Addiction Specialist
Lemuel Shattuck Hospital
Boston, Massachusetts

Contributors to the First Edition

Marguarette M. Bolton

Priscilla Ebersole

Barbara Edlund

Lisa Guadagno

Martha A. Huff

Diane Feeney Mahoney

Barbara Resnick

Marianne Shaughnessy

Marjorie Simpson

James Sterrett

Lin Zhan

Acknowledgments

The second edition of this book became a reality because of the dedicated and knowledgeable contributors who devoted their time and expertise to advance the important field of geropsychiatric and mental health nursing. I am amazed and humbled by the contributions of these nationally recognized gerontological and psychiatric mental health nursing leaders. The John A. Hartford Institute for Geriatric Nursing Scholars Program was instrumental in the initial search for knowledgeable experts, and the behind-the-scenes mentorship and guidance provided to a number of those contributors by Dr. Kitty Buckwalter was most appreciated. I am also indebted to Drs. Cornelia Beck, Kitty Buckwalter, and Lois Evans for the leadership they have provided in the development of geropsychiatric nursing competency enhancements through the American Academy of Nursing/Hartford Institute for Geriatric Nursing-funded Geropsychiatric Nursing Core Competency Workgroup.

For the past and present University of Massachusetts Lowell gerontological nurse practitioner students whom I have had the pleasure to teach, I thank you. Your enthusiasm, commitment, and motivation toward quality care for older adults have been a source of immense professional satisfaction. For the students completing the graduate Geropsychiatric and Mental Health Nursing Certificate, I wish to thank you for choosing this important program of study and for making an impact in the care settings where you will be applying this knowledge. For my faculty colleague in this course, Dr. Betty Morgan, thank you for sharing your expertise and for demonstrating how gerontological nursing and adult psychiatric mental health nursing do indeed blend into the needed geropsychiatric and mental health nursing specialty.

For my co-editor, Susan Crocker Houde, I continue to be truly blessed to work with a professional colleague, friend, and confidante whose knowledge, work ethic, attention to detail, perseverance, support, and conscientiousness are unrivaled by anyone with whom I have worked. From the initiation of the project through its development, and into this second edition, Susan has stood out as the kind of colleague that every professional should have the chance to work alongside.

Finally, my family deserves recognition for their support and encouragement throughout the process. To Bob, my husband, and our four adult children, Michael, Marc, Eric, and Kara—you have all offered your own unique perspectives and laughter when it was needed, and have always helped to ground me in this endeavor. To my parents, Bob and Helen Devereaux, who both died during work on this second edition—you have been and will continue to be an inspiration to me in both my professional and personal life. Your lives are a remarkable example of why I chose gerontological nursing as a specialty, and why I strive to influence others in the positive way you have impacted me.

To Jones & Bartlett Learning, who undertook this project, to Kevin Sullivan, the acquisitions editor who initially approached us about the project, to Rachel Shuster who helped to ensure the manuscript was prepared to launch, and to the copyediting staff, I thank you.

Karen Devereaux Melillo, PhD,
GNP, ANP-BC, FAANP, FGSA

I feel honored to have the opportunity to edit and contribute to the second edition of this textbook. The positive feedback from the first edition and the expansion in the literature of geropsychiatric and mental health nursing research has been an inspiration to incorporate into the second edition. Dr. Karen Devereaux Melillo, a nationally renowned leader in the field of gerontological and geropsychiatric and mental health nursing, continues to be a model collaborative writing partner. Her conscientious work ethic, organizational skills, keen mind for detail, dedication, and friendship continue to motivate me in my scholarly pursuits, and working on this book with her was a positive and rewarding experience. I continue to feel I am blessed to have found someone with such outstanding qualities with whom to share my career. I also appreciate the contribution of Jones & Bartlett Learning and their support throughout the revision of this book. We are also indeed fortunate to have contributors who are willing to share their knowledge and expertise as professionals with little reward other than the knowledge and satisfaction that they are helping to prepare the geropsychiatric and mental health nurses of tomorrow. The support and friendship of colleagues in the Department of Nursing at the University of Massachusetts Lowell has helped to make this text a reality. To my students—thank you for the inquisitive questions that keep me searching for answers in the important areas of research and gerontology. This book was written for you. I would like to express my appreciation to my family—Chuck, Courtney, and Katelyn—for tolerating my long hours at the computer and for the support and understanding I receive on a daily basis. Your presence and understanding help me to keep a healthy perspective in my life. It is my hope that this text will help you, the readers, to achieve your professional goals and to contribute to improved geropsychiatric and mental health nursing care of older adults and their families.

Susan Crocker Houde, PhD, ANP-BC

I

Overview of Aging and Mental Health Issues

1

Introduction and Overview of Aging and Older Adulthood

Karen Devereaux Melillo

A projected change in the demographics of aging is the impetus for the development of this textbook. It is predicted nationally that by 2010, the older population of persons 65 years and older will be 13% of the total population, whereas those older than 60 years will represent 18.4% of the U.S. population (Administration on Aging [AOA], 2009). Demographic projections are that 20% of the population will be 65 years and older by 2030, with phenomenal growth anticipated for older minority populations, from 16.4% of the elderly population in 2000 to 23.6% in the year 2020 (AOA, 2008). This growing older population will experience mental health issues and psychiatric disorders. For the gerontological nurse, this requires increasing knowledge and skills. In fact, *Mental Health: A Report of the Surgeon General* (U.S. Department of Health and Human Services [DHHS], 1999) notes "disability due to mental illness in individuals over 65 years old will become a major public health problem in the near future . . . In particular, dementia, depression, and schizophrenia, among other conditions, will all present special problems in this age group" (p. 85). Furthermore, the President's New Freedom Commission on Mental Health projects that by 2030, some 20% of persons older than age 65 years will have a major psychiatric disorder

(President's New Freedom Commission on Mental Health, 2003).

MENTAL HEALTH AND OLDER ADULTS

The promotion of mental health in older adults is of critical importance. "Mental health is a state of wellbeing in which the individual realizes his or her own abilities, can cope with the normal stresses of life, can work productively and fruitfully, and is able to make a contribution to his or her community" (World Health Organization [WHO], 2007, p. 1). Mental health promotion includes encouragement in the use of both individual and family resources and skills. It reflects a social ecology model of health and health promotion, recognizing that improvements in the socioeconomic environment are key.

This social ecology model of health promotion, including mental health, suggests the need for individually oriented behavior change strategies in the care and treatment of mental health and psychiatric disorders, and proposes health promotion activities that emphasize a social causation of disease requiring changes in both physical and social environments (McLeroy, Bibeau, Steckler, & Glanz, 1988). The ecological perspective implies a reciprocal relationship between the individual and the environment. The five levels of analysis in an ecological model for mental health promotion include the following (McLeroy et al., 1988; McLeroy, Steckler, Goodman, & Burdine, 1992):

1. Intrapersonal factors (psychological factors, values, personality, skills, knowledge, attitudes, behavior, self-concept, self-efficacy, self-esteem, and developmental history of the individual)
2. Interpersonal processes and primary groups (formal and informal social networks, social support, family, work group, friendship networks, peers, and neighbors)
3. Institutional and organizational factors (social institutions, schools, and work settings; organizational characteristics and culture; management styles; organization structure; communication networks; and rules and regulations)
4. Community factors (relationships among organizations, institutions, places of worship, voluntary associations, neighborhoods, area economics, community resources, social and health services, governmental structures, formal and informal leadership, and folk practices)
5. Public policy (local, state, and national laws; legislation; taxes; regulatory agencies and policies; political parties; citizen participation; and bureaucracies)

Each of these social–ecological levels must be considered when addressing mental health promotion for older adults. Gerontological nurses can be key in defining the impact of each level on behavior when assessing and providing care for older adults.

Globally, WHO has emphasized that mental health policies should enhance public awareness of mental illness while addressing broader issues that affect the mental health of all sectors of society. People with mental health disorders "are often subjected to social isolation, poor quality of care and increased mortality. These disorders are the cause of staggering economic and social costs"

(WHO, 2005, para. 3). A mental health promotion policy must include the social integration of severely marginalized groups, including refugees, disaster victims, the socially alienated, the mentally disabled, the very old and infirm, abused women and children, and the poor; furthermore, this policy must "promote positive mental health throughout the life course by providing information and challenging stereotypical beliefs about mental health problems and mental illness" (WHO, 2002, p. 59).

The U.S. Surgeon General's *Mental Health: A Report of the Surgeon General* summarized themes that are important to consider when promoting mental health in the older adult (U.S. Surgeon General, 1999, p. 381):

■ Important life tasks remain for individuals as they age. Older individuals continue to learn and contribute to society, in spite of physiological changes due to aging and increasing health problems;
■ Continued intellectual, social, and physical activity throughout the life cycle are important for the maintenance of mental health in late life;
■ Stressful life events, such as declining health and/or the loss of mates, family members, or friends often increase with age. However, persistent bereavement or serious depression is not "normal" and should be treated;
■ Normal aging is not characterized by mental or cognitive disorders. Mental or substance use disorders that present alone or co-occur should be recognized and treated as illnesses;
■ Disability because of mental illness in individuals over 65 years old will become a major public health problem in the near future because of demographic changes. In particular . . .
   ◆ Dementia produces significant dependency and is a leading contributor to the need for costly long-term care in the last years of life.
   ◆ Depression contributes to the high rates of suicide among males in this population.

♦ Schizophrenia continues to be disabling in spite of recovery of function by some individuals in mid to late life.

▪ There are effective interventions for most mental disorders experienced by older persons (for example, depression and anxiety), and many mental health problems, such as bereavement;

▪ Older individuals can benefit from the advances in psychotherapy, medication, and other treatment interventions for mental disorders enjoyed by younger adults, when these interventions are modified for age and health status;

▪ Treating older adults with mental disorders accrues other benefits to overall health by improving the interest and ability of individuals to care for themselves and follow their primary care provider's directions and advice, particularly about taking medications;

▪ Primary care practitioners are a critical link in identifying and addressing mental disorders in older adults. Opportunities are missed to improve mental health and general medical outcomes when mental illness is underrecognized and undertreated in primary care settings; and,

▪ Barriers to access exist in the organizing and financing of services for aging citizens. There are specific problems with Medicare, Medicaid, nursing homes, and managed care.

To initiate appropriate interventions in a timely manner, nurses should be vigilant in assessing how older adults respond to life events, transitions, and challenges to their physical and mental well-being (DHHS, 2001).

INTRODUCTION TO MENTAL HEALTH ISSUES AND DISORDERS

Overall, only one third of Americans with mental illness or mental health problems receive care. For older adults, only half who acknowledge mental health problems receive treatment from any healthcare provider, with only a fraction (3%) of those receiving specialty mental health services (American Association for Geriatric Psychiatry [AAGP], n.d.). Additionally, "older Americans account for only 7 percent of all inpatient mental health services, 6 percent of community based mental health services, and 9 percent of private psychiatric care, despite comprising 13 percent of the population. Reasons cited for this underutilization include: stigma, denial of problems, access barriers, funding issues, lack of collaboration and coordination between mental health and aging networks, and shortages of appropriate health professions" (AAGP, n.d., para. 3). Data on mental health visits to nurse practitioners and other providers, such as social workers and psychologists, are typically not captured by national surveys (Institute of Medicine, 2008), but the impact of these providers in meeting the mental health service needs of older adults is important to assess.

There is often a lack of clear terminology to define the experiences of those suffering from mental disorders. A mental disorder is "conceptualized as a clinically significant behavioral or psychological syndrome or pattern that occurs in an individual and that is associated with present distress (e.g., a painful symptom) or disability (i.e., impairment in 1 or more important areas of functioning) or with a significantly increased risk of suffering death, pain, disability or with an important loss of freedom. In addition, this syndrome or pattern must not be merely an expectable and culturally sanctioned response to a particular event, for example, the death of a loved one" (American Psychiatric Association [APA], 2000, p. xxxi).

Nearly 20% of the population 55 years and older experience specific mental disorders that are not part of normal aging (AOA, 2001; U.S. Surgeon General, 1999), including "depression, Alzheimer's disease, alcohol and drug misuse and abuse, anxiety, late-life schizophrenia, and other conditions" (DHHS, Surgeon General, 1999, para. 3). The National Institute of Mental Health (NIMH) has reported that 4 of the 10 leading causes of disability in the United States and other developed countries are mental disorders: major depression, bipolar disorder, schizophrenia, and obsessive-compulsive disorder (NIMH, 2001).

The Healthy Aging Program at the Centers for Disease Control and Prevention (CDC) and the National Association of Chronic Disease Directors (NACDD) released an Issue Brief on the *State of Mental Health and Aging in America* (CDC & NACDD, 2008). They urge that the zeal with which prevention of infectious and chronic diseases has been undertaken in the areas of public health and health promotion be applied to the field of mental health. They reported on the response by older adults to the Behavioral Risk Factor Surveillance System question, "Now thinking about your mental health, which includes stress, depression and problems with emotions, for how many days during the past 30 days was your mental health not good?" For those reporting 14 or more days of poor mental health, a definition of frequent mental distress was applied. Results indicated that only 9.2% of U.S. adults 50 years or older and 6.5% of those age 65 years or older experienced frequent mental distress; however, Hispanics had a higher prevalence of frequent mental distress (13.2%) compared to white, non-Hispanics (8.3%) or black, non-Hispanics (11.1%), with women reporting more frequent mental distress than men (CDC & NACDD, 2008, p. 5).

The National Council on the Aging (Cutler, Whitelaw, & Beattie, 2002) reported on interviews conducted by telephone with a nationally representative sample of 3,048 community-residing older adults. On the topic of health and aging, 11% of respondents reported being diagnosed with depression. As expected, there was disparity in those reporting depression by age, gender, education, and race. For the 65- to 74-year-old age group, 12% reported being diagnosed with depression, whereas 10% of those older than 75 years reported depression. A nursing doctoral dissertation similarly reported depression to be greatest in the 65- to 74-year-old age group versus oldest-old adults, suggesting that resilience and coping of advanced-age survivors may be a factor in

ameliorating the effects of depressive symptomatology (Butler, 2003).

Cutler et al. (2002) found that females reported depression more frequently than males (13% compared to 8%). High school graduates reported depression less frequently than those who did not graduate from high school (10% compared to 14%). Blacks reported depression more than white respondents (14% compared to 10%). Overall, depression ranked ninth in the number of diseases or medical problems diagnosed (following high blood pressure, arthritis, prostate problems, heart disease, diabetes, respiratory problems, cancer, and osteoporosis) (Cutler et al., 2002). These findings underscore the prevalence and impact of depressive disorders among older adults.

Relationship of Functional Status and Mobility Impairments to Mental Health

For gerontological nurses, the notion that the mind and body cannot be separated is widely recognized. Nurses have long viewed people in terms of wholeness of mind, body, and spirit, noting the interdependence of affective, behavioral, cognitive, social, and spiritual factors on physical well-being (Edmands, Hoff, Kaylor, Mower, & Sorrell, 1999). Chronic health problems are more common in older adults than in younger adults, and functional impairments often occur as a result. The Institute of Medicine (2008) reports that mental health conditions are more prevalent among community-dwelling older adults with limitations in activities of daily living (ADLs) and instrumental activities of daily living (IADLs), and prevalence rates are even higher among nursing home residents. Because of this, older adults may experience mental health issues and problems in combination with the burden of chronic disease and functional disability or impairment. Consideration of these combined issues is essential in providing effective nursing care for older adults.

In the United States, approximately 80% of persons 65 years and older have at least one chronic condition, and 50% have at least two.

These chronic conditions often translate into limitations of activities, either IADL or ADL, and this becomes increasingly so with age. Fifty-two percent of older persons in 2002 reported some type of disability (sensory disability, physical disability, or mental disability), with "37% of older persons report[ing] a severe disability and 16% reporting that they needed some type of assistance as a result" (AOA, 2008, p. 14). Specifically, 28% of community-resident Medicare beneficiaries over age 65 years in 2005 had difficulty in performing one or more ADLs (bathing or showering, dressing, eating, getting in or out of bed or chairs, walking, or using the toilet), and 12.9% reported difficulties with IADLs (preparing meals, shopping, managing money, using the telephone, doing housework, or taking medication) (AOA, 2008). Rates among persons 85 years and older are much higher than those for persons 65 to 74 years. In 2001, 26.1% of those 65 to 74 years reported a limitation, compared to 45.1% of those 75 years and older (AOA, 2003). For those older than 80 years, almost three fourths (73.6%) report at least one disability.

There is a strong relationship between disability status and reported health status such that 68% of those older than 65 years with a severe disability reported fair or poor health status (AOA, 2003). Severe disability presence is also associated with lower income and lower educational attainment. Campbell, Crews, Moriarty, Zack, and Blackman (1999) examined data representing individuals 65 years and older regarding activity limitations and sensory impairments for 1994 and health-related quality of life for 1993 to 1997. They found that 6.2% of respondents 65 years and older who reported poor mental health during the preceding 30 days also stated their physical or mental health was "not good" (Campbell et al., 1999).

Functional impairment with activity limitation is a common problem in the older adult population. In 2002, over 50% of the older population reported having at least one disability of some type (sensory disability, physical disability, or mental disability) (AOA, 2008). The presence of a disability can have a major impact on mental health. Physically disabled adults specifically report higher rates of mental health conditions (Institute of Medicine, 2008). There seems to be a strong relationship between mental health and physical health and perceived health status in the older adult population. Research by Manton and Gu (2001) has identified a decline in recent disability rates using statistics from the National Long-Term Care Survey of the American population. In fact, the age-standardized prevalence of those with disability fell from 26.2% to 19.7% between 1982 and 1999. The Administration on Aging (2008) reported that in 2005, 28% of community-residing Medicare beneficiaries older than age 65 years had difficulty performing one or more ADLs and an additional 12.9% reported difficulties with IADLs. Ninety-two percent of institutionalized Medicare beneficiaries were reported to have difficulties with one or more ADLs. The current emphasis on health promotion by health professionals and the American public may be responsible for this improvement.

Vulnerable Populations

Certain populations of older adults are at particular risk for mental health disorders and psychiatric illnesses. Some of these populations are highlighted next.

Serious and persistent mental illness. Serious and persistent mental illness refers to the experience of an individual who has a psychiatric disorder that persists over time with remissions and recurrence of severe and disabling symptoms (Scholler-Jaquish, 2004). "The term 'serious and persistent mental illness,' is the currently accepted term for a variety of mental health problems that lead to tremendous disability. Although commonly associated with the illness schizophrenia, the severely and persistently mentally ill include people with a variety of psychiatric diagnoses" (Spollen, 2003, para. 1), including mood disorders, delusional disorders, dementia,

FIGURE 1-1

Percentage of Medicare Enrollees Age 65 and Over Who Have Limitations in Activities of Daily Living (ADLs) or Instrumental Activities of Daily Living (IADLs), or Who Are in a Facility, Selected Years 1992–2005.

This chart—Functional Limitations—shows the percent of Medicare enrollees age 65 and over who have limitations in ADLs and IADLs from 1992 to 2005. The chart shows a decrease in the level of ADL and IADL limitations during these years.

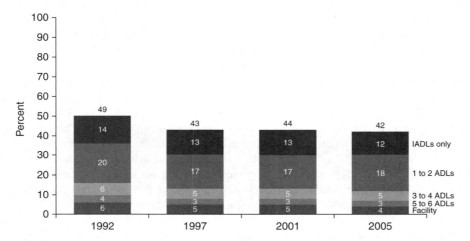

Note: The Medicare Current Beneficiary Survey has replaced the National Long Term Care Survey as the data source for this indicator. Consequently, the measurement of functional limitations (previously called disability) has changed from previous editions of *Older Americans*. A residence (or unit) is considered a long-term care facility if it is certified by Medicare or Medicaid; has 3 or more beds and is licensed as a nursing home or other long-term care facility and provides at least one personal care service; or provides 24-hour, 7-day-a-week supervision by a non-family, paid caregiver. ADL limitations refer to difficulty performing (or inability to perform for a health reason) one or more of the following tasks: bathing, dressing, eating, getting in/out of chairs, walking, or using the toilet. IADL limitations refer to difficulty performing (or inability to perform for a health reason) one or more of the following tasks: using the telephone, light housework, heavy housework, meal preparation, shopping, or managing money. Rates are age adjusted using the 2000 standard population. Data for 1992 and 2001 do not sum to the totals because of rounding.

Source: Federal Interagency Forum on Aging-Related Statistics (2008).

amnesia, and other cognitive or psychotic disorders (APA, 2000).

Persons with long-term or serious and persistent mental illness or psychiatric disabilities are particularly vulnerable, and meeting their care needs presents challenges for the geropsychiatric nurse. Gurland and Toner (1991) have suggested

the following quality-of-life criteria in identifying chronicity of mental illness:

(a) impairments of functional status in the performance of the basic and instrumental activities of daily life; and in such areas as social relationships, morale and life satisfaction, intellectual processes, communication skills, work, use of leisure time, initiative, and access to environmental and material resources;

(b) severity levels of symptomatic distress, or behaviors which are dangerous or disturbing to others because of the mental condition;

(c) the extent to which current impairments of the sufferer's functional status are the basis for planning and decisions respecting the future;

(d) the extent to which major options affecting quality of life, such as location of residence and degree of independence, have been predicated on the illness effects. (Gurland & Toner, 1991, p. 5)

Some older adults with severe and persistent mental illness have had mental illness for decades, whereas others may have been diagnosed later in life. In either case, the geropsychiatric nurse can play an important role. He or she can assist older adults by working with other multidisciplinary mental health team members in fostering access to coordinated care services and treatment programs that are geriatric-specific and by referring to agencies that can assist in ensuring appropriate care.

Older adults with mental retardation (MR) or developmental disabilities and their aging family caregivers. Individuals older than age 60 with lifelong intellectual and developmental disabilities numbered 641,000 in the United States in 2000. By 2030, these numbers are expected to double to 1,242,800 (Heller & Factor, 2004). The life expectancy of persons with intellectual disabilities was 66 years in 1993, up from 19 years in the 1930s and 59 years in the 1970s. For individuals with Down's syndrome, the life expectancy in 1993 was 56 years, compared to the average age at death in the 1920s of 9 years. Younger adults with MR (now labeled intellectual and developmental disabilities) can expect to live as long as their nonintellectually

and developmentally disabled peers, to 76.9 years (Fisher & Kettl, 2005).

Despite these significant demographic improvements, few nurses have been educated to anticipate the needs or provide care for this unique older adult population. Additionally, families are the primary providers of care for over two thirds of adults with intellectual and developmental disabilities who live at home, and 25% of these caregivers are themselves older than age 60 years (Heller, Janicki, Hammel, & Factor, 2002). Expanding life expectancy has created significant demands for residential services; advocates note that there are thousands on such waiting lists.

Individuals with Down's syndrome, the most common cause of MR in America, do suffer from dementia more often than their peers with other kinds of MR and have a much higher rate than the general population. At age 50, the prevalence of "dementia is found in 56% of those over age 60 with Down's syndrome, and in 67% by age 72" (Fisher & Kettl, 2005, p. 28). Fisher and Kettl (2005) report that older adults with Down's syndrome and dementia are more likely than their peers with MR and dementia to suffer from low mood, restlessness, disturbed sleep, and hallucinations, but are less likely to be aggressive than are other patients with dementia and MR.

A report has been generated with recommendations for new directions in research in policy that addresses promoting healthy aging, supporting families, and creating age-friendly communities for those aging with developmental disabilities. The recommendations included:

- Assess and conduct public health surveillance of the health status of adults aging with intellectual and developmental disabilities and track their healthcare experiences.
- Conduct research on the reciprocal relationships between mental and emotional status, physical health, and environmental factors, including poverty and abusive and stressful situations.
- Identify factors contributing to obesity and malnutrition, including nutritional status,

medication use, and physical activity for persons with varying conditions and syndromes through longitudinal studies.

■ Develop and evaluate health promotion programs encompassing health behavior education, nutrition, and physical activity, including analyses of differential effects for different syndromes and diagnostic groups, the impact on nontraditional exercise methods (e.g., Tai Chi), and methods of increasing exercise adherence (Heller et al., 2002, p. 10).

Furthermore, in the Report of the U.S. Surgeon General's Conference on Health Disparities and Mental Retardation, *Closing the Gap: A National Blueprint to Improve the Health of Persons with Mental Retardation* (DHHS, 2002), one of the goals identified is to improve the quality of health care for people with MR. Priority areas for achieving this goal include identifying, adapting, and developing evidence-based standards of care for use in monitoring and improving the quality of care for individuals with MR. Particularly, there is a need to address the cultural values of diverse communities in the diagnosis and treatment of emotional and behavioral disorders and mental illness, for which individuals with MR are at heightened risk. Age-appropriate health services, including geriatric, palliative, and end-of-life care, and the integration of standards of care for MR into the curricula for all health professions training must be addressed (DHHS, 2002).

Nursing has developed its own *Intellectual and Developmental Disabilities Nursing: Scope and Standards of Practice* (American Nurses Association [ANA], 2004). Few nurses have had any clinical experience in the care of this population, however, and nursing curricula do not adequately address this mental health area in the educational preparation of their graduates. This growing need, as evidenced by the demographic trends toward increasing life expectancy and community-based care settings, should be the basis for expanding model programs using nurses as pivotal care providers to adults and their caregivers.

Homeless. The National Alliance to End Homelessness (NAEH), *Alliance Online News* (March 25, 2008), reported on the results of a study by Shelter Partnership of the Los Angeles area elderly homeless population, defined as 62 years of age or older. "The study found that at least a third, and perhaps as many as half of those people are chronically homeless; that more than two-thirds are male; and that 62 percent have a physical or mental disability" (para. 1). Other researchers have noted that homeless individuals at age 50 years look and act like those 10 to 20 years older; thus, the older homeless population is often referred to as those age 50 years and older (Cohen, 1999; Cohen, Teresi, Holmes, & Roth, 1988). Estimates of the proportion of individuals 50 years and older in the homeless population range from 15% to 28% in shelter samples and up to 50% in street samples (DeMallie, North, & Smith, 1997). Obviously, locating and recruiting any homeless population for study can be quite difficult, and as a result older homeless people are especially neglected in the research literature.

Unfortunately, many people with serious mental illness are among the homeless. "At least 30% of homeless persons suffer from some type of mental disorder" (Hogstel, 1995, p. 314). In fact, five to six times as many people who are homeless suffer from serious mental illnesses compared to the general U.S. population (Substance Abuse and Mental Health Services Administration [SAMHSA], 2003). Reporting on the mental illnesses experienced by the homeless population, SAMHSA notes that as many as 50% have had a diagnosable substance abuse disorder at some point during their lives, and up to 50% have both substance use disorders and co-occurring mental illnesses, such as depression, bipolar disorder, schizophrenia, and severe personality disorders (SAMHSA, 2003).

In one large study of homeless individuals, 13% of 600 men and 3% of 300 women were in the older age group of 50 years or more, with a mean age of 57.1 ± 6.9, and a range of 50 to 82 (DeMallie et al., 1997). The study, designed to identify differences in psychiatric disorders between older and younger homeless subgroups, indicated that older subjects were more likely to be male and white, had lower incomes than their younger counterparts, and complained of worse health. Substance abuse history was present in 9 out of 10 older men with a psychiatric disorder. More than one third of the older population suffered from the following: schizophrenia, bipolar disorder, major depression, generalized anxiety disorder, panic disorder, posttraumatic stress disorder, organic mental disorder, antisocial personality disorder, or conduct disorder (DeMallie et al., 1997).

Older women are the least frequently studied group of homeless individuals and are estimated to be 20% of the older homeless population (Cohen, Ramirez, Teresi, Gallagher, & Sokolovsky, 1997). Unlike males, older women seem to have the best potential for finding housing, according to interviews conducted with 237 women. Using the SHORT-CARE instrument, 40% of the women sampled evidenced psychotic symptoms, including hallucinations, delusions, or disorganized thinking; 27% admitted to prior psychiatric hospitalizations; and 8% were moderate, heavy, or spree drinkers (Cohen et al., 1997). Not surprisingly, older participants who found housing were significantly less likely to exhibit psychotic symptoms. This research suggests that both individual risk factors and systemic factors related to the availability of low-cost housing contribute to the etiology of homelessness.

The NAEH (NAEH, 2007) reports that most who experience homelessness are single adults who enter and exit the homeless system fairly quickly. As reported by the United States Conference of Mayors (2007), the National Law Center on Homelessness and Poverty in 2004 found 25% of the homeless were ages 25 to 34 years; the same study found that 6% of persons aged 55 to 64 years were homeless. Males make up 67.5% of the single homeless population, and it is this single population that makes up 76% of the homeless populations surveyed (U.S. Conference of Mayors, 2007). In its 2006 survey of 25 cities, the U.S. Conference of Mayors found that the homeless population is estimated to be 42% African American, 39% white, 13% Hispanic, 4% Native American, and 2% Asian (U.S. Conference of Mayors, 2007).

Chronic homelessness is defined by the U.S. Department of Housing and Urban Development (n.d.) as "an unaccompanied homeless individual with a disabling condition who has either been continuously homeless for a year or more, or has at least four (4) episodes of homelessness in the past three (3) years. In order to be considered chronically homeless, a person must have been sleeping in a place not meant for human habitation (e.g., living on the streets) and/or in an emergency homeless shelter. A disabling condition is defined as a diagnosable substance abuse disorder, serious mental illness, developmental disability, or chronic physical illness or disability, including the co-occurrence of two or more of these conditions" (*Federal Register*, 2003, p. 4019). Reporting on a study of homeless people in New York City with serious mental illness, the NAEH noted that on average each homeless person used over $40,000 annually in publicly funded shelters, hospitals (including Veterans Administration hospitals), emergency departments, prisons, and outpatient health care. Much of the cost was for psychiatric hospitalization, which accounted for an average of over 57 days and nearly $13,000 (Culhane, Metraux, & Hadley, 2002). The public cost declined dramatically when individuals were placed in permanent supportive housing.

The National Coalition for the Homeless (2009) has published a fact sheet, *Mental Illness and Homelessness*, which recognizes from a policy and research perspective that homeless individuals with mental illnesses need to have both housing and access to continued treatment and services to achieve residential stability. Certainly forces and factors beyond the healthcare system strongly influence health, and programs and policies that emphasize personal lifestyle and behavioral factors ("victim blaming") overlook the broader determinants of health, especially mental health. Some of the determinants are biological (genetics, age, gender, and race or ethnicity), whereas others, termed "distal determinants of health" (Frankish, Bishop, & Steeves, 1999), include education, employment, income, housing, social support, and health-promoting behaviors. The population health approach to identifying and addressing the needs of older persons with mental illness in general, and homeless older persons in particular, is in keeping with the social ecology model of health promotion described earlier in this chapter.

Incarcerated. In a recent study on health and health care of U.S. prisoners (Wilper et al., 2009), the authors examined the prevalence of chronic illnesses, including mental illness, by analyzing the results of a large, nationally representative sample of the entire U.S. inmate population using the 2002 Survey of Inmates in Local Jails and the 2004 Survey of Inmates in State and Federal Correctional Facilities. Their findings revealed that, "Among inmates with a mental condition ever treated with a psychiatric medication, only 25.5% of federal, 29.6% of state, and 38.5% of local jail inmates were taking a psychiatric medication at the time of arrest, whereas 69.1%, 68.6% and 45.5% were restarted on a psychiatric medication after admission" (p. 4). The authors conclude that many of the prisons are "holding and treating many mentally ill people who were off treatment at the time of arrest" (p. 4).

Identifying and treating mental and psychiatric illness in this population seems to be a major focus of needed care in the prison setting, especially since the U.S. Department of Justice, Bureau of Justice Statistics, reported that more than half of all prison and jail inmates have mental health problems (U.S. Department of Justice, September 6, 2006), including 56% of state prisoners, 45% of federal prisoners, and 64% of local jail inmates. "Furthermore, prison and jail inmates older than age 55 years who had a mental health problem

included 39.6% in state prisons, 36.1% in federal prisons, and 52.4% in local jails" (U.S. Department of Justice, September 2006, p. 4).

The Pew Center on the States (2008) has published *One in 100: Behind Bars in America 2008* and notes that some states are "spending more and more on inmates who are less and less of a threat to public safety" (p. 13). They point out that the graying of the nation's prisons is causing costs to rise, particularly for the geriatric inmate, whose annual average cost is $70,000, which is two to three times more than that of a younger prisoner. They report that "between 1992 and 2001, the number of state and federal inmates aged 50 or older rose from 41,586 to 113,358, a jump of 173%" (Pew Center on the States, 2008, p. 12).

Dementia, palliative, and end-of-life care needs in prison populations, which are expected to increase with advancing age, present their own ethical and legal implications (Fazel, McMillan, & O'Donnell, 2002). Writing about the British prison population, these authors note that more than 1,000 men aged 60 years and older are in prisons, a level more than three times higher than the preceding decade. Rates of psychotic illnesses and major depression are two to four times higher than community samples of similar age (Fazel et al., 2002).

The Treatment Advocacy Center (TAC) Briefing paper, "Criminalization of Individuals with Severe Psychiatric Disorders" (TAC, 2007) has suggested that "the nation's jails and prisons have become, de facto, the nation's largest psychiatric hospitals" (p. 1). They purport that treating individuals in the community with needed psychiatric services and treatment programs would cost society 50% less than incarcerating those with severe psychiatric disorders. Furthermore, within these settings, access to mental health services of any kind may be seriously limited.

The ANA's *Nursing's Social Policy Statement* has proclaimed "human responses to actual or potential health problems are the phenomena of concern to nurses. Human responses include any . . . fact of interest to nurses, which may be the target of evidence-based nursing practice" (ANA, Congress on Nursing Practice and Economics, 2008, p. 6). Aging, mental illness, and incarceration are issues that combine to impact the psychiatric and mental health needs and care requirements of older prisoners. Gerontological and geropsychiatric nursing could be at the forefront in considering the psychiatric and mental health needs and concerns for this population and for conducting research that explores some of the "essential features of professional nursing—attention to the range of human experiences and responses to health and illness within the physical and social environments, and integration of . . . knowledge gained from an appreciation of the patient or group's subjective experience," and ultimately, "to influence social and public policy to promote social justice" (ANA, Congress on Nursing Practice and Economics, 2008, p. 5).

Overview Summary of Mental Health Problems Experienced by Older Adults

In the U.S. Surgeon General's *Mental Health: A Report of the Surgeon General* (1999), the annual prevalence of mental disorders among older adults (ages 55 years and older) was described as less well documented than that for younger adults, but estimates generated from the Epidemiological Catchment Area survey indicate that 19.8% of the older adult population have a diagnosable mental disorder during a 1-year period, with 4% of older adults having serious mental illness, and just under 1% having serious and persistent mental illness. None of these figures includes individuals with severe cognitive impairments, such as Alzheimer's disease (AD).

The AOA has reported on the following about mental health issues and older adults (AOA, 2001):

Age: Although suicide rates for persons 65 years and older are higher than for any other age group, the suicide rate for persons older than 85 years is the highest of all, nearly twice the overall national rate.

Gender: Women on average live 7 years longer than men and are much more likely than older men to be widowed, to live alone, to be institutionalized, to receive a lower retirement income from all sources, and to suffer disproportionately from chronic disabilities and disorders. However, white men older than 85 years have the highest suicide rate among older adults.

Older Gay Men and Lesbians: Social support, an important element of mental health for all older people, may be especially critical for older people who are gay, lesbian, or bisexual and who may have been exposed to prejudice, stigmatization, and anti-gay violence.

Marital Status: Emotional and economic well-being of older Americans is strongly linked to their marital status.

Minority Status: Minority populations, now representing 16% of the elderly population, are expected to represent 25% by 2030. Minorities face additional stressors, such as higher rates of poverty and greater health problems. In the mental health arena, it is important to note that Westernized mental health treatment emphasizes verbal inquiry, interaction, and response, which may not be compatible with minority cultural beliefs and practices.

Income: Poverty may be a risk factor associated with mental illness. Among older adults, women, African-Americans, persons living alone, very old persons, those living in rural areas, or those with a combination of these characteristics tend to be at greater risk for poverty.

Living Arrangements: Only a small percentage (4.2% or 1.43 million) of older persons live in nursing homes, but this percentage increases dramatically with age. Most nursing home residents have mental health disorders, including dementia, depression, or schizophrenia.

Physical Health: Most older persons have at least one chronic condition, and many have multiple problems. These chronic problems can result in functional limitations in the ability to carry out ADLs (bathing, eating, or transfer) or IADLs (shopping, managing money, housework, or taking medications). Functional limitations can contribute to mental health difficulties.

Many have suggested that underreporting of mental health problems in older adults is likely. Estimates that 8% to 20% of older adults in the community, and up to 37% of those who receive primary care, experience symptoms of depression have been reported (Hoyert, Kochanke, & Murphy, 1999). Approximately two thirds of nursing home residents suffer from mental disorders (Butler, Lewis, & Sunderland, 1998).

Although some older adults with mental health disorders have suffered from serious and persistent mental illness most of their lives, a substantial number of elders may experience a mental health problem for the first time in late adulthood. The morbidity from mental health problems can range from problematic to disabling to fatal. Assessment and diagnosis can be difficult with older adults because many present with different symptoms than younger people, emphasizing somatic complaints rather than psychological troubles (U.S. Surgeon General, 1999).

It is reported in *The State of Aging and Health in America* (Merck Institute of Aging & Health and the Gerontological Society of America [GSA], 2003) that of the 20% of older adults who experience mental disorders, many are never screened for or diagnosed with these illnesses, so they do not receive treatment. In fact, although constituting nearly 13% of the U.S. population, older adults use a disproportionately lower share of inpatient and outpatient mental health services, accounting for 7% of all inpatient mental health services, 6% of community-based mental health services, and 9% of private psychiatric care (Merck Institute & GSA, 2003). Barriers to this care-seeking include the mistaken belief that mental health problems are a normal part of aging or the stigma this cohort associates with seeking help for mental illness.

Provider barriers are also apparent, in which many primary care physicians and other healthcare providers associate depression with aging or believe that treatment for older adults is not effective. The often cited statistic that many older adults who committed suicide had visited a primary care provider very close to the time of the suicide (20% on the same day, 40% within 1 week, and 70% within 1 month of the suicide [Merck Institute & GSA, 2003]) should be impetus for including education in mental health assessment as part of gerontological assessment and nursing care.

INTRODUCTION TO GERONTOLOGY

Demographics and Population Characteristics

The United States is not the only country experiencing a demographic shift toward an aging society. Globalization of aging is apparent. The WHO reports a worldwide demographic revolution underway. In fact, the United Nations (UN) notes that the population of older persons is itself aging. In the publication *World Population Ageing 2007*, it was reported that among those 60 years or older, the fastest growing population is that of the oldest-old, those 80 years or older, with persons older than age 80 years accounting for about one in every eight older persons (60 or older). By 2050, the ratio is expected to increase to approximately 2 persons aged 80 or older among every 10 older persons (UN, 2007). In 2000, "the population aged 60 years or over numbered 600 million, with a growing rate of 2.6 percent per year as compared to the population as a whole which is increased at 1.1 percent annually. At least until 2050, the older population is expected to continue growing more rapidly than the population in other age groups. Such rapid growth will require far-reaching economic and social adjustments in most countries" (UN, 2007, p. xxvii). Both longer lives and declining birth rates contribute to this aging phenomenon. The projection of rapid population aging requires healthcare systems to accommodate the care required for this aging world. As the WHO notes, "Aging is a privilege and a societal achievement. It is also a challenge, which will impact on all aspects of 21st century society. It is a challenge that cannot be addressed by the public or private sectors in isolation; it requires joint approaches and strategies" (WHO, 2001, para. 4). Facts about world aging include the following (WHO, 2001, p. 1):

- "People aged 60 and over: about 600 million in 2000; 1.2 billion in 2025 and 2 billion in 2050
- About two-thirds of all older persons are living in the developing world, by 2025: 75%
- In the developed world, the very old (age 80+) is the fastest growing population group

- Women outlive men in virtually all societies; consequently in very old age the ratio of women/men is 2:1"

In the United States, the AOA releases its *A Profile of Older Americans* annually. The highlights of the 2009 profile are summarized in Box 1-1 (AOA, 2010). This important resource provides information for the gerontological nurse to understand the implications of current statistics for nursing practice.

Older Americans today represent about one of eight Americans; this number has increased by 3.4 million or 10% since 1996, and the number of Americans 45 to 64 years (the "baby boomers") who will reach 65 over the next two decades increased by 39% during this period (AOA, 2008). Women outnumber men, with the ratio of women

BOX 1-1   A PROFILE OF OLDER AMERICANS—2009 HIGHLIGHTS*

- The older population (older than 65 years) numbered 38.9 million in 2008, an increase of 4.5 million or 13% since 1998.

- The number of Americans aged 45 to 64, who will reach 65 years over the next two decades, increased by 31% during this decade.

- Over one in every eight, or 12.8%, of the population is an older American.

- Persons reaching age 65 have an average life expectancy of an additional 18.6 years (19.8 years for women and 17.1 years for men).

- Older women outnumber older men at 22.4 million older women to 16.5 million older men.

- In 2008, 19.6% of persons older than 65 years were minorities: 8.3% were African Americans; persons of Hispanic origin (who may be of any race) represented 6.8% of the older population; about 3.4% were Asian or Pacific Islander; and less than 1% were American Indian or Native Alaskan. In addition, 0.6% of persons older than 65 years identified themselves as being of two or more races.

- Older men were much more likely to be married than older women (72% of men versus 42% of women); 42% of older women in 2002 were widows.

- About 31% (11.2 million) of noninstitutionalized older persons live alone (8.3 million women, 2.9 million men).

- Half of older women (50%) over 75 years live alone.

(continues)

BOX 1-1   A PROFILE OF OLDER AMERICANS—2009 HIGHLIGHTS* *(continued)*

- About 471,000 grandparents aged 65 or more had the primary responsibility for their grandchildren who lived with them.

- The population 65 and older will increase from 35 million in 2000 to 40 million in 2010 (a 15% increase) and then to 55 million in 2020 (a 36% increase for that decade).

- The older than 85 years population is projected to increase from 4.2 million in 2000 to 5.7 million in 2010 (a 36% increase) and then to 6.6 million in 2020 (a 15% increase for that decade).

- Minority populations are projected to increase from 5.7 million in 2000 (16.3% of the elderly population) to 8 million in 2010 (20.1% of the elderly) and then to 12.9 million in 2020 (23.6% of the elderly).

- The median income of older persons in 2008 was $25,503 for men and $14,559 for women. Median money income (after adjusting for inflation) of all households headed by older people did not change in a statistically different amount from 2007 to 2008. Households containing families headed by persons older than 65 years reported a median income in 2008 of $44,188.

- Major sources of income for older people in 2007 were Social Security (reported by 87% of older persons); income from assets (reported by 52%); private pensions (reported by 28%); government employee pensions (reported by 13%); and earnings (reported by 25%).

- Social Security constituted 90% or more of the income received by 35% of all Social Security beneficiaries (21% of married couples and 44% of nonmarried beneficiaries).

- About 3.7 million elderly persons (9.7%) were below the poverty level in 2008, which is not statistically different from the poverty rate in 2007 (9.7%).

- About 11% (3.7 million) of older Medicare enrollees received personal care from a paid or unpaid source in 1999.

*Principal sources of data for the *Profile* are the U.S. Bureau of the Census, the National Center on Health Statistics, and the Bureau of Labor Statistics. The *Profile* incorporates the latest data available but not all items are updated on an annual basis.

Source: AOA (2010).

to men increasing with each passing decade. The ratio in 2006 was 138 women for every 100 men older than the age of 65 years, but the ratio increased to 213 women per 100 men for persons 85 years and older (AOA).

Life expectancy varies by gender. "In 2007, women reaching age 65 had an average life expectancy of an additional 19.8 years (84.8) while men's life expectancy had an average of 17.1 years (82.1)" (AOA, 2010, p. 4). There were 73,674 persons aged 100 or more in 2006 (0.19% of the total population), a 97% increase from 1990 (AOA, 2008). "Life expectancy at birth for a child born in 2007 was 77.9 years or 30 years longer than a child born in 1900" (AOA, p. 4). Interestingly, Hayflick (2000) reported that the dramatic changes in life expectancy occurred in the first 70 years of the 20th century, with only a 6-year increase in life expectancy from 1970 to 1997, suggesting an important but neglected area of aging research.

Patterns of future growth of older adults suggest the largest growth will be among minority populations, which are projected to increase to 20.1% of the elderly population in 2010 and are projected to represent 23.6% of the elderly population in 2020, up from 16.4% in 2000. "Between 2008 and 2030, the white [excludes persons of Hispanic origin] population 65+ is projected to increase by 64% compared with 172% for older minorities, including Hispanics (224%), African-Americans (120%), American Indians, Eskimos, and Aleuts (153%), and Asians and Pacific Islanders (199%)" (AOA, 2010, p. 5). Implications of these projections for the gerontological nurse include the need to create culturally competent assessments and nursing interventions.

Poverty statistics vary for different segments of the older adult population. In 2001, about 3.4 million elderly persons (10.1%) were below the poverty level. By 2006, about 3.4 million or 9% of the older population was living in poverty (Federal Interagency Forum on Aging-Related Statistics, 2008). "Poverty statistics are based on definitions originally developed by the Social Security Administration. These include a set of money income thresholds that vary by family size and composition. These thresholds are updated annually by the U.S. Census Bureau to reflect changes in the Consumer Price Index for all urban consumers" (Federal Interagency Forum on Aging-Related Statistics, 2002, p. 114). The 2009 DHHS Poverty Guidelines (used for determining financial eligibility for certain federal programs) for a family unit of one listed $10,830 and for a family unit of two listed $14,570 (DHHS, 2009). Another 2.2 million or 6.2% of older adults were classified as "near poor," whereby their income was between the poverty level and 125% of this level (AOA, 2008). Near poor older adults are challenged to meet their economic needs but may not be eligible for needs-based programs and services as a result of the definition of poverty.

Examination by race, ethnicity, and gender highlights the disparity in poverty among older adults. For elderly whites, 7% were poor in 2006, compared to 22.7% of elderly African Americans, 12% of Asians, and 19.4% of elderly Hispanics (AOA, 2008). Furthermore, in 2006 older women had a higher poverty rate (11.5%) than older men (6.6%). Those living alone or with nonrelatives were much more likely to be poor (16.9%) than were older persons living with families (5.6%) (AOA, 2008).

Poverty rates also vary by where older adults live. Compared with overall poverty rates of 9.4% for the older than 65 years population in general, higher rates were found among persons who lived in central cities (12.7%), those living in rural areas (11%), and those living in the South (11.7%). The highest poverty rates were experienced by older Hispanic women who lived alone (40.5%) and by older black women (37.5%) who lived alone, according to the AOA statistics (AOA, 2008).

The gerontological nurse recognizes that economic well-being is an essential component of overall quality of life for older adults. Without financial means, accessing needed resources for mental health and general well-being may be severely limited. Additionally, a lifetime exposure to financial hardships can add additional stress and burden in coping with age-related changes and access to health care for physical and mental health problems.

Theories of Aging

Gerontology is the multidisciplinary study of aging and older adults. Disciplines representing biology, psychology, and sociology were among the first to propose theories of aging based on research findings. These theories are an attempt to understand the phenomenon of aging as experienced by, and occurring within, older adults themselves and to enable professionals adequately to assess, plan, implement, and evaluate care, services, and policies that affect older adults. Although most nurses are familiar with a number of nursing models and theories, few have been exposed to gerontology as a formal course and are unfamiliar with how sociologists, psychologists, and biologists have viewed the structure and function of aging. An introduction to the most commonly cited theories of aging is presented next. This is not an exhaustive treatment of the subject, but rather an overview that frames the issues and concerns for the nurse in understanding and providing individualized geropsychiatric and mental health nursing care.

Biological Theories of Aging

The biological theories of aging explain the complex factors related to how and why aging occurs. These theories fall into two main groups: one emphasizes internal programmed biological clocks, and the other emphasizes external error or environmental forces that damage cells and organs until they can no longer function adequately (National Institute on Aging [NIA] & the National Institutes of Health [NIH], 2006). The programmed theories view aging as a predetermined, time phenomena. One of the first programmed theories, cellular aging, proposed by an internationally recognized researcher in cellular biology, Leonard Hayflick, described normal human cells as having a finite capacity for reproduction (approximately 50 doublings) and then dying. Other examples of programmed theories of aging include programmed senescence (where aging is the result of sequential switching on and off of certain genes, with senescence being defined as the time when age-associated deficits are manifested); endocrine theory (with biological clocks acting through hormones to control the pace of aging); and immunological theory (programmed decline in immune system functions leading to an increased vulnerability to infectious disease and thus aging and death) (NIA & NIH, 2006).

Error theories are thought to be randomly occurring events that accumulate over time. Among these theories are the wear and tear theory (where cells and tissues have vital parts that wear out); cross-linking theory (accumulation of cross-linked proteins damages cells and tissues, slowing down bodily processes); and free radical theory (where accumulated damage caused by oxygen radicals leads cells and eventually organs to stop functioning) (NIA & NIH, 2006). Antioxidant use, including vitamins E and C, beta-carotene, and selenium, represents the public's interest in attempting to reverse the damaging effects of free radicals on the aging process.

Another emerging error theory is caloric restriction. This theory, termed "rate of living" or "metabolic theory of aging," proposes that the greater an organism's rate of oxygen basal metabolism, the shorter its life span. Caloric restriction to reduce metabolism has been investigated in laboratory animals. The implications of this long-known phenomenon in laboratory animals are now being studied for its effect on human aging (Hadley et al., 2001).

With the mapping of the human genome, research is also underway to examine the relationship between DNA and the aging process. In a study by Puca et al. (2001), a genome-wide scan for linkage to human exceptional longevity identified a locus on chromosome 4. The authors propose that this might exert a substantial influence on the ability to achieve exceptional old age. This knowledge could lead to important insights on cellular pathways important to the aging process (Puca et al.). A second development is the discovery of telomeres, arms located at the ends of chromosomes, which may function as a cell's biological clock (Hayflick, 1998). The field of biological aging continues to evolve.

However, even with the knowledge of these biological aging theories, we continue to be perplexed by the social and psychological responses and processes that occur in the context of aging. Psychological and social theories of aging offer an important glimpse into these processes. This knowledge can enable the nurse to assist older adults in achieving self-defined "successful aging." For some, successful aging may be the ability to maintain the three key characteristics described by Rowe and Kahn (1998): "low risk of disease and disease-related disability, high mental and physical function, and active engagement with life" (p. 38). Others have suggested that positive spirituality is a fourth dimension that intersects with Rowe and Kahn's three key behaviors for successful aging (Crowther, Parker, Achenbaum, Larimore, & Koenig, 2002).

Psychological Theories of Aging

Psychological theories address how a person responds to age-appropriate developmental tasks (Madison, 2000). These theories recognize that both biology and sociology influence psychological responses. Examples of these psychological theories include Maslow's hierarchy of human needs, Jung's theory of individualism, Erikson's eight stages of life, and Peck's expansion on Erikson's theory.

Maslow's pyramid of human needs posits that basic physiological needs for air, food, elimination, sleep, activity, and comfort must be met before advancing to higher orders on the pyramid. Although illnesses and life crises may periodically require individuals to move up or down on the pyramid, the ultimate achievement for all humans is that of self-actualization. This can be achieved only when all basic needs for physiological integrity, safety and security, love and belonging, and ego strength and self-esteem are met. As a psychological theory for understanding aging and older adults, Maslow's top rung of self-actualization can be compared to Rowe and Kahn's successful aging.

Jung's theory of individualism suggests that human aging is accompanied by transcendence from the inner self to an emphasis on the external world and the need to contribute to the good of the larger society (Hooyman & Kiyak, 2002). Jung also noted that the psychological characteristics of anima/animus tend to be displayed in aging men and women. These characteristics enable older adults to adapt psychologically to aging and cope with age-related changes.

Erikson proposed eight stages of human development (Erikson, 1963). Achievement of each stage is required before higher-order stages can be met. Failure to achieve a stage renders the individual on the negative side of that stage's proposed dichotomy. In midlife, for example, if an individual cannot realize generativity in his or her chosen work, social roles, or life circumstances, then stagnation prevails versus generativity. For older adults who achieve the midlife developmental stage of generativity, Erikson proposes the final stage of ego integrity versus despair. For those who are able to review their life with a sense of inner peace, having made various life choices that, on reflection, were made with the best intentions and ability at the time, ego integrity can be achieved. Failing to see positives and suffering regrets over life decisions and outcomes renders the older adult with despair. Various psychosocial and psychotherapeutic therapies can enable older adults to gain insight into these negative perceptions and offer hope and provide opportunity for achieving ego integrity. Ego integrity is akin to Maslow's self-actualization, a psychological goal that all seek.

Peck expanded Erikson's original theory and divided the eighth stage, ego integrity versus despair, into additional stages occurring during middle age and older adulthood. The middle age stages consist of valuing wisdom versus physical powers; socializing versus sexualizing in human relationships (redefining men and women as individuals versus sexual objects); cathectic flexibility versus cathectic impoverishment (suggesting emotional flexibility in being able to reinvest emotions in other people and pursuits is necessary for emotional health); and mental flexibility versus mental rigidity (openness to new experiences versus reliance on fixed rules of behavior from prior experience). In older adults, Peck's theory includes ego differentiation versus work-role preoccupation (shift in value system from vocational roles to a broader range of role activities); body transcendence versus body preoccupation (transcending physical decline and discomforts and enjoying social and mental sources of pleasure); and ego transcendence versus ego preoccupation (inner contentment through children, contributions to the culture, and friendships as enduring signs of self-perpetuation after death). Peck suggests that stages in late life may be far less predictable in terms of chronological age than is true of the childhood stages proposed by Erikson (Peck, 1968).

Sociological Theories of Aging

Early sociological theories focused on social role losses as problems experienced by older adults and how individuals and society respond. Examples of these early theories, termed first-generation theories by some (Bengtson, Burgess, & Parrott, 1997), include disengagement theory (Cumming & Henry, 1961), activity theory (Neugarten, Havighurst, & Tobin, 1968), and subculture theory of aging. These reflect theories published between 1949 and 1969.

The controversial disengagement theory proposed that "social equilibrium is achieved by a mutually beneficial process of reciprocal withdrawal between society and older people" (Miller, 2004, p. 51). This theory places society's needs over individual needs, but also suggests that older adults desire this withdrawal and are satisfied with the disengagement process. Among the limitations of this proposed theory is that individuals who age successfully do not benefit by disengaging and withdrawing from social roles.

The essence of the activity theory of aging, however, suggests there is a positive relationship between activity and life satisfaction. Havighurst (1963, 1968) proposed the importance of social role participation for positive adjustment in old age. Other researchers examined activity in general, and interpersonal activity in particular, and noted that activity offers channels for acquiring role supports that sustain one's self-concept (Lemon, Bengtson, & Peterson, 1972). Thus, replacing roles lost is essential for maintaining life satisfaction in old age.

The subculture of aging theory suggests that there is a benefit derived for older adults who maintain involvement and activities with their similarly aged cohort. This cohort shares similar norms, expectations, beliefs, and habits and integrates better among themselves, compared to people from other age groups (Miller, 2004). This formation of a subculture is primarily a response of the loss of status resulting from old age in American society and the strength that can result from membership in a peer group.

In the second period of theory development, 1970 to 1985, new theoretical perspectives emerged that either built on or rejected earlier theories (Bengtson et al., 1997). Among these newer sociological theories are continuity theory (Atchley, 1972; Neugarten et al., 1968), exchange theory, life course, age stratification, and political economy of aging.

Neugarten and colleagues (1968) advanced the continuity theory because neither the activity nor the disengagement theory adequately explained successful aging. They proposed that personality characteristics, in place long before reaching older adulthood, continue. Those coping strategies used to adjust to changes throughout life are also used to adjust to aging. Their research demonstrated that personality type (identified as integrated, armored–defended, passive–dependent, and unintegrated–disorganized), extent of social role activity, and degree of life satisfaction more accurately reflect patterns of aging. Thus, the person's lifelong experience creates in him or her certain predispositions that will be maintained if at all possible.

Social exchange theories proposed that those who maintain an active contribution to and engagement with society, whether through paid or unpaid employment, volunteering, or community involvement, adapt most readily to aging. Thus, despite some older adults having fewer economic resources and skills to exert power in their social relationships, social exchange in the form of emotional support, wisdom, intergenerational transfers, and caring are valued by society (Hooyman & Kiyak, 2008; Markson, 2003). Social roles and social interactions and exchanges remain critical elements in adapting to age.

Age stratification theory was first proposed by Riley and colleagues in 1972 and "addresses the interdependencies between age as an element of the social structure and the aging of people and cohorts as a social process" (Miller, 2004, p. 52). This theory notes that aging people and society are constantly influencing one another. Societal expectations for each age strata differ from one another based on stage of life and historical events that have characterized that group's life.

The person–environment fit theory, put forth by Lawton (1982), considers the interrelationships between personal competence and the environment. Personal competence "involves ego strength, motor skills, biologic health, cognitive capacity and sensory–perceptual capacity" (Miller, 2004, p. 53). The individual interacts with an environment, which is viewed as having the potential for eliciting a behavioral response from that person. Lawton asserts that, for each level of competence, there is a corresponding level of environmental demand, or environmental press, which can best enable that person to function effectively. Those with lower-level competence can tolerate only lower levels of environmental press; those with higher levels of competence can respond well to higher levels of environmental press.

Political economy of aging theory suggests that power is in the hands of those who control the means of production or can influence the economy. Thus, in a social system where older adults are encouraged to retire, their power base is minimized. Estes (1979) pointed out that the "aging enterprise" in America benefits providers and practitioners more than older adults themselves, dispersing power among the owners of capital versus the elders for whom these programs, services, and agencies are intended to serve. Empowering older adults would change the balance of power; such organizations as AARP are intended to address this imbalance.

Theories described in the late 1980s to the present day include refinements of earlier proposed theories and newly developed theories. Reflecting the multidisciplinary scope in the field of gerontology, these theories represent the disciplines of sociology, psychology, history, and economics. Many of these theories encompass both individual and social structures as influencing behaviors or experiences of older adults. Included among these newer third-generation theories are social constructionist, feminist theories of aging, phenomenological, and critical gerontology.

Summary of Theories of Aging

The biological–physiological, psychological–developmental, and social–gerontological theories of aging continue to evolve and shape the thinking about gerontology. These varied theoretical perspectives make comparisons about theories of aging difficult, in part because many view the process and outcomes of aging from their own discipline-specific lens. Biologists, for example, are interested in predicting length of life or the viability of organ systems, whereas psychologists examine changes in a wide range of behavioral capacities, including learning, perception, and memory. Social scientists address theory as it relates to social status, life satisfaction, and adjustment to role changes associated with age, and include such concepts as culture, family, and cohort effects. As a result, there is no one integrated theory for examining and evaluating the complexities of aging and the aged. Instead, the value of an eclectic approach to the heterogeneous older adult population should be emphasized.

Each person ages in ways that are impacted by biological, psychological, and sociological factors. An understanding of the ways in which each of these factors affects the response by individuals and society to aging can be influential in the nurse's approach to geropsychiatric and mental health care. Ultimately, the goal of enhancing older adult well-being, quality of life, life satisfaction, and "successful aging" can be fostered when nursing assessments and interventions for older adults consider these factors. Knowledge of these theories in the practice of geropsychiatric and mental health nursing care can be helpful in enabling older adults to achieve the WHO definition of mental health.

Growth and Development in Old Age

As the various psychological and social theories of aging suggest, older adulthood is a dynamic period, and older adults themselves represent an extremely heterogeneous group of individuals. Research and clinical practice have long recognized that development and adaptation occur throughout life. Development, defined as learning to live with oneself as one changes, and adaptation, defined as learning to live in a particular way according to a particular set of values as one or as one's culture changes (Clark & Anderson, 1967; Matteson, McConnell, & Linton, 1997, p. 591), are necessary components in the quest for successful aging. Successful aging is possible for those experiencing chronic disease or functional limitations.

Rowe and Kahn's model of successful aging includes "absence of disease and disability, maintaining high cognitive and physical function, and active engagement with life" (1998, p. 39). Strawbridge, Wallhagen, and Cohen (2002) evaluated this model in their study of 867 Alameda County participants aged 65 to 99, and found that 50.3% of participants self-rated themselves as aging successfully compared to 18.8% when using the Rowe and Kahn criteria exclusively. The major differentiating factor in their study seemed to be that older adults with chronic conditions and functional difficulties still perceive their aging as successful. Thus, the high prevalence of chronic disease and functional limitations experienced by older adults need not be an obstacle toward the goal of successful aging and optimal mental wellness.

Other researchers have reexamined the Rowe and Kahn model and suggest the addition of a fourth factor to capture successful aging: positive spirituality. Incorporation of spirituality in interactions with older adults could strengthen efforts of healthcare providers and gerontological specialists to promote well-being in older adults (Crowther et al., 2002). The results of this research lend support for gerontological and psychiatric mental health nurses to incorporate positive spirituality in their assessment and interventions with older adults.

Holstein and Minkler (2003) have offered a critical perspective on aging that challenges the Rowe and Kahn view of successful aging. "If how we live determines how we age, and if how we live is shaped by many factors beyond individual choice, then success is far harder to come by for some than for others" (Holstein & Minkler, p. 791).

These authors suggest that the avoidance of disease and disability and the maintenance of high physical and functional capacity, as representing successful aging, are not inevitably under individual control. An elder who is disabled (because of a physical or mental illness or condition) is not so simply because he or she failed to try harder to make different health-promoting choices and decisions. As suggested earlier by the social–ecological model of health and mental health promotion, contextual factors, including economic conditions, physical and social environments, improvements in health, and healthcare access, most certainly shape the conditions of individual choice and must be foremost in the mind of the gerontological nurse in serving as an instrument of change.

Cognitive Changes with Age

"Perception, attention, learning, memory, thought, and communication—these are processes that are basic to much of our mental life and behavior, and they are all encompassed under the term cognition" (NIMH, 2000, para. 1). Nurses adept at conducting mental status evaluations with older adults are familiar with the testing and instruments needed to assess these dimensions of cognition.

> **Intelligence:** The theoretical limit of an individual's performance (Hooyman & Kiyak, 2008); the capacity to comprehend relationships, to think, to solve problems and to adjust to new situations (Taber's, 1993).
>
> **Attention:** "The power of concentration, the ability to focus on one specific thing without being distracted by many environmental stimuli" (Jarvis, 2004, p. 106).
>
> **Learning:** "The process by which new information (verbal and nonverbal) or skills are encoded, or put into one's memory" (Hooyman & Kiyak, 2008, p. 182).
>
> **Memory:** "The process of retrieving or recalling the information that was once stored.

Memory also refers to a part of the brain that retains what has been learned throughout a person's lifetime" (Hooyman & Kiyak, 2008, p. 182). An example is how to ride a bicycle. There are three types of memory: (1) sensory: information received through the sense organs and passed on to primary or secondary memory; it is stored for only a few tenths of a second (iconic [visual memory, such as remembering faces] and echoic [auditory memory, such as the sound of the ocean]); (2) primary memory: temporary stage or holding and organizing information, and does not necessarily refer to a storage area in the brain (i.e., most adults recall seven plus or minus two pieces of information for 60 seconds or less [local 7-digit phone numbers]; working memory that decides what information to be attended to or ignored); (3) secondary (long-term) memory: to retain information in permanent memory, it must be rehearsed or processed actively; requires cues to retrieve stored information (Hooyman & Kiyak, 2002). Thus, true learning implies that the material acquired through sensory and primary memories has been stored in secondary memory and can be retrieved.

Recall: the process of searching through secondary memory in response to a specific external cue (Hooyman & Kiyak, 2008).

Research has demonstrated the following age-related changes in cognition that are important to consider in caring for older adults. Intelligence is one aspect of cognition where there is controversy as to whether age-associated changes occur. It is well known that standardized testing and the time pressures associated with test-taking are more detrimental to older than younger persons. With these caveats in mind, certain age-associated changes have been identified. First, testing of fluid intelligence does demonstrate that older adults perform significantly worse on performance scales (Hooyman & Kiyak, 2008).

Fluid intelligence consists of skills that are biologically determined, independent of experience or learning, and may be similar to what is called "native intelligence." It includes spatial orientation, abstract reasoning, and perceptual speed. Crystallized intelligence, however, refers to knowledge and abilities that the individual acquires through education and lifelong experiences. As measured with the verbal scales of the WAIS-R, crystallized intelligence remains stable (Hooyman & Kiyak, 2008). These cognitive changes in intelligence, known as the "classic aging pattern," do hold up in both cross-sectional and longitudinal studies, with major changes generally not evident until the mid-70s.

Cohort effects may play a part in the results of these age-associated intelligence tests, including such factors as educational attainment; involvement in complex versus mechanistic work; cardiovascular disease; hypertension; sensory deficits; cognitive engagement (i.e., involvement in intellectual pursuits); nutritional deficiencies; and depression (Hooyman & Kiyak, 2008). Also reported in the literature is the rapid decline in cognitive function within 5 years of death, known as the "terminal drop," whereby test scores that are low may not be so much a function of age at testing as it is proximity to death (Kleemeier, 1962).

Age-related changes in memory are a source of significant concern for many older adults who fear this may be the onset of AD or a related dementia. "Normal aging does not result in significant declines in intelligence, memory and learning ability" (Hooyman & Kiyak, 2002, p. 199). However, the American Academy of Neurology guidelines have documented that mild cognitive impairment (MCI) is important to identify and monitor for progression to AD (Box 1-2). "MCI is a classification of persons with memory impairment who are not demented (normal general cognitive function; intact activities of daily living" (Peterson et al., 2001, p. 2). Other literature uses the terms "age-associated memory impairment" and "age-associated cognitive decline" to refer to the concept of increasing memory impairment with age compared to memory function in younger normal adult subjects.

According to the American Academy of Neurology, "between 6 and 25% of MCI patients progress to dementia or AD each year. Therefore, older adults with MCI should be evaluated regularly for progression to AD" (Peterson et al., 2001, p. 2). The NIA and NIH reported that in certain studies, about 40% of individuals with MCI develop AD within 3 years, whereas others have not progressed to AD, even after 8 years (NIA & NIH, 2002). More recently, the Alzheimer's Association notes that researchers are still investigating issues surrounding MCI and "how much memory impairment is too much to be considered more than normal for one's age and education" versus as a symptom of mild dementia. MCI "is a condition in which a person has a problem with memory, language or another essential cognitive function serious enough to be noticeable to others and to show up on tests, but not severe enough to interfere with daily life. Some, but not all, people with MCI develop dementia over time, especially when their primary area of difficulty involves memory" (Alzheimer's Association, 2007, p. 3).

The NIA and NIH (2002) *Progress Report on Alz-heimer's Disease 2001-2002* reported on a study that examined 404 people who had either mild memory loss (classified as MCI) or no memory problems. The 227 people with MCI were placed in one of three categories that reflected the researchers' degree of confidence that subtle signs of memory loss might indicate the onset of AD (fairly confident, suspicious, and uncertain) with volunteers being reassessed annually for up to 9.5 years. By the end of 9.5 years, all the volunteers with the most severe form of MCI had developed the clinical symptoms of AD. The findings were interpreted to mean that MCI is an early stage of AD (NIA & NIH, 2002). However, "not everyone with MCI develops Alzheimer's disease, and scientists have long been interested in determining indicators that might reliably predict which people with MCI will go on to develop Alzheimer's disease" (NIA & NIH, 2009, p. 29).

The American Psychiatric Association (2000) lists Age-Related Cognitive Decline (780.93) under other conditions that may be a focus of clinical assessment. According to the *Diagnostic and*

BOX 1-2   MILD COGNITIVE IMPAIRMENT CRITERIA

- Memory complaint, preferably corroborated by an informant
- Objective memory impairment
- Normal general cognitive function
- Intact activities of daily living
- Not demented

Source: Reproduced with permission of the American Academy of Neurology.

Statistical Manual of Mental Disorders. Text Revision: DSM-IV-TR (APA, 2000), this category is used when there is an "objectively identified decline in cognitive functioning consequent to the aging process that is within normal limits given the person's age. Individuals with this condition may report problems remembering names or appointments or may experience difficulty in solving complex problems" (APA, p. 741). It is assumed that a specific mental disorder or neurological condition has been ruled out as a cause for the cognitive impairment.

In contrast, dementia is described as "the development of multiple cognitive deficits that include memory impairment and at least one of the following cognitive disturbances: aphasia, apraxia, agnosia, or a disturbance in executive functioning. The cognitive deficits must be sufficiently severe to cause impairment in occupational and social functioning and must represent a decline from a previously higher level of functioning. A diagnosis of a dementia should not be made if the cognitive deficits occur exclusively during the course of a delirium" (APA, 2000, p. 148). Aphasia refers to difficulty expressing oneself when speaking, trouble understanding speech, and difficulty with reading and writing; apraxia (dyspraxia, if mild) is the loss of the ability to execute or carry out skills, movements, and gestures, despite having the desire and the physical ability to perform them; agnosia is the inability to recognize and identify objects or persons; and disturbance in executive functioning is demonstrated by impairment in planning, organizing, and sequencing (American Academy of Neurology, 2010).

Although research continues to determine the significance and impact of MCI on older adults, the gerontological nurse must recognize that the concerns and fears of older adults and their family members regarding any cognitive changes must be carefully assessed and support provided during the diagnostic processes.

SUMMARY

This chapter has introduced the field of aging and older adulthood. Current and projected future demographics of the aging population portray that society's needs for mental health and psychiatric care of older adults will continue to grow. There continue to be too many older adults who experience mental health issues and psychiatric disorders that go underdiagnosed and undertreated, in part because they fail to access needed services or are not seen as suffering by healthcare providers who dismiss the client's complaints as being normal aging. Knowledge about particularly vulnerable populations, including the developmentally disabled, the chronically and persistently mentally ill, the incarcerated, and the homeless, is essential for the gerontological nurse to adequately address patients' mental healthcare needs.

Although this chapter is not intended to be a comprehensive review of the field of gerontology, basic concepts to assist in the understanding of the life perspective of aging and older adults have been introduced. An introduction to the biological, social, and psychological theories of aging has been presented as an overview for the geropsychiatric nurse. Growth and development in old age, and the concept of successful aging, have been presented. A review of the cognitive changes occurring with age and their implications for the aged and the geropsychiatric nurse have also been included to provide a context for the assessment and treatment of mental health issues and psychiatric disorders that follow.

ACKNOWLEDGMENT

The author acknowledges the helpful critique of an earlier draft of this chapter in the first edition provided by Judith Conahan, RN, MS, PhD(c).

REFERENCES

Administration on Aging. (2001). *Older adults and mental health 2001: Issues and opportunities.* Retrieved June 24, 2004, from http://www.protectassets.ccm/ssa/Older-AdultsandMH2001.pdf

Administration on Aging. (2003). *A profile of older Americans: 2002.* Washington, DC: Author. Retrieved January 23, 2010, from http://www.aoa.gov/AoARoot/Aging_Statistics/Profile/index.aspx

Administration on Aging. (2008). *A profile of older Americans: 2007.* Washington, DC: Author. Retrieved January 23, 2010, from http://www.aoa.gov/AoARoot/Aging_Statistics/Profile/index.aspx

Administration on Aging. (2009). *A profile of older Americans: 2008.* Washington, DC: Author. Retrieved September 16, 2009, from http://www.aoa.gov/AoARoot/Aging_Statistics/Profile/2008/docs/2008profile.doc

Administration on Aging. (2010). *A profile of older Americans: 2009.* Washington, DC: Author. Retrieved January 18, 2010, from http://www.aoa.gov/AoARoot/Aging_Statistics/Profile/2009/2.aspx

Alzheimer's Association. (2007). *Every 72 seconds someone in America develops Alzheimer's. Alzheimer's disease facts and figures 2007.* Chicago: Author. Available at www.alz.org

American Academy of Neurology. (2010). The Brainmatters.org. Retrieved January 18, 2010, from http://www.thebrainmatters.org

American Association for Geriatric Psychiatry. (n.d.). *Health care professionals. Geriatrics and mental health—the facts.* Retrieved December 30, 2008, from http://www.aagponline.org/prof/facts_mh.asp.

American Nurses Association. (2004). *Intellectual and developmental disabilities nursing: Scope and standards of practice.* Silver Spring, MD: Nursesbooks.org

American Nurses Association's Congress on Nursing Practice and Economics. (2008). *Nursing's social policy statement: The essence of the profession.* Washington, DC. Retrieved January 19, 2009, from http://www.nursingworld.org /

American Psychiatric Association. (2000). *Diagnostic and statistical manual of mental disorders. Text revision: DSM-IV-TR* (text revision). Washington, DC: Author.

Atchley, R. C. (1972). *The social forces in later life.* Belmont, CA: Wadsworth.

Bengtson, V. L., Burgess, E. O., & Parrott, T. M. (1997). Theory, explanation, and a third generation of theoretical development in social gerontology. *Journal of Gerontology: Social Sciences, 52B*(2), S72–S88.

Butler, H. A. (2003). *Motivation: The role in diabetes self-management in older adults.* Ph.D. dissertation, University of Massachusetts, Lowell, MA.

Butler, R. N., Lewis, M. I., & Sunderland, T. (1998). *Aging and mental health: Positive psychosocial and biomedical approaches* (5th ed.). Boston: Allyn & Bacon.

Campbell, V. A., Crews, J. E., Moriarty, D. G., Zack, M. M., & Blackman, D. K. (1999). Surveillance for sensory impairment, activity limitation, and health-related quality of life among older adults: United States, 1993-1997. *Surveillance Summaries, 48*(SS08), 131–156. Retrieved January 23, 2010, from http://www.cdc.gov/mmwr/preview/mmwrhtml/ss4808a6.htm/

Centers for Disease Control and Prevention and the National Association of Chronic Disease Directors. (2008). *The state of mental health and aging in America. Issue brief #1; What do the data tell us?* Atlanta, GA: National Association of Chronic Disease Directors.

Clark, M., & Anderson, P. B. (1967). *Culture and aging.* Springfield, IL: Charles C Thomas.

Cohen, C. I. (1999). Aging and homelessness. *The Gerontologist, 39*(1), 5–14.

Cohen, C. I., Ramirez, M., Teresi, J., Gallagher, M., & Sokolovsky, J. (1997). Predictors of becoming redomiciled among older homeless women. *The Gerontologist, 37*, 67–74.

Cohen, C. I., Teresi, J. A., Holmes, D., & Roth, E. (1988). Survival strategies of older homeless men. *The Gerontologist, 28*, 58–65.

Crowther, M. R., Parker, M. W., Achenbaum, W. A., Larimore, W. L., & Koenig, H. G. (2002). Rowe and Kahn's Model of Successful Aging revisited: Positive spirituality—the forgotten factor. *The Gerontologist, 42*(5), 613–620.

Culhane, D. P., Metraux, S., & Hadley, T. (2002). Public service reductions associated with placement of homeless persons with severe mental illness in supportive housing. *Housing Policy Debates,* *13*(1), 107–163. Retrieved January 17, 2010, from http://repository.upenn.edu/cgi/viewcontent.cgi?articlew=1067&context=spp_papers/

Cumming, E., & Henry, W. E. (1961). *Growing old.* New York: Basic Books.

Cutler, N. E., Whitelaw, N. A., & Beattie, B. L. (2002). *2002 American perspectives of aging in the 21st century: A myths and realities of aging chartbook.* Washington, DC: The National Council on the Aging.

DeMallie, D. A., North, C. A., & Smith, E. M. (1997). Psychiatric disorders among the homeless: A comparison of older and younger groups. *The Gerontologist, 37*(1), 61–66.

Edmands, M. S., Hoff, L. A., Kaylor, L., Mower, L., & Sorrell, S. (1999). Bridging gaps between mind, body, spirit: Healing the whole person. *Journal of Psychosocial Nursing, 37*(10), 35–42.

Erikson, E. H. (1963). *Childhood and society* (2nd ed.). New York: W. W. Norton.

Estes, C. L. (1979). *The aging enterprise.* San Francisco: Jossey-Bass.

Fazel, S., McMillan, J., & O'Donnell, I. (2002). Dementia is prison: Ethical and legal implications. *Journal of Medical Ethics, 28*, 156–159.

Federal Interagency Forum on Aging-Related Statistics (as of 2000). (2002). *Older Americans 2000: Key indicators of well-being.* Hyattsville, MD: Author.

Federal Interagency Forum on Aging-Related Statistics. (2008). *Older Americans 2008: Key indicators of well-being.* Hyattsville, MD: Author. Retrieved January 23, 2010, from http://www.agingstats.gov/agingstatsdotnet/Main_Site/About/FAQ.aspx

Federal Register. (2003). Notice of funding availability for the collaborative initiative to help end chronic homelessness. *Federal Register, 68*(17), 4019. Retrieved January 17, 2010, from http://ftp.resource.org/gpo.gov/register/2003/2003_4019.pdf/

Fisher, K., & Kettl, P. (2005). Aging with mental retardation: Increasing population of older adults with MR require health interventions and prevention strategies. *Geriatrics, 60*(4), 26–29.

Frankish, C. J., Bishop, A., & Steeves, M. (1999). *Challenges and opportunities in applying a population health approach to mental health services: A discussion paper.* Institute of Health Promotion Research. University of British Columbia for the Health Systems Section of Health Canada.

Retrieved August 4, 2003, from www.ihpc.ubc.ca/pdfs/mentalhealthdraft.pdf

Gurland, B., & Toner, J. A. (1991). The chronically mentally ill elderly: Epidemiological perspectives on the nature of the population. In E. Light & B. D. Levowitz (Eds.), *The elderly with chronic mental illness* (chap. 1). New York: Springer.

Hadley, E. C., Dutta, C., Finkelstein, J., Harris, T. B., Lane, M. A., Roth, G. S., et al. (2001). Human implications of caloric restriction's effects on aging in laboratory animals: An overview of opportunities for research. *Journals of Gerontology: Biological Sciences and Medical Sciences, 56*, 5–6.

Hayflick, L. (1998). How and why we age. *Experimental Gerontology, 33*(7-8), 639–653.

Hayflick, L. (2000). The nature of ageing. *Nature, 408*, 267–269.

Havighurst, R. J. (1963). Successful aging. In R. Williams, C. Tibbits, & W. Donahue (Eds.), *Processes of aging* (Vol. 1). New York: Atherton Press.

Havighurst, R. J. (1968). Personality and patterns of aging. *The Gerontologist, 38*, 20–23.

Heller, T., & Factor, A. (2004). *Older adults with developmental disabilities and their aging family caregivers.* Rehabilitation Research and Training Center on Aging with Developmental Disabilities. University of Illinois at Chicago. Retrieved January 17, 2010, from http://www.rrtcadd.org/Resource/Publications/General/Brief/Info.html/

Heller, T., Janicki, M., Hammel, J., & Factor, A. (2002). *Promoting healthy aging, family support, and age-friendly communities for persons with developmental disabilities: Report of the 2001 Invitational Research Symposium on Aging with Developmental Disabilities.* Chicago: The Rehabilitation Research and Training Center on Aging with Developmental Disabilities, Department of Disability and Human Development, University of Illinois at Chicago.

Hogstel, M. O. (1995). *Geropsychiatric nursing.* St. Louis: Mosby.

Holstein, M. B., & Minkler, M. (2003). Self, society, and the "new gerontology." *The Gerontologist, 43*(6), 787–796.

Hooyman, N. R., & Kiyak, H. A. (2002). *Social gerontology: A multidisciplinary perspective.* Boston: Allyn & Bacon.

Hooyman, N. R., & Kiyak, H. A. (2008). *Social gerontology: A multidisciplinary perspective* (8th ed.). Boston: Allyn & Bacon.

Hoyert, D. L., Kochanke, K. D., & Murphy, S. L. (1999). Deaths: Final data for 1997. *National Vital Statistics Reports, 47*(9). Hyattsville, MD: National Center for Health Statistics.

Institute of Medicine of the National Academies, Committee on the Future Health Care Workforce for Older Americans Board on Health Care Services. (2008). *Retooling for an aging America: Building the health care workforce.* Washington, DC: The National Academies Press.

Jarvis, C. (2004). *Physical examination & health assessment* (4th ed.). St. Louis: Saunders.

Kleemeier, R. W. (1962). Intellectual changes in senium. *Proceedings of the Social Statistics Section of the American Statistical Association, 1,* 290–295.

Lawton, M. P. (1982). Competence, environmental press, and the adaptation of older people. In M. P. Lawton, P. G. Windley, and T. O. Byerts (Eds.), *Aging and the environment: Theoretical approaches* (pp. 33–59). New York: Springer.

Lemon, B., Bengtson, V. L., & Peterson, J. A. (1972). An exploration of the activity theory of aging: Activity types and life satisfaction among in-movers to a retirement community. *Journal of Gerontology, 27,* 511–523.

Madison, H. E. (2000). Theories of aging. In A. G. Lueckenotte, *Gerontologic nursing* (2nd ed., p. 21). St. Louis: Mosby.

Manton, K. G., & Gu, X. L. (2001). Dramatic decline in disability continues for older Americans. *Proceedings of the National Academy of Sciences* (May 8, 2001). National Institutes of Health, National Institute on Aging, NIH News Release. Retrieved July 2, 2003, from http://www.nia.nih.gov/news/pr/2001/0507.htm

Markson, E. W. (2003). *Social gerontology today: An introduction.* Los Angeles: Roxbury Publishing Company.

Matteson, M. A., McConnell, E. S., & Linton, A. D. (1997). *Gerontological nursing: Concepts and practice* (2nd ed.). Philadelphia: Saunders.

McLeroy, K. R., Bibeau, D., Steckler, A., & Glanz, K. (1988). An ecological perspective on health promotion programs. *Health Education Quarterly, 15*(4), 351–377.

McLeroy, K. R., Steckler, A., Goodman, R., & Burdine, J. N. (1992). Health education research, theory and practice: Future directions. *Health Educational Research: Theory and Practice, 7*(1), 1–8.

Merck Institute of Aging & Health and The Gerontological Society of America. (2003). *The state of aging and health in America.* Washington, DC: Authors.

Miller, C. A. (2004). *Nursing for wellness in older adults. Theory and practice* (4th ed.). Philadelphia: Lippincott Williams & Wilkins.

National Alliance to End Homelessness. (2007). *Chronic homelessness. Fact checker series.* Available at www.endhomelessness.org/

National Alliance to End Homelessness. (2008). *Alliance online news.* Retrieved March 25, 2008, from www.endhomelessness.org/

National Coalition for the Homeless. (2009). *Mental illness and homelessness.* Retrieved January 23, 2010, from http://www.nationalhomeless.org/factsheets/Mental_Illness.html/

National Institute on Aging and the National Institutes of Health. (2002). *Progress report on Alzheimer's disease, 2001-2002.* Washington, DC: Author.

National Institute on Aging and the National Institutes of Health. (2006). *Aging under the microscope: A biological quest.* Bethesda, MD: Author. Retrieved January 23, 2010, from http://www.nia.nih.gov/HealthInformation/Publications/AgingUnderTheMicroscope/default.htm/

National Institute on Aging and the National Institutes of Health. (2009). *2008 Progress report on Alzheimer's disease: Moving discovery forward.* Washington, DC: Author. Retrieved January 18, 2010, from http://www.nia.nih.gov/Alzheimers/

National Institute of Mental Health. (2000). *Cognitive research at the National Institute of Mental Health.* Retrieved January 18, 2010, from http://mentalhealth.about.com/library/rs/blcog.htm/

National Institute of Mental Health. (2001). *The numbers count: Mental disorders in America.* Retrieved June 24, 2004, from http://www.nimh.nih.gov/publicat/numbers/cfm/

Neugarten, B., Havighurst, R. J., & Tobin, S. S. (1968). Personality and patterns of aging. In B. L. Neugarten (Ed.), *Middle age and aging.* Chicago: University of Chicago Press.

Peck, R. (1968). Psychological determinants in the second half of life. In B. L. Neugarten (Ed.), *Middle age and aging.* Chicago: University of Chicago Press.

Peterson, R. C., Stevens, J. C., Ganguli, M., Tangalos, E. G., Cummings, J. L., & DeKosky, S. T. (2001). Practice parameter: Early detection of dementia: Mild cognitive impairment (an evidence-based review). Report of the Quality Standards Subcommittee of the American Academy of Neurology. *Neurology, 56*(Special Article), 1133–1142. Retrieved January 3, 2010, from http://www.neurology.org/cgi/reprint/56/9/1133.pdf/

Pew Center on the States. (2008). *One in 100: Behind bars in America 2008.* Retrieved January 21, 2009, from www.pewcenteronthestates.org/

President's New Freedom Commission on Mental Health. (2003). *Achieving the promise: Transforming mental health care in America. Final report.* Rockville, MD: DHHS Pub. No. SMA-03-3832. Retrieved September 17, 2009, from http://www.mentalhealthcommission.gov/reports/reports.htm/

Puca, A. A., Daly, M. J., Brewster, S. J., Matsie, T. C., Barrett, J., Shea-Drinkwater, M., et al. (2001). A genome-wide scan for linkage to human exceptional longevity identifies a locus on chromosome 4. *Proceedings of the National Academy of Sciences, 98*(18), 10505–10508.

Rowe, J. W., & Kahn, R. L. (1998). *Successful aging.* New York: Pantheon Books.

Scholler-Jaquish, A. (2004). Persons with severe and persistent mental illness. In K. M. Fortinash & P. A. Holoday Worret, *Psychiatric mental health nursing* (3rd ed., pp. 617–644). St. Louis: Mosby.

Spollen, J. J. (2003). Perspectives in serious mental illness. *Medscape Psychiatry & Mental Health, 8*(1). Retrieved January 12, 2009, from http://journal.medscape.com/viewarticle/455449_print/

Strawbridge, W. J., Wallhagen, M. I., & Cohen, R. D. (2002). Successful aging and well-being: Self-rated compared with Rowe and Kahn. *The Gerontologist, 42*(6), 727–733.

Substance Abuse and Mental Health Services Administration (SAMHSA), The Center for Mental Health Services. (2003). *Blueprint for change: Ending chronic homelessness for persons with serious mental illnesses and/or co-occurring substance use disorders.* Rockville, MD: Author. Retrieved August 27, 2004, from http://www.nrchmi.samhsa.gov/publications/default.asp/

Taber's cyclopedic medical dictionary (17th ed.). (1993). Philadelphia: Davis.

Treatment Advocacy Center. (2007). Briefing paper: Criminalization of individuals with severe psychiatric disorders. Retrieved January 19, 2009, from http://www.treatmentadvocacycenter.org/

United Nations. (2007). *World population ageing 2007.* New York: Author. Retrieved January 13, 2009, from www.un.org/esa/population/publications/WPA2007/wpp2007.htm/

United States Conference of Mayors. (2007). *A status report on hunger and homelessness in America's cities: A 23-city survey.* Washington, DC: Author. Retrieved September 18, 2009, from www.usmayors.org/HHSurvey2007/hhsurvey07.pdf/

U.S. Department of Health and Human Services. (1999). The fundamentals of mental health and mental illness. In *Mental Health: A Report of the Surgeon General* (pp. 45–49). Rockville, MD: U.S. DHHS, Substance Abuse and Mental Health Services Administration, Center for Mental Health Services, National Institutes of Health, National Institute of Mental Health.

U.S. Department of Health and Human Services. (2001). *National strategy for suicide prevention: Goals and objectives for action.* Rockville, MD: Author.

U.S. Department of Health and Human Services. (2002). *Closing the gap: A national blueprint to improve the health of persons with mental retardation.* Report of the Surgeon General's Conference on Health Disparities and Mental Retardation. Rockville, MD: U.S. DHHS, Public Health Service, Office of the Surgeon General.

U.S. Department of Health and Human Services. (2009). *The 2009 HHS poverty guidelines.* Retrieved January 17, 2010, from http://aspe.hhs.gov/09poverty.shtml/

U.S. Department of Housing and Urban Development. (n.d.). *Federal definition of homeless.* Retrieved January 13, 2009, from http://www.hud.gov/homeless/definition.cfm/

U.S. Department of Justice, Bureau of Justice Statistics, Office of Justice Programs. (2006, September 6). *Study finds more than half of all prison and jail inmates have mental health problems.* Press Release. Retrieved January 18, 2009, from www.ojp.usdoj.gov/bjs/pub/press/mhppjipr.htm/

U.S. Surgeon General. (1999). *Mental health: A report of the Surgeon General.* Rockville, MD: U.S. Department of Health and Human Services, Substance Abuse and Mental Health Services Administration, Center for Mental Health Services, National Institutes of Health, National Institute of Mental Health. Retrieved January 23, 2010, from http://www.surgeongeneral.gov/library/mentalhealth/

Wilper, A. P., Woolhandler, S., Boyd, J. W., Lasser, K. E., McCormick, D., Bor, D. H., et al. (2009). The health and health care of US prisoners: Results of a nationwide survey. *American Journal of Public Health, 99*(4), 1–7. Published ahead of print on January 15, 2009. Retrieved January 19, 2009, from http://www.ajph.org/cgi/doi/10.2105/AJPH.2008.144279/

World Health Organization. (2001). *Towards policy for health and ageing.* Retrieved January 23, 2010, from http://www.who.iint/mip2001/files/1991/TowardsPolicyforHealthandAgeing.pdf/

World Health Organization. (2002). *Active ageing: A policy framework.* Geneva. Retrieved December 26, 2008, from http://whqlibdoc.who.int/hq/2002/WHO_NMH_NPH_02.8.pdf/

World Health Organization. (2005). *Mental health policy, plans, and programmes.* Retrieved January 23, 2010, from www.who.int/mental_health/en/

World Health Organization. (2007). *Mental health: Strengthening mental health promotion. Fact sheet 220.* Retrieved January 23, 2010, from http://www.who.int/mediacentre/factsheets/fs220/en/

2

Geropsychiatric Nursing as a Subspecialty

Karen Devereaux Melillo
Lee Ann Hoff

All healthcare professionals, including nurses, receive insufficient geropsychiatric and mental health training and preparation. This fact can negatively affect individuals and families experiencing geropsychiatric and mental health issues. In the *Consensus Statement on the Upcoming Crisis in Geriatric Mental Health*, authors Jeste et al. (1999) acknowledge that a national crisis in geriatric mental health care is emerging. A myriad of factors are cited: inadequate research infrastructure, poor healthcare financing, lack of adequately trained mental healthcare personnel, and fragmented inadequate mental healthcare delivery systems that cannot meet the challenges posed by the increasing numbers of older adults, and of older adults needing psychiatric care. The *Consensus Statement* authors suggest there is a need for urgent action.

The Institute of Medicine (2008) notes that advanced practice nurses "represent a particularly important component of the workforce caring for older adults because of their ability to provide primary care as well as care for patients prior to, during, and following an acute care hospitalization and also to care for residents in institutional long-term care settings" (pp. 160–161). In fact, the Center for Health Workforce Studies (2005) reports 23% of office visits and 47% of outpatient visits with nurse practitioners (NPs) are made by people 65 years and older. As of April 2006, less than 1% of nurses in this country were American Nurses Credentialing Center (ANCC) certified as gerontological nurses. Even among the 70,000 to 80,000 advanced practice nurses, only 5% to 6% have been certified in gerontological nursing (American Academy of Nursing [AAN], 2002). There are roughly 4,300 master's prepared gerontological NPs and clinical nurse specialists (CNSs). These figures fall far short of national needs. In 2002, Mezey and Fulmer reported that only 63 programs nationwide prepared advanced gerontological nurses, and these programs graduated a mean of three students annually, making few available for the gerontological nursing care needed in healthcare settings. In 2004, some program growth was noted in that 62 master's NP and 56 post-master's NP programs prepared graduates to take the gerontological NP (GNP) certification examination, whereas 45 master's programs and 16 post-master's programs prepared graduates to take the gerontological CNS examination (American Association of Colleges of Nursing [AACN] & The John A. Hartford Foundation, 2004, pp. 2–3). The ANCC 2007 certification data reported that 182 GNPs and 13 gerontological CNSs successfully passed the certification examination in 2007

(ANCC, 2008). The Gerontological Advanced Practice Nurses Association (GAPNA, formerly called the National Conference of Gerontological Nurse Practitioners) reports there were 3812 GNPs holding ANCC GNP certification as of June 2008 (National Conference of Gerontological Nurse Practitioners [NCGNP], 2008).

Basic preparation in gerontology is often lacking for many practicing nurses and current nursing students. An online review of *Peterson's Guide*, which provides detailed profiles of more than 2100 colleges and universities in the United States and Canada, revealed that of 2- or 4-year schools, only 86 offered any gerontology coursework (*Peterson's Guide*, 2003). Formal programs in gerontology are increasing, with 147 bachelor's level aging studies programs reported by the Association for Gerontology in Higher Education (2009). This suggests that too few college graduates in any major, unless specifically focused on aging studies, may be equipped to understand the unique aspects of aging and older adults. This group of graduates includes nursing professionals.

Nurses have often been educated without the benefit of even a basic introductory undergraduate gerontology course. In 2004, a U.S. regional study that sampled 4-year baccalaureate nursing programs from the Northeast (12 schools), South (13 schools), West (15 schools), and Midwest (16 schools) reported that only 25% required courses in gerontology, whereas 97.4% reported gerontology to be integrated in course curricula, and as electives in 43.9% (Grocki & Fox, 2004). Even fewer have completed a nursing course dedicated to the nursing care of older adults. As for most nurses practicing today, whose average age is 46 years, with educational preparation likely occurring many years previously, even fewer may have had the opportunity to take a required course in geriatric or gerontological nursing.

In 1999, only 23% of baccalaureate nursing programs had a required geriatric or gerontological nursing course (Rosenfeld, Bottrell, Fulmer, & Mezey, 1999). Some improvement has been noted. Gilje, Lacey, and Moore (2007) conducted a national survey to examine gerontology and geriatric issues and trends in U.S. nursing programs, following the development of *Older Adults: Recommended Baccalaureate Competencies and Curricular Guidelines for Geriatric Nursing Care* (AACN & the John A. Hartford Foundation, 2000). Among the 202 survey respondents (36% response rate), 51% reported their curriculum offered a gerontology course and 49% reported integrating geriatric and gerontology content. For those offering a stand-alone course in gerontology, 76% required this course and 24% offered it as an elective (Gilje et al., 2007). In 2002, Kovner, Mezey, and Harrington described gerontology content as "woefully lacking in medical schools and nursing programs, and primary care and specialty health care professionals, who are likely to care for large numbers of older patients, continue to receive inadequate training" (para. 7). The Hartford Institute notes that "older people represent 60% of all adult primary care visits, 80% of home care visits, 46% of all hospital days and 85% of residents in nursing homes," and yet geriatric nursing is underrepresented at all levels of nursing practice and nursing education (The John A. Hartford Institute, Fast Facts, n.d.). However, improvements in gerontological integration are noted.

Within the specialty field of gerontological nursing, one must understand the unique mental health problems and specialized approaches to care for older adults that academic nursing programs have not fully addressed. To focus on these issues, nursing professionals with additional specialized knowledge and skills are needed.

Nurses are educationally prepared at the basic level for psychiatric mental health nursing. According to the American Psychiatric Nurses Association (APNA), basic level clinical practice of psychiatric mental health nursing includes registered nurses who "work with individuals, families, groups and communities, assessing mental health needs, and developing a nursing diagnosis and a plan of nursing care, implementing the plan and finally evaluating the nursing care" (APNA, 2009, para. 1). The assessment, diagnosis, treatment, and evaluation of older adults with geropsychiatric and mental health problems are seldom the primary focus of the educational preparation in generic baccalaureate nursing programs.

Unlike basic level psychiatric mental health nursing, geropsychiatric nursing is a master's level subspecialty within the adult psychiatric mental health nursing field. Subspecialization in a particular area of practice, according to Burgess (1997), "occurs during Master's and Doctoral preparation in nursing and/or through continuing professional education. Subspecialization is focused on the development of additional knowledge and skills for providing services to a population. Subspecializations within psychiatric mental health nursing are based on current and anticipated societal needs for various specialty nursing services. This subspecialization may be categorized according to a developmental period (e.g., child and adolescent, adult, geriatric); a specific mental/emotional disorder (e.g., addiction, depression, chronic mental illness); a particular practice focus (e.g., community, group, couple, family, individuals); and a specific role or function (e.g., forensic nursing, psychiatric consultation/liaison)" (Burgess, p. 21).

More recently, the APNA (2008) developed *Essentials of Psychiatric Mental Health Nursing in the BSN Curriculum*, in collaboration with the International Society of Psychiatric Mental Health Nurses. Among the core psychiatric mental health nursing content deemed essential for nursing preparation, with particular relevance to older adults, is "recognition of major disorders occurring in older age (depression, dementia, delirium)" (p. 4); "communication with patients experiencing common psychiatric symptoms such as disorganized speech, hallucinations, delusions, and decreased production of speech (for core communication theory and interpersonal relationship skills content)" (p. 5); "cultural, ethnic and spiritual concepts (including cultural issues and spiritual beliefs as they relate to psychiatric symptom expression)" (p. 7); "concepts of mental

health promotion and illness prevention (being able to describe populations at risk for psychiatric disorders)" (p. 7); and "symptom management with those who have co-occurring chronic conditions, and attention to vulnerable populations and health disparities in mental health care and outcomes (i.e., developmentally disabled, elders, and marginalized populations such as homeless and jailed)" (p. 8).

Currently, no certification examination for the geropsychiatric specialty is offered by the ANCC (Kovner et al., 2002; J. Stanley, personal communication, January 12, 2010). In 2003, Deirdre Thornlow, Director of the Gerontology Project with the AACN, reported knowing of only five programs that offer an MS Geropsychiatric CNS/NP degree, and among them are the University of Arkansas, University of Michigan, and Case Western Reserve University (D. Thornlow, personal communication, July 28, 2003). However, increasingly universities are offering the needed continuing professional education for this specialty. The University of Massachusetts Lowell, for example, offers a 12-credit postbaccalaureate certificate in geropsychiatric and mental health nursing, and several other such programs are available nationwide.

Fortunately, national specialty nursing groups and organizations are spearheading efforts to foster improved mental health promotion and psychiatric care for older adults. GAPNA identified, among its 2009 to 2010 *Health Affairs Agenda,* the need to "Expand access to home, community and long term care services for all older adults by partnering with groups that promote cost effective, accessible, quality health care reform" (GAPNA, 2009, p. 1). In 2003, the NCGNP specifically identified the need to "Advocate for improving the quality of mental health care for elders, especially those who reside in nursing homes" (NCGNP, 2003). The Hartford Foundation's Institute for Geriatric Nursing likewise identified strategies and tactics for the years 2001 to 2006. These included "important nursing education initiatives to assure that all advanced practice and baccalaureate nursing graduates are competent in geriatrics, to imbue best practice nursing care of older adults and their families across the continuum of care settings, to foster innovative clinical geriatric nursing research, and to shape the national agenda to improve nursing care to older adults" (The John A. Hartford Institute, n.d.).

The International Society for Education and Research in Psychiatric–Mental Health Nursing (SERPN) has established an Adult and Geropsychiatric–Mental Health Nurses Division to "identify, disseminate, and grow the unique body of knowledge that constitutes the scientific foundation for advanced practice psychiatric/mental health nurses who provide mental health care for adults, the elderly, their families, and communities" (International SERPN, n.d., para. 1). Among the goals identified for the division are to promote appropriate educational preparation for undergraduate and graduate level education of adult and geropsychiatric nurses (International SERPN). One key outcome has been the publication, with APNA, of *Essentials of Psychiatric Mental Health Nursing in the BSN Curriculum* (2008).

APNA describes itself as a professional organization representing the specialty practice of psychiatric–mental health nursing. It has more than 4000 members and is the largest national association of psychiatric nurses (www.apna.org). However, only 16% of psychiatric nurses have subspecialization in geriatrics (Bartels, 2003). A national online survey of graduate education in geropsychiatric nursing (Kurlowicz, Puentes, Evans, Spool, & Ratcliffe, 2007) found that 15 schools out of 206 responding reported offering a geropsychiatric nursing program, track, or minor. Interestingly, only 38% of the total of 60 schools that reported having a psychiatric mental health nursing graduate program identified that they include geropsychiatric nursing didactic or clinical content within the curriculum. The need is acute to address older adults' mental health care in the preparation of all nurses, at both undergraduate and graduate levels, with geropsychiatric and mental health nursing knowledge and skills.

In January 2008, The John A. Hartford Foundation awarded the AAN and the Universities of Arkansas, Iowa, and Pennsylvania funding for a 4-year collaborative project to enhance the cognitive and mental health of older Americans. The principal investigators are Drs. Cornelia Beck, Kathleen Buckwalter, and Lois Evans. "The Geropsychiatric Nursing Collaborative (GPNC) is designed to help improve the training of nurses for the care of elders suffering depression, dementia, and other mental health disorders. The collaborative effort will enhance extant competencies for all levels of nursing education, focusing them on older adults with mental health/illness concerns. The competency statements together with curriculum materials developed for basic, graduate, postgraduate, and continuing education nursing programs will be shared via [the] website" (AAN, 2009). Copies of the geropsychiatric competencies are available in Appendix A.

One definition of geropsychiatric nursing practice proposed by the AAN's Geropsychiatric Nursing Collaborative Work Group is, "Geropsychiatric nursing practice includes care of persons and their families approaching and/or experiencing developmental tasks and mental health concerns of later life. This care addresses the integration of biopsychosocial, functional, spiritual, cultural, economic, and environmental assessment in the mental health promotion and psychiatric treatment plans which are established, and emphasizes strengths-based assessment to support older adults and their families" (AAN, 2009, p. 1). Building on the National Organization of Nurse Practitioner Faculties *Domains and Core Competencies of Nurse Practitioner Practice* (2006) as a framework, members of the GPNC Competency Work Group have proposed geropsychiatric enhancements to the competencies for GNPs, psychiatric mental health NPs, adult NPs, family NPs, acute care NPs, and women's health NPs (see Appendix A). Entry-level geropsychiatric enhancements to the AACN and Hartford Institute for

Geriatric Nursing Gerontological Competencies have also been suggested. Additionally, members of the Geropsychiatric Mental Health Core Competencies Workgroup are serving on the newly combined Adult–Gerontology advanced practice nurse specialty groups developing competency statements (Diana Morris, PhD, RN, FAAN, FGSA, is serving on the Adult–Gerontology CNS Expert Panel; Karen Devereaux Melillo is serving on the Adult–Gerontology NP Expert Panel; and William Puentes, PhD, RN, is participating in the AACN and Hartford Institute for Geriatric Nursing process to revise the BSN Gerontological Competencies [Pamela Dudzik, personal communication, January 8, 2010]).

REVIEW OF STANDARDS

Geropsychiatric and mental health nursing is guided by a number of professional standards, beginning with the *ANA Standards of Clinical Nursing Practice* (1998), the *ANA Code of Ethics for Nurses with Interpretive Statements* (2001), the *ANA Social Policy Statement* (1996) and the *ANA Social Policy Statement* updated draft (2008). Standards serve as criteria on which to measure one's nursing practice. The American Nurses Association (ANA) notes "psychogeriatric nursing practice is a rapidly developing subspecialty that addresses the mental health needs of older adults" (ANA, 2001, p. 7). The practice of geropsychiatric and mental health nursing is also guided by two sets of practice guidelines: *Scope and Standards of Gerontological Nursing Practice* (ANA, 2001), currently under revision following posting for public comment (2009), and *Scope and Standards of Psychiatric-Mental Health Nursing Practice* (ANA, 2007).

The ANA has also published *Intellectual and Developmental Disabilities Nursing: Scope and Standards of Practice* (ANA, 2004), an important field in caring for older adults with disabilities. Nurses caring for older adults will likely be providing care to those with mental retardation and other developmental disabilities (e.g., cerebral palsy) and their family members. Current estimates by the American Association on Intellectual and Developmental Disabilities (formerly the American Association on Mental Retardation [AAMR]) suggest the numbers of adults age 60 and older with mental retardation will double to 1,065,000 by 2030 when the "baby boom" generation reaches their sixties (AAMR, 2002b). According to the former AAMR, mental retardation is neither a medical disorder nor a mental disorder. Rather, mental retardation is an important subcategory of developmental disabilities. Mental retardation, which originates before age 18, is defined as "a disability characterized by significant limitations both in intellectual functioning and adaptive behavior as expressed in conceptual, social, and practice adaptive skills" (AAMR, 2002a). Today, mental disability and mental retardation are often used to mean the same thing, although intellectual disability is gaining currency as the preferred term (American Association on Intellectual and Developmental Disabilities, 2009).

In its statement on the scope of practice (ANA, 1998), the ANA recognizes that persons with developmental disabilities or mental retardation are living longer. There is a need for both the nurse generalist and the advanced practice nurse to provide safe and effective care for this population using the Standards of Professional Performance, which reflect the role functions of nursing, and Standards of Care, which reflect many of the components of the nursing process (ANA, 1998). Both are described in the statement on the *Scope and Standards for the Nurse Who Specializes in Developmental Disabilities and/or Mental Retardation.* Table 2-1 provides an overview of standards of practice comparing gerontological nursing, psychiatric–mental health nursing, and intellectual and developmental disabilities (I/DD) nursing.

The ANA has published *Forensic Nursing: Scope and Standards of Practice* (2009), developed by the International Association of Forensic Nurses

TABLE 2-1

Standards of Practice Comparing Gerontological Nursing, Psychiatric-Mental Health Nursing, and Intellectual and Developmental Disabilities (I/DD) Nursing

Standard	Gerontological Nursing	Psychiatric–Mental Health Nursing	Intellectual and Developmental Disabilities Nursing
Assessment	The gerontological nurse collects patient health data	The psychiatric–mental health registered nurse collects comprehensive health data pertinent to the patient's health or situation	The registered nurse who specializes in I/DD collects comprehensive data pertinent to the patient's health or the situation
Diagnosis	The gerontological nurse analyzes the assessment data in determining the diagnosis	The psychiatric–mental health registered nurse analyzes the assessment data to determine diagnoses or problems, including level of risk	The registered nurse who specializes in I/DD analyzes the assessment data to determine the diagnoses or issues
Outcome identification	The gerontological nurse identifies expected outcomes individualized to the older adult	The psychiatric–mental health registered nurse identifies expected outcomes for a plan individualized to the patient or to the situation	The registered nurse who specializes in I/DD identifies expected outcomes for a plan individualized to the patient or the situation
Planning	The gerontological nurse develops a plan of care that prescribes interventions to attain expected outcomes	The psychiatric–mental health registered nurse develops a plan of care that prescribes strategies and alternatives to attain expected outcomes	The registered nurse who specializes in I/DD develops a plan that prescribes strategies and alternatives to attain expected outcomes
Implementation	The gerontological nurse implements the interventions identified in the plan of care	The psychiatric–mental health registered nurse implements the identified plan	The registered nurse who specializes in I/DD implements the identified plan
Evaluation	The gerontological nurse evaluates the older adult's progress toward attainment of expected outcomes	The psychiatric–mental health registered nurse evaluates progress toward attainment of expected outcomes	The registered nurse who specializes in I/DD evaluates progress toward attainment of outcomes

Source: Data from American Nurses Association and American Association on Mental Retardation (2004); American Nurses Association, American Psychiatric–Mental Health Nurses Association, & International Society of Psychiatric–Mental Health Nurses (2007); and American Nurses Association (2001). Reproduced with permission of the American Nurses Association.

and the ANA. Forensic nursing is defined as "the practice of nursing globally where health and legal systems intersect" (International Association of Forensic Nurses, 2008). Given the aging of some prison populations, and the U.S. Department of Justice, Office of Justice Programs, Bureau of Justice Statistics Special Report *Mental Health Problems of Prison and Jail Inmates* (James & Glaze, 2006), this forensic specialty within nursing is responsible for "providing age-appropriate care in a culturally and ethnically sensitive manner" (ANA, 2008, p. 28). For each reference to "health," "illness," "care," or "disease," emphasis should include both "physical" and "mental" in recognition of the significant impact mental health has on the populations served by the forensic nurse and the need to promote mental health and well-being for individuals, families, and communities.

THEORETICAL FOUNDATIONS FOR GEROPSYCHIATRIC AND MENTAL HEALTH NURSING

Gerontological nursing is a highly complex specialty, which has borrowed theories of aging from several disciplines, including psychology, biology, and sociology. Gerontological nursing has adapted these theories to the person, health, nursing, and environment paradigm in nursing. Eliopoulos has offered her interpretation of the information system needed by the gerontological nurse (Figure 2-1) (Eliopoulos, 2010, p. 74).

In addition to theories of aging, geropsychiatric nursing borrows theory from the interdisciplinary foundations of psychiatric and mental health nursing. Geropsychiatric nursing also draws on theories and concepts from psychiatry, the social and behavioral sciences, and the humanities. It recognizes the crisis in American psychiatry and heated debates between the neuroscientific and the psychodynamic or interpersonal approaches to understanding and treating psychiatrically disturbed older adults (Luhrmann, 2000; McHugh & Clark, 2006). Accordingly, the complexity of care for many older adults requires an interdisciplinary team approach that is attentive to neuropathology and the psychosocial facets of mental health care. Such an approach includes attention to the multifaceted conceptual roots of geropsychiatric nursing care. The following is an overview and critique of several disciplines' contribution to fulfilling the aims of this book, adapted and extended from Hoff, Hallisey, and Hoff (2009, chap. 1). It underscores the historical contributions of mental health theorists and psychotherapists whose ideals continue to inspire and guide psychiatric and mental health practice in a broad interdisciplinary healthcare arena. The section concludes with a case example illustrating the theoretical underpinnings of geropsychiatric care in the nursing paradigm.

Psychoanalytic and Personality Theories

Sigmund Freud was a pioneer in the study of human behavior in the late 1800s and early 1900s. His psychoanalytic theory focused on the behavior of disturbed individuals. It acknowledges and emphasizes the role of early childhood conflicts in the development of neurotic symptoms in later life. This approach is termed "determinism," a static concept that has been widely discredited. Nevertheless, many psychiatric nurses and others in psychotherapy roles appropriately inquire about a client's childhood experiences and their impact on later life, perhaps as a result of Freud's work.

Freud was the first to propose an unconscious level of mental functioning and the three-part system of personality: id, ego, and superego. He believed that one must maintain a balance (equilibrium) among the three parts to avoid psychopathology. Freud's psychoanalytical technique of listening is the mainstay of the therapeutic relationship. His insight into human behavior marked the beginning of modern psychiatry, and he has influenced the contemporary writings of theorists in the social and behavioral sciences.

The classic works of Harry Stack Sullivan (1947) and Erik Erikson (1963) reveal modifications of Freud's ideas toward less deterministic, more developmental theories for explaining human behavior. Sullivan, heavily influenced by sociology, focused on the social, interpersonal aspects of personality and one's cognitive representations of self and others, which he called "personifications." He believed that personality continues to develop well into adulthood, but he did not directly address the development in older adults.

FIGURE 2-1

Information System of the Gerontological Nurse.

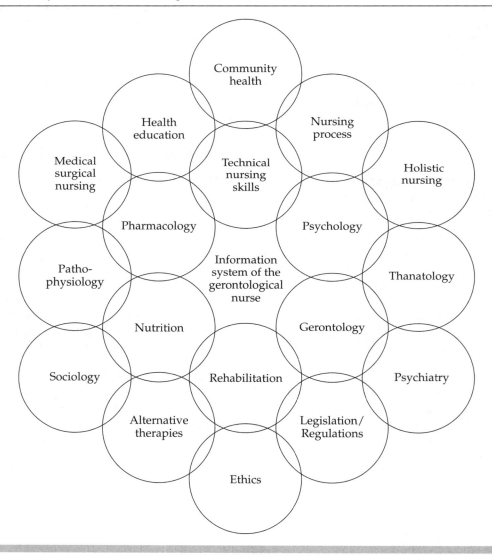

Erikson's theory of psychosocial development is the first theory to identify a stage of personality development in older adulthood, although his early work omitted the oldest-old. His theory has also been critiqued for its support of traditional family structures that produce increased stress for women who bear the burden of disproportionate caretaking roles over the lifespan (Crittenden, 2001; Waring, 1990). Despite these limitations, Erikson's theory offers valuable insights to the understanding of human development.

The theory of psychosocial development describes eight stages of development, each with two possible outcomes. The successful completion of each stage results in healthy personality development. As longevity becomes the norm, Erikson's ideas regarding "middle adulthood" (the successful completion of which results in generativity) may apply to individuals in their early retirement years. Ego integrity versus despair, the final stage, acknowledges the need for older adults to feel that they have led productive lives and that they have met their life goals. Unsuccessful completion of this stage can result in depression and despair. Interventions, such as intergenerational programs at nursing homes and senior centers, life review, and reminiscence groups, promote the development of ego integrity in the older adult.

Abraham Maslow's (1970) classic five-leveled hierarchy of needs has been widely used as a model to explain human behavior. Maslow stated that some needs (e.g., food and shelter) take precedence over others. Individuals must meet the needs of one level before moving onto the next, higher level of need. However, Maslow suggested that individuals with extreme problems at a particular level may become "fixated" on those needs for the rest of their life and regress to a lower level of need in response to life stress. For example, an older person traumatized by physical or sexual abuse as a child may never forget this history, but with skilled counseling can move beyond a "victim" identity to a satisfying life, whereas someone lacking such help can remain fixated on "victimhood" as an overarching life influence.

Spirituality, Stress, and Social Learning Theories

Viktor Frankl's ageless book, *Man's Search for Meaning* (1963), was in part a reaction to the reductionism of both medicine and psychology, demonstrated by their biological, mechanistic explanations of the mind and human behavior. Frankl sought a balance between physiology and humanity–spirituality. He emphasized the responsibility that an individual has for being human, and that one cannot be given meaning in life: meaning must be a lived experience. However, a therapist can assist people in their search for meaning. Frankl's writings about the existential search for meaning have relevance for psychiatric nursing in general, and in particular for geropsychiatric nurses helping clients come to terms with perhaps unresolved issues faced during life's final phase. In the spirit of logo (reading) therapy, another inspiring book for readers young and old is Sherwin Nuland's *The Art of Aging: A Doctor's Prescription for Well-Being* (2007).

In the existential framework, theories of the classical stress response are expanded to include values and meanings of people coping with life stressors. Hans Selye (1956), the founder of the concept of stress, proposed that failure to cope with stressors (whether positive or negative) can result in "diseases of adaptation," or can affect the body's capacity to respond to injury and disease.

Developed by Albert Bandura (1977, 1997), the theory of social learning and self-efficacy views individuals as self-organizing, proactive, self-reflecting, and self-regulating rather than as reactive organisms shaped by environmental forces or driven by unconscious impulses. From this theoretical perspective, human behavior is seen as the product of personal, behavioral, and environmental influences.

Antonovsky's (1980, 1987) research with concentration camp survivors and women in menopause led to his concept of "resistance resources," including social support and a concept of "sense of coherence," to explain differential responses to stressful situations. Sense of coherence includes the person's perception of events as comprehensible, manageable, and meaningful. Applied to the stress response, a person with a strong sense of coherence defines social stressors as social rather than assuming blame for trouble that did not originate from oneself. One's resistance resources can make the difference between positive or negative responses to developmental transitions or to extreme stress (which a clinician might define as "crisis"), such as an older person's loss of spouse and major source of support. Research with abused women (Hoff, 1990) supports these views and the interactional relationship between stress, crisis, and illness (physical, emotional, and mental) (Hoff et al., 2009).

One model, the progressively lowered stress threshold (PLST) (Hall & Buckwalter, 1987), has been offered as a conceptual foundation for the effects of stress on persons with Alzheimer's disease and related disorders. "The model is adapted from psychologic theories of stress, adaptation and coping – in addition to behavioral and physiologic research of Alzheimer's disease" (Hall & Laloudakis, 1999, para. 6). Dysfunctional behaviors are a direct result of four groups of symptom clusters: (1) the cognitive or intellectual losses, (2) affective or personality changes, (3) changes in ability to plan around losses that cause a predictable decline in activities of daily living abilities, and (4) the loss of stress threshold (Hall & Laloudakis). When any of six common triggers occurs (fatigue; change in environment, routine, or caregiver; misleading stimuli or inappropriate stimulus levels; affective responses to perceptions of loss; internal or external demands that exceed functional capacity; and physical stressors, such as pain, discomfort, infection, acute illness, or comorbid conditions), the patient's stress threshold is exceeded and dysfunctional behavior (problematic behaviors that may be upsetting for family members) or catastrophic events can occur (Hall & Laloudakis).

The PLST has been used in the design and evaluation of experimental interventions to assist caregivers in understanding and planning care for behavioral problems exhibited by patients (Gerdner, Buckwalter, & Reed, 2002) and in a caregiver training protocol for dementia management (Gerdner, Hall, & Buckwalter, 1996). PLST has been cited in an evidence-based protocol on wandering (Futrell, Melillo, & Remington, 2008), using expert opinion to offer this model as a basis for physical and psychosocial interventions to decrease wandering by eliminating stressors from the environment, including cold at night, changes in daily routines, and extra people at holidays (Hall & Laloudakis, 1999). The PLST model is a useful framework in applying theory to practice for geropsychiatric and mental health nursing.

Crisis Theory, Bereavement, and Preventive Psychiatry

The unique contribution of crisis theory, public health, and preventive psychiatry is the focus on identification and early intervention with vulnerable populations. Typically, the growing number of seniors requires more rather than fewer resources to maintain health and safety in chosen locales. Of particular note for older persons is Lindemann's (1944) classic work on loss, grief, and early support through mourning that is pivotal in avoiding the hazards of depression.

Lindemann's (1944) study of bereavement following the disastrous Coconut Grove fire in Boston defined the grieving process people went through after sudden death of a relative. Lindemann found that survivors of this disaster who developed serious psychopathologies had failed to go through the normal process of grieving. His findings are particularly relevant in the care of older people who typically have suffered many losses, but who often lack the assistance and social approval necessary for grief work following loss and instead may be offered only medication (Hoff et al., 2009, chaps. 4 and 10). Grief work consists of the process of mourning one's loss, experiencing the pain of such loss, and eventually accepting the reality of loss and adjusting to life without the loved person or object. Encouraging and supporting people to experience normal grieving can prevent depression and other negative outcomes of crises caused by loss.

Among the pioneers in crisis theory, public health, and preventive psychiatry, perhaps none is more outstanding than Gerald Caplan. In 1964, he developed a conceptual framework for understanding the process of crisis development. Caplan also emphasized a communitywide (i.e., public health) approach to crisis intervention. Public health includes education programs and consultation with various caretakers, such as geriatric care managers and community-based nurses, in preventing destructive outcomes of crises, such as suicide or abuse of others. In his classic work, *Principles of Preventive Psychiatry* (1964), Caplan's focus is on prevention, mastery, and the importance of social, cultural, and material "supplies" necessary to avoid crisis arising from stressful life events. This public health framework resonates with a current emphasis on human rights and the intrinsic connection between health and socioeconomic security and social justice for disadvantaged groups, such as older persons who are poor or homeless (Rodriguez-Garcia & Akhter, 2000).

Although Caplan's contribution to the development of crisis theory and practice is widely accepted, his conceptual framework is grounded in disease rather than health concepts (Brandt & Gardner, 2000; Hoff, 1990; Hoff et al., 2009), including some of the mechanistic concepts set forth by Freud (e.g., equilibrium between id, ego, and superego psychic functions). The static concept of homeostasis and maintaining equilibrium shortchanges the dynamic processes of growth, development, and creative integration of life experience that are so important during late stages of the life cycle. This limitation is offset, however, by Caplan's emphasis on prevention. A more dynamic interpretation of stressful events and the crisis experience corresponds with ego psychology and developmental theory, which emphasizes one's potential for growth and change through all stages of the life cycle (Erikson, 1963).

Crisis Care and Psychiatric Stabilization

Similar to the growing emphasis on primary health care is the integration of crisis approaches on behalf of those suffering from acute psychotic episodes. Typically, such persons are seen in the crisis unit of community mental health centers or in the emergency service of general hospitals where the emphasis is on triage and rapid disposition. However, such acute episodes also occur in long-term care facilities. Psychopharmacologic agents are often used to stabilize distressed people in these settings. The strong medical orientation in such situations warrants greater caution than usual by providers. Chemical stabilization should serve as a complement to rather than a mere substitute for skilled crisis intervention techniques. The aim is not only to restore acute upset persons to a state of "equilibrium" or homeostasis, but also to examine the environmental and interpersonal factors that may contribute to repeated upsets or abusive behavior of vulnerable clients.

For older people under stress or in acute crisis, overreliance on stabilization with psychotropic drugs is particularly hazardous. Chemical tranquilization practiced without humanistic crisis intervention is related to iatrogenesis (illness induced by physicians and other health providers) (McKinlay, 1990). Among some older persons with multiple social stressors and physical ailments or disabilities, it is all too easy to compound these problems by overmedication, failure to identify and prevent interactive side effects, and insufficient attention to contextual factors (such as economic status, social support, secure housing, and 24-hour access to help when needed—a pivotal element of comprehensive community mental health).

Community Mental Health

Caplan's concepts about crisis emerged during the same period in which the community mental health movement was born. An important influence on preventive intervention and crisis care during this era was the 1961 report of the Joint

Commission on Mental Illness and Health in the United States, *Action for Mental Health* (1961). This work documented through 5 years of study the crucial fact that people were not getting the help they needed, when they needed it, and where they needed it, close to their natural social setting. It underscores a key facet of healthy aging and the desires of older people needing mental health care: aging in place and receiving care at home or close to a familiar community and trusted social network, and coordinating such care with skilled medical and nursing interventions.

However, despite federal legislation and funding, the ideals of community-based mental health care are yet to be realized in the nationwide struggle for universal access, cost control, and insurance parity for mental health service. Community-based mental health service includes integration of mental health basics in primary care settings where most people are first seen, whether the presenting problem is medical or psychosocial (Hoff & Morgan, in press). But even among settings that include holistic approaches to care, emergency and other mental health services are often far from ideal. In these settings the growing numbers of clients are age 65 or older, whereas most primary care providers have minimal preparation in gerontology and geropsychiatric care.

Political and fiscal policies in past decades resulted in further departures from community mental health ideals worldwide (Hoff, 1993; Marks & Scott, 1990). In the United States, this can be traced in part to several historic themes: (1) the mind–body split in health practice (Edmands, Hoff, Kaylor, Mower, & Sorrell, 1999); (2) an individualistic versus population-based focus in health service delivery (Fee & Brown, 2000); and (3) continuing bias against and disparity in health insurance coverage for those with mental or emotional illness (Ustun, 1999).

Reform movements in Canada, Italy, and the United States, with support from the World Health Organization, have attempted to reverse this course and alleviate the global burden of mental illness (Kaseje & Sempebwa, 1989; Mosher & Burti, 1989; Rachlis & Kushner, 1994; Scheper-Hughes & Lovell, 1986; Ustun, 1999; World Health Organization, 2002). Despite some progress toward reform, cost-saving, and a community mental health ideal, debate continues about the patchwork system in the United States and leads to consideration of sociocultural and feminist factors influencing geropsychiatric care.

Sociologic, Diversity, and Feminist Influences

Discussion of theory influencing geropsychiatric nursing practice thus far suggests that the momentum has come largely from psychological, psychiatric, or community sources. Yet, sociology, anthropology, and feminist scholars offer invaluable insights into the understanding and practice of geropsychiatry. We are conceived, born, grow and develop, and die in a social context. We experience distress, illness, and crisis in our social milieu. People near us (friends, family, and the community) help or hinder us during stressful life events. Death, even for those who die alone and abandoned, demands some response from the society left behind.

Multidisciplinary research has supported a shifting emphasis from individual to sociocultural approaches in helping distressed people (e.g., Antonovsky, 1980, 1987; Hoff, 1990; McGoldrick & Hardy, 2008). Despite the prevalence of individual intervention techniques, overwhelming evidence shows that social networks and support are primary factors in a person's susceptibility to disease, the process of becoming ill and seeking help, the treatment process, and the outcome of illness, whether that is rehabilitation and recovery or death (e.g., Hoff et al., 2009, chap. 5; Loustaunau & Sobo, 1997). The work of clinicians during the golden age of social psychiatry supports the prolific social science literature on social approaches to distressed people (Hoff et al., 2009). Among earlier writers, psychiatrist Hansell (1976), building on Caplan's (1964) work, has done the most to stress social influences on preventive interventions with persons in distress and avoiding destructive outcomes of crisis, with particular application to the seriously and persistently mentally ill. His social–psychological approach to mental health theory and practice resonates with cross-cultural influences in the field.

Political, social, and technological developments have contributed to more permeable national boundaries, and at the same time have sharpened cultural awareness, unique ethnic identities, and sensitivity to diversity issues. These observations have implications for cross-cultural and diversity issues in the experience of crisis, and variance in response to older people in chronic or acute distress. The rich data on rites of passage marking human transition states in traditional societies are another significant contribution of cultural and social anthropology to the understanding of vulnerable populations in transition. These insights from other cultures are particularly relevant to older people who typically face the challenge of successfully navigating several transitions together or in rapid succession (e.g., a change in status from healthy to disabled, or a diagnosis of life-threatening illness; a move from home to institution; role change from spouse to widowed; and the final transition from life to death). Sadly, many older adults lack the support they need and deserve during these life-altering transitions (Hoff et al., 2009, Part II: Crises Related to Developmental and Situational Transition States).

Attention to and competency in caring for persons from diverse cultural groups are challenging for many providers as they face a multitude of languages and belief systems among their clients. Of central importance here is recognizing the wisdom and clinical relevance of a key principle in working with anyone different from ourselves: whatever our ethnic or cultural identity, we should never assume that—even with extensive study and exposure—we will ever be fully knowledgeable about a culture other than our own.

A helpful way of conveying respect for another's values and meaning system is to focus on a set of eight questions developed by medical anthropologist Arthur Kleinman and applied by Fadiman (1997, pp. 260–261) to a Hmong family's serious culture clash with medical practitioners in California who treated their daughter's seizures:

1. What do you call the problem?
2. What do you think has caused the problem?
3. Why do you think it started when it did?
4. What do you think the sickness does? How does it work?
5. How severe is the sickness? Will it have a short or long course?
6. What kind of treatment do you think the patient should receive? What are the most important results you hope are received from this treatment?
7. What are the chief problems the sickness has caused?
8. What do you fear most about the sickness?

To Kleinman's eight questions, we add: How do you think we (at this agency, clinic, or hospital) can best help you with this problem?

These generic questions can be adapted to any treatment situation or concern in which successful outcomes depend heavily on the nurse's attempt to understand the other's point of view, no matter how different from one's own or deviant from treatment protocols entirely foreign to the client. Such an approach embodies the essence of respect, which is fundamental to the interpersonal process of effective nursing care.

Complementing sociocultural influences, feminist theory offers important insights on the mental health status of older adults and a gender-sensitive response to their needs by geropsychiatric providers. Feminist influences mean taking gender into account in respect to theory, research, and geropsychiatric nursing practice with individuals and families. For example, the burden in caregiving roles falls disproportionately on women, despite some progress in gender equality and egalitarian relationships; marriage patterns result in more companionless women than men in old age with concomitant loss of sexual intimacy; traditional gender roles often leave widowed men at greater risk of depression and suicide than women; gender bias in paid and unpaid work roles typically leaves women with insufficient time for self-care and health-promoting leisure activity; and gender bias also results in women's greater risk of poverty and institutionalization in old age (Estes, 1995).

Nursing Theories

Geropsychiatric nursing practice has benefited greatly from the nursing theories developed by Dorothea E. Orem and Hildegarde E. Peplau, who began their careers in the early 1930s. Both nursing theorists continued to develop their concepts over many years. Orem's sixth edition of *Nursing: Concepts of Practice* was published in 2001. Peplau's original work, *Interpersonal Relations in Nursing* (originally published in 1952, last reprint 1991), is required reading in many nursing schools. Her psychodynamic nursing theory is particularly useful for psychiatric nurses.

Orem's (1980) self-care deficit nursing theory (SCDNT) establishes nursing as a practical science having a focus that is distinct from other disciplines. Orem's SCDNT is actually a model that encompasses three theories: self-care, self-care deficits, and nursing systems. Self-care is a human regulatory function that people either perform for themselves or have performed for them to maintain life, health, development, and well-being. The abstract term "self-care deficit" refers to the relationship between a person's capabilities and the need for care. Nursing is an intentional human action and includes operations of diagnosis, prescription, and regulation (Taylor et al., 1998). SCDNT provides a framework for understanding the nursing process in general, but it is particularly helpful when thinking of older clients who may be experiencing "deficits" as part of the normal aging process.

Hildegarde Peplau's psychodynamic nursing theory was influenced by Freud, Maslow, and especially Sullivan, with whom she studied. The

functions of psychodynamic nursing are "Being able to understand one's own behavior to help others identify felt difficulties, and to apply principles of human relations to the problems that arise at all levels of experience" (Peplau, 1991, p. xi). Peplau emphasized the importance of the nurse–patient relationship and identified four phases of that relationship: (1) orientation, (2) identification, (3) exploitation, and (4) resolution. During the relationship, both the patient and the nurse grow through experiences. Peplau stated that illness brings up feelings derived from prior experiences, and that the nurse–patient relationship is an opportunity for nurses to assist clients to finish developmental tasks.

Geropsychiatric nurses can use Peplau's phases of the interpersonal relationship to track their progress in guiding clients toward mutually agreed-on goals. Additionally, nurses can promote the positive resolution of the developmental tasks of later life.

THE NURSING PARADIGM APPLIED TO GEROPSYCHIATRIC NURSING

The overview of multidisciplinary theories and concepts underpinning gerontology and geropsychiatric nursing offers a rich source for bridging gaps between theory and practice. In the everyday demands of nursing practice, a firm grasp of theory and confidence in its application is sometimes short-changed. When that happens, desired outcomes of nursing interventions may be compromised. This section aims to bridge the divide between theory and practice.

The nursing paradigm with its key interrelated concepts is presented in Figure 2-2 (Hoff, 2009). Each of the paradigm's key concepts depicts the interdisciplinary theoretical underpinnings of the particular concept with reference to geropsychiatric nursing practice (Box 2-1).

The following case example illustrates the application and integration of the nursing paradigm's four concepts.

FIGURE 2-2

Nursing Paradigm.

This model illustrates the centrality of the four **key/anchor** concepts in the nursing paradigm: **nurse/provider, person/family, health, environment.** A few supporting concepts (especially those pertaining to geropsychiatric nursing) are illustrated as well; e.g., threat to safety, vulnerability, social isolation, coping (healthy and unhealthy).

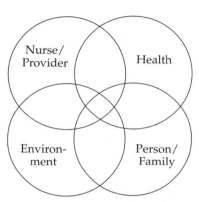

A. Key anchor concepts in the nursing paradigm: provider, person, health, environment

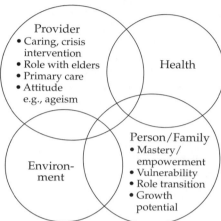

B. Beginning level: all concepts are introduced; provider and person are emphasized.

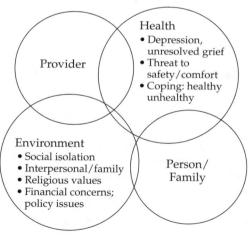

C. Mid-level: all concepts are elaborated; health, environment are emphasized.

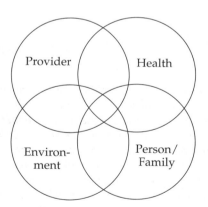

D. Expert level: all concepts are brought together/integrated.

Source: Reproduced with permission from Hoff (1994); Hoff (2009).

BOX 2-1   NURSING PARADIGM KEY CONCEPTS AND THEORIES

I. Person/Family
   a. Developmental, life-cycle theories
   b. Gender and role theories
   c. Personality theory
   d. Existential theory

II. Environmental
   a. Social stress
   b. Community mental health
   c. Sociocultural, feminist influences
   d. Socioeconomic theory

III. Health
   a. Psychoanalytic theory
   b. Crisis, public health theories
   c. Emotional stress
   d. Orem's self-care deficit theory
   e. Social support and preventive psychiatry

IV. Nurse/Provider
   a. Peplau's interpersonal relationship theory
   b. Attitudes, knowledge, and skills in caring for older adults

CASE STUDY

Frank Kelly, a 72-year-old widowed white man, presents at the emergency department of a community hospital complaining of chest pain. His daughter Kate, the youngest of three children, encouraged him to seek treatment and is with him. His cardiac workup is negative, but during the assessment he is tearful and says that he wishes he were dead so that he could be with his wife. She died 2 years ago, and since then, weekly visits from his children, who all live nearby, have been Frank's only social support. "I think about killing myself all the time, but I was raised Irish Catholic and I don't want to go to hell," he laments.

He admits feeling depressed most of his life, but never sought help, saying "Who would I have asked?" Kate states that Frank's sister is treated with citalopram for depression.

Frank and his wife sold their house 5 years ago and bought a condo unit in a complex for seniors. He never developed friendships with neighbors because he focused on his wife during her last 2 years. Since then he has remained isolated, and his only distraction is watching television. He has no hobbies, but previously enjoyed hunting and owns several guns. Frank smiles briefly and expresses pride in his career as a pipe fitter, which enabled him

CASE STUDY

to provide a comfortable lifestyle for his wife and children. His pension and Social Security income cover his living expenses now, but he is worried about escalating costs of his Medicare Part B coverage.

Frank admits that he has not seen his primary care physician since just after his wife died. At that time his physician suggested that he join a widower's support group, but he did not want to share his feelings at that point. Frank takes aspirin 81 mg, and hydrochlorothiazide daily for hypertension, but has called the office for refills without further evaluation. He has pain from osteoarthritis, which is "pretty bad most days," but does not take any medication for this. About every 4 months his right great toe swells and is tender; he states that at "one time a doctor said it was gout."

Frank has never smoked and quit drinking 20 years ago because his wife objected to it. However, 6 months ago he started drinking beer again. He currently has five to seven beers a day, three to four times a week. He drinks alone at home and notes, "It sort of dulls the arthritis pain, so I can sleep better. I nod off in front of the TV." Frank estimates that he sleeps a total of 7 to 10 hours a day, with many naps. He reports a fair appetite, but Kate thinks he has lost about 15 pounds in the last 2 years.

Application of Theory

Using the nursing paradigm, the nurse notes that Frank Kelly ("Person") is an older widowed white man who has not adjusted to his retired status or his role as widower. The nurse remembers that older white men as a group have the highest rate of suicide. Frank's difficulty in adjusting is interpreted considering developmental, life cycle, gender, and role theories. Additionally, existential theory relates to Frank's lack of meaning apart from his traditional, gender-specific role as a worker and provider. Accepting assistance from his children,

members of the "sandwich generation" (the generation caring for both children and parents), may threaten his self-esteem.

Environmental factors particular to this case include social isolation; unresolved grief with inappropriate coping (alcohol); ethnic and religious influences; financial concerns; and the general absence of community mental health services given current priorities in health care. Sociocultural and socioeconomic theories and the concepts of social stress and community mental health must be considered as the nurse assesses Frank's environment.

Evaluation of Frank's health is informed by psychoanalytical, crisis, and public health theories, and the concept of emotional stress. A suicide risk assessment would note that he has access to a lethal means of killing himself, and that his drinking (which increases impulsive behavior) increases his risk further. Orem's self-care deficit theory, social support, and concepts of preventive psychiatry should be considered as the nurse notes Frank's depression and weight loss, his arthritic pain, and his self-medication with alcohol. Assessment of his ability to live independently should include an assessment of social support. Current support (his children) may be inadequate to meet his present needs, as he attempts to cope with the loss of his wife. The nurse can provide Frank with information about accessing medical and mental health care.

The nurse/provider uses the interpersonal relationship (Peplau) as a therapeutic tool in working with Frank. Nurses must become aware of their own attitudes toward older adults and should develop interpersonal skills best suited for this population. Physical assessment is guided by the nurse's knowledge of normal changes associated with aging. Finally, application of mind–body concepts allows the nurse to integrate all data obtained, so as to provide holistic care.

ACKNOWLEDGMENTS

The author thanks Martha (Marti) A. Huff, who summarized the section on nursing theories for the 2005 edition of this book.

REFERENCES

American Academy of Nursing. (2002). *New initiative on geriatric nursing education issues formal report outlining goals and strategies* [Press release]. Retrieved February 22, 2002, from http://www.nursingworld.org/pressrel/2002/pr0204a.htm

American Academy of Nursing. (2009). *Geropsychiatric Nursing Collaborative (GPNC).* Retrieved January 18, 2009, from www.aannet.org/i4a/pages/index.cfm?pageid=3833

American Association of Colleges and Nursing and The John A. Hartford Foundation Institute for Geriatric Nursing. (2000). *Older adults: Recommended baccalaureate competencies and curricular guidelines for geriatric nursing care.* Washington, DC: Author. Retrieved August 7, 2009, from http://www.aacn.nche.edu/Education/gercomp.htm

American Association of Colleges of Nursing and The John A. Hartford Foundation. (2004). *Hartford Geriatric Nursing Initiative. Nurse practitioner and clinical nurse specialist competencies for older adult care.* Washington, DC: American Association of Colleges of Nursing.

American Association of Intellectual and Developmental Disabilities. (2009). *Definition of intellectual disability.* Retrieved August 7, 2009, from http://www.aamr.org/content_100.cfm?navID=21

American Association on Mental Retardation (2002a). *Definition of mental retardation.* Retrieved August 29, 2003, from http://www.aamr.org/Policies/faq_mental_retardation.shtml

American Association on Mental Retardation (2002b). *Fact sheet: Aging, older adults and their caregivers.* Retrieved August 29, 2003, from http://www.aamr.org/Policies/faq_aging.shtml

American Nurses Association. (1996). *Social policy statement.* Silver Spring, MD: Nursesbooks.org

American Nurses Association. (1998). *Standards of clinical nursing practice.* Silver Spring, MD: Nursesbooks.org

American Nurses Association. (2001). *Code of ethics for nurses with interpretive statements.* Washington, DC: Author.

American Nurses Association. (2001). *Scope and standards of gerontological nursing practice* (2nd ed.). Silver Spring, MD: Nursesbooks.org

American Nurses Association. (2004). *Intellectual and developmental disabilities nursing: Scope and standards of practice.* Silver Spring, MD: Nursesbooks.org

American Nurses Association. (2007). *Scope and standards of psychiatric-mental health nursing practice* (2nd ed.). Silver Spring, MD: Nursesbooks.org

American Nurses Association. (2008). *Social policy statement. Draft for public comment.* Washington, DC: Author. Retrieved January 19, 2009, from www.nursingworld.org

American Nurses Association. (2009). *Draft gerontological nursing: Scope and standards of practice. Prepared for posting for public comment, April 22, 2009.* Retrieved June 1, 2009, from www.nursingworld.org

American Nurses Association and American Association on Mental Retardation. (2004). *Intellectual and developmental disabilities nursing: Scope and standards of practice.* Silver Spring, MD: Nursesbooks.org

American Nurses Association, American Psychiatric-Mental Health Nurses Association, & International Society of Psychiatric-Mental Health Nurses. (2007). *Psychiatric-mental health nursing: Scope and standards of practice.* Silver Spring, MD: Nursesbooks.org

American Nurses Association and International Association of Forensic Nurses. (2009). *Forensic nursing: Scope and standards of practice.* Washington, DC: Author.

American Nurses Credentialing Center. (2008). *2007 ANCC Certification data.* Silver Spring, MD: Author. Retrieved January 18, 2009, from www.nursescredentialing.org

American Psychiatric Nurses Association. (2009). What do psychiatric mental health nurses do? Retrieved January 12, 2010, from http://www.apna.org/i4a/pages/index.cfm?pageid=3292#3

American Psychiatric Nurses Association and International Society of Psychiatric Mental Health Nurses. (2008). *Essentials of psychiatric mental health nursing in the BSN curriculum: Collaboratively developed by ISPN and APNA, 2007–2008.* Retrieved January 18, 2009, from www.apna.org/files/public/revmay08finalCurricular_Guidelines_for_undergraduate_Education_in_psychiatric_Mental_Health_Nursing.pdf

Antonovsky, A. (1980). *Health, stress, and coping.* San Francisco: Jossey-Bass.

Antonovsky, A. (1987). *Unraveling the mysteries of health.* San Francisco: Jossey-Bass.

Association for Gerontology in Higher Education. (2009). *Directory of educational programs in gerontology and geriatrics* (8th ed.). Washington, DC: Author.

Bandura, A. (1977). *Social learning theory.* Englewood Cliffs, NJ: Prentice Hall.

Bandura, A. (1997). *Self-efficacy: The exercise of control.* New York: W. H. Freeman.

Bartels, S. J. (2003). Improving the United States system of care for older adults with mental illness: Findings and recommendations for the President's New Freedom Commission on Mental Health (commentary). *American Journal of Geriatric Psychiatry, 11*(5), 486–497.

Brandt, A. M., & Gardner, M. (2000). Antagonism and accommodation: Interpreting the relationship between public health and medicine in the United States during the 20th century. *American Journal of Public Health, 90*(5), 707–715.

Burgess, A. W. (1997). *Psychiatric nursing: Promoting mental health.* Stamford, CT: Appleton & Lange.

Caplan, G. (1964). *Principles of preventive psychiatry.* New York: Basic Books.

Center for Health Workforce Studies. (2005). *The impact of the aging population on the health workforce in the United States.* Rensselaer, NY: Center for Health Workforce Studies, School of Public Health, University at Albany. Retrieved December 29, 2009, from http://chws.albany.edu/index.php?reportsid=11,0,0,1,00

Crittenden, A. (2001). *The price of motherhood: Why the most important job in the world is still the least valued.* New York: Metropolitan Books.

Edmands, M. S., Hoff, L. A., Kaylor, L., Mower, L., & Sorrell, S. (1999). Bridging gaps between mind, body and spirit: Healing the whole person. *Journal of Psychosocial Nursing, 37*(10), 1–7.

Eliopoulos, C. (2010). *Foundations of gerontological nursing* (7th ed.). Philadelphia: Lippincott Williams & Wilkins.

Erikson, E. (1963). *Childhood and society* (2nd ed.). New York: W. W. Norton.

Estes, C. L. (1995). Mental health services for the elderly. Key policy elements. In M. Gatz (Ed.), *Emerging issues in mental health and aging* (pp. 303–327). Washington, DC: American Psychological Association.

Fadiman, A. (1997). *The spirit catches you and you fall down.* New York: The Noonday Press.

Fee, E., & Brown, T. M. (2000). The past and future of public health practice. *American Journal of Public Health, 90*(5), 690–691.

Frankl, V. E. (1963). *Man's search for meaning: An introduction to Logotherapy* (I. Lasch, Trans.). New York: Washington Square Press.

Futrell, M., Melillo, K. D., & Remington, R. (2008). *Evidence-based protocol: Wandering.* Iowa City, IA: The University of Iowa Gerontological Nursing Intervention Research Center, Research Dissemination Core.

Gerdner, L. A., Buckwalter, K. C., & Reed, D. (2002). Impact of a psychoeducational intervention on caregiver response to behavioral problems. *Nursing Research, 51*(6), 363–374.

Gerdner, L. A., Hall, G. R., & Buckwalter, K. C. (1996). Caregiver training for people with Alzheimer's based on a stress threshold model. *Image: Journal of Nursing Scholarship, 28*(3), 241–246.

Gerontological Advanced Practice Nurses Association. (2009). *GAPNA Health affairs agenda, 2009–2010.* Retrieved January 12, 2010, from https://www.gapna.org/health-affairs.html

Gilje, F., Lacey, L., & Moore, C. (2007). Gerontology and geriatric issues and trends in U.S. nursing programs: A national survey. *Journal of Professional Nursing, 23*(1), 21–29.

Grocki, J. H., & Fox, G. E. (2004). Gerontology coursework in undergraduate nursing programs in the United States: A regional study. *Journal of Gerontological Nursing, 30*(3), 46–51.

Hall, G. R., & Buckwalter, K. C. (1987). Progressively lowered stress threshold: A conceptual model for care of adults with Alzheimer's disease. *Archives of Psychiatric Nursing, 1*, 399–406.

Hall, G. R., & Laloudakis, D. (1999). A behavioral approach to Alzheimer's disease. *Advance for Nurse Practitioners, 7*(7), 39–46, 81.

Hansell, N. (1976). *The person in distress*. New York: Human Sciences Press.

Hoff, L. A. (1990). *Battered women as survivors*. London and New York: Routledge.

Hoff, L. A. (1993). Review essay: Health policy and the plight of the mentally ill. *Psychiatry, 56*(4), 400–419.

Hoff, L. A. (1994). *Violence issues: An interdisciplinary curriculum guide for health professionals*. Ottawa, Canada: Health Programs and Services Branch.

Hoff, L. A. (2009). *Violence and abuse issues: Cross-cultural perspectives for health and social services*. http://www.routledge.com/textbooks/9780415465724

Hoff, L. A., Hallisey, B. J., & Hoff, M. (2009). *People in crisis: Clinical and diversity perspectives* (6th ed.). New York and London: Routledge.

Hoff, L. A., & Morgan, B. (in press). *Psychiatric & mental health essentials in primary care: An introduction for nurse practitioners*. New York and London: Routledge, Taylor and Francis.

Institute of Medicine of the National Academies, Committee on the Future Health Care Workforce for Older Americans Board on Health Care Services. (2008). *Retooling for an aging America: Building the health care workforce*. Washington, DC: The National Academies Press.

International Association of Forensic Nurses. (2008). *Forensic nursing: Definition*. Retrieved January 15, 2009, from www.iafn.org

International Society for Education and Research in Psychiatric-Mental Health Nursing. (n.d.). *Divisions. Adult and Gero-psychiatric mental health nurses*. Retrieved August 7, 2009, from http://ispn-psych.org/html/agpn.html

International Society of Psychiatric-Mental Health Nurses and the American Psychiatric Nurses Association. (2008). *Essentials of psychiatric mental health nursing in the BSN curriculum: Collaboratively developed by ISPN and APNA, 2007–2008*. Retrieved January 17, 2009, from www.apna.org/files/public/revmay08finalCurricular_Guidelines_for_undergraduate_Education_in_psychiatric_Mental_Health_Nursing.pdf

James, D. J., & Glaze, L. E. (2006). *Mental health problems of prison and jail inmates*. U.S. Department of Justice, Office of Justice Programs, Bureau of Justice Statistics, Special Report. Washington, DC: Author.

Jeste, D. V., Alexopoulos, G. S., Bartels, S. J., Cummings, J. L., Gallo, J. J., Gottlieb, G. L., et al. (1999). Consensus statement on the upcoming crisis in geriatric mental health: Research agenda for the next two decades. *Archives of General Psychiatry, 56*(9), 848–853. Retrieved August 7, 2009, from http://archpsyc.ama-assn.org/cgi/reprint/56/9/848

Joint Commission on Mental Illness and Health. (1961). *Action for mental health. Report of the Joint Commission on Mental Illness and Health*. New York: Basic Books.

Kaseje, D. C. O., & Sempebwa, E. K. N. (1989). An integrated rural health project in Saradidi, Kenya. *Social Science and Medicine, 28*(10), 1063–1071.

Kovner, C. T., Mezey, M., & Harrington, C. (2002). Who cares for older adults? Workforce implications of an aging society. *Health Affairs, 21*(5), 78–89.

Kurlowicz, L. H., Puentes, W. J., Evans, L. K., Spool, M. M., & Ratcliffe, S. J. (2007). Graduate education in geropsychiatric nursing: Findings from a national survey. *Nursing Outlook, 55*(6), 303–310.

Lindemann, E. (1944). Symptomatology and management of acute grief. *American Journal of Psychiatry, 101*, 101–148.

Loustaunau, M. O., & Sobo, E. J. (1997). *The cultural context of health, illness, and medicine*. Westport, CT: Bergin & Garvey.

Luhrmann, T. M. (2000). *Of two minds: The growing disorder in American psychiatry*. New York: Knopf.

Marks, I., & Scott, R. (Eds.). (1990). *Mental health care delivery: Innovations, impediments and implementation*. Cambridge: Cambridge University Press.

Maslow, A. (1970). *Motivation and personality* (2nd ed.). New York: Harper & Row.

McGoldrick, M., & Hardy, K. V. (Eds.). (2008). *Re-visioning family therapy: Race, culture, and gender in clinical practice*. (2nd ed.). New York: Guilford Press.

McHugh, P. R., & Clark, M. R. (2006). Diagnostic and classificatory dilemmas. In M. Blumenfeld & J. J. Strain (Eds.), *Psychosomatic medicine* (pp. 39–45). Philadelphia: Lippincott Williams & Wilkins.

McKinlay, J. B. (1990). A case for refocusing upstream: The political economy of illness. In P. Conrad & R. Kern (Eds.), *The sociology of health and illness: Critical perspectives* (3rd ed., pp. 502–516). New York: St. Martin's Press.

Mezey, M., & Fulmer, T. (2002). The future history of gerontological nursing. *Journal of Gerontology: Medical Sciences, 57A*(7), M438–M441.

Mosher, L. R., & Burti, L. (1989). *Community mental health: Principles and practice*. New York: W. W. Norton.

National Conference of Gerontological Nurse Practitioners (2003). *2002–2003 NCGNP health affairs agenda*. Retrieved November 26, 2002, from http://www.ncgnp.org/displaycommon.cfm?an=3

National Conference of Gerontological Nurse Practitioners. (2008). What is a GNP? Retrieved September 29, 2008, from https://www.ncgnp.org/about-ncgnp.html

National Organization of Nurse Practitioner Faculties. (2006). *Domains and core competencies of nurse practitioner practice*. Washington, DC: Author.

Nuland, S. B. (2007). *The art of aging: A doctor's prescription for well-being*. New York: Random House.

Orem, D. E. (1980). *Nursing: Concepts of practice*. New York: McGraw-Hill.

Orem, D. E., Taylor, S. G., & Renpenning, K. M. (2001). *Nursing: Concepts of practice* (6th ed.). St. Louis, MO: Mosby.

Peplau, H. E. (1952). *Interpersonal relations in nursing: A conceptual frame of reference for psychodynamic nursing*. New York: Putnam.

Peplau, H. E. (1991). *Interpersonal relations in nursing: A conceptual frame of reference for psychodynamic nursing*. New York: Springer.

Peterson's guide to colleges and universities. (2003). Retrieved June 27, 2003, from http://iiswinprd03.petersons.com/ugchannel/articles/asp

Rachlis, M., & Kushner, C. (1994) *Strong medicine: How to save Canada's health care system*. Toronto: Harper Collins.

Rodriguez-Garcia, R., & Akhter, M. N. (2000). Human rights: The foundation of public health practice. *American Journal of Public Health, 90*(5), 693–694.

Rosenfeld, P., Bottrell, M., Fulmer, T., & Mezey, M. (1999). Gerontological nursing content in baccalaureate nursing programs: Findings from a national survey. *Journal of Professional Nursing, 15*(2), 84–94.

Scheper-Hughes, N., & Lovell, A. M. (1986). Breaking the circuit of social control: Lessons in public psychiatry from Italy and Franco Basaglia. *Social Science and Medicine, 23*(2), 159–178.

Selye, H. (1956). *The stress of life*. New York: McGraw-Hill.

Sullivan, H. S. (1947). *Conceptions of modern psychiatry*. Washington, DC: Wm. Alanson White Psychiatric Foundation.

Taylor, S. G., Compton, A., Eben, J. D., Emerson, S., Gashti, N. N., Tomey, A. M., et al. (1998). Dorothea E. Orem: Self-care deficit theory of nursing. In A. M. Tomey and M. R. Alligood (Eds.), *Nursing theorists and their work* (pp. 175–197). St. Louis, MO: Mosby.

The John A. Hartford Foundation Institute for Geriatric Nursing. (n.d.). *Fast facts: Emphasis needed on geriatric nursing*. Retrieved June 22, 2004, from http://hartfordign.org

The John A. Hartford Foundation Institute for Geriatric Nursing. *The phase II renewal plan, strategies and tactics years 2001–2006*. New York: Author.

Ustun, T. B. (1999). The global burden of mental disorders. *American Journal of Public Health, 89*(9), 1315–1321.

Waring, M. (1990). *If women counted: A new feminist economics*. San Francisco: Harper San Francisco.

World Health Organization. (2002). *Global burden of mental illness*. Geneva: Author.

3

Comprehensive Mental Health Assessment: An Integrated Approach

Lisa A. Brown
Lee Ann Hoff

Assessment, the first step in the nursing process, lays the foundation for making a diagnosis, planning crisis intervention and treatment, implementing the plan, and evaluating results through follow-up strategies. Lack of progress in meeting treatment goals, unanticipated complications, and provider frustration or burnout can often be traced to inadequate or incomplete assessment. Such barriers to effective service delivery are compounded in the psychiatric and mental health practice arena by a key factor in one's experience of emotional distress or mental illness: subjectivity. As discussed in Chapter 2, the meaning that people attach to life events and their emotional, physical, and social sequelae often constitute a major influence on one's healthy or unhealthy response to life's hardships, challenges of role transition, and recovery from traumatic experiences.

In the physical realm, providers can rely on a variety of technological and other objective assessment and diagnostic tools. In the emotional and cognitive spheres, however, although structured assessment tools exist, they are never as accurate as those available for diagnosing physical phenomena precisely because of the subjectivity of people's emotional, cognitive, and spiritual response to life events. To illustrate, the indifferent attitude of a

provider ordering laboratory tests for diagnosing a physical problem does not affect the objective laboratory results, although it may exacerbate a client's distress, whereas an indifferent attitude of a provider aiming to ascertain a depressed person's risk of suicide may result in denial of suicidal plans and failure to obtain other data for assessing suicide risk. This means that, in addition to structured assessment guides, the nurse–patient relationship and the provider's communication skills constitute the most essential "tools" in the psychiatric and mental health assessment process (Peplau, 1993).

This chapter begins with an overview and critique of assessment methods and published instruments available to the geropsychiatric nurse: nursing diagnosis, Mini-Mental State Examination (MMSE), *Diagnostic and Statistical Manual of Mental Disorders* (DSM), International Classification of Diseases (ICD), and the Comprehensive Mental Health Assessment tool (CMHA). The use of these tools is then illustrated with a case example, with the major focus on the CMHA. This tool (Hoff, Hallisey, & Hoff, 2009) is highlighted for its close correspondence to the emphasis on functional assessment of older persons, whose welfare and treatment outcomes can be compromised by concentrating on pathology and psychiatric diagnostic labels at this stage of the life cycle. Also discussed is the CMHA's complementarity with psychiatrist McHugh's (2001) "essentials" approach to psychiatric diagnosis.

A service contract form illustrates a client and provider intervention framework that complements the CMHA tool. It lists the CMHA assessment items as a structured guide for a data-based crisis intervention and mental health service plan that emphasizes a collaborative nurse–patient relationship as a key factor in treatment outcomes. Continuing the client-empowerment focus of the CMHA, it spells out specific strategies that the client and provider will use to address the items identified.

OVERVIEW OF ASSESSMENT METHODS

The multifaceted process of aging complicates mental health assessment of older people. As with any age group, it is essential to rule out an organic cause for any mental status change before assigning a psychiatric diagnosis. Subsequent to ruling out all organic causes of changed mental status, a thorough psychiatric and mental health assessment is warranted.

Nursing Diagnosis

Nursing diagnosis addresses areas of life affected by an alteration in health status. Nursing diagnoses of mental health are grouped under the following categories of Gordon's functional health patterns: cognitive–perceptual pattern, self-perception–self-concept pattern, role–relationship pattern, sexuality–reproductive pattern, coping-stress tolerance pattern, value–belief pattern, and sleep–rest pattern. An example is "alteration in mental status related to postoperative procedure as evidenced by short-term memory loss, disorientation to time and place." The nursing diagnosis illustrates what the problem is and how it is manifesting itself. Registered nurses are educated to provide comprehensive, holistic assessments.

Because they practice in a multidisciplinary system, nurses should be familiar with medical diagnosis and treatment.

Diagnostic and Statistical Manual of Mental Disorders and International Classification of Diseases

The DSM is currently published in its fourth edition with revisions (DSM-IV-TR). The fifth edition (DSM-V) is expected to be released in the year 2012. Physicians, advanced practice psychiatric nurses, social workers, and psychologists use the DSM-IV-TR as a guide for diagnosing mental disorders. It is important for geropsychiatric nurses to be familiar with this tool, its benefits, and its limitations in practice.

The first DSM, published in 1952, was a compilation and description of diagnostic categories. Reflecting the influence of Adolf Meyer's psychobiologic approach, the word "reaction" was used to depict his belief that each disorder was a reaction to psychological, social, or biological factors, or a combination of these factors. The DSM-II was very similar to the first edition except that it eliminated the term "reaction," thereby removing discussion of "cause" and ultimately the mind–body connection.

The DSM-III, published in 1980, included explicit diagnostic criteria, a multiaxial system, and a "descriptive approach that attempted to be neutral with respect to theories of etiology" (American Psychiatric Association [APA], 2000, p. 26). One of the primary goals of creating the DSM-III was to provide a medical nomenclature for clinical providers and researchers. The DSM-IV was published in 1994, and the fourth edition with text revision in 2000.

The DSM-IV has been widely accepted in clinical and research settings. Significant controversy surrounded the development of the DSM-III and the revised text (Caplan, 1995; Cooksey & Brown, 1998; Luhrmann, 2000). This controversy seems to have abated with publication of the fourth edition with text revision (APA, 2000). Although there is dialog in the medical literature regarding the upcoming DSM-V, there is little thought-provoking discourse. The DSM-V is scarcely discussed in the nursing and social science literature.

The broad acceptance of the DSM-IV, often referred to as the "bible" of psychiatry, is evident in the lack of literature discussing its use, benefits, and limitations. This is most obvious in the area of nursing and the social sciences, including social work and clinical psychology. Dialogue is also limited in the medical arena; however, this is where most of the literature can be found.

Yet, new voices internationally and across disciplines raise questions about the validity and widespread acceptance of the DSM zeitgeist and its prominence in psychiatric and mental health assessment. For example, Marie Crowe (2006, p. 125), a senior lecturer in mental health nursing in New Zealand, cautions nurses: ". . . because psychiatric diagnosis often fails to describe the individual's experience of mental distress . . . while not necessarily intentionally, [it] serves to maintain oppressive power relations within society. It does this by establishing and maintaining the parameters of normality and abnormality in a manner that reflects particular gender, culture, and class biases." She goes on to discuss the societal implications of having a psychiatric diagnosis and the biases in the diagnostic process as outlined in the DSM-IV. She calls on nursing to stay true to the discipline with holistic assessments based on the patient's lived experiences versus their "diagnosis." Crowe's analysis resonates with research findings by Cooksey and Brown (1998), in which nurses criticized the DSM for its failure to provide adequate information about the client's individual experience. This is in direct contrast to a nursing diagnosis outlining an alteration in mental health. It is important for registered nurses to be familiar with the criteria for diagnosis and simultaneously complete a thorough biopsychosocial assessment of each client.

Clinical psychologist Gerald Rosen (2008) and his colleagues have questioned the DSM diagnosis of posttraumatic stress disorder, ridiculing the elaboration of this diagnosis to include "post traumatic embitterment disorder as a result of being insulted or humiliated." He challenges the DSM for "the cross-cultural medicalization of normal human emotions" (p. 4).

Psychiatrist Paul McHugh, a long-time opponent of the DSM, also speaks out about the diagnosis of posttraumatic stress disorder. McHugh and Treisman (2007) propose that this diagnosis moves the mental health field away from, rather than toward, a better understanding of the natural psychological responses to trauma. McHugh's work (1999, 2001) supports key concepts of crisis theory, rooted as it is in results of treating traumatized combat soldiers at the front lines with the aim of their rapid return to work, minus the disadvantage of a psychiatric "disorder" label as a precondition for receiving necessary services for the predictable psychosomatic symptoms resulting from extraordinary war trauma. Applied to geropsychiatric health care, the following geriatrician's request to primary care providers at a Harvard Medical School conference is apt: Would you please do a functional assessment and let 80-year-olds go to their grave without a DSM diagnosis?

Darrel Reiger (2007), vice-chair of the task force to develop the DSM-V, describes the DSM as "a dictionary of mental disorder diagnoses that describes the characteristic's of each mental disorder diagnosis" and notes that the DSM-V will pay greater attention to "measurement based care." He emphasizes the need for this tool for research, reminding us that although the DSM is used in clinical practice, the DSM-III, -IV, and -IV-TR were all designed primarily with research in mind. This point resonates with the research findings of Cooksey and Brown (1998), revealing that many clinicians find the several hundred page DSM tome cumbersome in everyday mental health practice. Another important goal of the DSM-V is to be more congruent with the ICD.

The ICD is currently in its 9th edition, with the 10th edition due for publication in 2014. The ICD is published by the World Health Organization (WHO) and used worldwide for morbidity and mortality statistics, reimbursement systems, and automated decision support in medicine. This system is designed to promote international comparability in the collection, processing, classification, and public presentation of these statistics.

The ICD includes a section classifying mental and behavioral phenomena. This has been developed alongside the DSM, and the two manuals seek to use the same codes. There are significant differences, however, such as the ICD including personality disorders on the same axis as other mental disorders, unlike the DSM. The WHO is revising its classifications in these sections as part of the development of the tenth edition.

Since the 1990s, the APA and WHO have worked to bring the DSM and the relevant sections of ICD into concordance, but some differences remain. An international survey of psychiatrists in 66 countries comparing use of the ICD and DSM-IV found that the ICD was more often used for clinical diagnosis, whereas the DSM was more valued for research (Mezzich, 2002).

The five axes of the multiaxis systems of the DSM-IV-TR are as follows (APA, 2000, p. 27; O'Brien, Kennedy, & Ballard, 1999, pp. 64–65):

Axis I Clinical disorders, such as major depression or schizophrenia, and other conditions, such as alcohol dependence, that may be a focus of clinical attention

Axis II Personality disorders and mental retardation

Axis III General medical conditions (e.g., HIV infection may cause dementia [Axis I], or alcohol dependence [Axis I] may cause cirrhosis [Axis III])

Axis IV Psychosocial and environmental problems; includes events and stressors that may precipitate, result from, or affect mental status and treatment outcomes

Axis V Global assessment of functioning; indicates the client's overall functional level, including psychologic, social, and occupational well-being on a scale of

1 to 100 (low numbers designating low-level functioning, and higher numbers revealing a higher functioning level)

Axis V of the DSM corresponds most closely to the CMHA for use in charting a client's progress from admission to discharge. However, although the Axis V assessment is "global" in its inclusion of psychological and social dimensions for scoring, it does not identify particular areas of functioning according to the urgency of a client's need for provider attention and intervention.

Despite its name, the growing critique of the DSM underscores the questionable clinical application of a tool designed primarily for research. In this respect, busy clinicians have long recognized the limitations of lengthy tools for use in clinical settings. This does not abrogate the importance of evaluating clinical tools for their validity and reliability. Rather, it is simply unrealistic to transfer into clinical protocols a tool like the DSM intended for research versus practice. Besides its limitation for clinical diagnosis, the DSM also fails to outline recommended treatment. Neither the DSM diagnosis nor the ICD code provides a format to obtain information regarding a particular individual's functioning in daily life.

Overall, mental health assessment tools are varied and usually are specific to certain elements of mental health. For example, there are mania scales, depression scales, suicide risk assessment scales, and so forth. Many of these were originally designed as research tools and may not be suitable for easy use in clinical practice, particularly in high-risk situations where time is of the essence. The average clinician, not to mention the client, cannot be expected to administer several scales (each requiring 5 to 10 minutes) with little time left in a typical 20-minute person-to-person session that should not shortchange attention to high-risk issues, such as suicide, violence, job loss, or similar items illustrated in the CMHA assessment tool discussed later in this chapter.

Further, let us suppose a client reluctantly discloses (or fails to disclose altogether) in a paper-and-pencil checklist a high-risk item, such as domestic violence, while in the waiting area, with limited time to discuss such a topic face-to-face with an empathic provider. Such a "mechanical" approach to The Joint Commission–required victimization screening in routine health history checklists might be counterproductive for a vulnerable client's readiness to disclose current risk, which is sometimes implied by presenting physical symptoms. The CMHA Initial Contact sheet and Assessment Worksheet offers an alternative in its Likert-like scale assessing for degree of urgency in contrast to the DSM approach to diagnosis, as in identifying "5 out of 7" or "7 out of 10" criteria for particular diagnoses with no rating of seriousness or its effect on a person's functioning. Clearly, although providing an outline of criteria for each diagnosis, the DSM-IV-TR does not offer a format for ascertaining disturbances or deficiencies in a person's psychosocial functioning in everyday life.

To summarize, mental health assessment tools are varied and generally are specific to certain elements of mental health. For example, there are mania scales, depression scales, suicide risk assessment scales, and so forth. Many of these were originally designed as research tools and are not always suitable for clinical assessment, particularly in high-risk situations where time is of the essence.

COGNITIVE ASSESSMENT TOOLS

Cognitive impairment is an important issue in aging patients. Early detection is imperative for safety and may also allow a person the time and opportunity to make important financial and health-related decisions before disease progression makes it impossible.

There are many tools available for brief cognitive assessment including the General Practitioner Assessment of Cognition, developed by Brodaty et al. (2002); Memory Impairment Screen, developed at the Albert Einstein College of Medicine, Bronx, NY (Buschke et al., 1999); the Mini-Cog designed at the University of Washington, Seattle, WA (Borson, Scanlon, Brush, Vitaliano, & Dokmak, 2000); and

the MMSE developed by Folstein, Folstein, and McHugh (1975).

The MMSE remains the most commonly used instrument (Brodaty, Low, Gibson, & Burns, 2006). The MMSE provides a brief assessment of an individual's cognitive function. It is simple, brief, and can be administered by a variety of disciplines with minimal training. The MMSE's use may be limited by the patient's individual presentation. To administer the examination correctly, the patient must possess the ability to interact verbally and read and write. Its use in assessing patients who may be blind or have limited education, for example, is tentative. The MMSE has been shown to be a reliable and valid tool for swift assessment of cognition. It has been translated into many languages and adapted to meet specific cultural needs without affecting validity and reliability.

As with any assessment tool, if the MMSE is administered in a mechanical way that contradicts the importance of interpersonal rapport and empathy as prerequisites for a thorough holistic assessment of a distressed human being, its findings will be limited. For example, item number eight in the CMHA refers explicitly to the cognitive function of decision making. Depending on a client's or family member's response regarding this question, the MMSE might be administered in the CMHA holistic assessment context. It is prudent never to lose sight of the cultural, social, educational, and medical–physical factors that may affect one's "mental status" (Peplau, 1993) (see Box 3-1 for sample questions from the MMSE tool).

COMPREHENSIVE MENTAL HEALTH ASSESSMENT TOOL

The CMHA was developed and tested in the 1970s in the Erie County Mental Health System, Buffalo, NY (Hoff & Rosenbaum, 1994). The description of this record system (Boxes 3-2 through 3-7; Table 3-1) is excerpted and adapted from Hoff et al. (2009, pp. 97–104 and p. 121) and reprinted here with permission of the authors. A major impetus for this tool came from the New York State

▌ BOX 3-1 MMSE SAMPLE ITEMS

Orientation time: "What is the date?"

Registration: "Listen carefully. I am going to say three words. You say them back after I stop. Ready? Here they are . . . HOUSE [pause], CAR [pause], LAKE [pause]. Now repeat those words back to me." [Repeat up to 5 times, but score only the first trial.]

Naming: "What is this?" [Point to a pencil or pen.]

Reading: "Please read this and do what it says. [Show examinee the words on the stimulus form.] CLOSE YOUR EYES.

Source: Reproduced by special permission of the Publisher, Psychological Assessment Resources, Inc., 16204 North Florida Avenue, Lutz, Florida 33549, from the Mini-Mental State Examination, by Marshal Folstein and Susan Folstein. Copyright 1975, 1998, 2001 by Mini Mental LLC, Inc. Published 2001 by Psychological Assessment Resources, Inc. Further reproduction is prohibited without permission of PAR, Inc. The MMSE can be purchased from PAR, Inc. by calling (800) 331-8378 or (813) 968-3003.

government's need for a record system to track the incidence of mental disorders, and the effectiveness of community-based services for a range of people in acute distress or with serious and persistent mental illness. The tool's origin coincided with a nationwide development of the community mental health system following Congressional legislation in 1963 and 1965. The entire CMHA record system consists of these forms[1]:

1. Initial contact sheet (includes crisis rating)
2. Client assessment worksheet

3. Significant other assessment worksheet
4. Comprehensive mental health assessment (summary of interview and worksheet data)
5. Termination summary
6. Interagency referral form
7. Consultation form
8. Follow-up assessment
9. Child screening checklist
10. Service contract

The CMHA forms provide a structured guide to the interview, assessment, and service planning process with clients. Their intended use is within a health service system that recognizes the intrinsic relationship between physical, emotional, and sociocultural factors affecting the mental health status of individuals. The underlying philosophy of this record system emphasizes three key assumptions: (1) the person in distress or crisis is a member of a social network; (2) the stability of

---

[1] The complete set of CMHA forms, including operational definitions of the 21 assessment items, is available by contacting author Lee Ann Hoff at leeann.hoff@comcast.net. Those interested in further research on the CMHA assessment tool can learn more from the Web site of Hoff et al., 2009: http://www.routledgementalhealth.com/people-in-crisis/ in the item "Crisis Research."

a person's social attachments and gratification of basic human needs strongly influences his or her physical, emotional, and mental health and one's related ability to function within the community; and (3) the provision of crisis prevention, early intervention, and social support services conserves costly health care dollars by restoring and maintaining people in noninstitutional settings and preventing readmission to psychiatric facilities whenever possible.

The original record system was designed specifically for clinical use by a psychiatric and mental health interdisciplinary team. It was tested in the 1970s with crisis and mental health workers and people receiving services in community mental health agencies in New York's six Erie County catchment areas that adopted the system. Included were most publicly funded programs serving urban, suburban, and rural communities in a metropolitan area with a population of 1.25 million. A client was considered an active partner in developing the record and had full access to the record. Examples of client feedback include the following:

"I'm not so bad off as I thought."

"This takes some of the mystery out of mental health."

"Getting help with a problem isn't so magical after all."

"Now I have a diary of how I worked out my problems and got better."

The current CMHA version builds on Hoff's (1990) research with abused women, in which the tool was used to assess mental health sequelae of violence and victimization (Hoff & Rosenbaum, 1994). Its updated edition was developed and pilot-tested for validity and interrater reliability in six comparable agencies in Massachusetts and in Ontario, Canada, by Lee Ann Hoff and psychiatric nursing graduate students at the University of Massachusetts Lowell (Hoff et al., 2009).

The CMHA assessment and planning tool emphasizes client-centered, goal-oriented treatment. It uses a five-point Likert-like scale (1 = excellent/very high functioning, 3 = fair; 5 = very poor/very low functioning) to ascertain client stress levels in 21 areas of biopsychosocial functioning through active collaboration with the client and significant others. It also allows for systematic evaluation of treatment outcomes and follow-up planning. The forms are designed to assist in the achievement of several objectives:

1. To provide health and mental health providers, clients, and collaborating agencies a standardized framework for gathering data, while including subjective, narrative-style information from the client and significant others that is relevant to mental health across the life cycle.

2. To organize this information in a way that sharply defines the client's level of functioning (emotional, cognitive, and behavioral) and life-threatening risk, and outlines complementary treatment goals and methods to evaluate progress toward desired outcomes in specified functional areas.

3. To assist in fostering continuity between service during acute crisis states and the longer-term mental health treatment needed by some clients (this objective is especially relevant vis-à-vis the issue of "socially constructed suicidality" that is sometimes used as the only "ticket" to psychiatric inpatient admission when health system economic factors supersede client need in clinical decision making).

4. To provide supervisory staff with the information necessary to monitor service and ensure quality and continuity of client care.

5. To provide administrative staff with information for monitoring and evaluating achievement of crisis intervention, counseling or psychotherapy, and related services for individual clients, and cumulative data revealing service outcomes in relation to agency objectives.

In an era of providing cost-effective health care without compromising the quality of care, this assessment and planning tool is especially relevant in its focus on client-centered, goal-oriented treatment and systematic evaluation of service outcomes. Its design depicting a person's functional level also avoids the negative effects of psychiatric labeling. Data concerning a client's "basic life attachments" and "signals of distress" (Hansell, 1976) offer a structured, holistic, humanistic framework for addressing a range of human experience and functioning affected by various life events and traumas and the emotional and mental illness or disabilities that may follow.

The 21 assessment items in the CMHA, with ratings from high to low functioning, can serve as a checklist to ensure that a thorough evaluation has been done. The scaled items evaluate a person's physical, mental, emotional, behavioral, spiritual, and social concerns allowing for prioritizing issues for action. The tool can facilitate meeting the demands of cost-effective service delivery, emphasis on community-based treatment, client empowerment, and evaluation of observable treatment outcomes as manifested by the functional level of the client and his or her quality of life.

The CMHA allows for varying techniques in collecting data and exemplifies the importance of obtaining collateral information from other healthcare providers and significant others. Depending on the clinical situation, the Client Self-Assessment Worksheet can be given to and completed by the client before formal interview or used as an interview guide. Either way it serves to reinforce the idea of the client's active involvement in the assessment process. The complete assessment protocol includes data collection from significant others on the same 21 items.

The structured five-point Likert-like scale allows for formal comparative assessment at (1) initial, (2) interim, and (3) termination phases of counseling or treatment. Besides prioritizing problems, immediate risks, and goals, it presents visually the potential progress in a client's strengths,

functional level, and stress reduction. The scales and descriptive comments also assist both client and mental health provider to remain focused and to chart progress toward meeting treatment goals. Finally, the tool is a guide for additional interventions or referrals that might follow from the crisis intervention or counseling process (see Boxes 3-2 through 3-7).

CMHA AND MCHUGH'S "ESSENTIALS": DESCRIPTION AND COMMONALITIES

Elements of the CMHA are complementary to the work of Dr. Paul McHugh of Johns Hopkins University. In his critique of psychiatric assessment tools, McHugh states: "At Johns Hopkins Department of Psychiatry we have long held that psychiatry needs a new conceptual structure that ties the mental disorders we treat to mental life as psychological science understands it today. Such a structure would insist on defining mental disorders by their essential natures rather than by their appearances alone" (McHugh, 2001, p. 2).

McHugh divides the 20th century of psychiatry into three segments, the first being Meyerian, based on the teachings of Adolf Meyer, who emphasized psychobiology. Psychobiology differs from biologic psychiatry by studying life from the psychologic perspective. Next, the psychoanalytic period emerged. The discovery of psychotropic medication in the 1950s put an end to this period, giving way to emphasis on the empirical. The focus of the empirical period is on the importance of reliability in diagnosis, revisiting comprehensive assessments as emphasized by Meyer; this led to the development of the current DSM. McHugh acknowledges advancements in the area of research while pointing out that the emphasis on reliability has neglected the validity of psychiatry.

McHugh takes issue with certain diagnoses, such as multiple personality disorder and chronic posttraumatic stress disorder. He requests psychiatry to give up "appearance driven" diagnosis, as did internal medicine many years ago. McHugh (1999) refers to the "weaknesses inherent in a system of classification based on appearances—and contaminated by self-interest advocacy." He calls for a new method that can "comprehend several interactive sources of disorder and sustain a complex program of treatment and rehabilitation" (McHugh, p. 38).

McHugh (2001) illustrates an alternative approach to categorizing and treatment planning for mental disorder. In a structure consisting of interactive perspectives of psychiatry, he reunites psychosocial components with biology. These interactive sources of disorder include four perspectives for assessment and diagnosis in psychiatric practice: (1) the disease perspective, encompassing pathophysiology and pathogenesis; (2) the dimensional perspective, including personality, life circumstances, and neurotic symptoms; (3) the behavioral perspective, including physiological drive, conditioned learning, and choice; and (4) the life story perspective, encompassing setting, sequence, and outcome.

McHugh (2001) and colleagues at Johns Hopkins hold that these four distinct but interrelated levels of expression constitute the hierarchical organization of human psychological life from the most basic neurological to the most highly developed psychological functioning. Assessment skill demands ascertaining the particular way a person's psychological functioning can go awry as defined by the four perspectives.

The dynamic interactive sources of disorder McHugh proposes for assessing psychological functioning are highly complementary to assessment factors depicted in the CMHA. In particular, McHugh's four perspectives underscore two key concepts framing the CMHA tool: basic life attachments and signals of distress, which are concepts from ego psychology, sociocultural theory, crisis theory, and preventive psychiatry (Caplan, 1964; Hansell, 1976; Hoff et al., 2009).

The complementarity of McHugh's perspective and the CMHA become more apparent in the following case example with application of the MMSE, nursing diagnosis, and DSM-IV-TR.

CASE STUDY

Frank Kelly, first introduced in Chapter 2, is a 72-year-old widowed white man. He presented to the emergency department of a community hospital complaining of chest pain. The cardiac workup was negative and evaluation revealed that Frank had been depressed and having thoughts of suicide. A psychiatric evaluation was ordered. The crisis team was called and a clinician proceeded with assessment. The clinician asked to speak with Frank and then his daughter. Unfortunately, his daughter needed to leave to care for her children and would return as soon as possible; therefore, the CMHA was conducted only with Frank.

Comprehensive Mental Health Assessment for Case Example

Boxes 3-2 through 3-4 illustrate the comprehensive mental health assessment for the case example.

(continues)

CASE STUDY *(continued)*

BOX 3-2 INITIAL CONTACT SHEET

Today's date: *September 2, 2009*   ID#: *9999*

Name: *Kelly, Frank*

Age: *72*   Relationship status: ❏ Married ❏ Single ☑ Widowed

Address: *7 Any Street, Anytown, USA*

Telephone: *555-1111*

Have you talked with anyone about this? ❏ No ☑ Yes

If yes, who? *Kate who is with him in ER*   Date of last contact: _____

Significant other (name and phone): *Kate Smith 555-2222 (daughter)*

Are you taking any medication now? ❏ No ☑ Yes

If yes, what? *ASA 81 mg daily, Hydrochlorothiazide 12.5 mg daily*

CRISIS RATING: 1   2   3   ④   5
                    Not urgent   Very urgent

Probability of engaging for counseling treatment contract (1 = high; 5 = low)
                    1   ②   3   4   5

Summary of presenting situation or problem and help-seeking goal:

Frank Kelly, a 72-year-old Caucasian, widowed male was brought to the emergency department by his daughter secondary to complaints of chest pain. The cardiac workup was negative. During his evaluation, a depressed mood and sad affect were observed and suicidal ideations were reported. Frank was cooperative with the mental health assessment but seemed surprised when the issue of counseling/mental health care was raised.

Date of next contact/appointment: _____

Signature (intake/triage person): _____ Date: _____

CASE STUDY (*continued*)

BOX 3-3 ASSESSMENT WORKSHEET

To be used as initial interview guide with client.

NOTE: Comments by client are italicized; comments by provider are [in brackets].

1. **Physical health:** How do you judge your physical health in general?

1	②2	3	4	5
Excellent	Good	Fair	Poor	Very poor

Comments: *Sometimes I have a lot of pain with the arthritis but most days it is tolerable.*

2. **Self-acceptance/self-esteem:** How do you feel about yourself as a person?

1	2	3	④4	5
Excellent	Good	Fair	Poor	Very poor

Comments: *I am proud of my marriage and we raised three good kids. I had a decent career as a pipe fitter. I am just not sure what to do with myself now.*

3. **Vocational/occupational (includes student, homemaker, volunteer):** How would you judge your work/school situation?

1	②2	3	4	5
Very good	Good	Fair	Poor	Very poor

Comments: *Retired, I guess I could use something to do.*

4. **Immediate family:** How would you describe your relationship with your family?

1	②2	3	4	5
Very good	Good	Fair	Poor	Very poor

Comments: *The kids come by to see me at least once a week. They have their own lives to lead now.* [Considerable low self-esteem and depression, he may feel unworthy of more attention.]

5. **Intimacy/significant other relationship(s):** Is there anyone you feel really close to and can rely on if you're very upset or in a life-threatening situation?

1	2	③3	4	5
Always	Usually	Sometimes	Rarely	Never

Comments: *I could call my kids if I needed them in an emergency. I don't want to call them up crying, though. I have no interest in meeting women.*

(continues)

CASE STUDY (*continued*)

6. **Residential/housing:** How do you judge your housing situation?

(1)	2	3	4	5
Excellent	Good	Fair	Poor	Very poor

Comments: *We sold our house five years ago and bought a condo unit in a complex for seniors.*

7. **Financial:** How would you describe your financial situation?

1	(2)	3	4	5
Very good	Good	Fair	Poor	Very poor

Comments: *I don't have any problems paying my bills and I have enough money so it won't cost the kids to bury me.*

8. **Decision-making ability:** How satisfied are you with your ability to make life decisions?

(1)	2	3	4	5
Always very satisfied		Somewhat dissatisfied		Always very dissatisfied

Comments: *I wish I had my wife to talk to like I used to but I can make decisions just fine.*

[Correlate with MMSE.]

9. **Problem-solving ability:** How would you judge your ability to solve everyday problems?

(1)	2	3	4	5
Very good	Good	Fair	Poor	Very poor

Comments: *Same thing—wish the wife was here but I can do it myself.*

[Although he prides himself on problem solving, suicidal ideation suggests desperation and unhealthy problem solving.]

10. **Life goals/spiritual values:** How satisfied are you with how your life goals (and things you value most) are working for you?

1	2	3	4	(5)
Always very satisfied		Somewhat dissatisfied		Always very dissatisfied

Comments: *My only goal now is to die and be with my wife. The problem is, if I kill myself I will go to hell and I will never be with her. I don't go to church as much as I used to with my wife. I still try to go. I do find it helpful; I feel better when I go.*

CASE STUDY (*continued*)

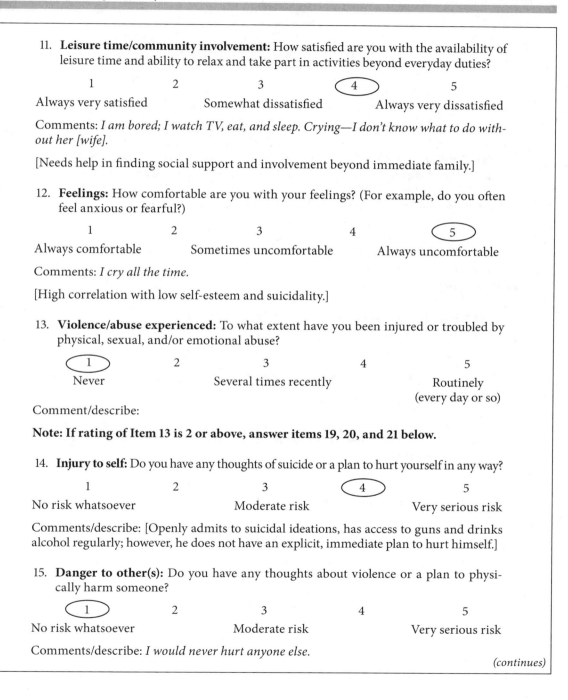

11. **Leisure time/community involvement:** How satisfied are you with the availability of leisure time and ability to relax and take part in activities beyond everyday duties?

1	2	3	4	5

Always very satisfied   Somewhat dissatisfied   Always very dissatisfied

Comments: *I am bored; I watch TV, eat, and sleep. Crying—I don't know what to do without her [wife].*

[Needs help in finding social support and involvement beyond immediate family.]

12. **Feelings:** How comfortable are you with your feelings? (For example, do you often feel anxious or fearful?)

1	2	3	4	5

Always comfortable   Sometimes uncomfortable   Always uncomfortable

Comments: *I cry all the time.*

[High correlation with low self-esteem and suicidality.]

13. **Violence/abuse experienced:** To what extent have you been injured or troubled by physical, sexual, and/or emotional abuse?

1	2	3	4	5

Never   Several times recently   Routinely (every day or so)

Comment/describe:

Note: If rating of Item 13 is 2 or above, answer items 19, 20, and 21 below.

14. **Injury to self:** Do you have any thoughts of suicide or a plan to hurt yourself in any way?

1	2	3	4	5

No risk whatsoever   Moderate risk   Very serious risk

Comments/describe: [Openly admits to suicidal ideations, has access to guns and drinks alcohol regularly; however, he does not have an explicit, immediate plan to hurt himself.]

15. **Danger to other(s):** Do you have any thoughts about violence or a plan to physically harm someone?

1	2	3	4	5

No risk whatsoever   Moderate risk   Very serious risk

Comments/describe: *I would never hurt anyone else.*

(continues)

16. **Substance use (alcohol and/or other drugs):** Does the use of alcohol and/or other drugs concern you or interfere with your life in any way (work, family)?

1	2	3	4	5
Never	Rarely	Sometimes	Frequently	Constantly

(4 is circled)

Comments/describe: *My wife hated me drinking so I quit about 20 years ago. I started drinking again six months after she died. I don't have a problem. I only drink at home. I don't drive after I have been drinking. [Reports consuming 6–8 beers 3–4x/week. Denies other drug use. Blood alcohol 0 today and drug screen negative.]*

17. **Legal:** What is your tendency to get into trouble with the law?

1	2	3	4	5
None	Slight	Moderate	Great	Very great

(1 is circled)

Comments/describe: *I haven't been in any trouble since I was 17 and even then it was drinking in public.*

18. **Agency use:** How satisfied are you with getting the help you need from doctors or other health providers?

1	2	3	4	5
Always very satisfied		Somewhat dissatisfied		Always very dissatisfied

(1 is circled)

Comments: *I have no complaints.*

19. **Relationship with abuser:** How would you describe your relationship with the person who has abused you?

1	2	3	4	5
No contact or conflict now		Occasional conflict		Great conflict and turmoil

Comments: _____

20. **Safety—self:** How safe do you feel now?

1	2	3	4	5
Very safe		Somewhat safe		Very unsafe

Comments: _____

CASE STUDY (*continued*)

21. **Safety—children (if there are children):** How safe do you think your children are?

1	2	3	4	5
Very safe		Somewhat safe		Very unsafe

Comments: _____

Additional items: Do you have any other issues, concerns, or problems that you wish to discuss with a counselor?

No, I told you everything.

Urgency/importance: Among the items noted, which do you consider the most urgent and/or in need of immediate attention?

I want to feel better.

BOX 3-4 CMHA ASSESSMENT WORKSHEET HIGHLIGHTS

Among the 18 functional items applicable to Mr. Kelly, the following should receive the most immediate attention and action, based on ratings between 3 and 5 (moderate to high stress). The number in parentheses ( ) indicates the rating for these priority items.

12: Feelings (5)

10: Life goals/spiritual values (5)

14: Injury to self (4)

16: Substance use (4)

11: Leisure time/community involvement (4)

2: Self-acceptance/self-esteem (4)

5: Intimacy/significant other relationships (3)

Of particular note among these priority ratings is their interrelationship; for example, Mr. Kelly does not know what to do with himself, he just wants to die and be with his wife, his risk for suicide, feeling reluctant to reach out to family, and coping with excessive use of alcohol. Planned actions (by provider and client) around these "basic life attachments" and "signals of distress" are illustrated in Table 3-1, the Service Contract.

(*continues*)

CASE STUDY *(continued)*

BOX 3-5 MINI-MENTAL STATE EXAMINATION

Score 24; poor concentration noted; difficulty with recall. Note: See Appendix B for a sample of MMSE questions and information for obtaining the complete form.

BOX 3-6 NURSING DIAGNOSES

1. Risk for violence toward self as evidenced by suicidal ideations, access to guns, and frequent use of alcohol.

2. Dysfunctional grieving related to loss of wife and career as evidenced by inability to establish new relationships, activities, and goals.

3. Knowledge deficit related to signs and symptoms of depression as evidenced by his difficulty in accepting the recommendation for counseling and mental health care.

4. Situational low self-esteem related to loss of marriage and career and evidenced by self-report, "I don't know what to do with myself now."

5. Family coping, potential for growth as evidenced by concern by children, regular visits, and opportunity to open up dialogue regarding increased needs of the family patriarch.

6. Social isolation as evidenced by lack of peers, time spent home alone drinking alcohol.

BOX 3-7 DIAGNOSTIC AND STATISTICAL MANUAL DIAGNOSIS

Axis I   Major depressive disorder, single episode, alcohol dependence

Axis II   Not applicable

Axis III   Hypertension, gout, arthritis

Axis IV   Death of wife, retirement, lack of peer support

Axis V   Global assessment of functioning (GAF) = 50

DATA-BASED SERVICE PLANNING

Table 3-1 illustrates a service contract developed with Frank Kelly from assessment data. Problems and issues identified for counseling and treatment correspond to the numbered items in the CMHA assessment tool. Numbers in parentheses indicate the stress rating for particular items. Note that of the 21 CMHA items, the seven functional areas with ratings of 3, 4, or 5 (indicating high stress or low functioning) included here illustrate priority areas for crisis intervention and treatment.

This service contract example suggests a cautionary note regarding suicide prevention. The "no-suicide contract" is a technique used by some health providers in which the client promises not to harm himself or herself between sessions. Although widely practiced (especially by providers without specialty training in crisis intervention), such contracts offer no special protection against suicide, or legal protection for the therapist or other provider. Any value the contract may have is only as good as the quality of the therapeutic relationship in which caring and concern for the client are conveyed. A no-suicide contract should never be used as a convenient substitute for time spent in empathic listening to and planning nonlethal alternatives with a suicidal person (Clark & Kerkhof, 1993; Hoff et al., 2009, pp. 343–345). The service contract with Frank Kelly highlights such alternatives, and attention to Mr. Kelly's losses, his unhealthy coping with alcohol, and other issues fueling his despair.

TABLE 3-1

Service Contract: Frank Kelly

Date: _____

Code

1. Physical health	8. Decision-making ability	15. Danger to other(s)
2. Self-acceptance/self-esteem	9. Problem-solving ability	16. Substance use/abuse
3. Vocational/occupational	10. Life goals/spiritual values	17. Legal
4. Immediate family	11. Leisure time/community involvement	18. Agency use
5. Intimacy/significant other relationship(s)	12. Feelings	19. Relationship with abuser
6. Residential/housing	13. Violence/abuse experienced	20. Safety—self
7. Financial security	14. Injury to self	21. Safety—children

Stress rating code: 1 = low stress/very high functioning   5 = high stress/very low functioning

Item/stress rating	Problem/issue specification	Strategies/techniques (planned actions of client and health provider)
12. Feelings (5)	"I cry all the time."	1. Provide supportive environment, allowing patient to express feelings freely 2. Provide education on depression 3. Explore role of unresolved grief of multiple losses (wife, career, health)

(continues)

TABLE 3-1

Service Contract: Frank Kelly *(continued)*

Item/stress rating	Problem/issue specification	Strategies/techniques (planned actions of client and health provider)
10. Life goals/spiritual values (5)	"My only goal now is to die and be with my wife." He believes he will "go to hell" and therefore not be with his wife if he takes his own life.	1. Explore openness to including pastoral counseling 2. Discuss opportunities to become active in his church
14. Injury to self (4)	Suicidal ideation, possesses guns, consumes alcohol on regular basis	1. Recommend immediate removal of firearms from home 2. Assess risk for suicide every visit 3. Confer with family and discuss suicide risk
16. Substance use (4)	Drinks 6–8 beers, 3–4x/wk	1. Assess if patient believes alcohol to be a problem 2. Provide education regarding alcohol and depression 3. Reevaluate frequently
11. Leisure time/ community involvement (4)	"I am bored, I watch TV, eat, and sleep."	1. Integrate above strategies to increase activity, decrease isolation therefore increasing self-esteem/acceptance, increase possibility of peer relationships and explore options to set goals and achieve them.
2. Self-acceptance/ self-esteem (4)	Was proud of marriage and career and both are now gone; "not sure what to do with myself now."	1. Explore areas of interest 2. Set small attainable goals to foster feeling of worth and accomplishment
5. Intimacy/ significant other relationships (3)	Has ongoing, reliable relationship with children but does not want to burden them. No peer support.	1. Discuss attending a grief support group 2. Explore social options available in his community 3. Explore having joint session with family as additional suicide prevention measure

Signatures:

Client _____

Crisis worker _____

REFERENCES

American Psychiatric Association. (2000). *Diagnostic and statistical manual of mental disorders* (4th ed., Rev.). Washington, DC: Author.

Borson, S., Scanlan, J., Brush, M., Vitaliano, P., & Dokmak, A. (2000). The Mini-Cog: A cognitive "vital signs" measure for dementia screening in multilingual elderly. *International Journal of Geriatric Psychiatry, 15*, 1021–1027.

Brodaty, H., Low, L. F., Gibson, L., & Burns, K. (2006). What is the best dementia screening instrument for general practitioners to use? *American Journal of Geriatric Psychiatry, 14*(5), 391–400.

Brodaty, H., Pond, D., Kemp, N., Luscombe, G., Harding, L., Berman, K., et al. (2002). The GPCOG: A new screening test for dementia designed for general practice. *Journal of the American Geriatrics Society, 50*(3), 530–534.

Buschke, H., Kuslansky, G., Katz, M., Stewart, W. F., Sliwinski, M. J., Eckholdt, H. M., et al. (1999). Screening for dementia with the Memory Impairment Screen. *Neurology, 52*, 231.

Caplan, G. (1964). *Principles of preventive psychiatry.* New York: Basic Books.

Caplan, P. (1995). *They say you're crazy.* Reading, MA: Perseus Books.

Clark, D. C., & Kerkhof, A. J. F. M. (1993). No-suicide decisions and suicide contracts in therapy. *Crisis, 14*(3), 98–99.

Cooksey, E. C., & Brown, P. (1998). Spinning on its axes: DSM and the social construction of psychiatric diagnosis. *International Journal of Health Services, 28*(3), 525–554.

Crowe, M. (2006). Psychiatric diagnosis: Some implications for mental health nursing care. *Journal of Advanced Nursing, 53*(1), 125–133.

Folstein, M. F., Folstein, S. E., & McHugh, P. R. (1975). Mini-mental state. A practical method for grading the cognitive state of patients for the clinician. *Journal of Psychiatric Research, 12*(3), 189–198.

Hansell, N. (1976). *The person in distress.* New York: Human Sciences Press.

Hoff, L. A. (1990). *Battered women as survivors.* London: Routledge.

Hoff, L. A., Hallisey, B. J., & Hoff, M. (2009). *People in crisis: Clinical and diversity perspectives* (6th ed.). New York and London: Routledge.

Hoff, L. A., & Rosenbaum, L. (1994). A victimization assessment tool: Instrument development and clinical implications. *Journal of Advanced Nursing, 20*(4), 627–634.

Luhrmann, T. M. (2000). *Of two minds: An anthropologist looks at American psychiatry.* New York: Vintage Books.

McHugh, P. R. (1999). How psychiatry lost its way. *Commentary, 108*(5), 32–39.

McHugh, P. R. (2001). Beyond DSM-IV: From appearances to essences. *Psychiatric Research Report, 17*(2), 1–5.

McHugh, P. R., & Treisman, G. (2007). PTSD: A problematic diagnostic category. *Journal of Anxiety Disorders, 21*(2), 211–222.

Mezzich, J. E. (2002). International surveys on the use of ICD-10 and related diagnostic systems. *Psychopathology, 3*, 72–75.

O'Brien, P. G., Kennedy, W. Z., & Ballard, K. A. (1999). *Psychiatric nursing.* New York: McGraw-Hill.

Peplau, H. (1993). *Interpersonal relations in nursing.* New York: Springer.

Reiger, D. (2007). Somatic presentation of mental disorders: Refining the research agenda for DSM-V. *Psychosomatic Medicine, 69*(9), 827–828.

Rosen, G., Spitzer, R., & McHugh, P. R. (2008). Problems with the post-traumatic stress disorder diagnosis and its future in DSM-V. *The British Journal of Psychiatry, 192*(1), 3–4.

4

Ethnic Elders

Jane Cloutterbuck

Dramatic changes in the nation's demographic and immigration patterns are rapidly transforming the United States into a multicultural, multiracial, and multilingual society. As the U.S. population ages and becomes more ethnically and culturally diverse, mental health providers will increasingly encounter ethnic elders in their practice. The growing presence of ethnic elders in the population, coupled with the high level of disparities that they experience in mental health care, places moral and ethical pressure on mental health planners, providers, and administrators to critically evaluate psychiatric assessment and management for these groups. The need to integrate concepts of culture and ethnicity into mental health services and provide culturally competent care to this chronically underserved and often clinically misunderstood population is both immediate and imperative.

DEMOGRAPHIC CHANGE

The older population in the United States is rapidly increasing in diversity. Since 1960, the number of ethnic elders has doubled with each census, and this trend is expected to continue well into the 21st century. Although white Americans comprise the largest segment of the older adult population in the United States today, ethnic elders are an increasingly substantial proportion of this population. Between 2007 and 2030, white elders are projected to increase by 68%, and the expected growth for ethnic elders will be 184%. Specifically, the projected percentage increase for African Americans will be 126%, for Asians and Pacific Islanders 213%, for Native American/Alaska Natives Indians 167%, and for Hispanics 244% (Administration on Aging, 2008).

Table 4-1 reports the racial composition of individuals age 65 and older in the year 2006 and projects changes through 2050 (U.S. Bureau of the Census, 2006). In 2006, 81% of older adults were white and 19.2% were minorities. Among older minorities, African American elders represented 8.5%, those of Hispanic origin 6.4%, and Asian or Pacific Islanders 3.2%. All other races in combination totaled 1.1%. By 2050, it is projected that white elders will have decreased to 60% of the older population and ethnic elders will have grown to 41.1% (U.S. Bureau of the Census, 2006). Some projections (Byrd, 2006) suggest that by 2050, ethnic elders may account for as much as 50% of the older adult population, with those who self-identify as Hispanic representing the fastest growing group.

TABLE 4-1

Population Age 65 and Older by Race and Hispanic Origin, 2006 Estimates and 2050 Projections

	2006 estimates		2050 projections	
	Number	*Percent*	*Number*	*Percent*
Total population 65 +*	37,260,352	100	86,705,637	100
Non-Hispanic white alone	30,187,588	80.8	53,159,961	61.3
Black alone	3,167,986	8.5	10,401,575	12.0
Asian alone	1,176,599	3.2	6,776,033	8.9
All other races in combination	413,355	1.1	2,328,390	2.7
Hispanic (of any race)	2,399,320	6.4	15,178,025	17.5

*The term "non-Hispanic white alone" is used to refer to people who reported being white and no other race and who are not Hispanic. The term "black alone" is used to refer to people who reported being black or African American and no other race. The term "Asian alone" is used to refer to people who reported only Asian as their race. The use of single-race populations in this report does not imply that this is the preferred method of presenting or analyzing data. The U.S. Census Bureau uses a variety of approaches. The race group "All other races alone or in combination" includes American Indian and Alaska Native, alone; Native Hawaiian and Other Pacific Islander, alone; and all people who reported two or more races. Reference population: These data refer to the resident population.

Source: U.S. Bureau of the Census (2006).

Another emerging subset of the ethnic elder population is older immigrants, admitted to the United States as relatives of citizens, permanent residents, and refugees (Gorospe, 2006).

WHO ARE ETHNIC ELDERS?

Ethnic elders in the United States are generally identified as belonging to four federally designated, non-European groups: African American, Asian American/Pacific Islander, Native American/ Alaskan Native, and Hispanic. The four major groups are comprised of many distinct subgroups, each characterized by a wide variety of cultural and linguistic differences. The African American category, for example, includes native-born descendants from Africans and free blacks who lived through the slavery era, and immigrants whose country of origin is a Caribbean island, Africa, or a South American country (Wikipedia, n.d.). The Asian/Pacific Islander group embraces at least 32 separate subgroups, including Chinese, Korean, Japanese, Filipino, and Samoan (Wikipedia, n.d.). The category Native American/Alaskan Native

includes American Indians, Aleuts, and Inuits from approximately 278 federally recognized reservations, 560 federally and 180 state recognized tribes, at least 100 nonfederally recognized tribes, and bands of native villages (Wikipedia, n.d.). The Hispanic category is classified as an ethnicity versus a race, because persons of Hispanic origin may be of any race. Although Hispanic subgroups are unified by linguistic and some cultural traditions, there are significant differences between Mexican American, Cuban, Puerto Rican, South American, and Central American populations (Wikipedia, n.d.). With the exception of the Native American/ Alaskan Native group, ethnic minority groups in the United States include a mix of native-born and immigrant individuals. "Approximately 6% of the black (African American) population is foreign born...There are more black immigrants in the United States [for example] than American Indians, Cuban Americans, Chinese, or Japanese. Blacks from the Caribbean constitute the largest subgroup of black immigrants" (Williams et al., 2007, p. 306).

Ethnic elders are further differentiated by a number of crosscutting factors that vary their life situations. Socioeconomic status, educational achievement, age cohort, geographic region or country of origin, family structure and dynamics, immigration status and level of acculturation, linguistic fluency and literacy level, cognitive and physical level of functioning, and personal experience with the healthcare system are examples of such crosscutting factors. In addition, each ethnic minority group has also been shaped by its own special history in the United States or country of origin. Compared to their white counterparts, ethnic elders have, in general, experienced a considerably greater level of social and material adversity across a lifetime, and many have less education, less money, less adequate housing, poorer health, and fewer years of life. They have collectively faced differential and unequal treatment in America and tend to perceive themselves as objects of discrimination and oppression because of their racial, ethnocultural, and linguistic characteristics (Barnes et al., 2004; Biegel & Leibbrandt, 2006; Hooyman & Kiyak, 2005), and for being old. This dual effect results in extra vulnerability for mental health problems (Atkinson, 2003), and places these groups at increased risk of mental disorders (Ong, Fuller-Rowell, & Burrow, 2009; Williams, Neighbors, & Jackson, 2003). It is essential for mental health providers to be familiar with the social and historical contexts that have shaped ethnic elders' life experiences and perspectives, and influenced their current patterns of health-related behavior and interactions (Primm, Levy, Cohen, & Bondurant, 2009). Providers must be knowledgeable about patterns and issues in ethnic elders' lives, but care must be taken to balance group indicators with individual biographies and avoid overgeneralization or stereotyping (Sellers, Jackson, & Hardison, 1998).

PREVALENCE RATE FOR MENTAL DISORDERS OF ETHNIC ELDERS

Earlier this decade, prevalence rates of mental disorders for ethnic elders who lived in the community were reported as comparable to those of community-dwelling older whites after controlling for differences in education, income, and marital status (Omotade, 2003; Tseng, 2001). More recent reports are mixed and indicate that mental health morbidity varies according to race and ethnicity across population groups (Agbayani-Siewert, Takeuchi, & Pangan, 2006; Breslau, Kendler, Su, Gaxiola-Aguilar, & Kessler, 2005; Harris, Edlund, & Larson, 2005; Hasin, Goodwin, Stinson, & Grant, 2005; Ojeda & McGuire, 2006; Skarupski et al., 2005; Sue & Chu, 2003; Williams et al., 2007). Miranda, McGuire, Williams, and Wang (2008) report, for example, that although minorities have fewer psychiatric disorders than do whites, both blacks and Hispanics are more likely to be persistently ill. Others report that ethnic minorities are as likely to experience at least as many mental health problems as European Americans, but a large proportion does not seek formal help and that the service needs of ethnic minorities may exceed those of whites (Snowden, 2003).

DISPARITIES IN MENTAL HEALTH CARE

According to a substantial body of evidence gathered over the last decade, much deeper disparities exist in mental health care for racial ethnic minorities compared to the general population (Atdjian & Vega, 2005; Cook, McGuire, & Miranda, 2007; Institute of Medicine [IOM], 2004; Miranda et al., 2008; Ruiz, 2008; U.S. Department of Health and Human Services (DHHS), 2001), constituting a major public health concern (Arean et al., 2005). Collectively, ethnic minorities experience a greater disability burden from mental illness than do whites. "This higher level of burden likely stems from minorities receiving less care and poorer care than from their illness being inherently more severe or prevalent in the community" (Thompson, 2006, pp. 163–164) and to the level and type of care received, including less primary prevention for and early identification of mental disorders (Miranda et al., 2008; Office of Minority Health and Health Disparities, 2008). Ethnic minorities have less access to mental health services than do whites. Foreign-born elders are less likely to have health insurance (Mold, Fryer, & Thomas, 2004; Sohn, 2004) or may not use Medicare benefits because they do not fully understand what services are covered (Pang, Jordan-Marsh, Silverstein, & Cody, 2003). Even when adequate insurance coverage and knowledge of its use are taken into account, ethnic elders are more likely than their white counterparts to delay or fail to seek mental health treatment (Gellis, 2006). Ethnic minorities who have insurance coverage and do use formal mental healthcare services commonly experience misdiagnosis, suboptimal treatment, premature termination of treatment, and other negative outcomes (Snowden & Yamada, 2005; Virnig et al., 2004).

KEY TERMINOLOGY: RACE, CULTURE, ETHNICITY, AND MINORITY GROUP

Before moving ahead, it is important to define the terms race, culture, ethnicity, and minority group, because they are central to discussion in this chapter. Universally agreed-on definitions for these terms do not yet exist. They are often used interchangeably and have different interpretations depending on the context in which they are used. Their meaning is continually transforming.

Race

Historically, race is a biological idea. Over time, scientific evidence has led to the conclusion that race has little explanatory power in human behavior and has even less use as a meaningful descriptor clearly to distinguish subgroups of humankind (Sue & Sue, 2007). Although race is now considered more as a sociological and political construct than a biological one (IOM, 2003), race still matters. The continuing concept of race as a biological idea is reflected when social groups continue to be treated as inferior or superior and have differing access to power and resources. Many health and human service organizations and the general public continue to associate

race with fixed genetic and behavioral features (Tyler, 2008). Despite the limitations inherent in the concept of race, federal agencies continue to require collection of data on racial groups for research, administrative, and political purposes. Race, sometimes used as a synonym for ethnicity, does not imply a social or cultural component (Ahmed & Kramer, 2004–2006).

Culture

Culture describes nonbiologically determined and socially learned attitudes and patterns of behavior that are transmitted from generation to generation and shared and understood by members of the same cultural group. "Culture is an integrated pattern of human behavior that includes thoughts, communications, languages, practices, beliefs, values, customs, courtesies, rituals, manners of interacting, roles, relationships, and expected behaviors of a racial, ethnic, religious or social group" (National Center for Cultural Competence, 2004, p. vii). Finally, culture determines one's worldview. Worldview is a cultural construction of reality, a framework through which an individual interprets and interacts with the world. It speaks to basic assumptions about the nature of reality that becomes the foundation for all actions and interpretations.

Ethnicity

The concept of ethnicity focuses attention on the social and historical context of individuals and groups rather than on questionable genetic and biological (racial) differences (Ahmed & Kramer, 2004–2006; Sellers et al., 1998). Ethnicity refers to one's identification with a broad population or social grouping based on presumptions of common ancestral descent, history, religion, geographic origin, language, or nationality. Individuals within an ethnic group consider themselves or are considered by others to share characteristics, beliefs, and behavioral norms that differentiate them from other collectives within society (Lu, Lim, & Mezzich,

2008; McGoldrick, Giordano, & Garcia-Preto, 2005). Ethnicity is closely linked to one's self-image, personal identity, and feelings of connectedness with other ethnic group members. Caution is needed to avoid making assumptions about clients' ethnicity or ethnic group membership based on such characteristics as language and appearance alone. Such assumptions, if incorrect, can lead to misunderstanding and possibly misdiagnosis (Gaw, 2001). Gaw also warns that the concept of ethnicity in mental health should not be exoticized and viewed as a subspecialty thought to apply only to ethnic minority groups. The concept has universal application across all population groups, including European Americans. Some authors (Verkuyten, 2004) point out to keep in mind that use of the more generic term "ethnicity" to describe groups formerly referred to as ethnic–racial minorities may cloud or ignore the significance of day-to-day realities of bias, racism, and discrimination that influence the delivery of health care.

Minority Group

This refers to a minority status rather than to a numerical population. From a social science perspective, minority groups are perceived as being different and having a lower status within society based on some characteristic, such as their race, ethnicity, or national origin (Weine & Siddiqui, 2009). Minority groups generally lack access to resources, power, wealth, or privilege (Bottero, 2005). They are evaluated less favorably than most of the population and tend to be stereotyped, disadvantaged, underprivileged, excluded, or exploited. In America, persons of color, women, the disabled, and the gay–lesbian–bisexual–transgendered population are typically thought of as minority groups.

THE SOCIOCULTURAL CONTEXT OF MENTAL ILLNESS

To provide effective mental health services to ethnic elders, mental health professionals must pay attention to the social, cultural, and historical context that shapes ethnic elders' worldview and within which mental disorders occur (Agbayani-Siewert et al., 2006; Carpenter-Song, Schwallie, & Longhofer, 2007a; Cole, Stevenson, & Rogers, 2009; Hwang, Meyers, Abe-Kim, & Ting, 2008; Uba, 2003). This context includes an individual's and the clinician's explanatory models of mental illness, the influence of family, stigma associated with mental illness, and level of trust in the healthcare system and its providers (Rosenberg & Rosenberg, 2006).

Explanatory Models of Mental Illness

An individual's subjective interpretation of the nature of the problem, its cause, its severity, prognosis, and treatment preference, and his or her response to a specific illness experience (Kleinman, Eisenberg, & Good, 1978; McCabe & Priebe, 2004) are influenced by social environment, culture, and ethnicity (Murray, 2001; Tseng, & Streltzer, 2004). In Western medicine, the origin of mental illness is attributed to two main sources: psychological–psychiatric stress or trauma; and organic causes, such as chemical imbalances in the brain that lead to the manifestation of a disease. Mental illness is generally conceptualized and characterized within this biomedical framework of scientific reductionism by a separation of mind and body (Lake, 2008; Sue & Sue, 2007; Thomas, Braken, & Yasmeen, 2007; Yeung & Kam, 2006). Therapies are based on monocultural, Western European and North American concepts, values, and beliefs, and view the client as autonomous, egalitarian, and rational. An intrapsychic etiology model is assumed and an open-verbal communication style that is self-assertive and self-aware (Ho, Rasheed, & Rasheed, 2003) is required. Ethnic minority groups, especially the less acculturated, may conceptualize the cause of mental problems and related behavior differently (Brown, Sellers, Brown, & Jackson, 2006; Constantine, Meyers, Kindaichi, & Moore 2004; Uba, 2003). They tend to have a nonlinear, more holistic view and approach to the world and are less likely than the general population to make clear distinctions between mental and physical health issues (Yeh, Hunter, Madan-Bahel, Chiang, & Arora, 2004). Although mental illness is thought by some to be caused by disease (a natural illness), mental problems may be attributed to wider socioreligious or metaphysical factors. Spirit possession, witchcraft, divine retribution, the breaking of religious taboos, the loss of a vital body essence, capture of the soul by a spirit, and disharmony in the biological, spiritual, family, or community realm number among them (Hwang et al., 2008; Versola-Russo, 2006). Mental problems in non-Western groups have also been attributed to a lack of personal willpower; character weakness; God's will; or as punishment for an evil committed by the individual in a former life, by a family member, or by ancestors (Dixon & Vaz, 2005). Until recently, explanations for mental disturbances attributed to etiologies outside of the Western biomedical model have received little attention in modern therapy. More needs to be known about how they are used by individuals to explain, organize, and manage episodes of impaired well-being.

Although rigorous methodological research in this area is lacking (DHHS, 2001), illustrations of alternative explanatory models appear in the literature. Tseng (2006) cites, for example, a Hispanic woman who presented for treatment with the problem of "losing her soul," and an American Indian woman who could not escape her "spirit song" (Tseng). Vedantam (2005, p. A01) cites the story of an African American truck driver who told a psychiatric resident that he frequently saw the devil sitting beside him suggesting that his life was about to take a turn for the worse. The resident, trained to pay attention to cultural issues and somewhat familiar with African American folklore, thought to ask the man about his religious beliefs. The truck driver explained that he had used an allegorical religious expression common to many southern communities in the United States. The resident realized that the truck driver's statement should not be taken literally, but rather be viewed within its cultural context. An uninformed clinician assessing these examples at face value might suspect psychosis or a delusional disorder. Misinterpretation of such behaviors in a cross-cultural clinical encounter can easily result. The risk of misconstruing client behavior is heightened when the provider fails to consider the unique meaning and the cultural context within which behavior occurs. Patcher's Awareness–Assessment–Negotiation Model (Patcher, 1994) may be useful when dealing with individuals whose presentation of symptoms does not fit a standard biomedical model. Its application calls for the clinician to (1) be familiar with the health beliefs and practices commonly held by individuals in the population served, (2) determine whether the individual subscribes to these common beliefs and practices, and (3) negotiate how to incorporate indigenous practices safely into a treatment plan that both the clinician and the individual see as being useful. The Cultural Influences on Mental Health Model (Hwang et al., 2008) is another resource that can help the mental health professional to understand culture's impact.

Idioms of Distress and Culture-Bound Syndromes

There is clear evidence of variation in the symptomatic expression of psychosocial suffering by culture and locality. Each culture has established a set of interpretive behaviors that its members can accept and use with each other to describe and cope with what is wrong (DHHS, 2001; Nichter, 1981). Idioms of distress can be thought of as culture-specific ways of accounting for misfortune or expressing distress. *Ataque de nerviosis*, an idiom of distress prominent among the Hispanic population from the Caribbean and other Hispanic groups, is thought to be a direct result of a stressful life event related to the family or significant others (Guarnaccia & Martinez, 2002; Guarnaccia, Rivera, Franco, Neighbors, & Allende-Ramos, 1996; Interian et al., 2005). A general feature experienced by most sufferers is feeling out of control. Symptoms associated with *ataque* commonly include attacks of crying, uncontrollable screaming, trembling, and becoming verbally or physically aggressive. The person may experience amnesia in relation to the *ataque* but otherwise quickly return to his or her usual level of functioning. These symptomatic or interpretive behaviors should not be confused with mental illness (Saint Arnault & Kim, 2008).

African Americans, Asian Americans, and Hispanics are more likely than non-Hispanic whites to express mental distress through physical symptoms (somatization). Somatization, the most common "idiom of distress" worldwide, describes symptoms caused by stress but experienced as bodily sensations that cannot be defined biomedically. Somatic symptoms are considered to be culturally acceptable expressions of mental distress and vary according to the ethnocultural group in which they exist. Care should be taken to differentiate somatization from psychosomatic disease, which has a verifiable physiological disturbance (Escobar, Hovos-Nervi, & Gara, 2002; Kroenke & Rosmalen, 2006). The most common somatic symptoms associated with mental distress are musculoskeletal pain, fatigue, stomach pain, chest pain, and dizziness. The mental distress that causes somatization may not be consciously conceptualized by an individual or may not be discussed because of the social stigma often associated with mental problems (Yeung & Kam, 2006). Some somatic symptoms may seem bizarre when encountered outside of a client's cultural context. A culturally uninformed primary care provider serving ethnocultural minority clients may miss the opportunity to refer them for further investigation and the root problem of the distress goes unexamined and untreated. Even on referral, a specialty provider who is unfamiliar with idioms of distress may mistakenly diagnose the behavior as delusional or a psychotic disorder.

The "culture-bound syndrome" is another important concept for mental health professionals who serve individuals from ethnocultural minority groups (Tseng, 2006). The American Psychiatric Association ([APA] 2000) defines culture-bound syndromes as "locality-specific patterns of aberrant behavior and troubling experience that do not occur worldwide." Similar to idioms of distress, they are culturally influenced expressions of mental distress and reflect the underlying values, morals, and traditions embedded in the social and cultural context within which they exist. Because these syndromes may not be linked with disorders listed in the *Diagnostic and Statistical Manual of Mental Disorders. Text revision, DSM-IV-TR* (APA), if not understood, they can be misdiagnosed as mental illness by the mental health professional (Flaskerud, 2009).

Koro and ghost sickness are two examples of culture-bound syndromes observed in certain cultural environments. Koro (genital retraction syndrome) occurs in China and Southeast Asia (Tseng, 2006). It is a sudden intense anxiety that the penis will recede into the body and possibly cause death. This phenomenon is explained as a sign of fatal exhaustion of the yang element within the framework of the yin–yang balance, and is attributed to guilt and anxiety over real or imagined sexual excess, especially autoerotic. Ghost sickness occurs among American Indian groups in the United States and is a preoccupation with death and the dead and is thought to be associated with witchcraft. Symptoms include loss of appetite, nightmares, weakness, fear and dread, anxiety and confusion, a sense of being suffocated, hopelessness, and fainting (Faison & Armstrong, 2003; Jackson, 2006).

Until fairly recently, Western mental health professionals have been generally unaware of or insensitive to ethnocultural differences in symptom expressions of emotional distress. They have tended to assume universal (etic) applications of their concepts and goals to the exclusion of culture-specific (emic) views (Sue & Sue, 2007). The APA's *DSM-IV-TR* (2000) brings better awareness of the importance of the cultural dimension of the client's clinical presentation in Appendix I of the Outline for Cultural Formulation (CF) and Glossary of Culture-Bound Syndromes (Borra, 2008). It calls attention to five distinct aspects of the cultural context of illness (Table 4-2). The CF

TABLE 4-2

Components of Cultural Formulation

Cultural formulation section	*Subheading*
Cultural identity of the individual	Individual's ethnic or cultural reference group(s)
	Degree of involvement with both the culture of origin and the host culture (for immigrants and ethnic minorities)
	Language abilities, use, and preference
Cultural explanations of the individual	Predominant idioms of distress through which illness symptoms, or the need for social supports, are communicated
	Meaning and perceived severity of the individual's symptoms in relation to norms of the cultural reference group(s)
	Local illness categories used by the individual's family and community to identify the condition
	Perceived causes and explanatory models that the individual and the reference group(s) use to explain illness
	Current preferences for and past experiences with professional and popular sources of care
Cultural factors related to psychosocial environment and levels of functioning	Culturally relevant interpretations of social stressors, available social supports, and levels of functioning and disability
	Stresses in the local social environment
	Role of religion and kin networks in providing emotional, instrumental, and informational support
Cultural elements of the relationship between the individual and the clinician	Individual differences in culture and social status between the individual and the clinician
	Problems that these differences may cause in diagnosis and treatment (e.g., difficulties in relating or eliciting symptoms and understanding their cultural significance, in determining whether a behavior is normal or pathologic, etc.)
Overall cultural assessment for diagnosis and care	Discussion of how cultural considerations specifically influence comprehensive diagnosis and care

Source: Adapted with permission from the *Diagnostic and Statistical Manual of Mental Disorders,* Text Revision, Fourth Edition. 2000. American Psychiatric Association.

supplements the multiaxial diagnostic assessment by helping the clinician to systematically evaluate and report the impact of the individual's context in the illness experience during the clinical encounter. Articles by Fernandez and Diaz (2002) and Bucardo, Patterson, and Jeste (2008) provide excellent, detailed clinical case studies that illustrate use of the CF. An updated version of the *Diagnostic and Statistical Manual of Mental Disorders*, the DSM-V, scheduled for publication in May 2012, will include a reformulated and expanded CF on the role of race, ethnicity, and culture in the diagnosis of illness (Page & Blau, 2006; Wintrob, 2008). The challenge for its authors is to "incorporate cultural information into the structure of the evolving DSM-V without benefit of an adequate research base to provide useful guidelines" (Vega et al., 2007, p. 386).

Stigma and Shame

Goffman (1963, p. 3) characterizes *stigma* as "an attribute that reduces the bearer from a whole and usual person to a tainted and discredited one." The American Heritage Dictionary of the English Language (2009) defines stigmas as "a mark of disgrace; a stain or reproach as on one's reputation." The association of stigma with mental illness in the United States is common (Link, Yang, Phelan, & Collins, 2004). Feelings about stigma are, however, much more pronounced among ethnic minority groups (Alvidrez, Snowden, & Kaiser, 2008; Gary, 2005; Grandbois, 2005; Guarnaccia, Martinez, & Acosta, 2005; Hsu et al., 2008; Newhill & Harris, 2007; Ojeda & McGuire, 2006; Page & Blau, 2006; Yang & Kleinman, 2008; Yang, Phelan, & Link, 2008). Ethnic minorities are more likely than the general population to view mental illness as something of which to be ashamed (Moreno-John et al., 2004; Primm, 2006; Primm et al., 2009). Stigma-related concerns in the general population are more related to individuals and what others will think of them if a mental health problem or diagnosis is uncovered. For ethnic minority groups, stigma-related concerns extend to the entire family. Public knowledge of a family member's mental disorder can result in shame and loss of face; bring disgrace by association to the entire family; and ruin their public image, reputation, and respect (Larson & Corrigan, 2008; Uba, 2003; Wynaden et al., 2005; Yang & Kleinman, 2008). It is assumed that the family has a bad genetic or hereditary link (Sadavoy, Meier, & Ong, 2004; Wynaden et al.), so the stigma associated with mental illness could extend to the family becoming marginalized or shunned within their own community and with chances for a good marriage or gainful employment in the community being greatly diminished. Understanding the intense degree

of stigma associated with mental illness among Asian American groups and other ethnocultural minorities may help explain help-seeking behavior and why stigma serves as a powerful barrier to the use of formal mental health services.

Level of Trust

"Trust is a measure of willingness to seek mental health services, to remain in treatment, and to be able to develop a therapeutic relationship with a counselor or clinician" (Fabian & Edwards, 2005, p. 230). Lack of trust in the healthcare system and its providers among ethnic elders is best documented in the older African American population born in the United States. Much of their early lives was spent under a separate but unequal system of segregated health care and many have been directly scarred by a history of discrimination and racism, especially during the pre-civil rights era (Ahmed & Kramer, 2004–2006; Byrd & Clayton, 2002; Cohen, Magai, Yaffee, & Walcott-Brown, 2005; Hwang et al., 2008; Kennedy, Mathis, & Woods, 2007; Moreno-John et al., 2004; Primm, 2006; Primm et al., 2009; Suite, La Bril, Primm, & Harrison-Ross, 2007; Washington, 2006). The Tuskegee syphilis study and other historical medical atrocities perpetrated on the African American community have left a lingering legacy of distrust (Armstrong, Karima, Ravenell, McMurphy, & Putt, 2007; Byrd & Clayton, 2002; Halbert, Armstrong, Gandy, & Shaker, 2006; Johnson, Saha, Arbelaez, Beach, & Cooper, 2004; Washington, 2006). Examples of historical distrust are also documented among other groups of ethnic elders (Gee & Ro, 2009; Taxis, 2006). Even today, encounters with the healthcare system are marked by disregard, disrespect, lack of access, and abuse (Boulware, Cooper, Ratner, LaVeist, & Powe, 2003; Choi & Gonzalez, 2005; Cloutterbuck & Mahoney, 2003; Dovido et al., 2008; Guadangnolo et al., 2009; IOM, 2003; Koroukian, 2009; Snowden & Yamada, 2005; Spencer & Chen, 2004; Washington, 2006). Having experienced lifelong humiliation and subordination in health care and in other societal venues, ethnic elders may hesitate to seek needed help within what they perceive to be a hostile environment. Feelings of fear and distrust may be especially pronounced for older immigrants who are undocumented or who have migrated to the United States from countries with oppressive, authoritarian governments. Older immigrants' lack of trust is further intensified when care is provided by persons who know little of their country of origin or migration history and who are or may be perceived to be biased against their language or culture (Aroian, Wu, & Tran, 2005; Barrio et al., 2008; Sentell, Schumway, & Snowden, 2007).

Family Influence

Until fairly recently, the concept of family in the United States has been synonymous with Western culture's nuclear structure, which is based on immediate family membership. Nuclear family structure comes out of an individualistic worldview (Concepcion, 2000; Loue & Sajatovic, 2009; Triandis, 1995) in that it values independence and personal goals taking preference over group (or family) goals. The ethnic minority family is characterized by a collectivist worldview that subordinates personal goals and holds high regard for in-group (family, community, and nation) norms that tend to favor extended family networks (Triandis; Yeh, Arora, & Wu, 2006). Familial obligation and a sense of duty toward in-group members generate emotional and instrumental support for family members in need (Anez, Paris, Bedregal, Davidson, & Grilo, 2005; Barrio et al., 2008; Weisman, Rosales, Kymalainen, & Armesto, 2005). Although very little research has been conducted on the causes and consequences of family determinants of minority mental health and wellness (Weine & Siddiqui, 2009), coping with mental problems within collectivist-oriented families is thought to serve as a major resource in assisting the affected family member to cope with life problems during times of need than it is among white families in the care of mentally ill members (Guarnacia et al., 2005; Lee & Mock, 2005; Wang et al., 2006;

Woodward et al., 2008). Generally speaking, family determinants can function as either risk or protective factors in different phases of a family member's mental illness (Weine & Siddiqui). A family strength can, ironically, also be a weakness. Ethnic minorities, for example, have higher tolerance for and tend to normalize aberrant behavior within the family (Cloutterbuck & Mahoney, 2003; Henderson & Traphagan, 2005; Weisman et al., 2005). They are also less likely to acknowledge or recognize mental disorders, such as depression (*Medical News Today*, 2008), and may hide a family member with a mental health disorder from the community and/or avoid seeking formal help. This interplay of strength and weakness can cause delay in seeking formal help and treatment for a family member with a mental disorder or condition when needed (Mahoney, Cloutterbuck, Neary, & Zhan, 2005). Conversely, a study by Willging, Salvador, and Kano (2006) provides an example of family proactivity in a poor, multiethnic, rural area of New Mexico. Hispanic and Native American families, who typically make every effort to provide support and care within the family, helped mobilize "secular (professional and lay) and sacred (indigenous and Christian) mental health care resources" (Willging et al., p. 871) for family members who belonged to sexual minorities. Of note, families tended to influence choice of services that were based in nonbiomedical or religious belief systems (Willging et al.). Choices made may have been a function of factors beyond the scope of the study, such as living in a medically underserved area, lack of knowledge about formal mental health services, or having meager financial resources or little or no health insurance coverage. Although families in the Willging et al. study were proactive, there was a delay in having their family member seek formal mental health services, if needed. Only a few reports in the literature empirically link family characteristics among ethnic minority groups to service use, but family influence is thought to exert a great influence on an individual's help-seeking behavior and pathway toward the use of formal mental health services (Ho et al., 2003).

Help-Seeking Behavior

Help seeking behavior for mental health problems is shaped by culture (Mallinckrodt, Shigeoka, & Suzuki, 2005) and influenced by illness-related beliefs and explanatory models (Snowden & Yamada, 2005). What triggers an individual to seek help for mental distress, when, and from whom is highly variable across ethnocultural groups (Fernandez & Diaz, 2002; Hwang et al., 2008; Morgan et al., 2005; Rogler & Cortez, 2008; Rudell, Bhui, & Priebe, 2008). Help-seeking behavior can be conceptualized as occurring in three stages: (1) an individual must first recognize that he or she has a problem, (2) must decide to seek help, and (3) must select a provider (Cauce et al., 2002; Versola-Russo, 2006). A typical help-seeking pathway toward obtaining formal mental health care services among ethnic minority groups is as follows: (1) no care is sought, (2) the problem is managed through personal coping or interfamilial support and intervention, (3) consultation is sought from trusted extended family and friends, (4) outside help is sought from an indigenous healer or from the faith-based community, and (5) presentation of a somatic complaint is made to a primary care provider (Abe-Kim et al., 2007; Kirmayer et al., 2007). According to this trajectory, help is finally sought from formal mental services only after multiple alternative attempts to address suffering have been tried but were unsuccessful. This help-seeking pattern explains in part why ethnic minorities in the United States are less likely than whites to seek formal mental health treatment, and why they may demonstrate patterns of delay and underrepresentation in formal mental health services (Burgess, Ding, Hargreaves, van Ryn, & Phelan, 2008; Neighbors et al., 2008; Sadavoy et al., 2004). Other social and ethnocultural factors include (1) poor proficiency in speaking or low health literacy, (2) fatalism, (3) lack of knowledge about services, (4) concern about confidentiality and adverse effects of medication, (5) fear of being hospitalized involuntarily, (6) lack of awareness of mental health services, (7) negative experience in the mental health service system, and (8) socioeconomic issues.

Sociostructural Context of Mental Health Care

Although the sociocultural context of mental health care significantly influences an individual's approach to and potential use of formal mental health services, the sociostructural context can also affect an individual's access to and receipt of quality mental health care. The sociostructural context is comprised of factors that exist within the healthcare environment that are external to the direct control of the individual. Selected factors for consideration are the financing and organization of healthcare services and institutional and provider characteristics. Zhan's Access Barrier Model (2003) depicts three major barriers for ethnic elders as they seek and use formal mental health services (Figure 4-1). The first two barriers, demographic and cultural, were addressed earlier in this chapter. The third, structural barriers, is extended here to include provider characteristics. In common with all older Americans, ethnic elders encounter the structural barriers of cost, system fragmentation, lack of available services (Jackson, 2006), limited hours of service, and varying degrees of difficulty navigating complex bureaucratic systems. Ethnic elders face the additional structural barrier of provider characteristics. Provider bias, prejudice (IOM, 2003), and provider-related factors, such as use of the Western disease (mental health) classification system to evaluate individuals from a different culture, may negatively affect the quality of care received.

ACCESS TO CARE

Access to health care refers to the timely use of personal health services when an individual seeks or needs them (Agency for Health Care Research and Quality [AHRQ], 2008; Millman, 1993; Shi & Singh, 2010). Almost a decade ago, *Mental Health,*

FIGURE 4-1

Zahn's Access Barrier Model (2003b).

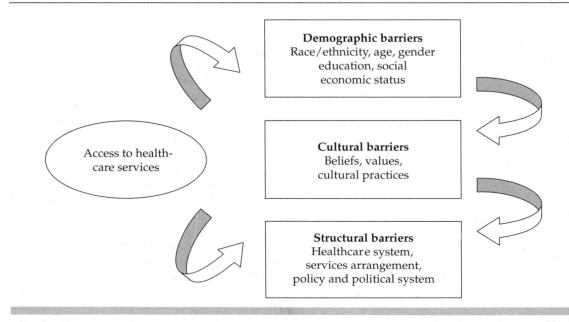

Culture, Race, and Ethnicity (DHHS, 2001), a watershed supplement to *Mental Health: A Report of the Surgeon General* (DHHS, 1999), reported that racial and ethnic minorities had less access to mental health services and were more unlikely to receive care when they needed it compared to the general population. It further reported that when care was received, it was likely to be substandard or sought too late (Virnig et al., 2004). Almost 10 years after the DHHS 2001 report was published, racial, ethnocultural, and linguistic minority groups continue to face similar problems (AHRQ, 2008; Atdjian & Vega, 2005; McGuire & Miranda, 2008; Office of Minority Health, 2008; Ruiz & Primm, 2009; Smedley, 2008). Alegria et al. (2008), for example, reported that an analysis of pooled data collected in 2007 on approximately 9,000 adults from three national surveys found significant differences in the access and quality of depression treatments among individuals with

any depressive disorder. Of those in the study who did not access any mental health treatment within the past 12 months, 40.2% were white, 58.8% African American, 63.7% Latino, and 68.7% Asian American. Access to care can be conceptualized as having two levels: primary and secondary (Jackson, 2006). Primary access is related to gaining entry into the healthcare system. Secondary access is related to the quality of care received by the individual once he or she has achieved primary access. Primary access alone or simply obtaining a service does not guarantee that, if received, it will be of high quality (Snowden & Yamada, 2005).

QUALITY OF CARE

Quality care in mental health can be measured by the degree to which services provided to individuals and populations increase the likelihood of desired outcomes (Clancy, 2008; Kilstrom, 1998). Although the quality of mental health care for all groups today is far from ideal, compared to the dominant culture, widespread differences are revealed in the quality, type, timing, intensity, and effectiveness of mental health care for racial, ethnocultural, and linguistic minorities (Pushkar & Marquis-Kerner, 2007; Sambamoorthi, Olfson, Wei, & Crystal, 2006; Schraufnagel, Wagner, Miranda, & Roy-Byrne, 2006; Stockdale, Lagomasino, Siddique, McGuire, & Miranda, 2008). Alegria et al. (2008) found, for example, that of persons who obtained treatment for depression in 2007, members of ethnic minorities were significantly less likely than whites to receive adequate care; 33% of whites received adequate care compared to 22% of Latinos, 13% of Asians, and 12% of African Americans. Sambamoorthi et al. found that "African Americans diagnosed with depression were less likely to receive antidepressant treatment and, if they did receive such treatment, [were] more likely to receive the older tricyclic drugs" (p. 141). Lower rates of antidepressant use in ethnic minorities compared to white patients can be attributed to a variety of factors that include differences in health insurance, provider–patient relationships, mistrust, and other cultural preferences (Blazer, Hybels, Fillenbaum, & Pieper, 2005; Chen & Rizzo, 2008; Schnittker, 2003).

Mechanisms thought to underlie disparities in quality of mental health care between minority and majority populations operate on two levels, the healthcare system and the clinical encounter (IOM, 2003; Jackson, 2006). Selected system-level factors include the location and type of setting where services occur, rate of referrals made to a mental health specialist, availability of interpreters, presence of screening and assessment tools developed or validated for use in minority populations, and the extent of an organization's commitment and ability to offer culturally responsive care (Alegria et al., 2007; Atdjian & Vega, 2005; Hernandez, Nesman, Mowery, Acevedo-Polakovich, & Callejas, 2009; Jackson, 2009; Miranda et al., 2008; Moon & Rhee, 2006; Newhill & Harris, 2007; Vedantiam, 2005). The second mechanism thought to underlie the quality of mental health services is the interaction

that occurs between the provider of care and the individual who seeks care. Within the clinical encounter, when the patient and provider are from dissimilar social, racial, ethnic, cultural, or linguistic backgrounds, each tends to interpret the behavior of the other within the context of his or her own cultural experience. Such considerations as the use of surnames, the appropriate degree of personal interaction, attitudes toward authority figures, education and class differences, language facility, and terminology usage are extremely important when establishing a therapeutic alliance. Providers who are unfamiliar with certain cultural values run the risk of offending, often resulting in poor interpersonal or therapeutic outcomes. Indirect evidence indicates that differences between the patient and provider can result in bias, prejudice, cultural distance, and clinical uncertainty (Alverson et al., 2007; Alvidrez et al., 2008; Balsa & McGuire, 2003; Fiske, 2002; IOM, 2003). This is especially so when the pressure of time to complete the clinical encounter is added to the equation (Sentell et al., 2007). Clinician bias during the clinical encounter is often unintentional and unconscious. It may be based on unfounded assumptions for reason of ageism or cultural distance, and emerge from unexamined racial stereotyping, class differences, or notions of racial superiority. Even when the provider and patient share a similar background, the diagnosis and identification of mental illness is challenging (Carpenter-Song, Schwallie, & Longhofer, 2007b; Yeung, 2008). When the dynamics of difference are at play, this challenge is heightened. Racial, ethnocultural, and linguistic minorities may define and express their problems differently than the general population because of cultural beliefs or behavioral patterns and communication styles.

Diagnostic assessment is complicated when a provider, unfamiliar with cultural frames of reference and culture-specific syndromes, uses the Western disease (mental health) system to evaluate individuals from a different cultural background. The quality of interaction during the clinical encounter can be further affected by limited verbal communication related to a lack of language proficiency, misunderstanding of nonverbal communication, different expectations of cultural norms for interpersonal behavior and style of interaction, and misunderstanding of symptom presentation (Alegria et al., 2007; Burgess et al., 2008; Cooper, Beach, Johnson, & Inui, 2006; Dixon & Vaz, 2005; Ghods et al., 2008; Jackson, 2006; Keating & Robertson, 2004; McGuire & Miranda, 2008; Miranda et al., 2008; Mui, 2001; Mui, Kang, & Domanski, 2007; Neighbors et al., 2008; Newhill & Harris, 2007; Noh, Kaspar, & Wickrama, 2007; Snowden, 2003; Spencer & Chen, 2004). An Asian American may, for example, present in a clinic setting complaining of vague physical symptoms that, on examination, have no discernible physiological basis. The patient may actually be depressed, but because the mind and body are considered inseparable, the individual may express emotional difficulties through somatic complaints (Kung & Lu, 2008). Yeung, Chang, Gresham, Nierenberg, and Fava (2004) found that of participants in their study who were identified by the Beck Depression Inventory as being depressed, 76% presented with somatic complaints. No participants complained of a depressed mood spontaneously. The most common symptoms experienced were fatigue, insomnia, headache, and pain. When asked to what their condition could be attributed, 55% reported that they did not know and 17% stated it was caused by a medical illness. Most patients were unaware they were suffering from depression and almost half reported that they had never heard of major depression. Somatic symptoms are more socially acceptable than psychological symptoms and carry a lower stigmatizing effect when care is finally sought. Most patients in the study sought help from primary care, lay help, or used alternative treatments.

Interestingly, Yeung et al. (2004) also found that somatization by some Chinese Americans may be influenced by their perception that healthcare professionals are more interested in physical, not psychological symptoms. Useful assessment starts with the presumption of what is normative behavior. What is considered normative in one population may not be so in another. African American patients with a mental disorder are, for example, less likely than white patients with the same symptoms to be diagnosed with mood disorders. African American patients, especially men, are disproportionately diagnosed with schizophrenia (Atdjian & Vega, 2005; Barnes et al., 2004; Fernandez & Diaz, 2002; Kirmayer, Groleau, Guzder, Blake, & Jarvis, 2003; Kirwin, 2009; Kunen, Smith, Niederhauser, Morris, & Brian, 2005; Mintzer, Endrie, & Faison, 2005; Strakowski et al., 2003; Whaley, 2004). Providers may misinterpret behavioral characteristics displayed within the clinical encounter. African American men may project "protective wariness" or "healthy paranoia" as a precaution against real or perceived physical or psychological exploitation, and score higher on measures of mistrust and paranoia on assessment tools developed for use in the dominant culture, but not validated with the African American population. From observed behavior and interpretation of screening results, a dominant culture provider may incorrectly arrive at the conclusion that the patient is experiencing pathological delusions rather than demonstrating protective cultural mechanisms (Strakowski et al.; Whaley).

Faulty interpretations of presenting symptoms can lead to overpathologizing or underpathologizing and misdiagnosis. Overdiagnosing, "misinterpreting culturally sanctioned behavior as pathological" (Leong & Lau, 2001, p. 207), and underdiagnosing, "attributing psychiatric symptoms to cultural differences" (Leong & Lau, p. 207), can lead to inappropriate, possibly harmful treatment and long-term implications. Underdiagnosing, leaving the underlying mental disorder untreated, can cause avoidable emotional suffering because many of the more common disorders, such as depression and anxiety, can respond well to psychotherapy and pharmacological interventions (Kunen et al., 2005). Some authors suggest that past racism and racist perspectives in biomedical and psychiatric practice may play a part in the differential application of quality mental health care (Suite et al., 2007).

Bevis (1921), who perceived African Americans as having a primitive psychic nature, represents the thinking of some psychiatrists in the early 1900s. Such thinking questioned whether black Americans could experience affective illness (Suite et al.). It is possible that a residual of such views may persist today and unconsciously cloud diagnostic decision making of some providers.

It is especially important for the provider to factor in the sociohistorical context and structural factors that shape an individual's experience (Trierweiler, Muroff, Jackson, Neighbors, & Munday, 2005; Yamada, Barrio, Morrison, Sewell, & Este, 2006; Yamada & Brekke, 2008). Care must be taken to avoid the use of screening and assessment instruments that were developed for use with the majority population, but not validated or standardized with racial, ethnocultural, and linguistic minorities (Atdjian & Vega, 2005; Huang, Chung, Kroenke, Delucchi, & Spitzer, 2006; Liu, Mezzich, Zapata-Vega, Ruiperez, & Yoon, 2008). Today, more screening instruments, such as the CES-D and the Beck Depression inventory, have been validated in African American populations and can assist in identifying affective illness in African Americans (Baker, 2001). This is also the case with other racial and ethnocultural groups (Huang et al.). The provider should also remember to take culture, language, and literacy issues into account in the application and analysis of diagnostic tools (Atdjian & Vega; Jackson, 2009; Vedantum, 2005). Clumsy, clueless, or inept handling of dynamics of difference within the clinical encounter runs the risk of engendering mistrust in the patient and leads to lack of faith in the treatment regimen, which lowers adherence, or to worse outcomes such as early dropout, often after the initial session (Atdjian & Vega; Barnes et al., 2004; Barnes et al., 2008). Few studies have attempted to empirically test mechanisms thought to affect quality mental health services for racial, ethnocultural, and linguistic minorities. Direct evidence bearing on the possible role of mechanisms thought to be associated with quality mental health care is not yet definitively available (IOM, 2003). More investigation is needed.

CULTURAL COMPETENCE

Cross, Bazron, Dennis, and Issacs' (1989) statement on cultural competence serves as the foundation for most definitions of cultural competence in use today. Cultural competence is generally defined as a set of cultural behaviors and attitudes integrated into the practice methods of a system, agency, or its professionals, that enable them to work effectively in cross-cultural situations (Cross et al.). It includes the integration and transformation of knowledge about individuals and groups of people into specific standards, policies, and practices, and attitudes used in appropriate cultural settings to increase the quality of services, thereby producing better outcomes (Davis, 1997). It is thought that increasing cultural competence in health and mental health care can contribute to better access, higher quality, and a reduction in existing disparities in mental health services (Hernandez et al., 2009; Lu & Primm, 2006). It is further thought to help in reducing risk management in terms of lawsuits and legal action, increasing patient satisfaction and the likelihood of parity within the mental healthcare system, and reflecting the fundamental value base of being responsive to individual needs and preferences (National Technical Assistance Center for State Mental Health Planning, 2004). Mental health services should ensure that care provided is congruent versus conflicting with cultural norms. "The goal of cultural competence is to create a health care system and workforce that is capable of delivering the highest quality care to every patient regardless of race, ethnicity, culture, or language proficiency" (Betancourt, Green, Carrillo, & Park, 2005, p. 499).

Part of striving to become a culturally competent agency or organization includes actively promoting a culturally diverse workforce and enhancing the cultural capability of the mainstream or dominant culture workforce through training in cultural competency. Training or education in cultural competency should be an integral part of undergraduate nursing education and continue at a higher level in masters and doctoral degree programs. One way of ensuring inclusion of cultural competency in healthcare content in undergraduate programs is to include it on the National Council Licensure Examination for nurses. Once formal schooling has been completed, training and ongoing information on cultural competence should be available through the workplace, in-service programs, courses offered at institutions of higher education, and through self-study. A number of excellent resources on cultural competence and mental health care are available on the Internet and in journal articles and textbooks.

Initially, begin to learn more about the culture of those patients you are most likely to see in your own practice. Several authors (Andrulis & Brach, 2007; Stone, 2005) recommend asking the "Kleinman Questions" (Kleinman et al., 1978; cited in Andrulis & Brach, 2007) to learn about the patient's explanatory model or meaning of their illness, including: "What do you think has caused the illness? What do you think the illness does? How does it work? What kind of treatment do you think you should receive? What are the most important results you hope you receive from this treatment?" Other authors, such as Rust et al. (2006), suggest using a shortcut way to remember the essential components of culturally competent health care and communicate effectively with diverse patient populations through the use of a mnemonic. Rust et al. developed the mnemonic CRASH for the following: consider *C*ulture, show *R*espect, *A*ssess/*A*ffirm differences, show *S*ensitivity and *S*elf-Awareness, and do it all with *H*umility. A number of similar mnemonics, such as LEARN, ETHNIC, and PRACTICE, are available in the literature. Useful conceptual models, such as Hwang et al.'s (2008) Cultural Influences on Mental Health Model, are also being developed for use as guides for practice and research. Cultural competence activities include the development of knowledge, attitudes, and skills through education and training; use of self-assessment for providers, organizations, and systems; and the implementation of objectives to ensure that governance, administrative policies, practices, and clinical skills are responsive to the culture and diversity within the populations served. Lastly, cultural competence, a process of continuous quality improvement, should be conceptualized as a journey, not a destination.

SUMMARY

Population demographics of the United States are rapidly changing. The growing numbers of older adults who are persons of color are creating an increasing demand for more services tailored to meet their needs, and a more diversified or better informed georopsychiatric and mental health workforce. Providers must become familiar with the historical, sociocultural, and sociostructural factors that influence ethnic elders' help-seeking patterns, behavior, and trajectory toward the use of formal mental healthcare services when needed. So, too, providers must become knowledgeable about the challenges older adults face in gaining access to formal mental health services and receiving quality care. It is well documented that persons from racial, ethnocultural, and linguistic backgrounds disproportionately experience disparities in mental health care compared to their dominant culture counterparts. The development of cultural competence is a critical element in the provision of effective and appropriate care. During the clinical encounter, practitioners who lack knowledge of cultural beliefs, behaviors, practices, and expectations often violate rules of cultural etiquette, ask fewer and less relevant questions, rely on stereotypes, may misinterpret unfamiliar expression of symptoms, and run the risk of making an incorrect diagnosis, which can compromise planning for appropriate treatment. Building cultural knowledge, which begins with self-awareness, has to do with forming attitudes and building skills that facilitate delivery of care that is congruent with the needs and preferences of older ethnic and linguistic adults. Culturally competent approaches and strategies help set the stage for positive outcomes of care. The culturally competent provider uses general information about ethnominority and cultural groups, but particularizes or individualizes that body of knowledge according to patient characteristics that make them unique. All of this must be incorporated into direct care and integrated into and supported by organizational practices and policies. Major gaps continue to exist in the nursing and mental health literature regarding best practices and effective models of care for ethnic elders. Investigation is needed to tease out or disentangle the relative importance of factors thought to affect the dynamics that occur within the clinical encounter, such as clinician bias. Such research will go a long way in establishing evidence-based pathways to care that go beyond trial and error and conjecture and result in positive outcomes.

CASE STUDY

Ms. Yeung is a 67-year-old Chinese woman who emigrated from Hong Kong 5 years ago with her husband to join their son, who lives in a city neighborhood that has a high concentration of Chinese and Chinese American families. Adjustment to living in a new country has been difficult because of poor English proficiency and loss of the status enjoyed in her country of origin. Being reunited with her son has, however, restored a sense of balance and harmony to Ms. Yeung's life. Six months ago, Ms. Yeung's husband died unexpectedly. Two months later, her son became engaged to an American-born woman from a prominent Chinese family that has lived in the community since the late 1900s. Recently, Ms. Yeung learned that her son has been offered an important job promotion, contingent on his moving to another state. Her son has accepted. After the wedding, which is imminent, her son and his new wife will be relocating. It has been decided that until they are settled, Ms. Yeung will not be joining them.

Ms. Yeung is increasingly concerned that her son, although respectful, has forgotten or possibly forsaken his parental duty and obligation to filial piety. She is also significantly dismayed about her soon-to-be daughter-in-law's lack of deference toward her. Ms. Yeung is harboring a growing worry that there may be no room in their new life for her.

In anticipation of her son's move, Ms. Yeung now occupies an apartment in an elderly high-rise located a few miles from the community where she had been living. She misses her friends in the old neighborhood, but because of her language limitation, she is apprehensive about using public transportation or taking a private taxi to visit them. Although she still sees her son, he has other commitments and his fiancé demands a lot of his time. The one person with whom Ms. Yeung can relate in the housing complex where she now lives is Annie Moi. Unlike Ms. Yeung, Ms. Moi is not a newcomer. She came to the United States from Hong Kong several years ago and is bilingual. They have only recently met and are tentatively building a friendship.

Ms. Yeung has not been sleeping well and feels tired all the time. She spends most of her days in bed with the Chinese television channel droning in the background. She is concerned about her increasing episodes of shortness of breath and palpitations. Because her stomach stays upset, she has little appetite. She is thinking if her son re-arranges the furniture in her apartment to be more in keeping with the principles of fung shui, her condition will improve. This change

(continues)

may also dispel the "inappropriate emotions" she has been feeling. Although she has tried self-control and determination to avoid dwelling on them, they have been difficult to manage. The Chinese herbs that Ms. Moi brought to her from the Chinese herbal emporium in the old neighborhood have not yet helped. If she can restore balance to her body, her mind also should settle. Ms. Yeung is thinking of seeing an acupuncturist, who uses moxibustion and will consult on balancing hot and cold foods, now that she is unable to shop at the Chinese market.

Ms. Yeung's son notices that his mother is losing weight, has less energy, and seems disinterested in participating in activities she used to enjoy. More alarming are her reports of shortness of breath and palpitations. He makes an appointment for her to be seen at a primary care clinic. Although Ms. Yeung does not think it will help, out of deference to her son, she consents to keep the appointment. On the day of the appointment, Ms. Yeung's son learns he cannot take off from work. As a last minute option, he asks Ms. Moi to accompany his mother to the clinic.

After a long wait, a young medical resident finally sees Ms. Yeung. The only Chinese interpreter available that day speaks Mandarin, not Cantonese. The clerk at the front desk asks Ms. Moi if she will translate. Ms. Moi is hesitant, but agrees. Ms. Yeung is similarly not eager because she does not know Ms. Moi that well. She "politely" acquiesces, because Ms. Moi may lose face if Ms. Yeung refuses. Besides, Ms. Yeung does not want to disappoint her son by not completing the visit. The resident enters the examination room without introducing himself and asks abruptly, "which one of you two is here to be seen?" Once it has been established

that Ms. Yeung is the patient, the resident begins questioning Ms. Yeung about her past medical history. He directs his questions to Ms. Moi almost exclusively, who relates them to Ms. Yeung and back. The resident seems rushed and barely looks at Ms. Yeung except while conducting a cursory physical examination. Out of deference to the doctor's status, Ms. Yeung keeps her eyes averted throughout the visit. The resident's first question to Ms. Yeung is why she has come to the clinic. When she answers that her son told her to come, the resident is put off by her nonspecific response and launches into a number of direct, rapidly fired questions (a low context style of communication). Ms. Yeung does not understand the terminology of many of the questions and is embarrassed about having to provide private information to persons outside of the family, the resident and Ms. Moi. In her accustomed style, Ms. Yeung answers the resident's question as best she can. He thinks her responses are vague, indirect, and meandering (high-context style communication). He is increasingly impatient because it is taking so long to elicit information from Ms. Yeung about her symptoms. At the end of the visit, the resident tells Ms. Yeung that he does not know what is wrong with her and gives her the option of returning for diagnostic testing. On his way out of the examination room, reflecting on Ms. Yeung's flat affect, lack of eye contact, and seemingly reluctant, convoluted responses, he turns and asks Ms. Yeung point blank, "Have you ever had any problems with your mental health? Are you sure you're not depressed?" Mortified, Ms. Yeung quickly dresses and does not wait to make a follow-up appointment. She has no plans to return. The bus ride home with Ms. Moi is deadly silent.

CASE STUDY (continued)

Discussion Questions

Consider your responses within the framework of what is generally known about Chinese and Chinese American culture and issues of mental health.

- Given her presenting symptoms at the primary care clinic, what, if anything, would suggest that Mrs. Yeung might have a mood disorder?
- Aside from the grief that Ms. Yeung may still be experiencing following her husband's death, what family and situational issues may be contributing to Ms. Yeung's growing sense of "depression?"
- Had the resident been tuned into Ms. Yeung's initial response, why would it have prompted him to take a social history? What might it have revealed that would help him with his assessment?
- Ms. Yeung displayed certain self-help and help-seeking behaviors before seeking formal care. What do they tell us about how Ms. Yeung may be conceptualizing the cause of her symptoms?
- If Ms. Yeung has developed a mood disorder, offer a few explanations as to why she is expressing it through physical symptoms?
- Would it be stereotyping Ms. Yeung to ask her if she uses traditional Chinese medicine? Why or why not?
- What are your thoughts on the choice of Ms. Moi to serve as interpreter for Ms. Yeung during the clinical encounter? If you think it was a good idea, why? If you disagree, what is your rationale?
- During the clinical encounter, what tenets of cultural etiquette did the resident violate with Ms. Yeung?
- Identify the cultural "red lights," breaches of cultural etiquette the resident committed during the clinical encounter? Why might they be offensive to Ms. Yeung?
- Aside from his display of cultural insensitivity, in what three behaviors did the resident engage that might reduce Ms. Yeung's level of confidence in his ability as provider?
- Why was Ms. Yeung mortified when, in the presence of Ms. Moi, the resident asked whether she (Ms. Yeung) had a history of mental illness and might be depressed?
- What additional worry might Ms. Yeung have, now that Ms. Moi knows that the doctor is questioning whether she (Ms. Yeung) might possibly have a mental disorder?
- How should this visit have been conducted? As a "culturally competent" provider, what would you have done differently at the beginning and throughout the clinic visit with Ms. Yeung? Include in your response what factors you would assess and factor into your initial "diagnostic" determination. Also, how might you keep Ms. Yeung engaged in the process after the initial visit?

REFERENCES

Abe-Kim, J., Takeuchi, D. T., Hong, S., Zane, N., Sue, S., Spencer, M. S., et al. (2007). Use of mental health-related services among immigrant and US-born Asian Americans: Results from the national Latino and Asian American study. *American Journal of Public Health, 97*(1), 91–98.

Administration on Aging. (2008). *A profile of older Americans 2007.* U.S. Department of Health and Human Services. Washington, DC: Government Printing Office.

Agbayani-Siewert, P., Takeuchi, D. T., & Pangan, R. W. (2006). Mental illness in a multicultural context. In C. S. Aneshensel & J. C. Phelan (Eds.), *Handbook of the sociology of mental health* (pp. 19–36). New York: Springer.

Agency for Health Care Research and Quality. (2008). *2008 National Health Care Disparities Report.* U.S. Department of Health and Human Services. Rockville, MD: Author.

Ahmed, I., & Kramer, E. (Eds.). (2004–2006). *Ethnic minority elderly curriculum.* Arlington, VA: American Psychological Association.

Alegria, M., Chatterji, P., Wells, K., Cao, Z., Chen, C., Takeuchi, D., et al. (2008). Disparity in depression treatment among racial and ethnic minority populations in the United States. *Psychiatric Services, 59,* 1264–1272.

Alegria, M., Mulvaney-Day, N., Woo, M., Torres, M., Gao, S., Oddo, V., et al. (2007). Correlates of 12-month service use among Latinos: Results from the National Latino and Asian American Study, *American Journal of Public Health, 97,* 76–83.

Alverson, H. S., Drake, R. E., Carpenter-Song, E. A., Chu, E., Ritsema, M., & Smith, B. (2007). Ethnocultural variations in mental illness discourse: Some implications for building therapeutic alliances. *Psychiatric Services, 58*(12), 1541–1546.

Alvidrez, J., Snowden, L. R., & Kaiser, D. M. (2008). The experience of stigma among Black mental health consumers. *Journal of Health Care for the Poor, 19*(3), 874–893.

American Heritage Dictionary of the English Language (4th ed.). (2009). Boston: Houghton Mifflin.

American Psychiatric Association. (2000). *Diagnostic and statistical manual of mental disorders. Text revision, DSM-IV-TR* (4th ed.). Washington, DC: American Psychiatric Association.

Andrulis, D. P., & Brach, C. (2007). Integrating literacy, culture, and language to improve health care quality for diverse populations. *American Journal of Health Behavior, 31,* S122–S133.

Anez, L. M., Paris, M., Bedregal, L. E., Davidson, L., & Grilo, C. M. (2005). Application of cultural constructs in the care of first generation Latino clients in a community mental health setting. *Journal of Psychiatric Practice, 11*(4), 221–230.

Arean, P. A., Ayalon, L., Hunckler, E., Lin, E. H. B., Tang, L., Harpole, L., et al. (2005). Improving depression care for older minorities in primary care. *Medical Care, 43*(4), 381–390.

Armstrong, K., Karima, L., Ravenell, M. S., McMurphy, S., & Putt, M. (2007). Racial/ethnic differences in physician distrust in the United States. *American Journal of Public Health, 97*(7), 1283–1289.

Aroian, K. J., Wu, B., & Tran, T. V. (2005). Health care and social Chinese immigrant elders. *Research in Nursing and Health, 28*(2), 95–105.

Atdjian, S., & Vega, W. A. (2005). Disparities in mental health treatment in U.S. racial and ethnic minority groups: Implications for psychiatrists. *Psychiatric Services, 56*(12), 1600–1602.

Atkinson, D. R. (2003). *Counseling American minorities* (6th ed.). New York: McGraw-Hill.

Baker, F. M. (2001). Diagnosing depression in African Americans. *Community Mental Health Journal, 37*(1), 31–38.

Balsa, A. I., & McGuire, T. G. (2003). Prejudice, clinical uncertainty and stereotyping as sources of health disparities. *Journal of Health Economics, 22*(1), 89–116.

Barnes, L. L., Mendes De Leon, C. F., Lewis, T. T., Bienias, J. L., Wilson, R. S., & Evans, D. A. (2008). Perceived discrimination and mortality in a population-based study of older adults. *American Journal of Public Health, 98*(7), 1241–1247.

Barnes, L. L., Mendes De Leon, C. F., Wilson, C. F., Bieneas, J. L., Bennett, D. A., & Evans, D. A. (2004). Racial differences in perceived discrimination in a community population of older blacks and whites. *Journal of Aging and Health, 16*(3), 315–337.

Barrio, C., Plainkas, L. A., Yamada, A. M., Fuentes, D., Cirado, V., Garcia, P., et al. (2008). Unmet needs for mental health services for Latino older adults: Perspectives from consumers, family members, advocates, and service providers. *Community Mental Health Journal, 44*(1), 54–74.

Betancourt, J., Green, A. R., Carrillo, J. E., & Park, E. R. (2005). Cultural competence and health care disparities: Key perspectives and trends. *Health Affairs, 24*(2), 499–505.

Bevis, M. W. (1921). Psychoanalytic traits of the Southern Negro with observations as to some of his psychoses. *American Journal of Psychiatry, 18,* 67–78.

Biegel, D. E., & Leibbrandt, S. (2006). Elders living in poverty. In B. Berkman (Ed.), *Handbook of social work in health and aging* (pp. 167–180). New York: Oxford University Press.

Blazer, D. G., Hybels, C. F., Fillenbaum, G. G., & Pieper, C. F. (2005). Predictors of antidepressant drug use among older adults: Have they changed over time? *American Journal of Psychiatry, 162*(4), 705–710.

Borra, R. (2008). Working with the cultural formulation in therapy. *European Psychiatry, 23,* S43–S48.

Bottero, W. (2005). *Stratification: Social division and inequality.* New York: Routledge.

Boulware, L. E., Cooper, L. A., Ratner, L. E., LaVeist, T. A., & Powe, N. R. (2003). Race and trust in the health care system. *Public Health Reports, 118,* 358–365.

Breslau, J., Kendler, K. S., Su, M., Gaxiola-Aguilar, S., & Kessler, R. C. (2005). Lifetime risk and persistence of psychiatric disorders across ethnic groups in the U.S. *Psychosocial Medicine, 35*(3), 317–327.

Brown, T. N., Sellers, S. L., Brown, K. T., & Jackson, J. S. (2006). Race, ethnicity, and culture in the sociology of mental health. In C. S. Aneshensel & J. C. Phelan (Eds.), *Handbook of the sociology of mental health* (pp. 167–182). New York: Springer.

Bucardo, J. A., Patterson, T. L., & Jeste, D. V. (2008). Cultural formulation with attention to language and cultural dynamics in a Mexican American psychiatric patient treated in San Diego, California. *Culture, Medicine and Psychiatry, 32,* 102–121.

Burgess, D. J., Ding, Y., Hargreaves, M., van Ryn, M., & Phelan, S. (2008). The association between perceived discrimination and underutilization of needed medical and mental health care in a multiethnic community sample. *Journal of Health Care for the Poor and Underserved, 19*(3), 894–911.

Byrd, L. (2006). *Health disparities affecting minority elderly populations.* Presented at the National Conference of Gerontological Nurse Practitioners (NCGNP) 25th Anniversary Conference, September 29, 2006, Ponte Vedra Beach, FL.

Byrd, M., & Clayton, L. A. (2002). *An American health dilemma: Race, medicine, and health care in the United States, 1900–2000.* Florence, KY: Routledge.

Carpenter-Song, E., Schwallie, M. N., & Longhofer, J. L. (2007a). Cultural competence reexamined: Critique and direction for the future. *Psychiatric Services, 58*(10), 1362–1365.

Carpenter-Song, E., Schwallie, M. N., & Longhofer, J. L. (2007b). Using care with culture. In S. Loue, M. Sajatovic, & J. L. Longhofer (Eds.), *Diversity issues in the diagnosis and treatment of mood* (pp. 3–16). New York: Oxford University Press.

Cauce, A. M., Domenech-Rodriquez, M., Paradise, M. M., Cochran, B. N., Shea, J. M., Srebnik, D., et al. (2002). Cultural and contextual influences in mental health help seeking: A focus on ethnic minority youth. *Journal of Counseling and Clinical Psychology, 70*(1), 44–55.

Chen, J., & Rizzo, J. A. (2008). Racial and ethnic disparities in antidepressant drug use. *Journal of Mental Health, Policy, and Economics, 11,* 155–165.

Choi, N. G., & Gonzalez. (2005). Geriatric mental health clinician's perceptions of barriers and contributors to retention of older minorities in treatment: An exploratory study. *Clinical Gerontologist, 28*(3), 3–25.

Clancy, C. M. (2008). *Measuring health care quality.* KaiserEDU.org. Washington, DC: U.S. Agency for Research and Health Care Quality. Retrieved December 9, 2009, from http://www.kaiseredu.org/tutorials/quality/player.html

Cloutterbuck, J., & Mahoney, D. F. (2003). African American dementia caregivers: The duality of respect. *Dementia, 2*(2), 221–243.

Cohen, C. I., Magai, C., Yaffee, R., & Walcott-Brown, L. (2005). Comparison of users and nonusers of mental health services among older, depressed, urban African Americans. *American Journal of Geriatric Psychiatry, 13*(7), 545–553.

Cole, E., Stevenson, M., & Rogers, B. (2009). The influence of cultural health beliefs on self-reported mental health status and mental health service utilization in an ethnically diverse sample of older adults. *Journal of Feminist Family Therapy, 21,* 1–17.

Concepcion, B. (2000). The cultural relevance of community support programs. *Psychiatric Services, 51,* 878–884.

Constantine, M. G., Myers, L. J., Kindaichi, M., & Moore, J. L. (2004). Exploring indigenous mental health practices: The roles of healers and helpers in promoting well-being in people of color. *Counseling and Values, 48,* 110–125.

Cook, B. J., McGuire, T., & Miranda, J. (2007). Measuring trends in mental health disparities, 2000–2004. *Psychiatric Services, 58,* 1533–1540.

Cooper, L. A., Beach, M. C., Johnson, R. L., & Inui, T. S. (2006). Delving below the surface: Understanding how race and ethnicity influence relationships in health care. *Journal of General Internal Medicine, 21,* S21–S27.

Cross, T. L., Bazron, B. J., Dennis, K. W., & Issacs, M. R. (1989). *Towards a culturally competent system of care: A monograph on effective services for minority children who are severely emotionally disturbed.* Washington, DC: National Technical Assistance Center for Children's Mental Health, Georgetown University Child Development Center.

Davis, K. (1997). *Exploring the intersection between cultural competency and managed behavioral health care policy: Implications for state and county mental health agencies.* Alexandria, VA: National Technical Assistance Center for State Mental Health Planning.

Dixon, C. G., & Vaz, K. (2005). Perceptions of African Americans regarding mental health counseling. In D. A. Harley & J. M. Dillard (Eds.), *Contemporary mental health issues among African Americans* (pp. 163–174). Alexandria, VA: American Counseling Association.

Dovido, J. F., Penner, L. A., Albrecht, T. L., Norton, W. E., Gaertner, S. L., & Shelton, J. N. (2008). Disparities and distrust: The implications of psychological processes for understanding racial disparities in health and health care. *Social Sciences and Medicine, 67*(3), 478–486.

Escobar, J. I., Hovos-Nervi, C., & Gara, M. (2002). Medically unexplained physical symptoms in medical practice: A psychiatric perspective. *Environmental Health Perspectives, 110*(Suppl. 4), 631–636.

Fabian, E. S., & Edwards, Y. V. (2005). Community mental health and African Americans. In D. A. Harley & J. M. Dillard (Eds.). *Contemporary mental health issues among African Americans* (pp. 36–47). Alexandria, VA: American Counseling Association.

Faison, W. E., & Armstrong, D. (2003). Cultural aspects of psychosis in the elderly. *Journal of Geriatric Psychiatry and Neurology, 16*(4), 225–231.

Fernandez, R. L., & Diaz, N. (2002). The cultural formulation: A method for assessing cultural factors affecting the clinical encounter. *Psychiatric Quarterly, 73*(4), 271–295.

Fiske, S. T. (2002). What we know about bias and intergroup conflict, the problem of the century. *Current Directions in Psychological Science, 11,* 123–127.

Flaskerud, J. H. (2009). What do we need to know about culture-bound syndromes? *Issues in Mental Health Nursing, 30*(6), 406–407.

Gary, F. (2005). Stigma: Barrier to mental health care among ethnic minorities. *Issues in Mental Health Nursing, 26*(10), 979–999.

Gaw, A. C. (2001). *A concise guide to cross cultural psychiatry.* Washington, DC: American Psychiatric Association.

Gee, G. C., & Ro, A. (2009). Racism and discrimination. In C. Trinh-Shevrin, N. S. Islam, & M. J. Rey (Eds.), *Asian American communities and health: Context, research, policy and action* (pp. 364–402). San Francisco: Jossey-Bass.

Gellis, Z. D. (2006). Older adults with mental and emotional problems. In B. Berkman and S. D'Ambruoso (Eds.), *Handbook of social work in health and aging* (pp. 129–139). New York: Oxford University Press.

Ghods, B. K., Roter, D. L., Ford, D. E., Larsen, S., Arbelaez, J. J., & Cooper, L. (2008). Patient-physician communication in the primary care visits of African Americans and whites with depression. *Journal of General Medicine, 23*(5), 600–606. Retrieved August 4, 2009, from http://www.ncbi.nlm.nih.gov:80/pmc/articles/PMC2324146/

Goffman, E. (1963). *Stigma: Notes on management of spoiled identity.* Englewood Cliffs, NJ: Prentice Hall.

Gorospe, E. (2006). Elderly immigrants: Emerging challenges for the U.S. healthcare system. *The International Journal of Healthcare Administration, 4*(1), 1–4.

Grandbois, D. (2005). Stigma of mental illness among American Indian and Alaska Native nations: Historical and contemporary perspectives. *Issues in Mental Health Nursing, 26,* 1001–1024.

Guadagnolo, B. A., Cina, K., Helbig, P., Molloy, K., Reiner, M., Cook, E. F., et al. (2009). Medical mistrust and less satisfaction with health care among Native Americans presenting for cancer treatment.

Journal of Health Care for the Poor and Underserved, 20(1), 210–226.

Guarnaccia, P. J., & Martinez, I. M. (2002). *Comprehensive in-depth literature review and analysis of Hispanic mental health issues*. Institute for Health Care Policy and Aging Research. Newark, NJ: Rutgers the State University of NJ.

Guarnaccia, P. J., Martinez, I., & Acosta, H. (2005). Mental health in the Hispanic community: An overview. *Journal of Immigration and Refugee Services, 3*(1/2), 21–46.

Guarnaccia, P. J., Rivera, M., Franco, F., Neighbors, C., & Allende-Ramos, C. (1996). The experiences of attaques de nervios: Towards anthropology of emotions in Puerto Rico. *Culture, Medicine, and Psychiatry, 20*, 343–367.

Halbert, C. H., Armstrong, K., Gandy, O. H., & Shaker, L. (2006). Racial differences in trust in health care providers. *Archives of Internal Medicine, 166*, 896–901.

Harris, K. M., Edlund, M. J., & Larson, S. (2005). Racial and ethnic differences in the mental health problems and use of mental health care. *Medical Care, 43*(8), 775–784.

Hasin, D. S., Goodwin, R. D., Stinson, F. S., & Grant, B. F. (2005). Epidemiology of major depressive disorder: Results from the national epidemiologic survey on alcoholism and related conditions. *Archives of General Psychiatry, 62*(10), 1097–1106.

Hendersen, J. N., & Traphagan, J. W. (2005). Cultural factors in dementia: Perspectives from the anthropology of aging. *Alzheimer's Disease and Associated Disorders, 19*(4), 272–274.

Hernandez, M., Nesman, T., Mowery, D., Acevedo-Polakovich, I. D., & Callejas, L. M. (2009). Cultural competence: A literature review and conceptual model for mental health services. *Psychiatric Services, 60*(8), 1046–1050.

Ho, M. K., Rasheed, J. M., & Rasheed, M. Z. (2003). *Family therapy with ethnic minorities*. Thousand Oaks, CA: Sage.

Hooyman, N. R., & Kiyak, H. A. (2005). *Social gerontology: A multidisciplinary perspective* (6th ed.). Boston: Allyn & Bacon.

Hsu, L. K. G., Wan, Y. M., Chang, H., Summergrad, P., Tsang, B. Y. P., & Chen, H. (2008). Stigma of depression is more severe in Chinese Americans than Caucasian Americans. *Psychiatry, 71*(3), 210–218.

Huang, F. Y., Chung, H., Kroenke, K., Delucchi, K. L., & Spitzer, R. L. (2006). Using the patient health questionnaire-9 to measure depression among racially and ethnically diverse primary care patients. *Journal of General Internal Medicine, 21*(6), 547–552.

Hwang, W. C., Meyers, H. F., Abe-Kim, J., & Ting, J. Y. (2008). A conceptual paradigm for understanding culture's impact on mental health: The cultural influences on mental health (CIMH) model. *Clinical Psychology Review, 28*, 212–228.

Institute of Medicine of the National Academies. (2003). *Unequal treatment: Confronting racial and ethnic disparities in health care*. Washington, DC: National Academy Press.

Institute of Medicine of the National Academies. (2004). *In the nation's compelling interest: Ensuring diversity in the health care workforce*. Washington, DC: National Academy Press.

Interian, A., Guarnaccia, P. J., Vega, W. A., Gara, M. A., Like, R. C., Escobar, J. I., et al. (2005). The relationship between *ataque de nervios* and unexplained neurological symptoms: A preliminary analysis. *The Journal of Nervous and Mental Disease, 193*(1), 32–39.

Jackson, V. (June 8–11, 2009). *Dimensions of racial and ethnic disparities in mental health services*. Conference Presentation at the Center for Mental Health Services, Substance, Abuse and Mental Health Services Administration, National Policy Summit on the Elimination of Disparities, New Orleans, LA.

Jackson, Y. K. (Ed.). (2006). *Encyclopedia of multicultural psychology*. Thousand Oaks, CA: Sage.

Johnson, R. L., Saha, S., Arbelaez, J. J., Beach, M. C., & Cooper, L. A. (2004). What explains racial and ethnic differences in patient ratings of cultural competence? *Journal of General Internal Medicine, 19*(2), 101–110.

Keating, F., & Robertson, D. (2004). Fear, Black people and mental illness: A vicious circle. *Health and Social Care in the Community, 12*(5), 439–447.

Kennedy, B. R., Mathis, C. C., & Woods, A. K. (2007). African Americans and their distrust of the health care system: Healthcare for diverse populations. *Journal of Cultural Diversity, 14*(2), 56–60.

Kilstrom, L. C. (1998). Mental health services research. In *Encyclopedia of Mental Health* (Vol. 2, pp. 653–663). Cleveland, OH: Academic Press.

Kirmayer, L. J., Groleau, D., Guzder, J., Blake, C., & Jarvis, E. (2003). Cultural consultation: A model of mental health service for multicultural societies. *Canadian Journal of Psychiatry, 48*(3), 145–153.

Kirmayer, L. J., Weinfeld, M., Burgos, G., Galbaud du Fort, G., Lasry, J. C., & Young, A. (2007). Use of health care services for psychological distress by immigrants in an urban multicultural milieu. *Canadian Journal of Psychiatry, 52*, 295–304.

Kirwin, D. (2009). *Testimony of the American Association for Geriatric Psychiatry on March 18, 2009 Before the Appropriations Subcommittee on Labor, Health and Human Services, and Education.* Washington, DC: U.S. Government Printing Office.

Kleinman, A., Eisenberg, L., & Good, B. (1978). Culture, illness and care: Clinical lessons from anthropologic and cross-cultural research. *Annals of Internal Medicine, 88*, 251–258.

Koroukian, S. M. (2009). Minority mental health and wellness: A perspective from health care systems. In S. Loue & M. Sajatovic (Eds.) *Determinants of minority mental health and wellness* (pp. 1–35). New York: Springer.

Kroenke, K., & Rosmalen, J. G. (2006). Symptoms, syndromes, and the value of psychiatric diagnosis in those patients who have functional somatic disorders. *Medical Clinics of North America, 90*(4), 603–623.

Kunen, S., Smith, P. O., Niederhauser, R., Morris, J. A., & Brian, D. (2005). Race disparities in psychiatric rates in emergency departments. *Journal of Consulting and Clinical Psychology, 73*(1), 116–126.

Kung, W. W., & Lu, P. (2008). How symptom manifestations affect help seeking for mental health problems among Chinese Americans. *The Journal of Nervous and Mental Disease, 196*, 46–54.

Lake, J. (2008). Nonconventional modalities. *Psychiatric Times, 25*(8), 10–12.

Larson, J. E., & Corrigan, P. (2008). The stigma of families with mental illness. *Academic Psychiatry, 32*(2), 87–91.

Lee, E., & Mock, M. R. (2005) Asian families: An overview. In M. McGoldrick, J. Giordano, & N. Garcia-Preto (Eds.), *Ethnicity and family therapy* (3rd ed., pp. 269–289). New York: Guilford Press.

Leong, L., & Lau, A. S. L. (2001). Barriers to providing effective mental health services to Asian Americans. *Mental Health Services Research, 3*(4), 201–214.

Link, B. G., Yang, L. H., Phelan, J. C., & Collins, P. Y. (2004). Measuring mental illness stigma. *Schizophrenia Bulletin, 30*(3), 511–541.

Liu, J. S., Mezzich, J. E., Zapata-Vega, M. I., Ruiperez, M. A., & Yoon, G. (2008). Development and validation of the Chinese version of the multicultural quality of life index. *Culture, Medicine and Psychiatry, 32*, 123–134.

Loue, S., & Sajatovic, M. (Eds.). (2009). *Determinants of minority mental illness and wellness*. New York: Springer.

Lu, F. G., Lim, R. F., & Mezzich, J. E. (2008). Issues in the assessment and diagnosis of culturally diverse individuals. In J. E. Mezzich & G. Caracci (Eds.), *Cultural formulation: A reader for psychiatric diagnosis* (pp. 115–148). Lanham, MD: Rowman and Littlefield.

Lu, F. G., & Primm, A. (2006). A mental health disparities, diversity, and cultural competence in medical student education: How psychiatry can play a role. *Academic Psychiatry, 30*, 9–15.

Mahoney, D. F., Cloutterbuck, J., Neary, S., & Zhan, L. (2005). African American, Chinese, and Latino family caregivers' impressions of the onset and diagnosis of dementia: Cross-cultural similarities and differences. *The Gerontologist, 45*(6), 783–792.

Mallinckrodt, B., Shigeoka, S., & Suzuki, L. A. (2005). Asian Pacific American students' acculturation and etiology beliefs about typical counseling center presenting problems. *Cultural Diversity and Ethnic Minority Psychology, 11*, 227–238.

McCabe, R., & Priebe, S. (2004). Explanatory models of illness in schizophrenia: Comparison of four ethnic groups. *The British Journal of Psychiatry, 185*, 25–30.

McGoldrick, M., Giordano, J., & Garcia-Preto, N. (Eds.). (2005). *Ethnicity and family therapy* (3rd ed.). New York: Guilford Press.

McGuire, T. G., & Miranda, J. (2008). New evidence regarding racial and ethnic disparities in mental health policy: Policy implications. *Health Affairs, 27*(2), 393–403.

Medical News Today. (2008, October 31). Disparities persist in mental health care. *Medical News Today*. Retrieved July 15, 2009, from http://www.medicalnewstoday.com/printerfriendlynews.php?newsid=127740

Millman, M. (Ed.). (1993). Committee to Monitor Access to Personal Health Care Services. *Access to health care in America*. Institute of Medicine. Washington, DC: National Academy Press.

Mintzer, J., Endrie, H., & Faison, W. (2005). Minority and sociocultual issues. In B. Sadock & V. Sadock (Eds.), *Comprehensive textbook of psychiatry* (pp. 3813–3822). New York: Lippincott Williams and Wilkins.

Miranda, J., McGuire, T. G., Williams, D. R., & Wang, P. (2008). Mental health in the context of health disparities. *American Journal of Psychiatry, 165*(9), 1102–1108.

Mold, J. W., Fryer, G. E., & Thomas, C. H. (2004). Who are the uninsured elderly in the United States? *Journal of the American Geriatrics Society, 52,* 601–606.

Moon, A., & Rhee, S. (2006). Immigrant and refugee elders. In B. Berkman & S. Dambruso (Eds.), *Handbook of social work in health and aging* (pp. 205–217). New York: Oxford University Press.

Moreno-John, G., Gachie, A., Fleming, C. M., Napoles-Springer, A., Mutran, E., Mason, S. M., et al. (2004). Ethnic minority older adults participating in clinical research: Developing trust. *Journal of Aging and Health, 16*(Suppl 5), 93S–123S.

Morgan, C., Mallett, R., Hutchinson, G., Bagalkote, H., Morgan, K., Fearon, P., et al. (2005). Pathways to care and ethnicity 2: Source of referral and help-seeking. *British Journal of Psychiatry, 186,* 290–296.

Mui, A. C. (2001). Stress, coping, and depression among elderly Korean immigrants. *Journal of Human Behavior in the Social Environment, 2*(3/4), 281–299.

Mui, A. C., Kang, S. K., & Domanski, M. D. (2007). English language proficiency and health-related quality of life among Chinese and Korean Immigrant Elders. *Health and Social Work, 32*(2), 119–127.

Murray, C. B. (2001). Culture as a determinant of mental health. In N. J. Smelser & P. B. Baltes (Eds.), *International encyclopedia of the social and behavioral sciences* (pp. 143–147). Amsterdam: Pergamon.

National Center for Cultural Competence. (2004). *Culture.* Washington, DC: Georgetown University, Center for Child and Human Development.

National Technical Assistance Center for State Mental Health Planning. (2004). *Final report. Cultural competency: Measurement as a strategy for moving knowledge into practice in state mental health systems.* Alexandria, VA: Author.

Neighbors, H. W., Woodward, A. T., Bullard, K. M., Ford, B. C., Taylor, R. J., & Jackson, J. S. (2008). Mental health service use among older African Americans: The national survey of American life. *American Journal of Geriatric Psychiatry, 16*(12), 948–956.

Newhill, C. E., & Harris, D. (2007). African American consumers' perception of racial disparities in mental health services. *Social Work Public Health, 23*(2-3), 107–124.

Nichter, M. (1981). Idioms of distress: Alternatives in the expression of psychosocial, distress. *Culture, Medicine and Psychiatry, 5,* 379–408.

Noh, S., Kaspar, V., & Wickrama, K. A. S. (2007). Overt and subtle racial discrimination and mental health: Preliminary findings for Korean immigrants. *American Journal of Public Health, 97*(7), 1269–1274.

Office of Minority Health and Health Disparities (2008). Mental health 101. *Office of Minority Health.* Washington, DC: U.S. Department of Health and Human Services.

Ojeda, V. D., & McGuire, T. G. (2006). Gender and racial/ethnic differences in use of outpatient mental health and substance use services by depressed elderly. *Psychiatric Quarterly, 77,* 211–222.

Omatade, A. O. (2003). SNMA's presidential initiative. Mental health and minority communities. *Journal of the American Medical Association, 95*(4), 296–297.

Ong, A. D., Fuller-Rowell, T., & Burrow, A. L. (2009). Racial discrimination and the stress process. *Journal of Personality and Social Psychology, 96*(6), 1259–1271.

Page, J., & Blau, J. (2006). Public mental health systems: Breaking the impasse in the treatment of oppressed groups. In J. Rosenberg & S. Rosenberg, *Community mental health: Challenges for the 21st century* (pp. 103–115). Portland, OR: C.R. Press.

Pang, E. C., Jordan-Marsh, M., Silverstein, M., & Cody, M. (2003). Health-seeking behaviors of Chinese Americans: Shifts in expectations. *The Gerontologist, 43,* 864–875.

Patcher, L. M. (1994). Culture and clinical care: Folk illnesses, beliefs and behaviors, and their implications for health care delivery. *Journal of the American Medical Association, 271*(9), 1096–1138.

Primm, A. (2006). Issues in the assessment and treatment of African American patients. In R. Lim (Ed.), *Clinical manual of cultural psychiatry* (pp. 35–68). Washington, DC: American Psychiatric Publishing.

Primm, A. B., Levy, R. A., Cohen, D., & Bondurant, A. (2009). *Improving outcomes for adult depression in ethnically and racially diverse populations.* Medscape CME/CE. Retrieved May 29, 2009, from http://cme.medscape.com/viewarticle/702891

Pushkar, K., & Marquis-Kerner, C. R. (2007). Minority group therapy and the advanced practice nurse. *Journal of Multicultural Nursing and Health Care, 13*(1), 37–42.

Rogler, L. H., & Cortez, D. E. (2008). Help-seeking pathways: A unifying concept. In J. E. Mezzich & G. Caracci (Eds.), *Cultural formulation: A reader for psychiatric diagnosis* (pp. 51–68). Lanham, MD: Rowman and Littlefield.

Rosenberg, J., & Rosenberg, S. (2006). *Community mental health: Challenges for the 21st century*. Portland, OR: C. R. Press.

Rudell, K., Bhui, K., & Priebe, S. (2008). Do alternative help-seeking strategies affect primary care service use? A survey of help-seeking for mental distress. *BMC Public Health, 8*, 207–217.

Ruiz, P. (2008). Taking issue: The persistence of disparities in mental health care. *Psychiatric Services, 59*(11), 1239.

Ruiz, P., & Primm, A. (Eds.). (2009). *Disparities in psychiatric care: Clinical and cross-cultural perspectives*. Philadelphia: Lippincott Williams & Wilkins.

Rust, G., Kondwani, K., Martinez, R., Dansie, R., Wong, W., Fry-Johnson, Y., et al. (2006). A crash-course in cultural competence. *Ethnicity and Disease, 16*(2, Suppl. 3), S3-29–S3-36.

Sadavoy, J., Meier, R., & Ong, A. Y. (2004). Barriers to access to mental health services for ethnic elders: The Toronto study. *Canadian Journal of Psychiatry, 49*, 192–199.

Saint Arnault, D., & Kim, O. (2008). Is there an Asian idiom of distress? Somatic symptoms in female Japanese and Korean students. *Archives of Psychiatric Nursing, 22*(1), 27–38.

Sambamoorthi, U., Olfson, M., Wei, W., & Crystal, S. (2006). Diabetes and depression care among Medicaid beneficiaries. *Journal of Health Care for the Poor and Underserved, 17*(1), 141–161.

Schnittker, J. (2003). Misgivings of medicine? African Americans' skepticism of psychiatric medication. *Journal of Health and Social Behavior, 44*, 506–524.

Schraufnagel, T. J., Wagner, A. W., Miranda, J., & Roy-Byrne, P. P. (2006). Treating minority patients with depression and anxiety: What does the evidence tell us? *General Hospital Psychiatry, 29*, 27–36.

Sellers, S. L., Jackson, J. S., & Hardison, C. B. (1998). Minority issues. In M. Henderson & V. B. Van Hasslet (Eds.), *Handbook of clinical geropsychology* (pp. 505–521). New York: Springer.

Sentell, T., Schumway, M., & Snowden, L. (2007). Access to mental health treatment by English language proficiency and race/ethnicity. *General Internal Medicine, 22*(Suppl. 2), 289–293.

Shi, L., & Singh, D. A. (2010). *Essentials of the U.S. health care system* (2nd ed.). Sudbury, MA: Jones and Bartlett.

Skarupuski, K. A., Mendes de Leon, C. F., Bienias, J. L., Barnes, L. L., Everson-Rose, S. A., Wilson, R. S., et al. (2005). Black–white differences in depressive symptoms among older adults over time. *The Journals of Gerontology Series B: Psychological Sciences and Social Sciences, 60*(3), P136–P142.

Smedley, B. D. (March/April, 2008). Moving beyond access: Achieving equity in state health care reform. *Health Affairs, 27*(2), 447–445.

Snowden, L. R. (2003). Bias in mental health assessment and intervention: Theory and evidence. *American Journal of Public Health, 93*(2), 239–243.

Snowden, L. R., & Yamada, A. M. (2005). Cultural differences in access to care. *Annual Review of Clinical Psychology, 1*, 143–166.

Sohn, L. (2004). The health and health status of older Korean Americans at the 100-year anniversary of Korean immigration. *Journal of Cross-Cultural Gerontology, 19*, 203–219.

Spencer, M. S., & Chen, J. (2004). The effect of discrimination on mental health service utilization among Chinese Americans. *American Journal of Public Health, 94*, 809–814.

Stockdale, S. E., Lagomasino, I. T., Siddique, J., McGuire, T., & Miranda, J. (2008). Racial and ethnic disparities in detection and treatment of depression and anxiety among psychiatric and primary health care visits, 1995-2005. *Medical Care, 46*, 668–677.

Stone, J. H. (2005). *Culture and disability: Providing culturally competent services*. Thousand Oaks, CA: Sage.

Strakowski. S. M., Keck, P. E., Arnold, L. M., Collins, J., Wilson, R. M., Fleck, D. E., et al. (2003). Ethnicity and diagnosis of inpatients with affective disorders. *Journal of Clinical Psychiatry, 64*(7), 747–754.

Sue, S., & Chu, J. Y. (2003). The mental health of minority groups: Challenges posed by the supplement to the Surgeon General's report on mental health. *Culture, Medicine and Psychiatry, 27*(4), 447–465.

Sue, D. W., & Sue, D. (2007). *Counseling the culturally diverse: Theory and practice* (5th ed.). Hoboken, NJ: Wiley.

Suite, D. H., La Bril, R., Primm, A., & Harrison-Ross, P. (2007). Beyond misdiagnosis: Misunderstanding and mistrust: Relevance of the historical perspective in the medical and mental health treatment of people of color. *Journal of the National Medical Association, 99*(8), 879–885.

Taxis, C. (2006). Attitudes, values, and questions of African Americans regarding participation in Hospice programs. *Journal of Hospice and Palliative Care, 8*(2), 77–85.

Thomas, P., Braken, P., & Yasmeen, S. (2007). Explanatory models for mental illness: Limitations and dangers in a global context. *Journal of Neurological Science, 176*, 176–181.

Thompson, M. L. (2006). Annotated primary documents: Excerpts for the 2nd U.S. Surgeon General's Report on Mental Health and Mental Illness. In *Mental illness.* Santa Barbara, CA: Greenwood Press.

Triandis, H. C. (1995). *Individualism and collectivism.* Bolder, CO: Westview Press.

Trierweiler, S., Muroff, J., Jackson, J. S., Neighbors, H. W., & Munday, C. (2005). Clinician race, situational variables, attributions, and diagnoses of mood versus schizophrenia disorders. *Cultural Diversity and Ethnic Minority Psychology, 11*(4), 351–364.

Tseng, W. S. (Ed.). (2001). *Handbook of cultural psychiatry.* San Diego, CA: Academic Press.

Tseng, W. S. (2006). From peculiar psychiatric disorders through culture-bound syndromes to culture-related specific syndromes. *Transcultural Psychiatry, 43*(4), 554–576.

Tseng, W. S., & Streltzer, J. (2004). Introduction: Culture and psychiatry. In W. S. Tseng & J. Streltzer (Eds.), *Cultural competence in clinical psychiatry* (pp. 1–20). Washington, DC: American Psychiatric Publishing.

Tyler, K. (2008). Ethnographic approaches to race, genetics and genealogy. *Sociology Compass, 2/6,* 1860–1877.

Uba, L. (2003). *Asian Americans: Personality, patterns, identity, and mental health.* New York: Guilford Press.

U.S. Bureau of the Census. (2006). Population age 65 and over and Hispanic origin in 2006 and projected 2050. *Population Estimates and Projections, 2006.* Washington, DC: U.S. Government Printing Office.

U.S. Department of Health and Human Services. (1999). *Mental health: A report of the Surgeon General.* Rockville, MD: U.S. Department of Health and Human Services, Substance Abuse and Mental Health Services Administration, Center for Mental Health Services, National Institutes of Health, National Institute of Mental Health.

U.S. Department of Health and Human Services. (2001). *Mental health: Culture, race, and ethnicity—A supplement to Mental health: A report of the Surgeon General.* Rockville, MD: U.S. Department of Health and Human Services, Substance Abuse and Mental Health Services Administration, Center for Mental Health Services, National Institutes of Health, National Institute of Mental Health.

Vedantam, S. (2005, June 26). Patients' diversity is often discounted: Alternatives to mainstream medical treatment call for recognizing ethnic, social differences. *The Washington Post,* A01.

Vega, W. A., Karno, M., Alegria, M., Alvidrez, J., Bernal, G., Escamilla, M., et al. (2007). Research issues for improving treatment of U.S. Hispanics with persistent mental disorders. *Psychiatric Services, 58,* 385–394.

Verkuyten, M. (2004). *The social psychology of ethnic identity.* London, England: Psychology Press.

Versola-Russo, J. M. (2006). Cultural and demographic factors of schizophrenia. *International Journal of Psychosocial Rehabilitation, 10*(2), 89–103.

Virnig, B., Huang, Z., Lurie, N., Musgrave. D., McBean, A. M., & Dowd, B. (2004). Does Medicare managed care provide equal treatment for mental illness across races? *Archives of General Psychiatry, 61*(2), 201–205.

Wang, P. C., Tong, H. Q., Liu, W., Long, S., Leung, L. Y. L., Yau, E., et al. (2006). Working with Chinese American families. In G. Yeo & D. Gallagher-Thompson (Eds.), *Ethnicity and the dementias* (2nd ed., pp. 173–188). New York: Routledge.

Washington, H. (2006). *Medical apartheid: The dark horse of medical experimentation on black Americans from colonial times to the present.* New York: Doubleday.

Weine, S., & Siddiqui, S. (2009). Family determinants of minority mental health and wellness. In S. Loue & M. Sajatovic (Eds.), *Determinants of minority mental illness and wellness* (pp. 221–255). New York: Springer.

Weisman, A., Rosales, G., Kymalainen, J., & Armesto, J. (2005). Ethnicity and family cohesion, religiosity and general emotional distress in patients with schizophrenia and their relatives. *Journal of Nervous and Mental Disease, 196*(6), 359–368.

Whaley, A. L. (2004). Ethnicity/race, paranoia, and hospitalization for mental health problems among men. *American Journal of Public Health, 94,* 78–81.

Wikipedia. (n.d.). *Ethnic groups in the United States.* Retrieved December 2008 from http://en.wikipedia.org/wiki/Ethnic_groups_in_the_United_States

Williams, D. R., Gonzales, H. M., Neighbors, H., Nesse, R., Abelson, J. M., Sweetman, J., et al. (2007). Prevalence and distribution of major depressive disorder in African Americans, Caribbean blacks, and non-Hispanic whites: Results from the National Survey of American Life. *Archives of General Psychiatry, 64,* 305–315.

Williams, D. R., Neighbors, J. S., & Jackson, J. S. (2003). Racial/ethnic discrimination and health: Findings from community studies. *American Journal of Public Health, 93*(2), 200–208.

Willging, C. E., Salvador, M., & Kano, M. (2006). Pragmatic help seeking: How sexual and gender minority groups access mental health care in a rural state. *Psychiatric Services, 57,* 871–874.

Wintrob, R. (2008, June 21). *Toward DSM-V: Outline for cultural formulation, cultural care formulation in psychiatry and medicine: Prospects and challenges.* Presentation at The Annual Meeting of the Society for the Study of Psychiatry and Culture, Promoting Interests in Cultural Aspects of Mental Health, San Francisco, CA.

Woodward, A. T., Taylor, R. J., Bullard, K. M., Neighbors, H. W., Chatters, L. M., & Jackson, J. S. (2008). Use of professional and informal support by African Americans and Caribbean blacks with mental disorders. *Psychiatric Services, 59,* 1292–1298.

Wynaden, D., Chapman, R., Orb, A., McGowan, S., Zeeman, Z., & Yeak, S. H. (2005). Factors that influence Asian communities' access to mental health care. *International Journal of Mental Health Nursing, 14,* 88–95.

Yamada, A. M., Barrio, C., Morrison, S. W., Sewell, D., & Este, D. V. (2006). Cross-ethnic evaluation of psychotic symptom content in hospitalized middle-aged and older adults. *General Hospital Psychiatry, 29*(2), 161–168.

Yamada, A. M., & Brekke, J. S. (2008). Addressing mental health disparities through clinical competence not just cultural competence: The need for assessment of socio-cultural issues in the delivery of evidence-based psychosocial rehabilitation services. *Clinical Psychology Review, 28,* 1386–1399.

Yang, L. H., & Kleinman, A. (2008). Face and the embodiment of stigma in China: The cases of schizophrenia and AIDS. *Social Science and Medicine, 67,* 398–486.

Yang, L. H., Phelan, J. C., & Link, B. J. (2008). Sigma and beliefs of efficacy toward traditional Chinese medicine and Western psychiatric treatment among Chinese-Americans. *Cultural Diversity and Ethnic Minority Psychology, 14*(1), 10–18.

Yeh, C. J., Arora, A. K., & Wu, K. A. (2006). A new theoretical model of collectivist coping. In T. P. Wong & L. C. J. Wong (Eds.), *Handbook of multicultural perspectives on stress and coping* (pp. 55–72). New York: Springer.

Yeh, C. J., Hunter, C. D., Mandan-Bahel, A., Chiang, L., & Arora, A. K. (2004). Indigenous and interdependent perspectives of healing: Implications for counseling and research. *Journal of Counseling and Development, 82,* 410–419.

Yeung, A. (2008). Ethical and cultural considerations in delivering psychiatric diagnosis: Reconciling the gap using MDD diagnosis delivery in less acculturated Chinese patients. *Transcultural Psychiatry, 45*(4), 531–552.

Yeung, A., & Kam, R. (2006). Recognizing and treating depression in Asian Americans. *Psychiatric Times, 23*(14), 50–58.

Yeung, S., Chang, D., Gresham, R. L., Nierenberg, A. A., & Fava, M. (2004). Illness beliefs of depressed Chinese Americans in primary care. *Journal of Nervous and Mental Disease, 192*(4), 324–327.

Zhan, L. (2003). Culture, health, and health practices. In L. Zhan (Ed.), *Asian Americans: Vulnerable populations, model interventions, and clarifying agendas* (pp. 3–18). Sudbury, MA: Jones and Bartlett.

5

Mental Health Promotion

Charles Blair

The number and proportion of the population age 65 years and older will grow rapidly after 2010 (U.S. Department of Health and Human Services [DHHS], 2000). As the nation ages, the growing mental health needs of older adults must be addressed. Mental health is a state of successful performance of mental functioning, resulting in productive activities, fulfilling relationships with other people, and the ability to cope with and adjust to the recurrent stresses of everyday living in an acceptable way. It is a state of balance that individuals establish within themselves and between themselves and their social and physical environments. Mental health is indispensable to personal well-being, family and interpersonal relationships, and one's contributions to community and society (DHHS).

To gain a deeper understanding of the meaning of mental health for older adults, Hedelin (2001) interviewed 16 women between the ages of 71 and 92. Participants in this study indicated that mental health is the experience of confirmation, trust, and confidence in the future, and a zest for life, development, and involvement in one's relationship to oneself and others.

Mental wellness is the capacity to perform well in any endeavor, to love and have friends, and to enjoy life with relative freedom from internal stress without causing stress to others. Promoting mental health is both any action to enhance the mental well-being of individuals, families, organizations, and communities, and a set of principles that recognize the mental health impact of how services, in the widest sense, are planned, designed, delivered, and evaluated. Mental health promotion works at three levels: (1) strengthening individuals or increasing emotional resilience through interventions designed to promote self-esteem, life skills, and coping skills (e.g., communicating, negotiating, and relationship skills); (2) strengthening communities by promoting social inclusion and participation, improving neighborhood environments, developing health and social services that support mental health, workplace health, community safety, and self-help networks; and (3) reducing structural barriers to mental health through initiatives to reduce discrimination and inequalities, and to promote access to education, meaningful employment, housing, services, and support for those who are vulnerable.

At each level, mental health promotion is relevant to the whole population, individuals at risk, vulnerable groups, and people with mental health problems. At each level, interventions may focus on strengthening factors known to protect mental health (e.g., social support, physical health) or to reduce factors known to increase risk (e.g., racial discrimination and loneliness). Mental health promotion has a role in preventing certain mental health problems in older adults, notably depression, anxiety, and substance abuse. Also, mental health promotion may foster recovery from mental illness and improve the quality of life of older adults with mental health problems (Hogstel, 1995).

STRESSORS IMPACTING MENTAL HEALTH

Older adults' lives are not free of stress. Stressors are events that either have a direct effect on the body or an indirect effect through various mediators. The individual's reaction to stressors is an attempt at adaptation, and if the stressors are not extreme or chronic, the attempt is usually successful. In that sense, stress reactions are good, in that they are a part of the homeostatic mechanism of the body to transient disruptions of equilibrium. If, however, the stressor becomes chronic, the individual's ability to successfully adapt is often compromised with resulting undesirable consequences, such as mental ill health. Stressors that may challenge the lives of older adults include physical health problems, financial issues, difficulty accessing social services, transportation barriers, isolation, and finding affordable long-term care services.

However, it makes little sense to speak of, or to consider, older adults as a homogeneous group. Cook and Kramek (1986) suggested that older adults could be viewed as two distinct groups: those who are both financially poor and subject to chronic illness, and those who are both physically and financially well off. Moreover, issues of gender, race, and ethnicity create further distinctions. Ruiz (1995) noted, for example, that old men and old women are treated differently in the United States, as are older adults of various races and ethnic backgrounds. What is of interest here is that each of these variables may be considered a stressor, and to some degree may affect

the mental health of older adults. From a mental health perspective, becoming aware of the basis of these stressors may be the first step toward mental health promotion and illness prevention.

Gender

Longevity and living arrangements have a significant impact on all older adults' quality of life and mental health, but more so on older women's. Because many more women than men survive into old age, the role of gender deserves special consideration in any discussion of mental health promotion in older adults. Women who reach age 65 can expect to live nearly 20 more years, whereas men at age 65 can expect only about 15 years (Moody, 2002). The typical fate is for men to die early and for women to survive with chronic disease. Because women tend to marry men who are older than they are, women are more likely to be widowed and live alone in old age than men. Because the family caregiving role of women often has the consequence of removing them from the paid labor force, they accumulate lower pension benefits than men. Retirement income for older women is on average only about 55% of what it is for older men, and nearly three out of four older Americans who fall below the poverty line are women (Moody).

Divorce is also becoming an increasingly prevalent influence on older women's living arrangements (Moody, 2002). Divorced women usually experience a sudden reduction in their financial circumstances and they, unlike men, are less likely to remarry. For older women, socioeconomic stressors, patterns of inequality involving social class, race, ethnicity, and gender reinforce one another. If women earn less than men, and if minority group members are subject to prejudice over their lifetime, it is not surprising that an older, divorced, or widowed woman, who is from a lower socioeconomic class and a member of a minority racial or ethnic group, would experience problems in the area of health status, income, and housing that could negatively affect her mental health.

Race and Ethnicity

The poor socioeconomic position of many individuals in minority ethnic populations in the United States is a major cause of poor mental health and highlights the need for policies and programs to reduce inequalities in mental health services between the majority and minority populations (Chow, Jaffee, & Snowden, 2003). In studies conducted in South London, based on contact with psychiatric services over a 10-year period, Boydell et al. (2001) and Sharpley, Hutchinson, Murray, and McKenzie (2001) found that the incidence of schizophrenia in nonwhite minority groups increased significantly as the proportion of such minorities in the local population fell. The authors concluded that the increase may have been caused by reduced protection against stress and life events because of isolation and fewer social networks. They suggested that people from minority racial and ethnic groups may be more likely to be singled out or to be more vulnerable when they are few in number or dispersed. These findings point to the importance of social factors as an explanation for the increased rate of schizophrenia among British-born minority racial and ethnic individuals.

Psychosocial factors may have particular significance for minority racial and ethnic populations because of the impact of racism and discrimination on individual and collective self-esteem. Racism affects mental well-being in two main ways. First, it contributes to mental distress and can lead to feelings of isolation, fear, intimidation, low self-esteem, and anger. Depression may be caused by feelings of rejection, loss, helplessness, hopelessness, and an inability to have control over external forces (Bhugra & Bahl, 1999). Second, it can act as a barrier to the access and provision of appropriate services. Minority racial and ethnic individuals may feel excluded from services because of direct discrimination by staff or through indirect discrimination, such as being unable to access services because of language barriers.

Challenges of Late Life

During their later years, adults are confronted with what are possibly the greatest number of challenges in their lives, often with their lowest level of emotional resources and financial means because of fixed and limited incomes. It is a time when they may feel psychologically and physically fragile, in the midst of what constitutes for many individuals a very difficult period: aging and impending mortality. Issues of loss, disability, and identity are just a few of the many biopsychosocial concerns that older adults need to address for a continued sense of well-being. In facing these issues, older adults often find their biological and social families fractured or missing because of death, illness, or relocation.

Changes or loss in health, family, society, and finances can foster psychological disequilibrium and promote stress in older adults. According to Neugarten and Datan (1975), the stressful impact of an event is less intense when change is expected as opposed to when it is not expected. For example, the sudden onset of illness can be traumatic and can result in older adults feeling that their health is out of their control, creating a very stressful experience. Seligman (1992) pointed out that generally, adults with limited emotional and financial resources who perceive their lives as having progressive and unexpected problems often experience their situation as unstable and unpredictable and are more inclined to become depressed.

Successful aging implies that individuals are satisfied or content with their lives; that is, they have found ways of maximizing the positives in their lives while minimizing the impact of inevitable age-related losses. Maintaining connections with others is an important aspect of adult life. Mitchell (1990) found that older adults often affirm themselves through interrelationships. Maintaining such connections can become increasingly difficult during older adulthood as significant others die or are relocated. Physical deficits that occur with aging may also limit access to others. Visual impairment may limit older adults' ability to travel independently outside their immediate surroundings, thereby reducing their ability to drive or use public transportation and thus reducing their opportunity to leave their homes.

Chronic Illness

Chronic illness, physical decline, and functional disability exert enormous strain on the mental health of older adults. Also, depressive symptoms are associated with many drugs used to manage chronic illness (Lueckenotte, 2000). Some chronic conditions, such as cataracts and hearing impairment, can be limiting but not life threatening. Other conditions, such as hypertension and heart disease, can lead to fatal disorders. Alzheimer's disease is probably one of the leading causes of disability and death afflicting people over age 65. Arthritis is the most familiar and the most prevalent chronic disease of later life, and it is the most important cause of physical disability in the United States (Moody, 2002). The joint and bone degeneration that occurs as a result of arthritis and osteoporosis is a major problem for many sufferers, causing a loss of strength, weakened bones that are more likely to break, and reduced ability to perform independent activities of daily living (ADLs), a major source of self-esteem for older adults (Blair, 1999). Parkinson's disease, characterized by a loss of control over body movements, affects mainly older people. Dementia is quite prevalent, and depression is common among people with Parkinson's disease. Cancer is overwhelmingly a disease of old age, and depressive symptoms occur as a side effect of the medications used to control the disease. Cardiovascular disease, which includes stroke and heart disease (Moody), is one of the leading causes of death among people over age 65. A stroke may cause immediate death or permanent disability including language or speech disturbance. For the disabled, the loss of quality of life can lead to frustration, anger, and depression. Alzheimer's disease involves progressive loss of the ability to think and remember. In its early stage, the symptoms of Alzheimer's disease may be

severe enough to interfere with usual ADLs, work, or social relationships, the consequence of which may be emotional distress and depression.

Financial Problems

Morgan and Kunkel (2001) noted that there have been striking improvements in the economic well-being of the average older American in the past three decades. However, many still remain near or below the poverty level. Being African American, Hispanic, or a female living alone is related to serious economic disadvantage. The rate of poverty for older African Americans and Hispanic Americans is about three times that of European Americans. Women of all racial and ethnic backgrounds have poverty rates almost twice the rate of their male counterparts. This difference in economic well-being is reflected in differences in psychological well-being, with those who are economically distressed showing greater signs of depression (Morgan & Kunkel).

Admission to Nursing Home

Despite a decline in health and functional ability, older adults prefer to remain and receive care in their own homes (Moody, 2002). Because of the high cost of healthcare services, however, many older adults are forced to depend on federally funded services purchased through the Medicare and Medicaid financing programs. For many, nursing home placement is seen as a negative experience and viewed as institutionalization. Reliance on Medicare and Medicaid for payment of nursing home services is also stressful for some older adults.

There is an increased and immediate sense of loss for older adults on admission to nursing homes. Relocation to such an institution can be fraught with emotional and psychological turmoil. As a result, depression is widespread among residents (Lueckenotte, 2000). Often this is caused by fear of losing one's identity, friends, possessions, lifestyle, history, and personal space. Allen (2003) noted that because residents live in an institutional setting, personal losses are inevitable. For many residents, the loss of control over their daily lives and the lack of decision-making opportunities constitute stressful living conditions. As far back as 1988, Phan and Reifler reported a high percentage of decreased interest, decreased energy, difficulty concentrating, feelings of helplessness and hopelessness, and psychomotor retardation in nursing home residents. Moody (2002) suggested that depression in nursing home residents may be a reaction to the fact that it is impossible for them to "start over" at this later stage of life.

COMPREHENSIVE MENTAL HEALTH ASSESSMENT IN CLINICAL PRACTICE

Nursing assessment calls for information about the nature and scale of clients' problems. The method in which assessment information is collected often depends on the problem involved. Because of the need to understand the "whole person," mental health nurses are required to assess all aspects of the person: biophysical, psychosocial, and spiritual. In this sense, mental health assessments may be formal or informal, but should always be rigorous and comprehensive (Campbell, 1995; Ritter & Watkins, 1997). Comprehensive assessment of older adults should identify not just weaknesses and problems, but also strengths and potentials. Comprehensive assessment of capabilities and incapacities, and social functioning and support systems, establishes a rational basis for the development of treatment plans tailored to the client's physical, psychological, and social needs. Accordingly, the essential components of comprehensive assessment should comprise physical functioning, mental and emotional functioning, family and social support, and living environmental characteristics.

Physical Functioning

A health history and assessment are essential to the psychiatric nursing assessment. Some physical problems can present with psychiatric complications. Similarly, some psychiatric disorders can present with physical problems. Loss of physical health has direct effects on the quality of life of older people. Bodily systems featured in the physical assessment include the cardiovascular, respiratory, endocrine, genitourinary, gastrointestinal, and musculoskeletal systems. Functional status is considered an important and significant component of an older adult's quality of life. Functional assessment determines the older person's capabilities in performing basic ADLs and the more complex instrumental ADLs (IADLs). Functional assessment also determines the person's nutritional status, ability to mobilize, sleep patterns, hearing and vision, and medication behavior. A widely used instrument for assessing ADLs is the Barthel Index (Mahoney & Barthel, 1965). A widely used instrument for assessing IADLs is the Instrumental Activities of Daily Living Scale (Lawton & Brody, 1969).

Pain history and assessment should be included in the assessment of physical functioning. Pain interferes with the proper physical functioning of older adults, especially their ability to mobilize, and this has a profound effect on perception of well-being. Pain correlates with less socialization with colleagues (Ritter & Watkins, 1997). The daily pain diary (McCaffery & Pasero, 1999) and the Self-Care Pain Management log (Ferrell & Ferrell, 1995) are useful tools for measuring pain in older adults.

Mental and Emotional Functioning

The mental status examination, one of the most important diagnostic screening measures available to nurses, is designed to assess the client's mental functioning level and estimate the effectiveness of the clients' mental capacity. The purpose of the mental status assessment in the older adult is to determine the client's level of cognitive functioning, the degree of cognitive impairment, and the effect of that impairment on functional ability. Cognitive functioning is the aspect of mental functioning most affected by aging (Moody, 2002).

"Cognition" refers to the mental organization or reorganization of information. Assessment of cognitive functioning is concerned with evaluating the older person's conscious processes: thoughts, memory, judgment, comprehension, reasoning, and problem-solving strategies used in daily living. Responses to cognitive demands may be tested in several ways. Abstract thinking, decision making, problem solving, and reasoning ability may be observed through such activities as budgeting, shopping, and other IADLs. Abstract reasoning involves the ability to think beyond a concrete way. Abstract reasoning may be tested by the interpretation of proverbs or the identification of similarities between items. Level of comprehension may be determined by the client's engagement and attentiveness to the interview and by the relevance and accuracy of the client's responses to questions and tasks. Memory may be tested in a simplistic way by asking the client to memorize and retrieve from memory a piece of information, such as a name or an address. Judgment is the end result of the client's ability to assess a situation, analyze it, come to an appropriate conclusion, and make sound decisions. Judgment can be assessed by listening as the client relates actual life events that required gathering and interpreting data, formulating a decision, and carrying out a plan. Judgment can be assessed by asking the client to make a decision about a hypothetical problem. Assessment of judgment also relies on observation and reports of informants who know the client well.

Older adults' cognitive functioning may be diminished by anxiety and worry, which may negatively influence recall and concentration (Morgan & Kunkel, 2001). Because of stereotypes of cognitive decline with aging that are held by society and the older adults themselves, mood and self-esteem of older adults are important factors to consider when measuring cognitive functioning. Ritter and Watkins (1997) noted that older clients tend to judge their memory as defective despite objective reports to the contrary. Consequently, self-report may not be a reliable way of estimating change in the cognitive functioning of older

adults. Also, because diminished cognitive function in older adults is associated with lower educational achievement and lower socioeconomic status (Luis, Loewenstein, Acevedo, Barker, & Duara, 2003), any assessment of an elderly person's cognitive ability should include independent information about family patterns and about the person's educational achievement, so that individual measures are interpreted within their true social context.

Although the mental status examination done by the nurse may provide good subjective evidence of the client's mental functioning, it provides only a baseline that identifies the need for the administration of one of the standardized mental status tests. The tests that nurses can use clinically include the Mini-Mental State Examination (Folstein, Folstein, & McHugh, 1975) and the Short Portable Mental Status Questionnaire (Pfeiffer, 1975).

Emotional Functioning

The feeling element is perhaps the most commonly recognized aspect of the emotional dimension. Emotion refers to affective states and feelings. Each individual has the capacity to experience the entire realm of feelings, which is meant to be experienced, not ignored. Feelings, such as joy, anger, sadness, and fear, occur most naturally in young children who are not yet restricted, through social learning, in expressing their feelings. Adults, however, often attach judgments to their feelings and consequently ignore uncomfortable ones.

As with the young, older adults are not passive receptacles of emotional experiences. A related social event can elicit and define the nature of a particular emotional experience, such as fear in response to a loss of power. The emotional status of the client is assessed in terms of affect, appropriateness of the affect to the situation, quality and stability of the mood, physical signs of emotion, and emotional response patterns. The appropriateness of affect to the situation is based on the congruency between the affect the client is displaying and the client's culturally expected affective response in a particular situation. Both affect and appropriateness of affect are in part culturally determined; also, emotional status is commonly altered in acute and chronic illness. Consequently, these circumstances must be considered in any interpretation by the nurse. Tools that may be used by nurses to measure affect include the Beck Depression Inventory, Short Form (Beck & Beck, 1972) and the Geriatric Depression Scale (Yesavage & Brink, 1983).

Family and Social Support

According to Morgan and Kunkel (2001), family members in all generations are involved in giving and receiving various types of assistance, including assistance during illness, child care, financial support, emotional support, and household management. Older adults who lack supportive ties on whom they can rely for assistance are at greatest risk for institutionalization when they can no longer care for themselves. Dwyer (1995) estimated that 80% of informal care to frail and disabled elders is provided by family caregivers. However, there are differences in the quality and quantity of support given to older adults by family members from different race, class, and ethnic groups.

The quality of life an older person experiences is closely linked to social functioning. Social support needs of older adults tend to increase with advancing years and functional limitations as a result of declining health. Although most older adults are assisted by family, many depend on friends and nonfamily social networks to maintain their independence and decrease loneliness and social isolation. Because many elderly individuals confront most of life's difficulties by seeking out information, advice, and support from trusted others, the contributions of this social support can positively influence their performance of everyday functional activities. Social interactions may also have negative consequences for the older adult. Interactions that are unwanted or unpleasant may be detrimental to social relationships.

Because social factors can be so influential in the mental health status of older adults, it is important that nurses take an adequate social history. The nurse must be careful to consider both familial and nonfamilial sources of social support when assessing older adults' social systems. Neff (1996) suggested nurses assess the client's living environment characteristics to determine how it is perceived by the client, and whether it is conducive to maximum functional abilities. The client's financial resources should also be assessed for change in income and ability to meet needs for food, clothing, shelter, recreational activities, or trips. The client's daily, weekly, and regular contacts should be noted. The client's verbalized insights into needs for services are also important. Client and family integration into the community should also be noted. Methods of transportation and the way the client spends a typical day should be assessed. Screening tools that nurses can use to assess clients' family and social support include the Family APGAR (Smilkstein, Ashworth, & Montano, 1982) and the OARS Social Resource Scale (Duke University Center for the Study of Aging and Human Development, 1988).

ASSERTIVENESS AND PROBLEM-SOLVING SKILLS TRAINING AS PART OF SOCIAL SKILLS TRAINING

Assertiveness is the ability to express one's needs and desires directly to the appropriate person in an appropriate manner. It involves standing up for personal rights and expressing thoughts, feelings, and beliefs, and making requests in direct, honest, and appropriate ways that respect the rights of others. It involves assuming responsibility for one's self and one's emotions and not projecting these onto others. In older adults, lowered interpersonal assertiveness has been found to be correlated with depression (Donohue, Acierno, Hersen, & Van Hasselt, 1995).

Because older adults with little or no effective interpersonal behaviors may be at risk of becoming depressed, it is incumbent on the nurse to help them gain the skills or make a referral for skills training to develop effective interpersonal behaviors and increased interpersonal assertiveness. Skills training may be provided by clinicians including nurses, psychologists, and social workers who have been trained in behavioral principles and procedures. Skills training may involve anything from teaching clients how to shake hands to practicing conversational skills. Evidence of effective interpersonal functioning includes being goal-directed, showing signs of perception and integration of social signals, self-presentation, ability to take the role of others, use of appropriate social behavior, and ability to provide feedback to others.

Teaching older adults to behave in a highly assertive yet appropriate manner through social skills training may reduce their chances of developing depression. Specific techniques of assertiveness training include repeated modeling of appropriate skills, role playing, high levels of descriptive verbal reinforcement, and in vivo rehearsal-based homework assignments that require that the individual rehearse assertiveness in assigned real-life situations, rather than in his or her imagination. The outcome of assertiveness training may be an increase in the perceived, if not the actual, level of control in interpersonal relationships.

LATE LIFE CHALLENGES THAT CAN CONTRIBUTE TO MENTAL HEALTH PROBLEMS

Caregiving Role and Stressors

Increasingly, older adults are taking on informal caregiving roles for individuals who become dependent or need assistance because of physical or mental effects of chronic illness. One notable chronic illness is that caused by HIV infection. Research conducted in the past decade suggests that of the many adults living with HIV infection, half depend on older relatives for financial, physical, medical, or emotional support (Allers, 1990; Ory & Zablotsky, 1989). An estimated 50,000 to 100,000 adult Americans with AIDS receive help from older caregivers. In addition, there is a growing population of orphans whose caregiving parents have died, who are cared for by grandparents

through standby adoption or guardianship (Goodkin et al., 2003). About 80% of the youths who are orphaned by HIV infection are people of color, and most older caregivers are members of minority ethnic groups. An estimated 70% of these caregivers are women, with 35% older than 65 years. As informal caregivers, older minority women face the multiple disadvantages of racial or ethnic inequities, compromised health status, poverty, aging, and sexism (Goodkin et al.). Despite the obvious benefits to care recipients, and regardless of their race, the stress experienced by most elderly caregivers often decreases their physical and psychological health (Given, Kozachik, Collins, DeVoss, & Given, 2001).

Dysphoria

Dysphoria is a disorder of affect characterized by distress and depression. Generally, the individual is in this state for understandable reasons. In older adults, the reasons may include the many losses and subsequent changes with which they are struggling to cope. The loss of physical health and independence, employment and income, family and friends, or house and comfortable environment are difficult to accept, especially if they all occur within a relatively short period. These losses may overwhelm some older adults, causing them to worry and preventing them from feeling in control of their lives. This type of disorder usually calls for major psychosocial intervention (Sadock & Sadock, 2000).

Loneliness and Isolation

Loneliness is a strong indicator that an individual is feeling isolated from others. A number of conditions support the notion that loneliness is more widespread among older adults. Social isolation and loneliness negatively affect older adults' physical and psychological well-being. Behaviors and symptoms associated with loneliness are similar to those of mild depressive mood and include isolation, constipation, weight loss, insomnia, fatigue, and loss of appetite (Allen, 2003).

Death of family and friends, retirement, relocation, and other life changes can reduce opportunities for social contacts and place older adults at risk for social isolation. Physical limitations, such as sensory deficits that limit communication or mobility, may prevent the visiting of friends and family. In studying the impact of loneliness on older adults, Pinquart and Sorensen (2001) noted that the old–old and oldest–old tend to experience the highest levels of loneliness because of physical and sensory decrements and loss of their spouse and friends; and older women, because of their higher risk of widowhood, tend to experience more loneliness than older men. Opportunities for social interaction also decrease with widowhood.

Lack of a social network may lead to nursing home admission. Pinquart and Sorensen (2001) found that older adults in nursing homes are lonelier than those in community dwellings. Allen (2003) noted that loneliness has a profound effect on the mental health of nursing home residents.

Role Loss, Change, and Coping

The mental, emotional, and physical health of people of all ages is related to their ability to cope with and adapt to the changes in their lives. Most changes in early life are often voluntary and involve assumption of greater responsibility. For the older adult the opposite is true (Bunten, 2001). Change in this group often represents a loss, and some interpret it as a role loss. Such losses as leaving a valued position in the workforce, losing parental authority as children leave home, losing physical ability because of chronic illness, and experiencing bereavement with the death of family and friends can create problems for those who are unable successfully to grieve their losses and establish new resources of morale and satisfaction (Moody, 2002).

Burden of Illness and Disability

Compared with the general population, older people on average have twice as many days in which activities are restricted because of chronic conditions, such as arthritis and heart conditions. Living with a chronic illness affects a person's lifestyle and interactions with others. Many chronically ill older adults become homebound, and this decreases contact with the community and leads to social isolation. As with other age groups, older adults with chronic illnesses typically have repeated hospitalization to treat exacerbations of their illnesses. Inability to control an illness or disability produces feelings of powerlessness, especially when there is realization of a loss of function and the loss of one's former self. Feelings of powerlessness can lead to a loss of hope and depression.

Common Maturational and Situational Crises of Older Adults

A crisis is an internal imbalance that results from a perceived threat to one's well-being. Crises are usually precipitated by situations of loss, transition, or change. When such situations arise, a series of behaviors are activated that lead either to mastery of the situation or to crisis. Blazer (1990) noted that some degree of cognitive and physical loss is expected as one matures into old age. These losses may provoke anxiety and depression in older adults whose coping resources are taxed beyond their customary capacity. As one slips into old age, occasional forgetfulness, especially of the recent past, and an increase in the time needed for processing information may occur. Likewise, older adults may take longer to respond to questions and requests, and to process multiple stimuli. Decrease in physical strength and changes in physical appearance, such as graying of the hair, wrinkled skin, and sagging bodies, may be difficult for some older adults to accept. Hearing difficulty is both the most common and the most disabling sensory problem of aging: a decrease in both pitch discrimination and hearing acuity may occur. Decreased visual acuity, accommodation, and adaptation to darkness, and increased sensitivity to glare are likely to occur. Presbyopia is one of the most common visual problems; however, age-related macular degeneration, cataracts, and glaucoma are more serious. Decline in cognitive and physical ability may lead to other problems, such as lessened ability to perform ADLs and IADL tasks independently, including driving and shopping, and may increase the chance of social isolation.

A situational crisis may be thought of as a sudden unexpected threat to or loss of basic resources or life goals. In the older adult, these crises may be more common than the maturational ones. Much of the depression and anxiety in older adults is caused by situational factors in the environment, such as the deaths of family and friends, loss of or relocation from home, and loss or decline in economic stability. Such losses as the death of a spouse, or a divorce, are commonly accompanied by a transition to being single. Loss of a job or retirement may mean the loss of not only financial resources, but also companionship and a major source of pride and self-esteem.

THERAPEUTIC INTERVENTIONS TO ADDRESS MENTAL HEALTH PROMOTION AND WELLNESS

Counseling and Support

Counseling is the act of providing advice and guidance to clients. The task of counseling is to give the client an opportunity to explore, discover, and clarify ways of living more resourcefully and toward greater well-being. Minardi and Hays (2003a) noted that an important aspect of counseling is the formation of a unique therapeutic relationship with the client in which an agreement is made as to the type of psychological work that will take place. Counseling involves using skills, such as active and attentive listening, paraphrasing, questioning, and responding in such a way as to demonstrate to the client that the counselor is genuine, empathetic, and trying to understand the client's concerns, while not supporting unhealthy behaviors the client may exhibit. Because counseling is not therapy (Minardi & Hays), and does not require specialized training, geriatric nurses are amply qualified to use counseling skills within their work settings to assist older adults in the

process of reminiscence, and to deal with their numerous losses. Through counseling, older adults can be helped to face the reality of the losses, deal with the effects, break down barriers to readjusting to those losses, and make healthy choices in selecting replacements or substitutes for them.

Crisis Intervention

Crisis intervention is an active entering into the life situation of the client who is experiencing the crisis, to decrease the impact of the crisis event, and to assist the individual to mobilize his or her resources and regain equilibrium (Jacobs, 1989). Although related to it, crisis intervention is not psychotherapy. It is the provision of short-term help by crisis workers, including nurses. The goal of crisis intervention is to resolve the most pressing problems within the shortest possible time through focused, directed intervention aimed at helping the older adult develop new adaptive coping methods. No attempt is made at in-depth analysis.

Older adults in crisis situations need to be provided immediate attention by therapists. Nothing will raise these clients' hope more than an immediate offer of help. An essential characteristic of a crisis is the highly motivated nature of clients. No one has to persuade them to accept help. Often, they plead for it and uncritically accept it when it is offered. Such trust among older adults allows maximum caregiver–client interaction.

The purpose of crisis intervention is to restore in the person the level of functioning that existed before the current crisis. Burgess (1998) suggests five therapeutic goals. (1) The first deals with safety and security. If there is danger of suicide, the family or significant others need to be informed and urged to exercise vigilance. In situations where the chance of self-harm is significant, the patient should be referred for emergency admission into the nearest hospital with an inpatient psychiatric service. Victims of crises often experience such intense turmoil that they fear they are going insane. (2) For this reason, the second goal is to allow victims the opportunity to ventilate and to have their reactions validated. (3) A third goal is to assist the individual to examine the circumstances related to the crisis and help him or her to prepare for dealing with similar situations in the future. Individuals should be encouraged to talk or write about the crisis experience and to identify a person to whom he or she could turn in the event of impending disaster. (4) A fourth goal is to practice role-playing responses to a variety of calamitous scenarios. This is considered a practical way to plan for future events. (5) The fifth goal is to provide educational opportunities for the individual through writing and reading assignments, self-assessment exercises, crisis intervention and supportive counseling, and peer support groups.

Pharmacological Therapies

Pharmacotherapy is the use of substances to alleviate symptoms, maintain improvements, and prevent relapse in psychiatric clients. Psychotropic agents can be used to control violence and dangerous or destructive behavior, improve the client's subjective feelings, shorten inpatient treatment time, and hasten the recovery of some clients. Because many nursing home residents have diagnosed psychiatric problems, psychotropic medications are more likely to be prescribed for this group of older adults. Psychotropic agents used with the older adult population include neuroleptics or major tranquilizers, antidepressants, and sedative–hypnotics.

Appropriate indications for neuroleptic prescriptions include treatment of psychoses, such as schizophrenia, paranoia, major depression, mania, and psychotic symptoms, such as hallucinations and delusions, which may occur in other conditions. Because of the potentially severe side effects of these medications, they should be prescribed only where a clear need exists.

Antidepressants are used to treat depressive symptoms in clients. Three major groups of these medications are used: (1) tricyclic antidepressants, (2) selective serotonin reuptake inhibitors, and (3) monoamine oxidase inhibitors. The choice

of antidepressant is dependent on its side-effect profile. Those with minimum potential for orthostatic hypotension, sedation, and anticholinergic effects are preferred. Antidepressants may be prescribed for dysthymia in older adults. For those with minor depression, it is suggested that antidepressants be given only when there is evidence of severe impairment as demonstrated by clients' need to make significantly increased effort to accomplish near-normal functioning in social, occupational, or other important areas of life.

Sedatives or antianxiety medications are used primarily to reduce anxiety in older adults. The major group of antianxiety agents is the benzodiazepines, which are also used to treat acute alcohol withdrawal and impending delirium tremens. Some benzodiazepines are used primarily to induce sleep and not to treat anxiety. Because of accumulation of their active metabolites, older adults may be more sensitive to toxic effects of these medications, and they are generally prescribed the lowest possible dosages and for time-limited periods. Selective serotonin reuptake inhibitors may also be used in the treatment of anxiety in older adults.

Individual, Group, and Family-Focused Interventions and Treatment Modalities

Nurses are well placed to use psychosocial interventions therapeutically with older adults in institutional and community settings to promote mental health and wellness. Many psychosocial interventions (the psychotherapeutic interventions) are designed to help clients alter dysfunctional relationship patterns and to develop more effective problem-solving skills. Development of insight or awareness of factors that motivate feelings, thoughts, and behavior is generally seen as a necessary precondition for change. Because older adults' capacity for insight may vary, some psychosocial interventions may serve to stimulate change without the active participation of clients in the process. Minardi and Hays (2003a, 2003b) point to several individual and group psychosocially based therapies available for use with older adults. These include psychotherapy; psychodynamic therapy; cognitive–behavioral therapy; reminiscence therapy; validation therapy; and the activity-based therapies of music, art, dance, drama, and exercise. Some of these psychosocial interventions are clearly within the nurse's role, whereas psychotherapies require advanced training to conduct. Minardi and Hays noted that, in using these interventions, nurses must establish a therapeutic relationship with older clients so that the clients feel psychologically safe enough to participate freely. An important aspect of using these therapies is the need for nurses to recognize the relationship boundaries between themselves, the clients, and the clients' significant others as they move in and out of the different interventions.

Psychotherapy, psychodynamic therapy, and cognitive–behavioral therapy may be provided in either group or individual formats. The facilitators are trained therapists and the sessions are structured with precise start and end times. However, the principles on which these therapies are based can be accommodated easily by nurses, because they already possess some of the necessary skills and knowledge.

The activity-based therapies, such as music, art, dance, and exercise therapies, may be delivered formally or informally, as when they are incorporated into interventions to promote relaxation or increase self-esteem and a sense of achievement. These therapies may be used in individual or group formats. When used formally, it may be necessary to leave interpretations of client's behaviors to qualified therapists, who are more competent to examine and interpret issues in depth.

Reminiscence therapy may be used by nurses to assist older adults to reexamine the life they have lived. It may be useful in helping clients to remember their accomplishments, their failures, and their contribution to society. It may be an important process for boosting the client's self-esteem. Validation therapy is used with demented older adults to relieve the client's distress and restore self-worth (Feil, 1992, 1999). Validation is a communication process. When using this therapy, the nurse focuses on the client's verbal and nonverbal communication and, rather than making interpretations based on the factual information presented in that communication, the nurse attempts to interpret only the emotions expressed in the communication. If the client's communication on a particular topic is repetitious, the nurse explores the client's feelings about the topic by prompting and shaping the client's communication on the topic. Minardi and Hays (2003b) noted that by not allowing factual errors to interrupt meaningful dialogue, nurses may use validation therapy to help demented older adults review their past and express feelings that may have been buried for a long time.

Complementary and Alternative Therapies

Older adults are taking herbal and other types of dietary supplements in record numbers (National Council for Reliable Healthy Information Newsletter, 2000). Although traditional therapies are the backbone of mental health care, botanical and nonbotanical complementary and alternative therapies, along with nontraditional psychosocial therapies, provide a break from the more regimented programs. These therapies encourage many of the same goals as traditional therapies and are thought to provide sensory and mental stimulation along with therapeutic benefits. According to McCabe (2002), an estimated one in three adults in the United States, including older adults, use botanical and nonbotanical complementary and alternative therapies to help promote mental well-being.

Botanical and Nonbotanical Therapies

Botanical agents include St. John's wort, a common weed that grows in the United States, which is frequently used for the treatment of depression. Despite its questionable efficacy, many take it on a regular basis. Ginkgo biloba comes from the leaves of a decorative tree. It is indicated for memory problems, and for this reason its common psychiatric use is with demented clients. Kava, a psychoactive derivative of the pepper plant, is used most often to treat anxiety and on some occasions insomnia. Ginseng has no focused use, but rather is indicated broadly for improved quality of life and generalized well-being. Valerian, grown abundantly in most parts of the world, may be used as a sedative and hypnotic (Hodges & Kam, 2002; McCabe, 2002). Passion flower, a compound derived from the dried flowers of the passion flower plant, is used as a mild sedative and antianxiety agent (McCabe, 2002; Starbuck, 1999). Nonbotanical mineral–vitamin agents include the dietary supplement S-adenosylmethionine, an amino acid compound used widely as an antidepressant, and omega-3 fatty oils, which are thought to promote mood stability and decreased aggression (McCabe).

Nontraditional Psychosocial Therapies

Pet and Plant Therapy

This approach, dubbed the "Eden Alternative" (Thomas, 1994), is an effort to address the three major plagues of nursing home life: loneliness, helplessness, and boredom. Birds, dogs, cats, rabbits, and plants are introduced to the nursing home environment. Here, the residents have the opportunity to gain physical, emotional, spiritual, sensory, and intellectual benefits while experiencing natural, living things. Plants and animals not only provide the older residents a link with nature, but also create an opportunity for a more meaningful, homelike atmosphere.

Dance and Movement Therapy

Dance and movement can allow older adults to improve mobility, circulation, and self-esteem. They also strengthen the body, making it easier to deal effectively with mental and physical stressors. Dance and movement may help participants to experience an inner awareness of self while having open interaction with the environment. This interaction provides a therapeutic self-help process that can release tension and anxiety, reduce

confusion, stimulate memory, decrease depression, and rechannel anger and frustration.

Music and Art Therapy

Music therapy is one of the most popular alternative therapies that allow older adults with various levels of cognition to experience many happy memories. Art therapy gives them the chance to express themselves and their emotions whether they can or cannot verbalize those emotions.

Consultation and Referral

Consultation in the mental health field involves the collaborative activity of professionals in the management of mental health problems. Generally, the problems presented for consultation are complex and potentially expensive. Caplan's (1970) model of mental health consultation identifies four types of consultation: (1) program-centered administrative consultation, (2) consultee-centered administrative consultation, (3) client-centered case consultation, and (4) consultee-centered case consultation. The latter two are the most relevant to this discussion.

The essence of consultation is personal and professional respect. The consultant's expertise in a specific area is sought by the consultee who needs help or advice to manage a client's mental health problem. The consultant and consultee may or may not be mental health professionals.

Referral in the mental health field is the process by which clients are introduced to other professionals for mental health–related services. Referral of clients may be from one mental health professional to another, from a non–mental health professional to a mental health specialist, or from a mental health professional to a non–mental health professional. Many psychiatric mental health nurses have a specialty focus to their work, and there is a wide range of medical settings (including critical care and burns units) and long-term care settings for older adults (including nursing homes and assisted living facilities) where consultant mental health nurses can use their expertise directly or indirectly to promote mental health care of older adults.

Education

Nurses are in a prime position to use education as a method of promoting mental health of older adults. Individual, family, and community-focused education intervention programs can be used to forge a partnership between mental health professionals, individuals, families, and communities, and thereby facilitate improved long-term mental health outcomes. Major objectives of these programs should be increasing knowledge of mental health promotion and illness prevention of the community at large, and supporting the self-care and daily management of mentally ill older adults by families.

Some educational interventions may be offered as formal stand-alone educational programs on mental health–related issues. Focus areas may include (1) coping needs that result from the decrements that occur naturally in the process of aging, (2) support systems, (3) socioeconomic changes caused by retirement and decreased earning ability, (4) ageism, and (5) community resources for the prevention or treatment of mental disorders. Some educational interventions may be imbedded in treatment programs for mentally ill clients, or physically ill clients at risk of mental illness. Emphasis should be placed on clients' and significant others' strengths rather than their weaknesses. Presentation formats may involve oral presentations, question-and-answer periods, discussion, and distribution of written materials. With the widening and almost universal availability of electronic media, presentation formats should include audiovideo formats, such as television, and the Internet.

FAMILY AND COMMUNITY RESOURCES TO ENHANCE MENTAL WELLNESS

The presence of a family has a positive influence on coping with aging. Family relationships are not only salient, but the support available within them is a key variable predicting well-being in older persons (Qualls, 2000). Often family members provide instrumental and intangible support to their elderly members, including assistance with ADLs,

transportation, finances, and so forth. Social support systems, such as the family, can buffer the negative effects of stress on the mental health status of older adults, thus reducing their vulnerability to mental illness and institutionalization.

The community approach to mental health promotion in older adults requires an appropriate mix of resources and service (Buckwalter, Weiler, & Stolley, 1995). Community resources and services may be professional or nonprofessional in nature. Nonprofessional services may be offered by voluntary or state-funded agencies and include home-delivered meals, transportation services, and home upkeep services. Private-pay services include geriatric day care and assisted living centers. Professional resources include personnel, such as physicians and nurses, psychologists, social workers, and academic educators who provide appropriate health, psychological, social, and academic services. Structural resources for supporting mental health promotion include hospitals, psychiatric day care centers, nursing homes, community colleges and universities, senior centers, and places of worship. Ideally, professional and nonprofessional services should complement each other and strive to satisfy the service needs of older adults.

CLINICAL RESEARCH PERTAINING TO MENTAL HEALTH PROMOTION IN OLDER ADULTS

Clinical Issues

Silvera and Allebec (2001) conducted face-to-face interviews with 28 male Somali immigrants, aged 60 years and older, to explore views on mental health and well-being and identify sources of stress and support so as to gain a greater understanding of factors leading to life satisfaction and depression in this population. Social isolation, low level of control over one's life, helplessness, ageism, perceived racial or religious discrimination, and racial harassment were identified in people who were depressed. Family support was the main buffer against depression.

Reijneveld, Westhoff, and Hopman-Rock (2003), in a randomized clinical trial, assessed the effect of eight, 2-hour long sessions consisting of health education and physical exercises on the health of 126 elderly Turkish immigrants living in the Netherlands. Results showed an improvement in the mental health of the subjects in the intervention group.

In a 6-month-long program, Matuska, Giles-Heinz, Flinn, Neighbour, and Bass-Haugen (2003) taught 65 older adults from three senior apartment complexes the importance to the quality of their lives of participation in meaningful social and community work. As a result, subjects had significantly higher scores on vitality, social functioning, and mental health over baseline. Participants reported increased frequency of social and community participation. Participants who benefited the most were older, attended more classes, and were nondrivers.

Watt and Cappeliez (2000) tested the effectiveness of integrative and instrumental reminiscence therapies, implemented in a short-term group format, and active socialization on decreasing depression in 26 older adults. Evaluation of the clinical significance of the results showed that both reminiscence therapies led to significant improvements in the symptoms of depression at the end of the intervention.

■ CASE STUDY*

Mrs. Mabel L. is an 81-year-old, 98-lb, 5′7″ white woman, living alone following the admission 2 years ago of her husband of 62 years, Arthur, to a long-term care facility a 20-minute drive away. Her husband suffers from Alzheimer's disease and severe mobility impairment. Mabel's entire life has been devoted to being a homemaker, wife, and mother. Her four children live within a 1-hour's drive and usually visit or call at least weekly. A caring young family lives next door and provides assistance with snow removal and yard work. She has no other social supports or involvement with her community, other than her church. Mabel's own health problems include long-standing hypertension, osteoarthritis affecting bilateral knees and shoulders, osteoporosis, and glaucoma and she has had a cataract extraction with intraocular lens implants bilaterally. Her corrected vision is 20/100 OU with her glasses. Medications include atenolol, 50 mg orally daily; alendronate, 70 mg once a week; multivitamin with calcium and vitamin D once every day; and latanoprost, 0.005% ophthalmic solution, one drop once daily in the evening. Mabel is a nonsmoker. She denies current or past use of over-the-counter or herbal medications or therapies other than extra strength acetaminophen, two 500-mg tablets once or twice a day, 2 to 3 days per week. She is independent in ADLs and IADLs, although she expresses concern that her "memory is not what it used to be." She limits driving to daytime use because of concerns she has about her vision with nighttime driving. She enjoys caring for her cat, visits to the nursing home to see her husband nearly every other day, and several television programs. Religion, prayer, and church attendance on Sunday are strong sources of support for Mabel.

Case Study Analysis

How can the nurse practitioner (NP) address mental health promotion for this client within the overall context of health promotion? One helpful framework is to consider the nursing paradigm with its key interrelated concepts: person–family, environment, health, and nursing. The

(continues)

CASE STUDY* *(continued)*

NP would assess the current state of mental well-being based on Mabel's self-report. A number of instruments and tools are available to conduct a formalized assessment. However, Hoff and Brown (2005) have described a detailed comprehensive mental health assessment method with an emphasis on functional assessment that is particularly relevant for older persons. In it, basic life functions (physical health, self-acceptance and self-esteem, vocational and occupation, immediate family, intimacy and significant others, residential and housing, financial security, decision-making ability, problem-solving ability, life goal and spiritual values, leisure time and community involvement, and feeling management) are addressed. Additionally, signals of distress (violence experienced, injury to self, danger to others, substance use, legal issues, agency use) are assessed. Such a detailed assessment can serve as a significant guide to the treatment plans that will follow. For Mabel, the NP must determine what the loss of her long-time companion and husband of 62 years, Arthur, to the nursing home has meant and continues to mean to her. The following are examples of the questions that should be considered:

- What have her past coping mechanisms been in dealing with life stressors and are these now effective?
- What personal goals does she have for her own present and future?
- Where in her life does she derive social support, and how satisfied is she with this currently?
- Have her feelings and beliefs about her self-identify and self-concept changed, and if so, how?
- How have these changes in her roles, especially that of primary caregiver, and relationships impacted her?
- How does she describe her current level of life satisfaction?

- What immediate or future goals can she envision, and does she see these as achievable through her present activities or involvement?
- Does she have a confidante to whom she can turn?
- Has she ever had any interest in community service involvement?
- What current community service interests does she have that might substitute for her prior caregiving role?
- Does she find a sense of purpose and fulfillment in her current situation?
- Would she consider involvement in church or animal shelter volunteering, for example?

The environment is a major component of the nursing paradigm, and it has numerous dimensions that can impact the health and mental well-being of older adults. Mabel's NP needs to identify what living alone in a single-family home means to the client. For instance, is Mabel fearful about her surroundings or community? Too often, well-meaning providers and families alike observe a living situation and apply their own personal value judgment or beliefs about "what would be best" for another individual. Asking Mabel herself about her environment and living situation is a key. With that information collected, the NP will be better able to determine next steps, either the offer of needed supports and community services to maintain this living arrangement or the provision of needed information about and referrals to alternative housing or living arrangements that may be available to Mabel, depending on her financial means and desired interests.

Source: Melillo, K. D. (2007). Mental health promotion. Part II. In *Gerontology topics: Essentials of health promotion for aging adults* (Vol. 1, pp. 13–19, 23–24). Developed by the American Academy of Nurse Practitioners Foundation in collaboration with the Fellows of the American Academy of Nurse Practitioners; with permission.

REFERENCES

Allen, J. E. (2003). *Nursing home administration* (4th ed.). New York: Springer.

Allers, C. T. (1990). AIDS and the older adult. *Gerontologist, 30,* 405–407.

Beck, A. T., & Beck, R. W. (1972). Screening depressed patients in family practice: A rapid technique. *Postgraduate Medicine, 52*(6), 81–85.

Bhugra, D., & Bahl, V. (1999). *Ethnicity: An agenda for mental health.* London: Gaskell.

Blair, C. E. (1999). Effect of self-care ADLs on self-esteem of intact nursing home residents. *Issues in Mental Health Nursing, 20,* 559–570.

Blazer, D. (1990). *Emotional problems in later life: Intervention strategies for professional caregivers.* New York: Springer.

Boydell, J., Van Os, J., McKenzie, K., Allardyce, J., Goel, R., McCreadie, R. G., et al. (2001). Incidence of schizophrenia in ethnic minorities in London: Ecological study into interactions with environment. *British Medical Journal, 322,* 1336.

Buckwalter, K. C., Weiler, K., & Stolley, J. (1995). Community programs. In M. O. Hogstel (Ed.), *Geropsychiatric nursing* (2nd ed., pp. 341–365). St. Louis, MO: Mosby.

Bunten, D. (2001). Normal changes with aging. In M. Maas, K. Buckwalter, M. Hardy, T. Tripp-Reimer, M. Titler, & J. Specht (Eds.), *Nursing care of older adults: Diagnoses, outcomes & interventions.* St. Louis, MO: Mosby.

Burgess, A. W. (1998). *Advanced practice psychiatric nursing.* Stamford, CT: Appleton & Lange.

Campbell, J. M. (1995). Assessment. In M. O. Hogstel (Ed.), *Geropsychiatric nursing* (2nd ed., pp. 73–95). St. Louis, MO: Mosby.

Caplan, G. (1970). *The theory and practice of mental health consultation.* New York: Basic Books.

Chow, J. C., Jaffee, K., & Snowden, L. (2003). Racial/ethnic disparities in the use of mental health services in poverty areas. *American Journal of Public Health, 93,* 792–797.

Cook, F. L., & Kramek, L. M. (1986). Measuring economic hardship among older Americans. *The Gerontologist, 26,* 38–47.

Donohue, B., Acierno, R., Hersen, M., & Van Hasselt, V. B. (1995). Social skills training for depressed, visually impaired older adults. *Behavior Modification, 19,* 379–424.

Duke University Center for the Study of Aging and Human Development. (1988). *OARS multidimensional functional assessment questionnaire.* Durham, NC: Duke University.

Dwyer, J. W. (1995). The effects of aging on the family. In R. Blieszner & V. H. Bedford (Eds.), *Handbook on aging and the family* (pp. 401–421). New York: Greenwood Press.

Feil, N. (1992). Validation therapy with late-onset dementia populations. In G. M. Jones & B. M. Miesen (Eds.), *Care-giving in dementia: Research and applications* (pp. 199–218). New York: Routledge.

Feil, N. (1999). Current concepts and techniques in validation therapy. In M. Duffy (Ed.), *Handbook of counseling and psychotherapy with older adults* (pp. 590–613). New York: Wiley.

Ferrell, B. R., & Ferrell, B. A. (1995). Pain in the elderly. In D. B. McGuire, C. H. Yarbro, & B. R. Ferrell (Eds.), *Cancer pain management* (2nd ed., pp. 273–287). Sudbury, MA: Jones and Bartlett.

Folstein, M. F., Folstein, S. E., & McHugh, P. R. (1975). Mini-Mental State: A practical method for grading the cognitive state of patients for the clinician. *Journal of Psychiatric Research, 12,* 189–198.

Given, B. A., Kozachik, S. L., Collins, C. E., DeVoss, D. N., & Given, C. W. (2001). Caregiver role strain. In M. L. Mass, K. C. Buckwalter, M. A. Hardy, T. Tripp-Reimer, M. G. Titler, & J. P. Specht (Eds.), *Nursing care of older adults: Diagnoses, outcomes, & interventions* (pp. 679–695). St. Louis, MO: Mosby.

Goodkin, K., Heckman, T., Siegel, K., Linsk, N., Khamis, I., Lee, D., et al. (2003). "Putting a face" on HIV infection/AIDS in older adults: A psychosocial context. *JAIDS, 33*(Suppl. 2), S171–S184.

Hedelin, B. (2001). The meaning of mental health from elderly women's perspectives: A basis for health promotion. *Perspectives in Psychiatric Care, 37,* 7–14.

Hodges, P. F., & Kam, P. C. (2002). The peri-operative implications of herbal medicines. *Anaesthesia, 57,* 889–899.

Hoff, L., & Brown, L. (2005). Comprehensive mental health assessment: An integrated approach. In K. D. Melillo & S. C. Houde (Eds.), *Geropsychiatric and mental health nursing* (pp. 45–67). Sudbury, MA: Jones and Bartlett.

Hogstel, M. O. (1995). *Geropsychiatric nursing* (2nd ed.). St. Louis, MO: Mosby.

Jacobs, L. S. (1989). Crisis screening and diversion services. *Hawaii Medical Journal, 48,* 73.

Lawton, H. P., & Brody, E. M. (1969). Assessment of older people: Self maintaining and instrumental activities of daily living. *Gerontologist, 9,* 179–186.

Lueckenotte, A. G. (2000). *Gerontologic nursing* (2nd ed.). St. Louis, MO: Mosby.

Luis, C. A., Loewenstein, D. A., Acevedo, A., Barker, W. W., & Duara, R. (2003). Mild cognitive impairment: Directions for future research. *Neurology, 61,* 438–444.

McCabe, S. (2002). Complementary herbal and alternative drugs in clinical practice. *Perspectives in Psychiatric Care, 38,* 98–107.

McCaffery, M., & Pasero, C. (1999). *Pain: Clinical manual* (2nd ed.). St. Louis, MO: Mosby.

Mahoney, F. I., & Barthel, B. W. (1965). Functional evaluation: The Barthel Index. *Maryland State Medical Journal, 14,* 61–65.

Matuska, K., Giles-Heinz, A., Flinn, N., Neighbour, M., & Bass-Haugen, J. (2003). Outcomes of a pilot occupational therapy wellness program for older adults. *American Journal of Occupational Therapy, 57,* 220–224.

Minardi, H., & Hays, N. (2003a). Nursing older adults with mental health problems: Therapeutic interventions—Part 1. *Nursing Older People, 15*(6), 22–28.

Minardi, H., & Hays, N. (2003b). Nursing older adults with mental health problems: Therapeutic interventions—Part 2. *Nursing Older People, 15*(7), 20–24.

Mitchell, G. J. (1990). The lived experience of taking life day-by-day in later life: Research guided by Parse's emergent method. *Nursing Science Quarterly, 3,* 29–36.

Moody, H. R. (2002). *Aging: Concepts and controversies.* Thousand Oaks, CA: Sage.

Morgan, L., & Kunkel, S. (2001). *Aging: The social context* (2nd ed.). Boston: Pine Forge Press.

National Council for Reliable Health Information [NCRHI] Newsletter (2000). The herbal hype of dietary supplements among the elderly. *NCRHI Newsletter, 23*(4), 1–2.

Neff, D. F. (1996). Gerontological counseling. In S. Lego (Ed.), *Psychiatric nursing: A comprehensive reference* (pp. 165–174). Philadelphia: Lippincott.

Neugarten, B. L., & Datan, N. (1975). Sociological perspectives on the life-cycle. In P. B. Baltes & K. W. Schaie (Eds.), *Lifespan developmental psychology: Personality and socialization* (pp. 53–69). New York: Academic Press.

Ory, M. G., & Zablotsky, D. (1989). Notes for the future: Research, prevention, care, public policy. In M. W. Riley, M. G. Ory, & D. Zablotsky (Eds.), *AIDS in an aging society: What we need to know* (pp. 202–216). New York: Springer.

Pfeiffer, E. (1975). A short portable questionnaire for the assessment of organic brain deficit in elderly patients. *Journal of the American Geriatrics Society, 23,* 433–441.

Phan, T. T., & Reifler, B. V. (1988). Psychiatric disorders among nursing home residents. *Clinical Geriatric Medicine, 4,* 601–611.

Pinquart, M., & Sorensen, S. (2001). Influence on loneliness in older adults: A meta-analysis. *Basic and Applied Social Psychology, 23,* 245–266.

Qualls, S. H. (2000). Therapy with aging families: Rationale, opportunities and challenges. *Aging & Mental Health, 4,* 191–199.

Reijneveld, S. A., Westhoff, M. H., & Hopman-Rock, M. (2003). Promotion of health and physical activity improves the mental health of elderly immigrants: Results of a group randomized controlled trial among Turkish immigrants in the Netherlands aged 45 and over. *Journal of Epidemiology and Community Health, 57,* 405–411.

Ritter, S., & Watkins, M. (1997) Assessment of older people. In I. J. Norman & S. J. Redfern (Eds.), *Mental health care for older people* (pp. 99–130). New York: Churchill Livingstone.

Ruiz, D. S. (1995). Demographic and epidemiological profile of the ethnic elderly. In D. K. Padgett (Ed.), *Handbook of ethnicity, aging, and mental health* (pp. 3–21). Westport, CT: Greenwood Press.

Sadock, B. J., & Sadock, V. A. (2000). *Kaplan and Sadock's comprehensive textbook of psychiatry* (7th ed.). Baltimore: Williams & Wilkins.

Seligman, M. E. P. (1992). *Helplessness: On depression, development and death.* San Francisco: Freeman.

Sharpley, M. S., Hutchinson, G., Murray, R. M., & Mc Kenzie, K. (2001). Understanding the excess of psychosis among the African-Caribbean population in England: Review of current hypotheses. *British Journal of Psychiatry, 178*(Suppl. 40), 60–68.

Silvera, E., & Allebec, P. (2001). Migration, ageing, and mental health: An ethnographic study on perceptions of life satisfaction, anxiety and depression in older Somali men in East London. *International Journal of Social Welfare, 10,* 309–320.

Smilkstein G., Ashworth, C., & Montano, M. A. (1982). Validity and reliability of the Family APGAR as a test of family functioning. *Journal of Family Practice, 15,* 303–311.

Starbuck, J. J. (1999). Calming herbs. *Better Nutrition, 61*(2), 50–52.

Thomas, W. (1994). *The Eden alternative: Nature, hope, and nursing home.* Cherburne, NY: Eden Alternative.

U.S. Department of Health and Human Services. (2000). *Healthy people 2010* (2nd ed., two vols.). Washington, DC: U.S. Government Printing Office.

Watt, L. M., & Cappeliez, P. (2000). Integrative and instrumental reminiscence therapies for depression in older adults: Intervention strategies and treatment effectiveness. *Aging & Mental Health, 4* (2), 166–177.

Yesavage, J. A., & Brink, T. L. (1983). Development and validation of a geriatric depression screening scale: A preliminary report. *Journal of Psychiatric Research, 17,* 37–49.

6

Psychopharmacology

Geoffry Phillips McEnany

Psychiatric illness among older adults is common-place and is a considerable factor in determining the quality of life in those older than 65 years of age. A number of factors contribute to the lowered vulnerability to episodes of mental illness including psychosocial stressors, medical comorbidities, and the life changes that accompany aging. Some older adults are able to reduce the risk of an episode of illness with such techniques as easy access to healthcare resources, use of social support systems, and healthy coping skills. Others are less fortunate in the absence of these resources and are at greatest risk for either an initial episode of illness or a relapse of an existing illness. Depression, anxiety, substance abuse, sleep dysregulation, and cognitive disorders are among some of the common culprits negatively impacting the mental health of older adults. Although the awareness of mental health issues among older adults is improving, the need for accurate identification of target symptoms and correct diagnosis is critical to positive clinical outcomes. Included in this treatment plan are pharmacological options that aim to alleviate symptoms, reduce risk, and facilitate healing and well-being.

In 2000, an estimated 9 million older adults suffered from some form of mental illness. This number is expected to increase to 20 million by the middle of this century given the aging demographics (U.S. Bureau of the Census, 2000). In 2010, the U.S. Census Bureau conducted another major census of the American populace allowing for a snapshot of the accuracy of these predictions in the first decade of the 21st century. It is reported that nearly 20% of those 55 years and older experience mental health disorders that are not part of normal aging. The common disorders in order of prevalence are anxiety, severe cognitive impairment, and mood disorders. There is concern that mental disorders in older adults are underreported. The rate of suicide is highest among older adults compared to any other age group, and the suicide rate for persons 85 years and older is the highest of all at twice the overall national rate (Metlay, 2008).

The composition of the population 65 years and older continues to shift to a more ethnically, racially, and culturally diverse group of older adults because of significant growth in minority populations. These factors combined will become the foundation for shifts in clinical practice aimed at both mental health maintenance and psychiatric disease prevention in the aging sector of the American population. Nurses continue to be a critical dimension in the health care of older adults, and the practice of nursing will be contoured by the factors influencing the care of this group.

Older adults often deal with a multiplicity of medical and psychiatric problems, and commonly part of the treatment regimen includes prescription and nonprescription medications. Older adults constitute just 13% of the U.S. population but consume 35% of all prescription drugs (Metlay, 2008). Psychotropics are the second most commonly prescribed class of drugs in geriatric patients and the most frequently associated with adverse drug reactions (Ives, 2001). Symptoms that become the focus of treatment include insomnia, agitation, aggression, and other disruptive behaviors. Commonly treated syndromes or disorders include anxiety, depression, mood cycling, psychosis, and cognitive disorders with associated dysregulations in sleep across all of these disorders (Blanchette et al., 2009; Pariente et al., 2008; Thomas, 2009).

Older adults commonly combine prescription and nonprescription medications, often unaware of the potentially negative impact that these combinations can produce. Recent research-based information on the combination of prescription and over-the-counter medications by Qato et al. (2008) revealed that among community-dwelling older adults, prescription and nonprescription medications were often used together, with nearly 1 in 25 individuals potentially at risk for a major drug–drug interaction. Given the commonplace use of herbal preparations among the general population and older adults in particular, clinicians often need a reliable source of reference in understanding the implications of these compounds. A resource such as the *Physician's Desk Reference for Herbal Medicines* (Kush et al., 2007) is a helpful compendium of information that can serve as a guide to clinicians who have questions related to the use of these medications separately or in combination with other drugs.

Undiagnosed and untreated mental illness can lead to unnecessary and costly procedures and hospitalizations, increased disability, premature death, increased morbidity, increased risk of institutionalization, and a significant decrease in quality of life for older adults. Changing demographics, combined with the disproportionate rate at which older adults use medical resources and the pressures to contain costs, will require that healthcare providers become increasingly knowledgeable in the care of a diverse older population (Edlund, 2004) and vigilant in diagnosing and treating mental illness in this population. It is essential that clinicians working with older adults aggressively address the mental health issues of this population to meet the goals for *Healthy People 2010*, which seek to increase quality years of life and eliminate health disparities (U.S. Department of Health and Human Services, 2000).

CHALLENGES IN PRESCRIBING FOR OLDER ADULTS

Mental health problems in older adults often differ in clinical manifestations, pathogenesis, and pathophysiology from mental health problems of younger adults (Sadock & Sadock, 2009). Thus, the diagnosis and treatment of older adults can present more difficulties. Factors contributing to such difficulties include normal age-related changes, the coexistence of chronic medical problems and disabilities, the use of multiple medications, and the presence of cognitive impairment (Nixdorff et al., 2008). In addition, the signs and symptoms of health problems in the older adult may not be as obvious as in the younger adult, given the complexities presented by medical comorbidities and natural changes incurred in the course of aging. There may also be differences in the quantity and quality of symptoms with older persons. Older adults may present with vague versus specific complaints. For example, lightheadedness may be the only symptom reported by an older adult experiencing anxiety, or multiple general somatic complaints may be the predominant presentation if experiencing depression. Older adults may also hesitate to mention changes in their bodies associated with health problems, because they perceive these changes as normal aging (Leff & Sonstegard-Gamm, 2006).

Clearly, changes need to be explored to determine whether there is underlying disease or whether the changes are age-related and normal. Additionally, older adults often perceive their health based on their ability to function rather than on the number of health problems. This population is unique in that they may be diagnosed with two or more chronic diseases, take a number of medications, and still function at a high level of health (Kane, Ouslander, & Abrass, 2004). These cohort-related trends may reflect both cultural and generational patterns of response.

Prescribing a psychotropic drug for an older adult should be based on a thorough assessment, target symptoms, stages and progression of illness, provider's knowledge of drug choices, and the pharmacokinetic and pharmacodynamic changes that accompany aging. In addition, a review of current medications that may interact with or contribute to adverse drug reactions should be conducted. A dose appropriate for the older adult should be prescribed in a dosing schedule that enhances compliance. Individualizing treatment plans that include psychoeducation and evaluating responses to drug interventions are essential because of the great deal of variability among the older adult population (American Nurses Association, 2001). Box 6-1 references several Web-based resources that may be helpful sources of information for clinicians working with elders who have diagnosed psychiatric conditions.

FACTORS INFLUENCING PHARMACO-THERAPY IN OLDER ADULTS

Pharmacotherapy in older adults may be complicated by multiple factors, among them the pharmacokinetic (drug absorption, distribution, metabolism, and excretion) and pharmacodynamic changes associated with aging (Box 6-2). These changes involve altered receptor response.

Pharmacokinetics is a source of concern from a variety of perspectives for clinicians who work with older adults. The sections that follow assist clinicians

BOX 6-1 WEB-BASED RESOURCES: GERIATRIC PSYCHIATRY AND GERONTOLOGY

The Gerontological Society of America (www.geron.org). This is an excellent resource that disseminates research-based information on many topics related to gerontology. Full text journals are accessible from the Web page.

National Institute on Aging (www.nih.gov/nia). This site contains an impressive compilation of information for the public on broad issues related to aging, and biomedical, behavioral, and social research related to aging. A variety of publications for professionals are available through this site.

Drug Interactions (http://www.drugs.com/drug_interactions.html). This is a particularly helpful Web site that offers the clinician some pragmatic information related to potential drug interactions. Drug–drug interactions can be checked on an interactive program.

American Psychiatric Association (www.psych.org). This Web site is an excellent resource for the clinician who is seeking information related to practice guidelines and evidence-based approaches to the treatment of psychiatric illnesses.

BOX 6-2 AGE-RELATED PHARMACOKINETIC CHANGES

Absorption	**Metabolism**
Delayed gastric emptying	Decreased liver size
Increased gastric pH	Decreased hepatic blood flow
Decreased intestinal motility	Decreased level of drug metabolizing enzymes
Decreased mucosal surface area	
Distribution	**Excretion**
Decreased lean body (muscle) mass	Decreased blood flow
Increased body fat	Decreased glomeruli
Decreased total body water	Decreased glomerular filtration
Decreased albumin	Decreased tubular secretion
Decreased α1-acid glycoprotein	Decreased creatinine production
	Decreased creatinine clearance

Source: Adapted from Kane, Ouslander, & Abrass, 2004; Keltner & Folks, 2005.

in the understanding of such pharmacokinetic-based concerns, and address these issues according to the categories of absorption, distribution, metabolism, and excretion.

Absorption

Although there is an age-related decrease in small bowel surface and an increase in gastric pH, changes in drug absorption seem to be the pharmacological parameter least affected by increasing age (Kane et al., 2004). In contrast, the distribution of a drug is influenced by age-related changes in body composition of water (total and intracellular) and lean body mass relative to body fat. Specifically, the percentage of total body water decreases by 10% to 15% between the ages of 20 and 80 years. This relative decrease in total body water leads to a higher blood and tissue concentration of some water-soluble drugs. In addition, the ratio of lean mass to body fat decreases with age. Thus, a drug distributed only in lean tissue, such as lithium, should be given in a lower dose because of the decrease in lean body mass with aging (Lueckenotte, 1996).

Distribution

Although the percentage of lean body mass to body fat decreases with age, the percentage of body fat increases from 18% to 36% in men and from 33% to 45% in women. An increase in total body fat increases the volume of distribution for lipophilic drugs, such as the long-acting benzodiazepines, diazepam (Valium), and chlordiazepoxide hydrochloride (Librium). Thus, many lipid-soluble psychotropic drugs are distributed more widely, prolonging the action of the drug and increasing the likelihood of serious adverse consequences (Keltner & Folks, 2005; Stahl, 2008).

In addition to changes in total body water and body fat, the distribution of drugs into the peripheral circulation and tissues is influenced by serum albumin (protein binding) and α1-acid glycoprotein levels. With age, there may be a decrease in serum albumin levels. This results in increased fractions of free drug (not bound to protein) circulating in the body. This is of great importance because the unbound, free drug is what is pharmacodynamically active. In contrast to decreasing levels of serum albumin, α1-acid glycoprotein levels increase with age, resulting in the increased binding of drugs that normally bind to this protein. An increase in α1-acid glycoprotein levels may affect the distribution of a number of psychotropic drugs, such as the tricyclic antidepressants (TCAs), resulting in a prolonged half-life of these drugs. However, the clinical consequences of an increase in α1-acid glycoprotein have not been well studied in older adults (Keltner & Folks, 2005; Stahl, 2008).

Metabolism

Drug metabolism in the older adult is complex, difficult to predict, and affected by age-related hepatic changes. These include a decrease in liver size, blood flow, and hepatic microsomal enzyme (cytochrome [CYP] P-450) activity. In addition, a variety of other factors can influence hepatic drug metabolism, such as caffeine; tobacco; foods that act as CYP P-450 inducers or inhibitors, such as grapefruit juice, cruciferous vegetables, or charbroiled meats; alcohol; current disease state; nutritional status; gender; genetic determinants; and lifelong exposure to various chemicals (Stahl, 2008). There is evidence that the first phase of drug metabolism declines with age, whereas the second phase seems to be less affected. An older adult with normal liver function tests may not be able to metabolize drugs as efficiently as a younger

individual, given normal changes in the hepatic system that occur with aging.

Excretion

Excretion of drugs by the kidneys is better understood than hepatic drug metabolism in the older adult. Age-related changes in renal function include decreases in renal blood flow, glomerular filtration rate, production of creatinine, and creatinine clearance. Because of an age-related decline in muscle mass resulting in the decreased production of creatinine, a serum creatinine level is not a reliable marker of renal function in the older adult. The serum creatinine, however, is used to calculate the creatinine clearance, a more accurate reflection of renal function in this patient population. A drug that depends on renal excretion for its elimination, such as lithium, is likely to accumulate to potentially toxic levels unless the dosage is adjusted to a lower dose in light of clinical monitoring of both therapeutic and potentially adverse effects (Keltner & Folks, 2005). Other factors, such as intrinsic renal disease, state of hydration, and cardiac output, also can affect the renal clearance of a drug. Thus, it is important to calculate a baseline estimate of creatinine clearance before initiating drug therapy in older adults.

In addition to the pharmacokinetic changes that occur with aging, pharmacodynamic changes also occur. These changes impact an individual's responsiveness to the concentration of a given drug (altered receptor response). It is known that an age-related sensitivity to both the therapeutic and toxic effects of many medications, especially centrally acting medications, increases. This sensitivity is heightened in the very frail and the very old individual. Kane et al. (2004) noted that this sensitivity was true for certain drugs, such as sedating medications, but not true for other drugs, such as blood pressure medications mediated by β-adrenergic receptors, which seem to decline with age. Although considerably less is known about the pharmacodynamic changes that occur with aging, increased sensitivity to the concentration of a particular drug must be considered, particularly when the medication has serious adverse side effects.

It is also important to understand the types of drug interactions to prevent the potential detrimental effect from two or more drugs that can interact with each other. One type of interaction occurs when a drug interferes with another drug's ability to interact with the receptor responsible for effect. Another example of a potential drug–drug interaction occurs when one drug enhances another's therapeutic or adverse effect by stimulation of the receptor by both drugs. For example, two agents that have properties of lowering blood pressure, when combined, may lead to greater chances of hypotension. The other general type of drug interaction occurs when one medication affects the plasma concentration of another medication by affecting absorption, distribution, metabolism, or elimination. This is termed a "pharmacokinetic interaction."

The CYP P-450 isoenzymes are located mostly in the liver and the small intestine. They are responsible for the first phase of biotransformation, the rate-limiting step in drug clearance. A CYP P-450 drug interaction occurs when a drug either speeds up (induction) or slows down (inhibition) enzymatic activity. The most clinically relevant isoenzymes include CYP1A2, CYP2C9, CYP2C19, CYP2D6, and CYP3A4 (Stahl, 2008). Competitive inhibition of the CYP P-450 hepatic isoenzymes is an example of this type of interaction and is common in psychotropic drug use. Visit www.drug-interactions.com for a review of the rudiments of the P-450 system and pragmatic information related to assessment for potential drug interactions. An additional resource can be found at http://www.preskorn.com/. This is the Web site of Sheldon Preskorn, MD, a renowned scientist in the area of drug metabolism and P-450-driven drug interactions. His site is informative, user friendly, and contains an extensive collection of clinical resources related to the implications of P-450 in practice.

The choice, dose, and dosing frequency of a medication for an older adult must be carefully planned in light of the pharmacokinetic and pharmacodynamic changes that occur with aging. This is true for all medications prescribed for this population but is even more critical for the prescription of psychotropic medications, the second most common category of drugs prescribed for older adults after cardiac medications. Psychoactive drugs are prescribed for 65% of nursing home residents, with some residents using three or more psychoactive drugs concurrently (Beers & Berkow, 2004).

Forty-eight medications or classes of medications to avoid in older adults have been identified by a national expert panel charged with updating widely used criteria for potentially harmful medications in older adults (Fick et al., 2003). A study of adverse drug effects found that 35% of ambulatory older adults experienced an adverse drug effect, and 29% required healthcare services (physician, emergency department, or hospitalization) for the adverse drug effect. Some two thirds of nursing facility residents have adverse drug effects over a 4-year period. Of these adverse drug effects, one in seven results in hospitalization (Fick et al.). Geriatrician Mark Beers (1997) is the developer of a well-documented list of medications to avoid in older adults, known as the "Beers Criteria," which continues to be a reliable guide to clinicians who provide treatment to this population. A complete list of the medications included in the Beers Criteria can be found at http://www.dcri.duke.edu/ccge/curtis/beers.html.

Voyer, Cohen, Lauzon, and Collin (2004) point out that the prevalence of psychotropic drug use among community-dwelling older persons (usually defined as those 65 years and older) varies from about 20% to 48%, and that many of these older adults use the psychotropic medications for more than 6 months. This time period may often exceed the time period for which the drug is needed (e.g., benzodiazepines). Along with the protracted use of these drugs may be the associated liabilities that are common to drug accumulation in older adults, caused by changes in pharmacokinetics. Such trends are noteworthy from the perspective that the use of these drugs may fall outside of evidence-based recommendations, and as such create liabilities for both the patient and the clinician who prescribes the drugs.

Bartels et al. (2003) noted that until recently there has been little information available to guide the practitioner in choosing appropriate psychotropic interventions for older adults. Recent advances in mental health treatment have led to the development of an evidence base specific to older adults (Bartels et al.). Thus, prescribing a psychoactive medication for an older adult with multiple comorbidities, who is taking an average of four to five medications, requires a thorough knowledge of the psychotropic drug and the latest consensus data specific for prescribing for this population, particularly in light of the pharmacokinetic and pharmacodynamic issues addressed previously.

To accomplish successfully the goal of maximizing outcomes while minimizing adverse events requires a multifactorial approach to prescribing psychotropic agents in older adults. The practitioner must consider medical comorbidity and polypharmacy, age-related physiological changes, cognitive ability, caregiver status, and psychosocial factors. Medical comorbidity and polypharmacy (nine or more medications or 12 or more doses per day) are common in the geriatric population. Polypharmacy has been shown to be a risk factor for developing adverse drug events in the older adult (Peterson et al., 2005). Proper education of patients and caregivers and monitoring medication regimens are important for early identification of adverse events and adherence problems. Equally important is the communication between different prescribers to avoid drug interactions and maximize outcomes.

Among older adults, as is the case with large numbers of the adult population in the United States, both over-the-counter medications and herbal supplements are commonly used to relieve symptoms (McEnany, 2001). Unfortunately, what many consumers do not realize is that "herbal" or "naturopathic" remedies are not benign substances, and are often cleared through hepatic metabolism, specifically by P-450 mechanisms. As

such, the potential for drug interactions with prescribed medications is significant and merits the attention of the prescriber. The clinician needs to assess usage patterns of both over-the-counter and herbal remedies closely to reduce the chances of a drug interaction and associated adverse events for the patient.

To ensure adherence feasibility the assessment of medication cost and insurance coverage is an important factor to consider. Sometimes the prescriber is forced to make medication choices based on external factors, such as insurance formularies or restrictions, and on the patient's ability to pay for medications. It is essential for clinicians to recognize that good prescribing practice is a multifaceted process as depicted in Figure 6-1.

Clinicians may find the Web site https://www.pparx.org/Intro.php helpful when dealing with patients who are uninsured or who have limited resources available for medications. This is an online resource that contains all of the details for how to access patient assistance programs for medications free of cost to the medically disadvantaged or indigent. The site has direct links to many of the pharmaceutical companies offering patient assistance programs, along with detailed descriptions of the procedures related to ordering medications.

Although psychiatric conditions are often underdiagnosed in the older adult, healthcare providers should carefully examine the necessity of pharmacotherapy before prescribing new medications. In addition, the necessity and compatibility of all long-term medications should be periodically reexamined. If deemed necessary, prescriptions, dosages, and intervals should be based on the patient's age, renal and hepatic function, and concomitant diseases and medications. To increase the quality of care and limit the inappropriate use of psychotropic medications in residents of long-term care facilities, the Omnibus Budget Reconciliation Act (OBRA) was passed in 1987. The interpretive guidelines enforcing OBRA were implemented in 1990 and updated in 1999. Because proper documentation of necessity and attempted withdrawal trials of medications

FIGURE 6-1

Multifaceted Process for Prescribing Psychiatric Medication in the Elderly.

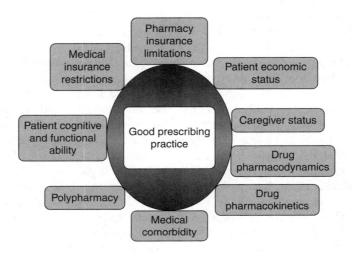

became requirements, the outcome of OBRA has been increased attention to appropriate prescribing of psychotropic medication in such a fashion as to minimize adverse events and detrimental effects on physical and cognitive function.

PSYCHOTROPIC DRUGS

Psychotropic drugs can be broadly categorized as antidepressants, anxiolytics, sedative-hypnotics, antipsychotics, and mood stabilizers. These categories of drugs, their characteristics, and the drugs included in each class are listed in Table 6-1. Each category of psychotropic drug is discussed in detail with recommendations for their use in older adults.

Antidepressants

The goal of antidepressant therapy includes improving and maintaining mood, physical and social daily functioning, and quality of life while minimizing side effects. Doses should be started low and titrated slowly to the desired effect. Antidepressants typically take 2 to 4 weeks before benefits can be discerned in the younger population, but 6 to 12 weeks in the older adult population. Titration should be adjusted based on tolerability of side effects and effectiveness.

Antidepressants can be subdivided into four categories: (1) TCAs, (2) monoamine oxidase inhibitors (MAOIs), (3) selective serotonin reuptake inhibitors (SSRIs), and (4) non-SSRI second-generation antidepressants (Table 6-2). The latter category includes serotonin-norepinephrine reuptake inhibitors (SNRIs) and a dopamine-norepinephrine reuptake inhibitor.

Although the older TCAs are effective for treating depression, most should be avoided in the older adult because of their substantial side-effect profile, which includes excessive sedation; anticholinergic effects (dry mouth, constipation, urinary

TABLE 6-1

Categories of Psychotropic Drugs

Category	Characteristics	Drug Classes
Antidepressants	Equally effective but differ based on side-effect profile and potential for drug interactions	Tricyclic antidepressants Monoamine oxidase inhibitors Selective serotonin reuptake inhibitors Nonselective serotonin reuptake inhibitor second-generation antidepressants (dopamine reuptake inhibitors, 5HT2 antagonists) Serotonin-norepinephrine reuptake inhibitors
Anxiolytics	Short-acting agents without active metabolites preferred in older adults to minimize lasting adverse events	Short-acting benzodiazepines Long-acting benzodiazepines Buspirone
Sedative-hypnotics	Should be avoided because of side-effect profiles	Barbiturates Miscellaneous hypnotic/sedatives Melatonin agonists (may provide a safer alternative)
Antipsychotics	Second-generation agents in low doses preferred because of less anticholinergic and extrapyramidal system side effects BLACK BOX WARNING in relation to the use of these medications in persons with dementia	First-generation antipsychotics Second-generation antipsychotics
Mood stabilizers	Both on-label and off-label uses of medications aimed to stabilize mood	Lithium carbonate Divalproate Lamotrigine Others

Source: Adapted from Bezchlibnyk-Butler, Jeffries, & Virani (2007).

retention, blurred vision, and confusion); and cardiovascular effects (orthostasis, tachycardia, and electrocardiogram changes). Because of their cardiovascular effects, TCAs are lethal in overdose, which is always a serious concern in depressed patients. If the decision is to use a TCA, then the best choices are desipramine and nortriptyline, because these agents have the least anticholinergic side-effect profile. Interestingly, the TCAs have fallen out of fashion as first-line agents for the treatment of depression. However, their use is on the rise in off-label applications in the treatment of migraines, chronic pain, sleep disturbances, and various neuropathic pain syndromes. The concern related to use in depression also applies to use off-label.

TABLE 6-2

Categories of Antidepressants and Mode of Action

Drug Class	Mode of Action
Tricyclic antidepressants	Increases the synaptic concentration of serotonin or norepinephrine in the central nervous system by inhibition of their uptake by the presynaptic neuronal membrane
Monoamine oxidase inhibitors	Inhibits the monamine oxidase A and B enzymes responsible for the intraneuronal metabolism of norepinephrine and serotonin
Reversible inhibitors of monoamine oxidase, type A (not available in the United States)	Selectively inhibits monoamine oxidase type A
Selective serotonin reuptake inhibitors	Inhibits central nervous system neuronal reuptake of serotonin
Nonselective serotonin reuptake inhibitor second-generation antidepressants	Variety of modes of action, including effects on serotonin, norepinephrine, and dopamine

Source: Adapted from Bezchlibnyk-Butler, Jeffries, & Virani (2007).

Although MAOIs, such as phenelzine (Nardil) and tranylcypromine (Parnate), have been found to be useful for some patients with atypical depression and in those resistant to the other antidepressants, they do have significant drug and food interactions and potentially can cause serious side effects. They can lead to a life-threatening rise in blood pressure, especially if combined with certain foods containing tyramine, such as wines, cheeses, smoked fish, beef or chicken liver, sausage, yeast, or certain bean pods. MAOIs also can potentiate many categories of drugs, such as central nervous system stimulants and sympathomimetics, and lead to hypertensive crisis. They are additive to the effect of sulfonyureas and can lower blood sugar to dangerous levels. Combining with other antidepressants has the potential to cause either seizures or serotonin syndrome, which may result in nausea, anxiety, tremor, or difficulty sleeping. MAOIs, therefore, are generally avoided in elderly patients because of their significant side-effect profile and food–drug and drug–drug interactions.

There are two types of monoamine oxidase inhibitors (types A and B) and each of these enzymes is involved with the breakdown of neurochemicals in the synaptic cleft. The conventional MAOIs in use in the United States target type B. A more recently developed MAOI includes a selective and reversible MAOI that specifically targets monoamine oxidase type A. Examples of these drugs include moclobemide and brofaromine, but this class of antidepressants has not been approved for use in the United States. Lotufo-Neto, Trivedi, and Thase (1999) completed a meta-analysis on the effectiveness of these drugs and found them to have equal efficacy with tricyclics and to be well tolerated.

The SSRIs, noted in Table 6-3, create a more attractive alternative, although not without flaws. On a positive note, they have good efficacy data and because of an extended half-life, an advantage to adherence is once-daily dosing. However, they can cause a serious adverse event, such as serotonin syndrome, syndrome of inappropriate antidiuretic hormone (hyponatremia), and withdrawal

TABLE 6-3

Common SSRIs: Dosing and Hepatic Enzyme Affected

Medication	Starting Dose in Older Adults Per Day (mg)	Maintenance Dose in Older Adults Per Day (mg)	Oral Solution Available	Hepatic Enzyme Affected
Citalopram (Celexa)	10	20 to 40	Yes	Minimal
Escitalopram (Lexapro)	5	5 to 20	No	Minimal
Fluoxetine (Prozac)	10	20 to 40	Yes	CYP2C9, CYP2C19
Fluvoxamine (Luvox, Solvay)	50	50 to 200	No	CYP1A4, CYP2C9, CYP2C19
Paroxetine (Paxil, Paxil CR)	10	20 to 30	Yes	CYP2D6
Sertraline (Zoloft)	25	50 to 150	Yes	Minor CYP2D6, CYP3A4, CYP2C19

Source: Adapted from Bezchlibnyk-Butler, Jeffries, & Virani (2007).

syndrome, if cessation is not titrated at an appropriate rate during the discontinuation of the drug. Discontinuation effects are more likely to occur with drugs in the SSRI class that have shorter half-lives (e.g., citalopram) versus those with longer half-lives (e.g., fluoxetine). Tolerability can be adversely affected by gastrointestinal effects, sexual dysfunction, and sleep disturbances. Although side effects tend to be an effect of the class of medication, drug–drug interactions are more individualized. Sleep disturbance, weight gain, and sexual dysfunction are very common to these agents.

The non-SSRI second-generation agents listed in Table 6-4 include venlafaxine (Effexor, Effexor XR); desvenlafaxine (Pristiq); duloxetine (Cymbalta); bupropion (Wellbutrin, Wellbutrin SR, Wellbutrin XL, Zyban); mirtazapine (Remeron); trazodone (Desyrel); and nefazodone (Serzone). In 2004, Bristol-Myers Squibb, the manufacturer of nefazadone, made the decision to remove this drug from the market because of issues of hepatotoxicity

(Choi, 2003). Two newer SNRI antidepressants have been introduced to the market: duloxetine and desvenlafaxine. Each agent has unique characteristics relevant to prescribing in the older adult. Venlafaxine inhibits the reuptake of serotonin and with higher doses, norepinephrine. Venlafaxine is available in both immediate and extended-release preparations, and documentation states that the extended-release form of the medication has an improved side-effect profile, which may enhance adherence (Nemeroff, 2003). Both venlafaxine and desvenlafaxine are similar in action to the older TCAs but without the anticholineric side effects of the TCAs. Venlafaxine has been approved for use in both depression and generalized anxiety disorder, whereas desvenlafaxine is only indicated for the treatment of depression. Like other antidepressants that interfere with serotonin reuptake, venlafaxine may interact pharmacodynamically with other serotonergic agents (e.g., tryptophan or dextromethorphan) and should be avoided because

TABLE 6-4

Non-SSRIs: Dosing and Hepatic Enzyme Affected

Medication	Starting Dose in Older Adults (mg)	Maintenance Dose in Older Adults Per Day (mg)	Hepatic Enzyme Affected
Venlafaxine (Effexor, Effexor XR)	25 BID; XR, 37.5 QD	75 to 150	CYP2D6, CYP2E1
Duloxetine (Cymbalta)	20 BID	Up to 30 BID	CYP1A2, CYP2D6
Desvenlafaxine (Pristiq)	50 QD	50 QD	Minimal, if any
Bupropion (Wellbutrin, Wellbutrin SR, Wellbutrin XL)	37.5 BID; SR, 100 QAM; XL, 150 QAM	100 to 150	CYP2B6, CYP2D6
Mirtazapine (Remeron, Remeron SolTab)	7.5 QHS	15 to 30	CYP1A2, CYP2D6, CYP3A4
Trazodone (Desyrel)	25 QHS	25 to 50	CYP3A4
Nefazodone (Serzone [no longer available in the United States])	50 BID	200 to 400	CYP3A4, CYP2D6

Source: Adapted from Bezchlibnyk-Butler, Jeffries, & Virani (2007); Package insert, Pristiq, Wyeth (2008).

of potential serotonin syndrome. Side effects with venlafaxine are similar to the SSRIs with the addition of dose-related elevated blood pressure. Proper monitoring of blood pressure should be performed initially and at follow-up visits because of the prevalence of hypertension and cardiovascular diseases in the older adult. Elevated serum levels and toxicity can occur if combined with either CYP2D6 (paroxetine, amiodarone, cimetidine, and quinidine), or CYP3A4 (clarithromycin, erythromycin, diltiazem, grapefruit juice, and ketoconazole) inhibitors (Semla, Beizer, & Higbee, 2003). Although dosage adjustment for age alone is unnecessary, dosing should be started low and increased gradually (Wyeth-Ayerst, 2003). A 25%

decreased dosage adjustment is required with renal impairment and 50% with moderate hepatic impairment (Semla, Beizer, & Higbee).

Desvenlafaxine is the newcomer to the market as of 2008 (Wyeth, 2008), and it has some differences from venlafaxine on some salient points. The most important difference is in the lack of interference with other drugs metabolized through the P-450 enzyme system. This is an important feature for older adults who are likely to be on a number of prescription and over-the-counter medications. It has a once-daily dosing recommendation, which may enhance adherence.

Desvenlafaxine has been indicated by the Food and Drug Administration (FDA) for the treatment of major depressive disorder (Wyeth, 2008). However, it has been used in a number of off-label applications in the treatment of fibromyalgia and neuropathic pain (Stahl, 2008). This medication requires adjustment in dosing in older adults who have hypertension, hypercholesterolemia, history of clotting factor disorder, seizures, stroke, glaucoma, and renal or hepatic disease. It is contraindicated with concomitant use of MAOIs.

Duloxetine is an SNRI that has been indicated by the FDA for the treatment of major depression, generalized anxiety disorder, fibromyalgia, and diabetic neuropathic pain. This medication may be administered in either a once-daily or twice-daily schedule, depending on the tolerability of the medication. It is contraindicated with concomitant use of MAOIs. Potential adverse effects with this medication are not dissimilar to other SNRIs and include potential for hepatotoxicity, orthostasis, abnormal bleeding, seizures, hyponatremia, and urinary hesitation and retention (Eli Lilly, 2004). Coadministration of duloxetine with potent CYP1A2 inhibitors should be avoided. Because CYP2D6 is involved in duloxetine metabolism, concomitant use of duloxetine with potent inhibitors of CYP2D6 results in higher concentrations (on average of 60%) of duloxetine. Use of duloxetine concomitantly with heavy alcohol intake may be associated with severe liver injury. For this reason, duloxetine should ordinarily not be prescribed for patients with substantial alcohol use (Eli Lilly).

Bupropion is a weak SNRI, and it has some dopamine reuptake inhibition (Glaxo SmithKline, 2003). It offers the advantages of no sedative side effects, no cardiotoxicity, and no sexual side effects. Buproprion, however, can increase agitation, headache, tremor, insomnia, and anorexia. The primary safety issue with bupropion is its ability to cause seizures. Coadministration of bupropion with drugs that lower the seizure threshold, such as typical antipsychotics, TCAs, fluoroquinolones, theophylline, and any drug that can increase buproprion levels or toxicity (2D6 substrates, levodopa, MAOIs), should be avoided because of the seizure

risk. Dosage adjustment must be made because of hepatic or renal disease. Bupropion is available in immediate-release, sustained-release, and once-a-day formulations. There is some evidence in the literature that the extended-release formulation may have a more tolerable side-effect profile, possibly contributing to greater adherence (Nemeroff, 2003). Both the immediate-release and sustained-release formulations of these drugs require twice-daily dosing, whereas the once-a-day version is given in a single dose.

Mirtazapine is different than the SNRIs in that it antagonizes α_2-adrenergic receptors, blocks two serotonin receptor subtypes, and has a strong affinity for histaminic receptors. It causes somnolence, particularly at lower doses, which relates to its affect on antihistamine receptors and should therefore be dosed at bedtime. Mirtazapine has low risks of drug interactions and no cardiotoxicity. It also has been associated with weight gain and can therefore be useful in depressed anorexic older patients. In rare instances, it can cause agranulocytosis. It is important to monitor WBC and neutrophil counts if the patient presents with associated signs or symptoms, such as infection or fever. Mirtazipine clearance is decreased up to 40% in older adults, particularly with males, compared to younger males, so dosing should be started low (Organon, 2002). Nicholas and colleagues (2003) have documented the possibility of elevated total cholesterol with the use of this agent.

Trazodone and nefazodone hydrochloride are serotonin reuptake inhibitors and serotonin 5-HT2 receptor antagonists. Trazodone causes significant sedation without significant anticholinergic activity and should therefore be reserved for use at bedtime for patients with insomnia. Nefazodone has less sedative effect but has significant drug interactions, and has also been known to cause hepatic failure. Nefazodone inhibits the CYP3A4 isoenzyme and also increases blood levels of digoxin, a drug with a narrow therapeutic index (Bristol-Myers Squibb, 2001). Because of concerns of hepatotoxicity, the sale of the brand name antidepressant Serzone was discontinued by the manufacturer in 2003. Since the drug's introduction in 1994, there have been 51 Canadian reports of adverse hepatic events, including jaundice, hepatitis, and hepatocellular necrosis. In two of these cases the patients subsequently underwent liver transplantation (Choi, 2003). The drug remains available in the generic form as nefazodone.

Discontinuing antidepressants too quickly can lead to a withdrawal syndrome. Antidepressant withdrawal syndromes have been reported with the TCAs, the SSRIs, and the SNRIs (Perahia, Kajdasz, Desaiah, & Haddad, 2005; Stahl, 2008). The syndrome can consist of a cluster of symptoms that may include headaches; nausea; dizziness; unstable moods; gastrointestinal upset; recurrence of depression; bizarre dreams; strokelike symptoms; abnormal sensations of burning, prickling, or tingling; or auditory hallucinations. TCA-related withdrawal also can include cardiac arrhythmias (Dilsaver, Greden, & Snider, 1987). Some investigators have discussed atypical symptoms of antidepressant discontinuation, including discontinuation-associated mania (Andrade, 2004), although this is very rare in clinical practice. What is clear from the body of literature is that clinicians need to be well-informed of these potential manifestations of discontinuation syndrome to ensure comfort and safety during antidepressant withdrawal. It is critical to address the issue of potential for discontinuation syndrome with patients before prescribing the medication and during the course of the medication trial. This strategy may help to reduce a negative experience in the course of the medication trial and possibly enhance adherence to the prescribed regimen.

Although it is important to recognize the individual differences between the classes and individual antidepressants, it should be understood there are no clear directives for choosing an antidepressant based on the summary of current clinical trials in the older adult population (Alexopoulos, Katz, Reynolds, Carpenter, & Docherty, 2001). All antidepressant classes demonstrate superiority over placebo in the older adult population. The provider's responsibility in prescribing, therefore, is to choose the best particular antidepressant based primarily on the potential for adverse effects, drug–drug interactions, and cost for each individual patient.

One topic that merits some attention from clinicians is the issue of tachyphylaxis related to the use of antidepressants. This phenomenon is best described as a precipitous or insidious loss of therapeutic effect from the use of the antidepressant. It is not well-understood and there have been no studies published to document predictors of this loss of effect. Clinicians are well-advised to review the practice guidelines available from the American Psychiatric Association, including the guideline on the treatment of depression (www.psych.org) (American Psychiatric Association, 2000). These guidelines offer evidence-based guidance related to the community standard for the treatment of select psychiatric disorders, including depression.

FDA Warnings on Antidepressant Use and Suicide Risk

In 2004, the FDA issued a black box warning on antidepressants regarding the risk of suicidal thinking and behavior (Cipriani, 2005). According to the FDA, use of antidepressants in a child or adolescent must balance this risk with the clinical need. Patients who are started on therapy should be observed closely for clinical worsening, suicidality, or unusual changes in behavior, particularly in the first 2 months of therapy (National Institute of Mental Health, 2009). This warning was updated in 2007 to also include language stating that scientific data did not show this increased risk in adults older than 24, and that adults ages 65 and older taking antidepressants have a decreased risk of suicidality. The warning statements emphasize that depression and certain other serious psychiatric disorders are themselves the most important causes of suicide (FDA, 2007) rather than particular drug-related responses. A set of guidelines from the FDA on the use of antidepressants and clinical monitoring recommendations can be found at http://www.fda.gov/cder/drug/antidepressants/antidepressants_MG_2007.pdf.

Antipsychotics

FDA Black Box Warning on the Use of Antipsychotic Medications in Those with Dementia

In April 2005, the FDA informed healthcare professionals and the public about the increased risk of mortality in elderly patients receiving second-generation (atypical) antipsychotic drugs to treat dementia-related psychosis. At that time, the analyses of 17 placebo-controlled trials that enrolled 5377 elderly patients with dementia-related behavioral disorders revealed a risk of death in the drug-treated patients of between 1.6 to 1.7 times that seen in placebo-treated patients. Although the causes of death were varied, most of the deaths seemed to be either cardiovascular (e.g., heart failure or sudden death) or infectious (e.g., pneumonia) in nature. Based on this analysis, the FDA requested that the manufacturers of second-generation antipsychotic drugs include information about this risk in a boxed warning and the warnings section of the drugs' prescribing information. Although the initial warnings were related to second-generation antipsychotic medications, in 2005 the warning was extended to include both conventional and second-generation antipsychotic medications (Kuehn, 2005). The specifics of the 2005 Health Advisory can be found at http://www.fda.gov/cder/drug/advisory/antipsychotics.htm, and the 2008 information for healthcare professionals is also available on the FDA Web site at http://www.fda.gov/cder/drug/InfoSheets/HCP/antipsychotics_conventional.htm.

Experts recommend antipsychotics in several geriatric psychiatric disorders, such as late-life schizophrenia, delusional disorder, and psychotic mood disorders (Alexopoulos, Streim, Carpenter, & Docherty, 2004). Providers must assess if symptoms presenting as these disorders are the result of treatable etiologies. These etiologies may include the use of pharmacological agents, such as ß-blockers, anticholinergics, or steroids; dosage additions or changes of other medications; or conditions, such as fluid or electrolyte loss, or infections. Correction by addressing the underlying cause, such as removing offending agents or treating a

disease state, should be the primary goal of therapy. If symptoms continue, an antipsychotic may be temporarily considered. Frequent attempts to withdraw the agent at appropriate intervals based on the disease state are important (Alexopoulos et al.). Gradual reduction is a key regarding attempts to discontinue antipsychotics. Abrupt discontinuation can lead to cholinergic rebound, withdrawal dyskinesias, and relapse or rebound syndrome.

Both conventional and second-generation antipsychotics have been clinically evaluated with older adults. The two classes of antipsychotics differ in both side-effect profiles and documented efficacy and can be considered for use in the older population. However, second-generation agents have generally been considered first line because of what previously was believed to be a more favorable side-effect profile than that of the conventional antipsychotics (Bartels et al., 2003). The second-generation agents include clozapine (Clozaril), risperidone (Risperdal), olanzapine (Zyprexa), quetiapine (Seroquel), ziprasidone (Geodon), and aripiprazole (Abilify). These drugs, with dosing schedule and adverse effects, are featured in Table 6-5. The drug interactions of the second-generation antipsychotics and geriatric considerations are noted in Table 6-6. The conventional agents include haloperidol, fluphenazine, trifluoperazine, chlorpromazine, and thioridazine.

The conventional antipsychotics offer a relatively poor benefit-to-risk ratio because of significant side effect, drug–drug, and drug–disease interaction profiles in the older adult population (Kastrup, 2004). They have considerable anticholinergic and sedative properties, both of which raise serious concerns in older adults. They can lead to falls, fractures, weight loss, pressure ulcers, incontinence, urinary tract infections, and decreased cognition. In addition, they are associated with movement disorders, such as tardive dyskinesia (TD) and extrapyramidal symptoms (EPS). TD is a troubling side effect characterized by involuntary and abnormal movements. EPS can cause patients to experience restlessness, an inability to sit still, or muscle rigidity. Conventional

TABLE 6-5

Second-Generation Antipsychotics: Dosing and Adverse Effects*

Medications	Starting Dose	Maintenance Dose	Adverse Effects
Clozapine (Clozaril)	25 mg/day	Up to 300 to 450 mg/day over slow titration	Agranulocytosis, anticholinergic side effects, cognitive and motor impairment, orthostasis, tachycardia
Risperidone (Risperdal)	0.25 to 0.5 mg once or twice daily	0.75 to 1.5 mg/day	Extrapyramidal symptoms, anticholinergic effects, orthostasis, sedation (all increased at higher dosages), slight increased risk of stroke
Olanzapine (Zyprexa)	5 mg/day	10 to 20 mg/day	Hyperprolactinemia, dose-related somnolence, headache, diabetes, dyslipidemia, slight increased risk of stroke
Quetiapine (Seroquel)	25 mg twice daily	150 to 750 mg/day	Somnolence, dyslipidemia, diabetes, slight increased risk of stroke, seizures, thyroid dysfunction, orthostasis
Ziprasidone (Geodon)	20 mg twice daily	20 to 80 mg twice daily	QT prolongation, cognitive and motor impairment, rash, orthostasis
Aripiprazole (Abilify)	5 mg daily	10 to 30 mg/day	Headache, orthostasis, anxiety, and insomnia

*Neuroleptic malignant syndrome has been reported with all second-generation agents.
Source: Adapted from Bezchlibnyk-Butler, Jeffries, & Virani (2007).

agents also cause increased prolactin secretion, which can lead to such problems as sexual and reproductive dysfunction, breast pathology, bone demineralization, depression, memory deficits, and damage to the cardiovascular endothelium (Bezchlibnyk-Butler et al., 2007).

Although the newer second-generation antipsychotics have become an attractive alternative, they are not devoid of side effects. Each drug in the class has slightly different characteristics, all of which are important to consider in the older adult population. Possible adverse effects of this class include headache, orthostatic hypotension, falls, cardiovascular effects, weight gain, dyslipidemia, diabetes, and to a lesser extent TD and EPS. As a class, however, the second-generation agents have a lower affinity for the dopamine D_2 receptor, which accounts for the relatively low incidence

of EPS, TD, and prolactinemia. The faster the drug dissociates from the D_2 receptor, the lower the rates of these treatment-induced D_2-related side effects. Clozapine and quetiapine have fast dissociation from the D_2 receptor. Olanzapine and risperidone have slower dissociation, and the conventional antipsychotics have even slower dissociation. Therefore, the conventional agents have the highest dopamine D_2-related side effects, followed by olanzapine and risperidone. The dopamine-related side-effect profiles of some second-generation agents are dose-dependent because of loss of specificity. For example, increasing doses of olanzapine, risperidone, and ziprasidone raise relative D_2 occupancy and can begin to resemble side-effect profiles of conventional agents at higher dosages. In older adults, this can be more problematic and occur at lower dosages than in younger age groups (Jeste, 2004).

TABLE 6-6

Second-Generation Antipsychotics: Drug Interactions and Geriatric Considerations

Medications	Drug Interactions	Geriatric Considerations*
Clozapine (Clozaril)	Benzodiazepines, antihypertensives, anticholinergics, CYP1A2	Not recommended for nonpsychotic patients
Risperidone (Risperdal)	CYP2D6 and CYP3A4, increased hypotension with antihypertensives, decreased levels with inducers, St. John's wort	Oral solution can be mixed with water, orange juice, or low-fat milk but not with cola, grapefruit juice, or tea
Olanzapine (Zyprexa)	CYP1A2, CYP2D6, increased hypotension with antihypertensives, decreased levels with inducers, St. John's wort	Half-life 1.5 times that of younger adults
Quetiapine (Seroquel)	CYP3A4, clearance increased with phenytoin	No oral solution available
Ziprasidone (Geodon)	Increased hypotension with antihypertensives, other agents that affect QTc prolongation	No dosage adjustment recommended; start low and titrate slowly based on response, avoid in patients with cardiac disease
Aripiprazole (Abilify)	CYP2D6, CYP3A4, highly protein bound	Once-daily dosing, does not cause weight gain or electrocardiogram changes

*Metoclopramide (Reglan), because of its affinity for dopamine, increases extrapyramidal symptoms, whereas the effects of levodopa may be antagonized by antipsychotics.

Source: Adapted from Desai (2003); Semla, Beizer, & Higbee (2003).

Second-generation antipsychotics have been studied much more extensively in younger populations than in older age groups and have been found to differ from conventional agents in that they have greater ability to treat negative symptoms. In 2004, Marder et al. published a consensus paper on physical health monitoring with persons treated with second-generation antipsychotics. This paper discusses the potential problems with lipid dysregulation, insulin resistance, and potential for type 2 diabetes in conjunction with these agents. In many ways, these problems are the equivalent of what TD was to the conventional antipsychotic agents, and needs to be addressed by any clinician who is working with patients receiving these agents as part of their treatment plan. There are specific guidelines for monitoring weight, lipids, and glucose, and these guidelines have become a dimension of the community standard of practice to which all clinicians are accountable. Additionally, the FDA requires that second-generation antipsychotic medications carry a warning related to risk of hyperglycemia and diabetes (Rosack, 2003). Such changes carry significant implications for the monitoring of older adults who are treated with these agents.

A great deal has been learned since 2004 because of a more concerted effort to understand the metabolic effects of the second-generation antipsychotic medications. It seems that the only medication from this generation of medications that holds significantly less liability for metabolic adverse effects is aripiprazole (Stahl, 2008). The remainder of the agents in this class have vulnerabilities associated with risks for metabolic dysregulation. Stahl uses the analogy of a highway when looking at the trajectory of liabilities associated with second-generation antipsychotic medications. He discusses that the entrance ramp for the metabolic highway is increased appetite and weight gain associated with these medications, and how these factors combined may cause an increase in body mass index to > 25. As one moves down the highway, the process continues with obesity, insulin resistance, and dyslipidemia coupled with increases in fasting triglyceride levels. The end of the road is marked with hyperinsulinemia, leading to pancreatic beta cell failure, prediabetes, and finally diabetes.

The American Diabetes Association (ADA) in conjunction with the American Psychiatric Association, the American Association of Clinical Endocrinologists, and the North American Society for the Study of Obesity examined the evidence related to metabolic dysregulation and put forth recommendations for clinical monitoring (ADA et al., 2004). The guidelines recommend that before the start of a second-generation antipsychotic medication a comprehensive family history of diabetes, cardiovascular disease, obesity, dyslipidemia, and hypertension needs to be taken. Weight must be checked at baseline and then at 4, 8, and 12 weeks and quarterly thereafter. Waist circumference must be measured at baseline and annually. Blood pressure and fasting glucose should be monitored at baseline, 12 weeks, and annually. Finally, fasting lipid monitoring should occur at baseline, 12 weeks, and then at 5-year intervals, providing that the results are normal. A PDF file of the monitoring recommendations can be found at http://www.ohsu.edu/medicine/residency/handouts/pharmpearls/Psychiatry%20CNS%20Neuro/MonitoringTheMetabolicEffectsOfAtypicalAntipsychotics.pdf

Clozapine has been studied for the treatment of psychotic symptoms, including those associated with dementia, and demonstrates overall benefit in over half of the older adult patients treated, especially at low doses. It has minimal effect in the striatal area, which explains its relative low potential for extrapyramidal side effects. Clozapine, however, does have other serious potential side effects in the older adult, such as seizures, hypotension, and potent anticholinergic effects. Even more limiting is the potential of clozapine-induced agranulocytosis, which can have an incidence as high as 1.3% per year (Novartis, 2002) but more commonly is cited in the range of 0.8% of patients treated with this medication, and agranulocytosis may occur in patients even after years of uneventful treatment (Sedky, Shaughnessy, & Hughes, 2005). The risk of fatal agranulocytosis requiring frequent blood monitoring makes it more restrictive to use than other second-generation antipsychotic medications. Clozapine may be considered in older adults refractory to all other choices and possibly in patients with Parkinson's disease, because it does not increase the motor symptoms, like many of the other antipsychotic agents.

Risperidone affects serotonin and dopamine and has been shown to improve both negative and positive symptoms of psychoses while reducing the incidence of EPS (Jeste, Okamoto, Napolitano, Kane, & Martinez, 2000). Risperidone should be dosed as low as possible to maintain efficacy and prevent dose-related D_2 motor side effects. Risperidone has been evaluated in several open-label studies and case studies, and one large randomized controlled trial in older adults with positive benefit (De Deyn et al., 2005).

Olanzapine is thought to work through an antagonism of both dopamine and serotonin receptors. It does affect muscarinic, histamine, and α_1-receptors to a degree that explains potential anticholinergic side effects, sedation, and hypotension. Studies of olanzapine use in the older adult have shown therapeutic effects across a number of conditions not related to dementia, particularly with delirium (Ozbolt, 2008). Olanzapine can increase the potential for development of diabetes and associated problems. Olanzapine can also contribute to the development of dyslipidemia. Therefore, proper monitoring for these two conditions is necessary.

Quetiapine is thought to work through a combination of dopamine and serotonin antagonism. It has no appreciable affinity for muscarinic or benzodiazepine receptors but does cause some blockade at histamine and α_1-receptors. Therefore, quetiapine can cause somnolence and orthostatic hypotension. Quetiapine does have a good EPS tolerability profile across the entire dose range (AstraZeneca Pharmaceuticals LP, 2004). The most common adverse events exhibited across placebo-controlled trials included headache, somnolence, and dizziness (Tariot, Salzman, Yeung, Pultz, & Rak, 2000). Quetiapine has been shown to be effective in the treatment of psychosis in older adults and in patients with Parkinson's disease. Effective doses are often lower when used in older adults (Friedman & Factor, 2000).

Ziprasidone and aripiprazole are two antipsychotic medications that have been used in the treatment of older adults with psychiatric illnesses. In general, there is no indication of any different tolerability of ziprasidone or for reduced clearance of ziprasidone in older adults compared to younger adults. However, dosages should still be started low and titrated slowly to therapeutic response with careful monitoring of potential side effects, such as orthostasis (Pfizer, 2002). Aripiprazole, another new antipsychotic, has common side effects of somnolence and orthostatic hypotension (Bristol-Myers Squibb, 2003; Burris et al., 2002). Aripiprazole is the first antipsychotic agent on the market whose mechanism of action includes dopamine partial agonism and serotonin antagonism. This unique mechanism of action places it in a class by itself, and it may be the first "atypical" second-generation antipsychotic agent. The alleged benefits of aripiprazole include an absence of hyperprolactinemia, reduced risk for weight gain and type 2 diabetes, and absence of dyslipidemia (Davies, Sheffler, & Roth, 2004).

It is important to note that the misuse of antipsychotics in older adults, particularly in long-term care settings, prompted the passage of OBRA in 1987 with modifications in 1990. This act mandated nursing home reform. Among its many stipulations, it stated that residents had the right to be free from chemical and physical restraints imposed for the purpose of convenience or discipline and not required to treat a medical condition. Further, there must be documented need for the use of this category of drugs to treat a specific condition. This act focused on improving quality of life and eliminating the unnecessary use of antipsychotic, anxiolytic, and sedative-hypnotic drugs as a means of chemically restraining older adults in long-term care settings.

Anxiolytics

Proper treatment of anxiety in older adults requires proper diagnosis by addressing organic causes, comorbid psychiatric conditions, or a medication that causes anxiety-related side effects. There are very little evidence-based data to guide anxiolytic therapy (Bartels et al., 2003). However, antianxiety medications should be prescribed based on the suitability of the drug for an individual patient, taking into account potential side effects and compatibility with the existing medication profile (Stahl, 2008). Antidepressants may be recommended as first-line therapy for anxiety disorders, but a short course of a benzodiazepine sometimes is considered (Alexopoulos et al., 2004). If a benzodiazepine is prescribed, it is important to appreciate the potential risks associated with its use.

Benzodiazepines have a side-effect profile particularly dangerous in older adults. Benzodiazepines are likely to cause sedation and a decrease in hand-eye coordination. The outcome of benzodiazepine use at modest doses impairs driving performance in the older driver to a level similar to the legal definition of alcohol intoxication (Beers & Berkow, 2004). Ataxia, slurred speech, impaired coordination, confusion, poor concentration, memory loss, sleep disturbances, and depressive symptoms also may occur. Patients should be monitored closely for adverse effects.

OBRA guidelines for benzodiazepine use with residents of long-term care facilities are fairly specific related to use with proper diagnoses, which drugs to avoid, duration of treatment, attempts at withdrawal of medication, and maximum daily dose (OBRA, 1987). Generally, geriatric patients experience fewer adverse effects from shorter-acting drugs without active metabolites, such as alprazolam, lorazepam, and oxazepam. Longer-acting drugs, such as diazepam and chlordiazepoxide, should be avoided. Short-acting benzodiazepines are listed in Table 6-7 with the recommended dosing schedule. It is generally recommended to use low regularly scheduled doses, but as-needed dosing (prn) may be beneficial in certain patients. Clinicians need to consider when and how to discontinue the antianxiety medications once they are started. A brief period of 4 to 6 weeks may be all that is required for treatment, but benzodiazepines may require an additional 3 to 4 weeks to be gradually tapered. Older adults should be aware of the need for short-term treatment with these agents, to prepare them better for proper titration off the drug at the appropriate time. Tapering a benzodiazepine too quickly can lead to rebound anxiety or even a withdrawal syndrome with possible seizures.

An alternative to benzodiazepines is buspirone (Buspar). Buspirone is less sedating than the benzodiazepines and is not addicting. Efficacy and safety of this drug are reported to be equal in older adults compared to younger adults (Semla et al., 2003). The initial dose is 5 mg twice daily and titrated by 5 mg daily up to an average dose of 20 to 30 mg divided into two or three doses per day. Buspirone takes longer to show subjective benefit than benzodiazepines; it usually begins to show benefit after 2 weeks and maximum benefit after 4 weeks of continuous therapy. Because of this delay in effect, patients who have used benzodiazepines in the past may be resistant to using buspirone. Concomitant use of benzodiazepines with buspirone reduces the effectiveness of buspirone.

TABLE 6-7

Preferred Benzodiazepines and Dosing Schedule*

Medication (Short-Acting Benzodiazepines)	Initial Dose (mg)	Recommended Maximum Daily Dose (mg)*	Dosing in Hepatic and Renal Disease	Dosage Forms
Alprazolam (Xanax)	0.125 to 0.25 BID	0.75	Decrease 50% in hepatic impairment, avoid in cirrhosis, caution in renal disease	Tablet, liquid
Lorazepam (Ativan)	0.25 to 0.5 BID	2	Caution if renal or hepatic disease	Tablet, liquid, intramuscular injection
Oxazepam (Serax)	10 BID	30	Avoid in hepatic disease, caution yet safer option in renal impairment	Tablet, capsule

* Per HCFA guidelines for residents of long-term care facilities.

Source: Adapted from Bezchlibnyk-Butler, Jeffries, & Virani (2007).

SUMMARY

Psychotropic medications are the second most commonly prescribed class of drugs in the geriatric population and the class most frequently associated with adverse drug reactions (Ives, 2001). It is essential for clinicians to recognize that good prescribing practice is a multifaceted process. This process not only involves the clinician's knowledge of pharmacotherapeutics but also takes into account patient and caregiver status, and financial concerns and insurance restrictions. The treatment of mental illness in older adults, as noted in this chapter, presents challenges unique to this patient population. By carefully considering and weighing the many factors that influence the treatment of mental illness in older adults, clinicians will evidence the very best prescribing practice as they address the mental health needs of older adults.

REFERENCES

Alexopoulos, G. S. Katz, I. R., Reynolds, C. F., Carpenter, D., & Docherty, J. P. (2001). Pharmacotherapy of depressive disorders in older patients. The Expert Consensus Guideline Series. A special report. *Postgraduate Medicine, 113*, 1–82.

Alexopoulos, G. S., Streim, J., Carpenter, D., & Docherty, J. P. (2004). Introduction: Methods, commentary, and summary. *The Journal of Clinical Psychiatry, 65*(Suppl. 2), 5–19.

American Diabetes Association, American Psychiatric Association, American Association of Clinical Endocrinologists, & North American Association for the Study of Obesity. (2004). Consensus Development Conference on Antipsychotic Drugs and Obesity and Diabetes. *Diabetes Care, 27*, 596–601.

American Nurses Association. (2001). *Psychiatric mental health nursing psychopharmacology project.* Washington, DC: American Nurses Publishing.

American Psychiatric Association. (2000). *Practice guideline for the treatment of patients with major depression.* Washington, DC: Author.

Andrade, C. (2004). Antidepressant-withdrawal mania: a critical review and synthesis of the literature. *Journal of Clinical Psychiatry, 65*(7), 987–993.

AstraZeneca Pharmaceuticals LP. (2004). *Seroquel* [product insert]. Wilmington, DE: Author.

Bartels, S., Dums, A., Oxman, T., Schneider, L., Areán, P., & Alexopoulos, G., et al. (2003). Evidence-based practices in geriatric mental health care: An overview of systematic reviews and meta-analyses. *The Psychiatric Clinics of North America, 26*, 971–990.

Beers, M. H. (1997). Explicit criteria for determining potentially inappropriate medication use by the elderly. *Archives of Internal Medicine, 157*, 1531–1536.

Beers, M., & Berkow, R. (Eds.). (2004). *Merck manual of geriatrics.* Whitehouse Station, NJ: Merck Research Labs.

Bezchlibnyk-Butler, K. Z., Jeffries, J. J., & Virani, A. S. (Eds.). (2007). *Clinical handbook of psychotropic drugs.* Cambridge, MA: Hogrefe Publishing.

Blanchette, C. M., Simoni-Wastila, L., Shaya, F., Orwig, D., Noel, J., & Stuart, B. (2009). Health care use in depressed, elderly, cardiac patients and the effect of antidepressant use. *American Journal of Health-Systems Pharmacy, 66*(4), 366–372.

Bristol-Myers Squibb. (2001). *Serzone* [package insert]. Princeton, NJ: Author.

Bristol-Myers Squibb. (2003). *Abilify* [package insert]. Princeton, NJ: Author.

Burris, K., Molski, T., Xu, C., Ryan, E., Tottori, K., & Kikuchi, T. (2002). Aripiprazole, a novel antipsychotic, is a high-affinity partial agonist at human dopamine D2 receptors. *The Journal of Pharmacology and Experimental Therapeutics, 302*(1), 381–389.

Choi, S. (2003). Nefazodone (Serzone) withdrawn because of hepatotoxicity. *Canadian Medical Association Journal, 169*(11), 29.

Cipriani, A. (2005). Suicide, depression and antidepressants. *British Medical Journal, 330*, 373–374.

Davies, M. A., Sheffler, D. J., & Roth, B. L. (2004). Aripiprazole: A novel atypical antipsychotic drug with a uniquely robust pharmacology. *CNS Drug Review, 10*(4), 317–336.

De Deyn, P. P., Katz, I. R., Brodaty, H., Lyons, B., Greenspan, A., & Burns, A. (2005). Management of agitation, aggression, and psychosis associated with dementia: A pooled analysis including three randomized, placebo controlled double blind trials in nursing home residents treated with respiradone. *Clinical Neurology and Neurosurgery, 107*(6), 497–508.

Desai, A. (2003). Use of pharmacologic agents in the elderly. *Clinics in Geriatric Medicine, 19*(4), 697–719.

Dilsaver, S. C., Greden, J. F., & Snider, R. M. (1987). Antidepressant withdrawal syndromes: Phenomenology and pathophysiology. *International Clinical Psychopharmacology, 2*, 1–19.

Edlund, B. (2004). Medication use and misuse. *Journal of Gerontological Nursing, 30*(7), 4.

Eli Lilly. (2004). *Cymbalta* [package insert]. Indianapolis, IN: Author.

Fick, D. M., Cooper, J. W., Wade, W. E., Waller, J. L., Maclean, J. R., & Beers, M. H. (2003). Updating the Beers criteria for potentially inappropriate medication use in older adults: Results of a US consensus panel of experts. *Archives of Internal Medicine, 163*, 2716–2724.

Food and Drug Administration. (2007). Antidepressant use in children, adolescents and adults. Retrieved April 5, 2009, from http://www.fda.gov/Drugs/DrugSafety/InformationbyDrugClass/UCM096273

Friedman, J. H., & Factor, S. A. (2000). Atypical antipsychotics in the treatment of drug-induced psychosis in Parkinson's disease. *Movement Disorders, 15*(2), 201–211.

Glaxo SmithKline. (2003). *Wellbutrin XL* [package insert]. Research Triangle Park, NC: Author.

Ives, T. J. (2001). Pharmacotherapeutics. In R. Ham, P. Sloane, & G. Warshaw (Eds.), *Primary care geriatrics: A case-based approach* (pp. 137–148). St. Louis: Mosby.

Jeste, D. V. (2004). Tardive dyskinesia rates with atypical antipsychotics in older adults. *Journal of Clinical Psychiatry, 65*(Suppl. 9), 21–24.

Jeste, D. V., Okamoto, A., Napolitano, J., Kane, J. M., & Martinez, R. A. (2000). Low incidence of persistent tardive dyskinesia in elderly patients with dementia treated with risperidone. *American Journal of Psychiatry, 157*, 1150–1155.

Kane, R., Ouslander, J., & Abrass, I. (2004). *Essentials of clinical geriatrics*. New York: McGraw-Hill.

Kastrup, E. (2004). *Drug facts and comparisons*. St. Louis, MO: Kluwer Health.

Keltner, N., & Folks, D. (2005). *Psychotropic drugs* (4th ed.). St. Louis, MO: Mosby.

Kuehn, B. M. (2005). FDA warns that antipsychotic drugs are risky for elders. *JAMA, 293*, 2462.

Kush, R. D., Bleicher, P., Raymond, S., Kubich, W., Marks, R., & Tardiff B. (2007). *PDR for Herbal Medicines* (4th ed.). Chicago, IL: Thompson.

Leff, E. W., & Sonstegard-Gamm, J. (2006). The home care team approach to self-neglecting elders. *Home Health Nurse, 24*(4), 249–257.

Lotufo-Neto, F., Trivedi, M., & Thase, M. E. (1999). Meta-analysis of the reversible inhibitors of monoamine oxidase type A moclobemide and brofaromine for the treatment of depression. *Neuropsychopharmacology, 20*, 226–247.

Lueckenotte, A. (1996). *Gerontological nursing*. St. Louis, MO: Mosby.

Marder, S. R., Essock, S. M., Miller, A. L., Buchanan, R. W., Casey, D. E., Davis, J. M., et al. (2004). Physical health monitoring of patients with schizophrenia. *American Journal of Psychiatry, 161*(8), 1334–1349.

McEnany, G. W. (2001). Herbal psychotropics (Part 4): Focus on gingko biloba, L-carnitine, lactobacillus/acidophilus & ginger root. *Journal of the American Psychiatric Nurses Association, 7*(1), 22–25.

Metlay, J. P. (2008). Medication comprehension and safety in older adults. *LDI Issue Brief, 14*(1), 1–4.

National Institute of Mental Health. (2009). *Antidepressant medications for children and adolescents: Information for parents and caregivers*. Retrieved May 6, 2009, from http://www.nimh.nih.gov/health/topics/child-and-adolescent-mental-health/antidepressant-medications-for-children-and-adolescents-information-for-parents-and-caregivers.shtml

Nemeroff, C. B. (2003). Improving antidepressant adherence. *Journal of Clinical Psychiatry, 64*(Suppl. 18), 25–30.

Nicholas, L. M., Ford, A. L., Esposito, S. M., Ekstrom, R. D., & Golden, R. N. (2003). The effects of mirtazapine on plasma lipid profiles in healthy subjects. *Journal of Clinical Psychiatry, 64*(8), 883–889.

Nixdorff, N., Hustey, F. M., Brady, A. K., Vaji, K., Leonard, M., & Messinger-Rapport, B. J. (2008). Potentially inappropriate medications and adverse drug effects in elders in the ED. *American Journal of Emergency Medicine, 26*(6), 697–700.

Novartis. (2002). *Clozaril* [package insert]. East Hanover, NJ: Author.

Omnibus Budget Reconciliation Act. (1987). *Subtitle C, nursing home reform: PL100-203*. Washington, DC: National Coalition for Nursing Home Reform.

Organon. (2002). *Remeron SolTab* [package insert]. West Orange, NJ: Author.

Ozbolt, L. B. (2008). Atypical antipsychotics for the treatment of delirious elders. *Journal of American Medical Directors Association, 9*(1), 18–22.

Pariente, A., Dartigues, J. F., Benichou, J., Letenneur, L., Moore, N., & Fourrier-Réglat, A. (2008). Benzodiazepines and injurious falls in community dwelling elders. *Drugs and Aging, 25*(1), 61–70.

Perahia, D. G., Kajdasz, D. K., Desaiah, D., & Haddad, P. M. (2005). Symptoms following abrupt discontinuation of duloxetine treatment in patients with major depressive disorder. *Journal of Affective Disorders, 89*(1), 207–212.

Peterson, J. F., Gilad, J., Kuperman, G. K., Shek, C., Patel, M., Avorn, J., et al. (2005). Guided prescription of psychotropic medications for geriatric inpatients. *Archives of Internal Medicine, 165*, 802–807.

Pfizer. (2002). *Geodon* [package insert]. New York: Author.

Qato, D. M., Alexander, G. C., Conti, R. M., Johnson, M., Schumm, P., & Lindau, S. T. (2008). Use of prescription and over-the-counter medications and dietary supplements among older adults in the United States. *JAMA, 300*(24), 2867–2878.

Rosack, J. (2003). FDA to require diabetes warning on antipsychotics. *Psychiatric News, 38*(20), 1.

Sadock, B., & Sadock, A. (2009). *Synopsis of psychiatry*. Philadelphia: Lippincott Williams & Wilkins.

Sedky, K., Shaughnessy, R., & Hughes, T. (2005). Clozapine-induced agranulocytosis after 11 years of treatment. *American Journal of Psychiatry, 162*, 814.

Semla, T. P., Beizer, J. L., & Higbee, M. D. (2003). *Geriatric dosage handbook* (8th ed.). Hudson, OH: Lexi-comp.

Stahl, S. M. (2008). *Essential psychopharmacology: Neuroscientific basis and practical applications* (3rd ed.). Cambridge: Cambridge University Press.

Tariot, P. N., Salzman, C., Yeung, P. P., Pultz, J., & Rak, I. W. (2000). Long-term use of quetiapine in elderly patients with psychotic disorders. *Clinical Therapeutics, 22*(9), 1068–1084.

Thomas, K. W. (2009). Antipsychotics and the elderly. *American Journal of Nursing, 109*(3), 13.

U.S. Bureau of the Census. (2000). *Demographic data*. Available at: www.census.gov

U.S. Department of Health and Human Services. (2000). *Healthy People 2010: Understanding and improving health*. Retrieved March 16, 2004, from http://www.health.gov/healthtypeople/

Voyer, P., Cohen, D., Lauzon, S., & Collin, J. (2004). Factors associated with psychotropic drug use among community-dwelling older persons: A review of empirical studies. *BMC Nurs, 3*(1), 3.

Wyeth-Ayerst. (2003). *Effexor* [package insert]. Philadelphia: Author.

Wyeth. (2008). *Pristiq* [package insert]. Philadelphia: Author.

II

Psychopathology of Late Life

7

Nursing Assessment and Treatment of Depressive Disorders of Late Life

Eve Heemann Byrd
Nancie A. Vito

Depression is a disorder of mood, so mysteriously painful and elusive in the way it becomes known to the self—to the mediating intellect—as to verge close to being beyond description. It thus remains nearly incomprehensible to those who have not experienced it in its extreme mood, although the gloom, "the blues" which people go through occasionally and associate with the general hassle of everyday existence are of such prevalence that they do give many individuals a hint of the illness in its catastrophic form.

William Styron, *Darkness Visible: A Memoir of Madness* (1990)

The President's New Freedom Commission on Mental Health (2003) has recognized that mental health is essential to overall health. The World Health Organization's (WHO) definition of health, which has not been amended since 1948, is stated in the WHO Constitution as follows: "Health is a state of complete physical, mental and social well-being and not merely the absence of disease or infirmity" (WHO, 2006, p. 1). Little more than a decade ago the U.S. Department of Health and Human Services (DHHS) Report of the Surgeon General declared that, "The mind and body are inseparable" (1999, p. 5).

Depression is one of the most common, often the most debilitating, yet the most treatable illnesses seen in older adults. The WHO has declared that depression is one of the leading causes of disability. Unipolar depression ranks fourth in the leading causes of disability adjusted life years and it is projected to rise to the second cause of disability and second "most burdensome" worldwide by 2020 (WHO, 2009). According to the Agency for Healthcare Research and Quality (AHRQ, 2007), major depressive disorder is the most common of the depressive disorders. It is estimated that between 1% and 5% of older adults living in the community experience major depression. The percentage increases to 11.5% of elderly hospital patients and 13.5% who require home health care (Hybels & Blazer, 2003). Older adult women are almost twice as likely to suffer from depression as older adult men.

CONSEQUENCES OF DEPRESSION

There is increasing evidence that depression is associated with other physical illnesses. Many people with chronic diseases suffer from depression and other mental disorders, which worsens their physical condition and hinders their ability to follow a prescribed healthcare regimen (WHO, 2003). Kessler et al. (2003) note that major depressive disorder is usually associated with "substantial symptom severity and role impairment" (p. 3095). Despite knowledge that depression frequently co-occurs with many other medical illnesses and although there is evidence that more persons with depression are being diagnosed by their primary care providers, most cases remain either untreated or undertreated (Wang et al., 2005).

Untreated depression is associated with poorer quality of life, higher use of medical care, increased medical costs, and increased disability (Centers for Disease Control and Prevention [CDC], 2005; Nemeroff, Musselman, & Evans, 1998). According to the WHO (2003), the burden of disease from mental disorders is expected to increase significantly over the next 20 years. The WHO reports that depression has a high prevalence–cost ratio and that "investing in mental health today can generate enormous returns in terms of reducing disability . . ." (p. 6). Pearson and colleagues (1999) confirmed a strong association exists between depression and an increased use of general medical services, such as outpatient visits, hospitalizations, and total hospital days.

Depression is not only disabling, but there is increasing evidence that depression is a fatal illness in older adults. Depression is the leading risk factor for suicide. The suicide rate for persons 65 years and older is greater than any other age group. In 2004, just over 12% of the U.S. population was older adults, and older adults accounted for 16% of all suicides (CDC, 2008). The highest frequency is found among white males 75 years and older at 14.7 per 100,000 (CDC).

Depression in older adults costs the nation an estimated $43 billion per year, not including the pain, suffering, and poor quality of life that results from depression (American Association of Geriatric Psychiatry, 2001). Furthermore, in one recent study, older adults with depression were found to incur twice as many Medicare costs as older adults who were not depressed (Unützer et al., 2009). Ours is an aging society and as the average age of the population increases, there will be an increased cost to the American public as a result of unnecessary

disability and mortality should late-life depression go undiagnosed and inadequately treated.

GLOBAL AND NATIONAL INITIATIVES FOR MENTAL HEALTH

Mental health is one of the top 10 leading health indicators of *Healthy People 2010* (DHHS, 2000). One of the major goals of *Healthy People 2010* is to improve access to mental health treatment. Other *Healthy People 2010* objectives for mental health include improving treatment access by increasing mental health screening and assessment in primary care offices, increasing the proportion of adults with mental disorders who receive treatment, and increasing recognition of depression in adults over the age of 18. As recommended by the WHO in 2007, providing mental health treatment in primary care offers the greatest promise of reducing the mental health global burden of disease. Furthermore, the final July 2003 report issued by the President's New Freedom Commission on Mental Health creates the vision for the United States as ". . . a future when everyone with mental illness will recover . . . , mental illnesses are detected early . . . , and everyone with a mental illness at any stage of life has access to effective treatment and supports . . ." (p. 1). The six goals of this report are as follows (p. 5):

1. Americans understand that mental health is essential to overall health.
2. Mental health care is consumer and family driven.
3. Disparities in mental health services are eliminated.
4. Early mental health screening, assessment, and referral to services are common practice.
5. Excellent mental health care is delivered and research is accelerated.
6. Technology is used to access mental health care and information.

The Mental Health Atlas published by the WHO (2005) notes "geographic disparities in mental health services delivery" exist, with a shortage of mental health services, especially in rural areas of the United States. The report also recognizes the fact that there is not currently a program in place that regularly provides training to primary care providers on the topic of mental health. Another barrier to mental health services for older adults is the combined stigma associated with being old and having a mental illness. Nurses are in a position to play a significant role in educating their patients and the community, decreasing stigma, and decreasing older adult disability and mortality. However, nurses must first assess their own prejudices toward persons with mental illness. Ageism and the stigma associated with depression are among the underlying reasons for the numerous barriers that older adults encounter in attempting to receive treatment for depression.

Older adults think depression is a normal part of aging. According to *Mental Health America* (2006), 58% of people 65 years of age and older believe it is normal for persons to get depressed as they get older. American culture and healthcare delivery perpetuate this belief. For decades Medicare has reimbursed only 50% of the Medicare allowable amount for psychological health services. In October 2008, the Mental Health Parity and Addiction Equity Act was signed into law in the United States, which will help decrease a barrier to mental health treatment. Once fully implemented and mental health services are reimbursed by Medicare at a rate similar to other medical illnesses, the financial burden of receiving mental health services will be lessened and the implication that mental health services are less needed or less worthy of reimbursement will be eliminated.

The *Surgeon General's Report* (DHHS, 1999) states that the only way the mental health needs of America will be met is for "nonmental health professionals" to be educated and participate in the mental health care of persons suffering from mental illness. The *World Health Report of 2006* (WHO, 2006) recognized that because there is a shortage of mental health providers, a shift needs to occur to include mental health services in community-based care and in primary care. In this report it is noted, ". . . the new emphasis on multidisciplinary and intersectoral approaches means changing roles for staff as well . . . . The challenge for health workers is to embrace change as an opportunity for further learning and personal and professional development . . ." (p. 26). Furthermore, Demyttenaere et al. (2004) note that reallocation of resources could help the unmet need of the treatment of mental disorders.

Nurses must educate themselves regarding depression and its treatments and must recognize that frequently they are the healthcare provider who spends the most time with an older client; therefore, nurses are often in a key position to assess for symptoms of depression. Nurses need to advocate for healthcare services and environments aimed at prevention and early recognition of depression. Finally, nurses must also advocate for adequate treatment. The nurse's goal in treating an older adult with depression is full remission from the illness.

Depression is insidious. It invades all aspects of the older adult's life: physical, mental, social, and spiritual. Symptoms of depression, such as loss of interest in activities, social withdrawal, irritability, anxiety, chronic aches and pains that do not respond to treatment, and increased dependency, are often incorrectly explained as a normal part of aging. Older adult women have described depression as "the reexperiencing of a severe personal insult" that results in feelings of worthlessness, increased vulnerability or insecurity, a loss of self-respect, and feelings of inferiority or incompetence (Hedelin & Strandmark, 2001, p. 407). The symptoms of depression are also too often attributed to neurological or other physical illnesses by both physicians and patients. Neurovegetative symptoms, such as sleep disturbances, loss of appetite, poor concentration, and low energy, are frequently explained as symptoms of a comorbid illness. There is a growing body of evidence that depression not only contributes to poor medical outcomes because of unhealthy behavior but it is also an etiologic factor in such illnesses as cardiovascular disease, stroke, cancer, and epilepsy (Evans et al., 2003). Depression, the "unwanted cotraveler," a phrase coined at the March 2001 National Institute of Mental Health Forum, also affects the progression of chronic illnesses, such as cardiovascular, cerebrovascular, and neurological disorders; diabetes; cancer; and HIV–AIDS (Evans et al.). Therefore, a strong case can be made for the development and implementation of depression prevention, early detection, and adequate treatment strategies.

ETIOLOGY

Typically, depression is multifactorial in origin and requires a biopsychosocial evaluation. Depression in late life can either be the recurrence of an illness experienced earlier or it can show up for the first time later in life, after the age of 55. Depression in older adults is most frequently associated with physiological changes or abnormalities of the brain (Lebowitz et al., 1997). These changes are thought to be of vascular origin or the result of early changes caused by dementing illnesses, such as Alzheimer's disease or vascular dementia. These physiological changes affect synaptic activity, causing fewer serotonin receptor sites or impaired receptor response (Blazer, 2003).

Despite some contradictory findings, most studies demonstrate the potential for neuroimaging (both structural and functional magnetic resonance imaging) to serve as an important diagnostic biomarker for late-life depression. Steffens argues that neuroimaging should be the gold standard in diagnosing vascular depression (Steffens, 2004). Vascular depression seems to exhibit different clinical characteristics including apathy and psychomotor changes, poorer response to antidepressant therapies, and association with a greater risk of cognitive decline and mortality (Alexopoulous et al., 1997; Steffens & Krishnan, 1998; Vaishnavi & Taylor, 2006). Although neuroimaging may be useful in diagnosing vascular depression, the findings do not provide information that will guide treatment and improve treatment outcomes in

vascular depression, and thus neuroimaging is not currently used as a diagnostic tool. The ability to quantify the brain's function with the use of both structural and functional neuroimaging is necessary to provide optimal targeted treatment (Mayberg, 2003).

Hormonal changes have also been associated with depression. Low levels of estrogen and dehydroepiandrosterone in women and low levels of total testosterone in older men have been shown to be associated with depressive symptoms; however, the efficacy of treating either has not been established (Blazer, 2003; Lebowitz et al., 1997; Tweedy, Morrison, & DeMichele, 2002).

In addition to the biological etiology of depression in older adults, there are clearly psychological contributing factors. The older adult's life events and the interpretation and response to the events contribute to the risk for developing depression. The predominant life events that put an older adult at risk for depression, and contribute to the older adult's experience and receptiveness to treatment for depression, are medical illness, bereavement or death of a loved one, disability, trauma, and impaired social support (Bruce & Pearson, 1999). These risk factors do not necessarily individually cause depression; rather, it may be the chain of events that results in depression (Bruce & Pearson). Risk factors, coupled with behavioral, psychodynamic, and negative thoughts surrounding life events, seem to contribute to late-life depression (Blazer, 2003). For instance, older adults' interpretation of their situation may be that no matter what they do, bad things continue to happen or they continue to experience losses, so they assume a helpless position. Older adults also may not adapt to physical changes that occur with aging and may have unrealistic expectations and feel as if they continue to fail (Blazer). The current culture that places value on one's accomplishments or one's physical ability to "do," versus an individual's contribution to the greater good, may compound the older adult's feelings of inadequacy. Impaired social support is also associated with depression in older adults (Blazer).

ASSESSMENT AND SCREENING OF LATE-LIFE DEPRESSION

Most older adults fall into one or more at-risk groups for depression. Many, however, do not recognize their symptoms as depression and do not request an evaluation. As previously mentioned, older adults may be resistant to seeking treatment because of the stigma of mental illness. As a result, all older adults should be screened for depression whether they present in a primary care office, hospital, long-term care home, or community senior center. Screening for major depression and other mental health disorders implemented in clinics at the local level is one of the six goals of the President's New Freedom Commission on Mental Health (2003). Likewise, the U.S. Preventive Services Task Force recommends "screening adults for depression in clinical practices that have systems in place to assure accurate diagnosis, effective treatment, and follow-up" (AHRQ, 2002). It has been shown that screening for depression is cost-effective (Nease & Maloin, 2003).

The first two questions of the Patient Health Questionnaire (PHQ)-9 (Figures 7-1a and 7-1b) have been shown to be valid in detecting depressive symptoms, with a sensitivity of 83% and a specificity of 92% for major depression with a PHQ-2 score of 3 or greater (Kroenke, Spitzer, & Williams, 2003). This two-item questionnaire (PHQ-2) is a short version of the original nine-item questionnaire, which is comprised of the symptoms of depression listed in the *Diagnostic and Statistical Manual of Mental Disorders IV* ([DSM-IV] American Psychiatric Association [APA], 2000). A meta-analysis of 22 studies revealed that two to four question tools can accurately detect depression (Mitchell & Coyne, 2007). The two questions on the PHQ-2 are comprised of the two key or hallmark symptoms of depression, which are related to mood (feeling blue, down, or sad) and anhedonia (having little interest or pleasure in doing things). The U.S. Preventive Services Task Force notes that asking these two questions may be as effective as using longer instruments

(AHRQ, 2002). These two questions can easily be added to a primary care health history questionnaire. Each question has an answer range of zero to three, with a possible total of six. When a patient answers positively one (or two) of the questions to obtain a score of three or above, the staff member could then either administer the nine-item questionnaire (the PHQ-9) to complete a full screening or refer to an outside resource for a full evaluation. If a patient completes the nine-item questionnaire and the score (greater than five) indicates the patient is experiencing symptoms of depression, a more thorough evaluation is indicated.

The Geriatric Depression Screening tool (Yesavage & Brink, 1983) is a valid and useful self-rated screening instrument (Figure 7-2). It is used frequently for detecting depression in older adults who have co-occurring medical illness and in older adults with mild to moderate cognitive impairment. A score of greater than 10 out of 30 yes-or-no questions is considered to be significant for depression and warrants a more thorough evaluation. There is also a 15-item or short form version of this tool. One drawback of the Geriatric Depression Screening is that it does not include a question on suicidal thought or intent.

Another screening instrument recommended for use in persons with dementia is an interviewer-rated scale called the Cornell Scale for Depression in Dementia (Figure 7-3) (Alexopoulos, Abrams, Young, & Shamoian, 1988; Alexopoulos, Katz, Reynolds, Carpenter, & Docherty, 2001). This is a 19-item questionnaire that takes approximately 20 to 30 minutes to administer. A score of 12 or greater indicates depression.

The need to gather information regarding the patient's symptoms from a caregiver for the purpose of diagnosing an older adult with depression has been accepted for years. There are emerging data that suggest as many as 27% of older adults who are not cognitively impaired and have depression living in residential facilities would go unidentified if collateral information regarding symptoms was not gathered from nursing staff (Davison, McCabe, & Mellor, 2009). Older adults

FIGURE 7-1a

Two-Question Screen for Depression: Patient Health Questionnaire 2 (PHQ-2).

During the last two weeks have you often been bothered:

- By having little interest or pleasure in doing things?   ❑ Yes   ❑ No
- By feeling down, sad, or hopeless?   ❑ Yes   ❑ No

If the client answers **YES** to either question, administer the PHQ-9 below.

FIGURE 7-1b

Patient Health Questionnaire (PHQ-9).

Read each item carefully and circle the client's response. Use a response card as necessary.

Over the last 2 weeks, how often have you been bothered by any of the following problems? (Repeat this as needed.)	Not at All	Several Days	More Than Half the Days	Nearly Every Day
1. Little interest or pleasure in doing things	0	1	2	3
2. Feeling down, depressed, or hopeless	0	1	2	3
3. Trouble falling asleep, staying asleep, or sleeping too much	0	1	2	3
4. Feeling tired or having little energy	0	1	2	3
5. Poor appetite or overeating	0	1	2	3
6. Feeling bad about yourself—or that you are a failure or have let yourself or your family down	0	1	2	3
7. Trouble concentrating on things, such as reading the newspaper or watching television	0	1	2	3

(continues)

FIGURE 7-1b

Patient Health Questionnaire (PHQ-9). *(continued)*

Over the last 2 weeks, how often have you been bothered by any of the following problems? (Repeat this as needed.)	Not at All	Several Days	More Than Half the Days	Nearly Every Day
8. Moving or speaking so slowly that other people could have noticed. Or the opposite—being so fidgety or restless that you have been moving around more that usual	0	1	2	3
9. Thoughts that you would be better off dead, or of hurting yourself in some way	0	1	2	3
Totals	___	___	___	___

10. If you have checked off *any* problems, how difficult have these problems made it for you to do your work, take care of things at home, or get along with other people?

Not Difficult at All	Somewhat Difficult	Very Difficult	Extremely Difficult
0	1	2	3

Suicide Risk: For any positive response to #9 above, ask this question and adhere to your agency's suicide protocol:

Do you feel these thoughts are a problem for you or something you might act on?   ❏ Yes ❏ No

PHQ-9 Scoring: ≤ 4—suggests that the patient may not need depression treatment; ≥ 5 to 14—physician uses clinical judgment about treatment, based on patient's duration of symptoms and functional impairment; ≥ 15—warrants treatment for depression, using antidepressant, psychotherapy, or combination of treatment. A functional health assessment is reflected in question 10 on the PHQ-9, which asks the patient how emotional difficulties or problems impact work, things at home, or relationships with other people. Patient responses can be one of four (see question 10). A response of very difficult or extremely difficult suggests that the patient's functionality is impaired.

FIGURE 7-2

Geriatric Depression Screening Tool.

	Yes	No	
1.	X	❑	Are you basically satisfied with your life?
2.	❑	X	Have you dropped many of your activities and interests?
3.	❑	X	Do you feel that your life is empty?
4.	❑	X	Do you often get bored?
5.	X	❑	Are you hopeful about the future?
6.	❑	X	Are you bothered by thoughts that you can't get out of your head?
7.	X	❑	Are you in good spirits most of the time?
8.	❑	X	Are you afraid that something bad is going to happen to you?
9.	X	❑	Do you feel happy most of the time?
10.	❑	X	Do you feel helpless?
11.	❑	X	Do you often get restless and fidgety?
12.	❑	X	Do you prefer to stay at home, rather than going out and doing new things?
13.	❑	X	Do you frequently worry about the future?
14.	❑	X	Do you feel you have more problems with your memory than most?
15.	X	❑	Do you think it is wonderful to be alive now?
16.	❑	X	Do you often feel downhearted and blue?
17.	❑	X	Do you feel pretty worthless the way you are now?
18.	❑	X	Do you often worry a lot about the past?
19.	X	❑	Do you find life very exciting?
20.	❑	X	Is it hard for you to get started on new projects?
21.	X	❑	Do you feel full of energy?
22.	❑	X	Do you feel that your situation is hopeless?
23.	❑	X	Do you think that most people are better off than you are?
24.	❑	X	Do you frequently get upset over little things?
25.	❑	X	Do you frequently feel like crying?
26.	❑	X	Do you have trouble concentrating?
27.	X	❑	Do you enjoy getting up in the morning?
28.	❑	X	Do you prefer to avoid social gatherings?
29.	X	❑	Is it easy for you to make decisions?
30.	X	❑	Is your mind as clear as it used to be?

The boxes indicate response indicating depressive symptom and each is equivalent to 1. Score of ≥ 10 indicates an evaluation for depression is indicated.

Source: Yesavage, J. A., & Brink, T. L. (1983). Development and validation of a geriatric depression scale: A preliminary report. *Journal of Psychiatric Research, 17*, 37–49. Reprinted with permission.

FIGURE 7-3

Cornell Scale for Depression in Dementia.

Scoring system: a = unable to evaluate; 0 = absent; 1 = mild or intermittent; 2 = severe.

A. Mood-Related Signs

1.	Anxiety: anxious expression, ruminations, worrying	a	0	1	2
2.	Sadness: sad expression, sad voice, tearfulness	a	0	1	2
3.	Lack of reactivity to pleasant events	a	0	1	2
4.	Irritability: easily annoyed, short-tempered	a	0	1	2

B. Behavioral Disturbance

5.	Agitation: restlessness, hand-wringing, hair-pulling	a	0	1	2
6.	Retardation: slow movement, slow speech, slow reactions	a	0	1	2
7.	Multiple physical complaints (score 0 if GI symptoms only)	a	0	1	2
8.	Loss of interest: less involved in usual activities (score only if change occurred acutely, i.e., in less than 1 month)	a	0	1	2

C. Physical Signs

9.	Appetite loss: eating less than usual	a	0	1	2
10.	Weight loss (score 2 if greater than 5 lb. in 1 month)	a	0	1	2
11.	Lack of energy: fatigues easily, unable to sustain activities (score only if change occurred acutely, i.e., in less than 1 month)	a	0	1	2

D. Cyclic Functions

12.	Diurnal variation of mood: symptoms worse in the morning	a	0	1	2
13.	Difficulty falling asleep: later than usual for this individual	a	0	1	2
14.	Multiple awakenings during sleep	a	0	1	2
15.	Early morning awakening: earlier than usual for this individual	a	0	1	2

E. Ideational Disturbance

16.	Suicide: feels life is not worth living, has suicidal wishes, or makes suicide attempt	a	0	1	2
17.	Poor self-esteem: self-blame, self-depreciation, feelings of failure	a	0	1	2
18.	Pessimism: anticipation of the worst	a	0	1	2
19.	Mood congruent delusions: delusions of poverty, illness, or loss	a	0	1	2

Ratings should be based on symptoms and signs occurring during the week prior to interview. No score should be given if symptoms result from physical disability or illness. Scores of 12 or greater indicate probable depression.

Source: Alexopoulos, G. S., Young, J. R., and Shamoian, C. A. (1988). Cornell Scale for Depression in Dementia. *Biological Psychiatry, 23,* 271–284. Reprinted with permission from the Society for Biological Psychiatry.

typically underreport symptoms of depression. Depressed mood and diminished interest in pleasurable activities (PHQ-2) and appetite disturbance or weight loss, loss of energy, worthlessness, and suicidal ideation are commonly denied by older adults (Davison et al.). Therefore, it should be noted that all of the tools discussed simply serve as screening tools and do not take the place of a full diagnostic evaluation of the older adult, which includes an extensive assessment of symptoms including information gathered from a reliable informant.

DIAGNOSIS OF MOOD DISORDERS

DSM-IV (APA, 2000) outlines the criteria for major depression, dysthymia, and minor depression. A diagnosis of major depression requires that for a 2-week period the individual either exhibits a sad, depressed mood or a loss of interest or pleasure in usual activities, and five or more of the following symptoms: significant weight loss or an increase or decrease in appetite; insomnia or hypersomnia nearly every day; psychomotor agitation or retardation observable by others nearly every day; fatigue or loss of energy nearly every day; feelings of worthlessness or excessive guilt; diminished ability to think or concentrate or make decisions nearly every day; or recurrent thoughts of death (not just fear of dying or developmentally appropriate thoughts of death as a part of growing old); recurrent suicidal ideation without a specific plan or a suicide attempt; or a specific plan for committing suicide (APA, 2000).

The diagnostic criteria for dysthymia is exhibiting a depressed mood for more days than not for 2 years and two or more of the following: poor appetite or overeating, insomnia or hypersomnia, low energy or fatigue, low self-esteem, poor concentration or difficulty making decisions, or feelings of hopelessness (APA, 2000).

In recent years, more attention has been paid to the importance of diagnosing and treating subsyndromal or minor depression. It is diagnosed with the occurrence of one or more periods of depressive

symptoms that are identical to major depressive periods in duration but involve fewer symptoms and less impairment. A minor depressive episode includes either a period of sad or "blue" mood or a loss of interest in activities and at least two additional depressive symptoms (APA, 2000).

There is growing evidence that supports aggressive treatment of minor depressive episodes. Twenty-five percent of persons with minor depression go on to experience a major depressive episode (Lyness, King, Cox, Yoediono, & Caine, 1999; Oxman, Barrett, & Gerber, 1990). Parmelee, Katz, and Lawton (1992) demonstrated that over time nursing home residents who exhibited minor depressive symptoms went on to develop major depression at a greater rate than those who did not exhibit depressive symptoms.

The DSM-IV criteria for major depression, dysthymia, and minor depression do not capture symptoms distinctive of geriatric depression. Older adults tend to have more somatic and cognitive complaints (Alexopoulos et al., 2002). They may not report a sad feeling but instead complain of a lack of feeling or emotion, apathy, or fatigue. Anxiety, nervousness, and increased worry are also common complaints of older adults experiencing depression. This presentation may be described as "depression without sadness" (Gallo & Rabins, 1999). For example, the primary complaint of an older adult may be anxiety or difficulty with concentration or memory. When evaluated further, additional symptoms are present, which add up to a diagnosis of depression.

The DSM-IV criteria for depression require that for a diagnosis of major depression, dysthymia, or minor depression, symptoms are not the result of a medical condition (e.g., hypothyroidism or vitamin deficiency) or a substance (e.g., medication or alcohol). Assessing depression in older adults is complicated by the fact that more frequently than not, the older adult is also experiencing the symptoms of chronic illnesses or symptoms of dementia.

Brown, Lapane, and Luisi (2002) found that nursing home residents with several diagnoses, including cancer, were all less likely to receive pharmacological treatment for depression. The tendency is to attribute symptoms of depression to other physical conditions because of the stigma associated with a depression diagnosis. Residents of nursing homes who were female, black, or cognitively impaired were less likely to receive treatment (Brown et al., 2002).

If an older adult screens positive for depression or if a screening tool is not used and a more "inclusive" approach to diagnosing is used, in which all depressive symptoms are indicative of depression and not disregarded as symptoms of another illness, then a thorough medical psychiatric evaluation is indicated. The medical evaluation for depression includes an extensive medical, psychiatric, and psychosocial history and a thorough evaluation of the causes for the depressive symptoms guided by a review of systems, a physical examination, including a neurological examination, and laboratory work. The laboratory examination should include, but not be limited to (depending on findings in the review of symptoms), serum electrolytes, complete blood count with platelets, thyroid panel with thyroid-stimulating hormone, vitamin B_{12}, and folate. The evaluation for depression includes an evaluation of medical conditions that contribute to depressive symptoms (Box 7-1) and medications that can cause depressive symptoms (Box 7-2).

SUICIDE

Untreated depression is a risk factor for suicide. The National Institute of Mental Health has recognized that suicide is a major but preventable public health problem (2008). The WHO (2003) reported nearly a million people commit suicide each year, and according to the CDC's National Center for Health Statistics, the number of suicides in the United States in 2005 was nearly 33,000 (CDC, 2008). A person dies by suicide every 16 minutes in the United States, and 90% of those who commit suicide have a diagnosable psychiatric disorder at the time of their death (American Foundation for Suicide Prevention, 2009). Therefore, early recognition and adequate treatment of mental illness will help prevent suicide.

Older adults who are widowed, live alone, have poor sleep quality, lack someone in whom they can confide, are grieving, are experiencing family discord, perceive themselves to be physically ill, suffer from chronic depression, or who have a history of prior suicide attempts are at high risk for suicide (Blazer, 2003; Conwell, Duberstein, & Caine, 2002). The consensus of expert clinicians is that the severity of the depressive illness, the presence of psychosis, alcoholism, a recent loss or bereavement, abuse of sedatives or hypnotics, and the development of disability are the greatest risk factors for suicide in older adults (Alexopoulos et al., 2001). "Older adult suicides give fewer warnings to others of their suicide plans, use more violent and potentially deadly methods to commit suicide, and apply those methods with greater planning and resolve" (Conwell et al., p. 194). It is imperative that nurses assess for suicidal ideation or intent, keeping in mind that noncompliance with medical recommendations may be suicidal behavior (Conwell et al.). A patient who speaks of wanting to die, who states he or she would be better off dead, or who exhibits behavior that indicates he or she is preparing for imminent death, including not following medical treatment, must be further assessed by asking poignant questions that determine the older adult's intentions. The nurse must be open to hearing and seeing this behavior among older adults, because there is great reluctance among nurses to ask patients if they are suicidal. As healthcare providers, nurses must assess their own beliefs and prejudices surrounding suicide because these can interfere with the ability to provide a complete assessment of a patient suffering from a potentially life-threatening illness. Furthermore, it is a myth that asking someone if he or she has thoughts of suicide is condoning the behavior or encouraging the persons to carry out his or her thoughts. In fact, asking with genuine concern if someone has suicidal thoughts or intent can instill hope during a time of crisis.

Metabolic disturbances
  Dehydration
  Azotemia, uremia
  Acid–base disturbances
  Hypoxia
  Hyponatremia and hypernatremia
  Hypoglycemia and hyperglycemia
  Hypocalcemia and hypercalcemia

Endocrine disorders
  Hypothyroidism and hyperthyroidism
  Hyperparathyroidism
  Diabetes mellitus
  Cushing's disease
  Addison's disease

Infections
  Viral: pneumonia, encephalitis
  Bacterial: pneumonia, urinary tract, meningitis, endocarditis
  Other: tuberculosis, brucellosis, fungal, neurosyphilis

Cardiovascular disorders
  Congestive heart failure
  Myocardial infarction, angina

Pulmonary disorders
  Chronic obstructive lung disease
  Malignancy

Gastrointestinal disorders
  Malignancy (especially pancreatic)
  Irritable bowel
  Other organic causes of chronic abdominal pain, ulcer, diverticulosis, hepatitis

Genitourinary disorders
  Urinary incontinence

Musculoskeletal disorders
  Degenerative arthritis
  Osteoporosis with vertebral compression or hip fractures
  Polymyalgia rheumatica
  Paget's disease

Neurological disorders
  Cerebrovascular disease
  Transient ischemic attacks
  Stroke
  Dementia (all types)
  Intracranial mass: primary or metastatic tumors
  Parkinson's disease

Other illnesses
  Anemia (of any cause)
  Vitamin deficiencies
  Hematologic or other systemic malignancy

Source: Kurlowicz, L. H., & NICHE Faculty. (1997). Nursing standard of practice protocol: Depression in older adult patients. *Geriatric Nursing, 18*(5), 192–199. Reprinted with permission from Elsevier.

BOX 7-2 DRUGS THAT CAUSE SYMPTOMS OF DEPRESSION IN OLDER ADULTS

Antihypertensives
  Reserpine
  Methyldopa
  Propranolol
  Clonidine
  Hydralazine
  Guanethidine
  Diuretics (by causing dehydration or electrolyte imbalance)

Analgesics
  Narcotics
  Morphine
  Codeine
  Meperidine
  Pentazocine
  Propoxyphene

Nonnarcotic
  Indomethacin

Antiparkinsonian agents
  L-Dopa

Antimicrobials
  Sulfonamides
  Isoniazid

Cardiovascular agents
  Digitalis
  Lidocaine (toxicity)

Hypoglycemic agents (by causing hypoglycemia)

Steroids
  Corticosteroids
  Estrogens

Others
  Cimetidine
  Cancer chemotherapeutic agents

Source: Kurlowicz, L. H., & NICHE Faculty. (1997). Nursing standard of practice protocol: Depression in older adult patients. *Geriatric Nursing, 18*(5), 192–199. Reprinted with permission from Elsevier.

Having a suicide protocol in place that clearly defines how the nurse will intervene should the nurse receive an affirmative response to the questions "Do you have thoughts of ending your life?" or "Do you have a plan and intend to carry it out?" will increase the nurse's comfort in completing a full assessment of the depressed patient. The protocol must include the involvement of others responsible for the care of the patient, such as the physician, nursing supervisor, family members, and others with whom the patient has a trusting relationship, such as a clergy person. If the patient has the intent to commit suicide and a plan to carry it out, then he or she must undergo constant supervision until hospitalization and the potential for carrying out the intent has been eliminated. If there is suicidal thought or ideation, then the nurse must, in conjunction with other healthcare providers, including a psychiatrist, develop a plan for keeping the patient safe. Involving someone in whom the patient feels comfortable confiding is important. The plan should include removing all lethal weapons or other means of suicide; consistent companionship or day treatment, if hospitalization is not possible; and close monitoring of the depression by a mental health specialist or the healthcare provider.

TREATMENT OPTIONS

Kessler et al. (2003), who examined the results of the National Comorbidity Survey Replication, recommended that "emphasis on screening and expansion of treatment needs to be accompanied by a parallel emphasis on treatment quality improvement" (p. 3095). The treatment options for depression are pharmacological, psychotherapeutic, and psychosocial interventions, and electroconvulsive therapy (ECT). Novel treatment options, such as transcranial magnetic stimulation and deep brain stimulation, are currently being investigated. The most effective treatment to date is a combination of pharmacological therapy and psychotherapy (DHHS, 1999). The goal of treatment is for the patient to return to his or her baseline before the depression episode or to where the residual physiological symptoms are clearly related to a chronic illness.

The AHRQ's National Guideline Clearinghouse (2008, Section I, para. 1) offers the following evidence-based recommendations: "For patients with mild to moderate Major Depressive Disorder (MDD), use either antidepressant medication or psychotherapy (Interpersonal Therapy, Cognitive Behavioral Therapy, or Problem-Solving Therapy) as first-line treatment." For the antidepressant medication strategy, the AHRQ's National Guideline Clearinghouse (2008, Recommendations section, para. 3) also recommends "Frequent initial visits. Patients require frequent visits early in treatment to assess response to intervention, suicidal ideation, side effects, and psychosocial support systems; Continuation therapy. Continuation therapy (9–12 months after acute symptoms resolve) decreases the incidence of relapse of major depression."

Recovery or obtaining a remission is not immediate. It may take longer for older adults to respond to treatment (Nelson, 2001). Generally, medications take 4 to 6 weeks to be effective and frequently 8 to 10 weeks in older adults and several additional months once a therapeutic dosage is reached to eliminate residual symptoms. The treatment of depression may require several different medication trials where the therapeutic dosage is prescribed for 8 to 10 weeks. A combination of medications (e.g., selective serotonin reuptake inhibitor [SSRI] and buproprion) aimed at relieving all symptoms or achieving the individual's baseline may be indicated only when a therapeutic trial of the initially started medication results in significant symptom reduction with residual symptoms of depression that are not responding to the initial medication. Frequently, patients are the last to recognize their gradual improvement despite family members being able to see positive changes; therefore, reassurance and identification and discussion of areas of improvement with the older adult may be beneficial and facilitate continuation of treatment. Older adults may blame a relapse or the recurrence of symptoms on other physical illnesses or life situations, continuing to deny their psychiatric illness. On the other hand, because of the pain and disability experienced when depressed, some patients become hypersensitive to their mood by becoming concerned that they are becoming depressed again whenever they have a "down" day or two as the result of normal life experiences. Patients need to be taught and reminded of the signs and symptoms of depression and their own presentation. They also may need to be reminded of the self-care strategies they have learned and when to seek professional care. Depression is a recurring illness and the use of a combination of treatments, such as medications, psychotherapy, and the adoption of positive psychosocial behaviors, helps prevent relapse and assists the client and his or her family to detect relapse early.

PHARMACOLOGICAL TREATMENT OPTIONS

Recommendations for pharmacotherapy in older adults are based on expert consensus because most clinical trials are conducted in younger patients (Alexopoulos et al., 2001). Clinicians treating older adults must apply what is known from clinical trials to a population of patients who generally have a number of coexisting medical conditions, metabolize medications more slowly, and are taking other medications that contribute to their depressive symptoms (Alexopoulos et al.). Antidepressant medications most frequently used in older adults include the SSRIs; serotonin and norepinephrine reuptake inhibitors or modulators (SNRIs); and unicyclic aminoketone (e.g., bupropion). Medications used less frequently in older adults include piperazine (e.g., trazodone and nefazodone); tricyclic antidepressants (TCAs); and monoamine oxidase in-hibitors (MAOIs). Although individuals respond differently to medications, all of the medications are 60% to 80% effective (McDonald, 2000).

The Expert Consensus Guideline Series (Alexopoulos et al., 2001) supports the use of SSRIs or venlafaxine XR (Duloxetine was not on the market at the time) in combination with psychotherapy as the first line of treatment for unipolar nonpsychotic major depression (Table 7-1). This is largely because of the presumed low side-effect profile of the SSRIs.

TABLE 7-1

Medication and Treatment Selection Strategies for Unipolar Nonpsychotic Major Depression (Mild and Severe) and Unipolar Psychotic Major Depression

Preferred	Alternate
Mild Depression	
Antidepressant medication and psychotherapy	Antidepressant medication alone or psychotherapy alone
SSRI	Bupropion
Venlafaxine XR	Mirtazapine
Severe Depression	
Antidepressant medication and psychotherapy	ECT
Antidepressant medication alone	
Psychotic Depression	
Antidepressant (SSRI or venlafaxine XR) plus antipsychotic (risperidone, olanzapine, quetiapine) or electroconvulsive therapy	Medication plus psychotherapy
	Antidepressant: TCA
	Antipsychotics: ziprasidone or aripiprazole*

*Ziprasidone had just been released at the time of the Expert Consensus Guidelines survey and aripiprazole had not yet been released.

Source: Adapted from Alexopoulos, G. S., Katz, I. R., Reynolds, C. F., Carpenter, D., and Docherty, J. P. (2001). The expert consensus guideline series: Pharmacotherapy of depressive disorders in older adults. In *A postgraduate medicine special report.* Minneapolis, MN: McGraw-Hill.

The currently available data, particularly that which pertain to older adults, do not support the use of hypericum perforatum (St. John's wort) or other herbals and botanicals over standard clinical care for the treatment of depression (Alexopoulos et al., 2001; Davidson et al., 2002; Desai & Grossberg, 2003). Table 7-2 provides an overview of the antidepressants and dosing most commonly recommended for older adults.

The familiar geriatric axiom "start low, go slow" holds true when prescribing antidepressants. However, a common mistake is to undertreat by not titrating to the recommended therapeutic dosage or not raising the dosage to its higher limits to eliminate all depressive symptoms and obtain full remission. Anxiety is a common residual symptom of depression, and it is recommended that the dose of antidepressant medication, other than TCAs, be raised to its highest therapeutic level to treat the anxiety (Alexopoulos et al., 2001). The patient should be maintained on the dose of the medication that adequately treated the depressive illness for at least 1 year if it is the first episode of depression (Alexopoulos et al.). Experts vary in their

TABLE 7-2

Dosing and Duration of Medication

Antidepressant	Average Starting Dose (mg/day)	Average Target Dose After 6 Weeks of Treatment (mg/day)	Usual Highest Final Acute Dose (mg/day)
SSRIs			
Citalopram	10–20	20–30	30–40
Fluoxetine	10	20	20–40
Escitalopram*	5–10	10	20
Paroxetine	10–20	20–30	30–40
Paroxetine CR	12.5	25–37.5	50
Sertraline	25–50	50–100	100–200
SNRI			
Venlafaxine XR	25–75	75–200	150–300
Duloxetine			
Others			
Bupropion SR	100	150–300 (in divided doses)	300–400 (in divided doses)
Bupropion XR	150	300	450
Mirtazapine	7.5–15	15–30	30–45
TCA			
Nortriptyline†	10–30	40–100	75–125
Desipramine†	10–40	50–100	100–150

Dosages given are based on pharmaceutical recommendations.

* Was not on the market at the time of the Expert Consensus Survey. Dosages given are based on pharmaceutical recommendations.

† Recommended target blood levels:
   Nortriptyline: 50–150 ng/ml
   Desipramine: 115–200 ng/ml

Source: Adapted from Alexopoulos, G. S., Katz, I. R., Reynolds, C. F., Carpenter, D., & Docherty, J. P. (2001). The expert consensus guideline series: Pharmacotherapy of depressive disorders in older adults. In *A postgraduate medicine special report.* Minneapolis, MN: McGraw-Hill.

recommendations as to how long a patient should be maintained on the antidepressant if it is the second or third depressive episode. Alexopoulos et al. note that in addition to the number of depressive episodes, other factors, such as severity of the illness and how well the illness responded to treatment, play a role in the decision to continue treatment for 3 years or longer.

For patients with symptoms of minor depression or dysthymia, which have persisted for 2 to 3 months, the first line of treatment is medication with psychotherapy or medication or psychotherapy alone (Alexopoulos et al., 2001). Watchful waiting and psychoeducation or psychotherapy is recommended for patients who exhibit dysthymia or minor depressive symptoms for a few weeks or more.

The most common side effects of the SSRIs are mild nausea, stomach upset, and a slight jittery feeling similar to what caffeine may cause. These common but mild side effects usually go away in 7 to 10 days and are minimized by slow titration of dosage. Serotonergic drugs can cause a "serotonin syndrome," which can be mild to severe nausea, tremor, difficulty sleeping, and anxiety. This occurs most frequently when a medication is started, possibly at too high of a dose, or when added to another serotonergic medication, such as L-tryptophan, hypericum (St. John's wort), MAOIs, or lithium (McDonald, 2000). This should be addressed by decreasing or eliminating a serotonergic medication. More notable side effects indicating a need to discontinue the medication include rash, agitation, headaches, insomnia, and loss of appetite. The SSRIs are not associated with cardiac effects and they do not potentiate medications that are central nervous system depressants. SSRIs should not be abruptly discontinued. When stopped abruptly, the patient can experience flu-like symptoms.

The SNRI venlafaxine (Effexor) does not have any effect on seizure threshold or cardiac side effects. It has a low incidence of sexual dysfunction and drug-induced anxiety that is sometimes seen when starting an SSRI, and it has a more rapid onset of effectiveness (McDonald, 2000). Similar to the SSRIs, such side effects as nausea, difficulty sleeping, or mild headaches can be minimized by starting the medication at a low dose and titrating up slowly. In some patients, SSRIs and venlafaxine are stimulating and therefore should be given in the morning. If a patient finds the medications to be a little sedating, then they should be dosed in the evening. Venlafaxine should be used with caution in persons with uncontrolled hypertension, because it is associated with dose-related hypertension. The patient's blood pressure should be monitored each time the dose is increased. Duloxetine (Cymbalta) is also an SNRI and indicated for diabetic peripheral neuropathy (Goldstein, Lu, Detke, Lee, & Iyengar, 2005; Raskin et al., 2005).

Bupropion and mirtazapine are considered high second-line alternatives (Alexopoulos et al., 2001). Bupropion (Wellbutrin), a unicyclic aminoketone, has a side-effect profile similar to the SSRIs. Unlike the SSRIs, it does not cause sexual dysfunction. The medication can be somewhat activating or stimulating; therefore, it should not be dosed in the evening because it could interfere with sleep. Bupropion is associated with an increased risk of seizure. The risk of seizure has been significantly decreased with the newer sustained-release and extended-release formulas.

Mirtazapine (Remeron), a piperazinoazepine or serotonin and norepinephrine reuptake modulator, also does not have significant sexual or cardiac side effects. Mirtazapine can cause weight gain. It also is sedating at lower doses. Dosing is counterintuitive with Remeron in that it is more sedating at lower starting doses than at target doses. Remeron is often selected as a treatment because of its side effects of weight gain and sedation, which can be helpful in an older adult with a poor appetite, weight loss, and difficulty sleeping.

Although more difficult to use in older adults because of their side-effect profile, TCAs may be considered an option when treating depression that is unresponsive to the newer antidepressants (e.g., SSRIs and SNRIs) that have a more favorable side-effect profile and are better tolerated in older adults (Alexopoulos et al., 2001). The Expert Consensus agrees with research showing the SSRIs are as effective as the TCAs with a better side-effect profile (Alexopoulos et al., 2001). TCAs are associated with anticholinergic side effects, including dry mouth, tachycardia, increased or decreased sweating, impaired visual accommodation or blurred vision, constipation and urine retention, orthostatic hypotension, and sedation (McDonald, 2000). Older adults are at risk of an anticholinergic-induced delirium in which the patient becomes confused, agitated, or more withdrawn. This could be confused with a worsening of depression. Most importantly, TCAs can cause heart block and arrhythmias. A TCA overdose is likely to be fatal.

MAOIs are effective antidepressants but are not used often in older adults because of the risk of severe drug interactions. As with TCAs, close monitoring for drug interaction is recommended when prescribing MAOIs (Alexopoulos et al., 2001). Hypertensive crisis can occur when MAOIs are taken with foods that contain tyramine, sympathomimetic medications, narcotics, TCAs, nefazodone (Serzone), and SSRIs.

Finally, piperazines, nefazodone, and trazodone (Desyrel) are not frequently used with older adults because they cause orthostatic hypotension and sedation at doses that are needed to have an antidepressant effect. Trazodone, however, may be used as a treatment for insomnia (Alexopoulos et al., 2001) and can be helpful in decreasing agitation in older adults (McDonald, 2000). When these medications are used, the patient needs to be carefully assessed for hypotension and instructed regarding the risk of falls. Neither medication is associated with cardiotoxicity or sexual dysfunction.

There is considerable evidence that supports augmentation using low doses of atypical antipsychotics in treatment-resistant depression (Blier & Szabo, 2005; Thase, 2002). However, *Expert Con-sensus Guidelines for Using Antipsychotic Agents in Older Patients* does not support the use of antipsychotic agents in the treatment of non-psychotic major depression (Alexopoulos, Streim, & Carpenter, 2005). The reason for this opinion is the unfavorable risk–benefit ratio; the high risk of adverse effects primarily caused by disease–drug and drug–drug interactions outweighs the limited documented benefit of use of atypical antipsychotics in the treatment of depression in older adults (Alexopoulos et al.). Expert consensus does recommend the use of atypical antipsychotics in the treatment of psychotic major depression in an older adult. Based on the evidence of the effectiveness of antipsychotics in treatment-resistant depression, the clinician must consider the risk–benefit in the use of atypical antipsychotics in the treatment of an older adult who is treatment resistant.

PSYCHOTHERAPY

The Expert Consensus Guidelines (Alexopoulos et al., 2001) consider cognitive–behavioral therapy, supportive psychotherapy, problem-solving psychotherapy, and interpersonal therapy to be first-line psychotherapy options for older adults. The two forms of psychotherapy that have been studied the most and have been shown to be the most effective in treating depression are cognitive–behavioral therapy and interpersonal therapy (Arean & Cook, 2002; Blazer, 2003). There is some evidence that brief dynamic therapy and reminiscence therapy are somewhat effective in treating late-life depression (Arean & Cook). Cognitive–behavioral therapy has also been shown to help prevent relapse and improve psychosocial functioning in younger patients (Fava, Grandi, Zielenzny, Canestrari, & Morphy, 1994; Paykel et al., 1999; Scott et al., 2000). Psychotherapy is effective for individuals or in groups. Group therapy is one way of providing a peer group for older adults who have lost their social network or support.

The skilled psychotherapist can treat almost all of the symptoms of depression and the resulting behaviors associated with depression (i.e., hopelessness, anhedonia, anxiety, interpersonal problems, treatment compliance, poor energy, and negative thoughts). However, a moderate to severe depressive episode, which may include sleep disturbance, change in appetite, suicidal thoughts, or psychosis, almost always requires pharmacotherapy. Licensed therapists, such as clinical nurse specialists, psychiatric nurse practitioners, psychologists, licensed clinical social workers, licensed professional counselors, licensed marriage and family counselors, pastoral counselors, and psychiatrists, are all psychotherapists. However, not all specialize in the therapies proven to be effective in treating depression and not all are skilled at working with older adults.

All advanced practice nurses treating older adults with depression can use cognitive–behavioral therapy techniques (when a therapist is not available or in collaboration with a therapist) with the goal of altering negative behaviors and thought patterns. The basic premise of behavioral therapy is to influence or change behavior that contributes negatively to an individual's depression. Someone who suffers from depression for any length of time adopts behaviors that exacerbate or perpetuate the symptoms of depression. A hallmark symptom of depression is loss of interest in activities that were pleasurable (anhedonia). Clearly, the depressed person who no longer enjoys things over time loses social contacts and becomes less physically active. Being separated from others socially and becoming less physically active contribute to depressive symptoms. Persons who have been cut off from family and friends and who are inactive because of their depression frequently need to be provided guidance and support to change behaviors. Chronically depressed persons or older adults who are transitioning from work to retirement, or from living independently to assisted living, may need assistance in identifying activities they enjoy and that provide them with a sense of satisfaction. Likewise, the changing of roles that is the result of retirement, loss of a spouse or friend, or a change in lifestyle can be facilitated with cognitive therapy by assisting with thoughts or perceptions of changing roles and contributions.

One behavioral therapy strategy is activity scheduling (France & Robson, 1997). Activity scheduling requires the patient to keep a diary of the activities he or she was involved in over the week (e.g., watching television, bathing, and grocery shopping). Once the nurse has a clear picture of the patient's level of activity, the patient should be asked to evaluate the activities, as to whether they are considered an achievement or a pleasurable experience. This information, in addition to the patient's psychosocial history, is used to help the patient identify which activities affect mood positively and to set goals for increasing those activities. During this process, the older adult might identify numerous barriers to assuming an active lifestyle (e.g., immobility, pain, or lack of transportation). Here lies the challenge to the nurse. These barriers should be discussed and the nurse can provide valuable guidance to the older adult in identifying ways to overcome the barriers or alternative activities that will be enjoyable to that individual. The nurse must make certain that the goals for changing behavior are the patient's and not the nurse's goals. Identification of the patient's goals is a key in problem-solving therapy and behavioral activation, both psychotherapeutic strategies shown to be effective in changing behaviors and decreasing depressive symptoms in older adults.

While implementing the "activity scheduling" technique, the nurse is certain to identify the depressed patient's negative or fatalistic attitudes. These negative thoughts are a hallmark of depression. Frequently, depression contributes negatively to the patient's self-esteem and the negativity becomes a conditioned or an automatic response. Cognitive therapy helps the depressed person recognize his or her negative thoughts and challenges those thoughts with a positive response (France & Robson, 1997). What one thinks about or how one interprets life's events affects mood. France and Robson suggest that even though a thought may be fleeting, the mood it creates may linger. The same is true with a negative interpretation of events.

One cognitive therapy strategy is a "negative automatic thoughts record" (France & Robson, 1997). The patient is instructed to keep a record of negative thoughts, including the negative meaning he or she has assigned to events and images and their mood during that day. The nurse can help the patient evaluate how thoughts correlate with moods. The patient is challenged to think about automatic thoughts regarding an event, if his or her response (thought) is rational, and if not what is a rational response. A plan to carry out the more positive rational response is developed.

ELECTROCONVULSIVE THERAPY

ECT is a highly effective treatment for major depression. Published research and expert clinicians support the safety and efficacy of ECT in older adults (Alexopoulos et al., 2001; Salzman, Wong, & Wright, 2002). ECT is most appropriate in psychotic depression when depression has failed to respond to an antidepressant and antipsychotic medication or in a severe depression that has failed to respond to adequate trials of two antidepressants (Alexopoulos et al.). It is also appropriate for severe depression with acute suicidal risk that may include refusing medication and food (Alexopoulos et al.). Unfortunately, ECT is postponed or not considered a viable treatment option by many patients, families, and clinicians because of its historical negative depiction. Likewise, there are persons who have had negative experiences with ECT and are opposed to the use of ECT. However, similar to many medical procedures, ECT has been developed over past years such that side effects are minimized. The most common side effect of ECT is disturbance of memory around the time of the course of treatment and possibly loss of memory of isolated events. Cognition is closely monitored during the course of treatment.

Before being treated with ECT, the patient undergoes a full medical evaluation including laboratory work, electrocardiogram, and a CT scan of the brain. A recent stroke is a contraindication for ECT. With close monitoring, persons with severe cardiovascular disease can be treated suc-cessfully with ECT (Zielinski, Roose, Devanand, Woodring, & Sackeim, 1993).

ECT is administered while the patient is asleep and the muscles are totally relaxed using medication. An electrical stimulus that causes a seizure is administered through the electrodes placed on the depressed person's head. The patient does not feel any pain. The patient awakes approximately 5 to 10 minutes following the seizure. The patient is closely monitored for confusion, agitation, headache, and changes in cognition or memory. Any changes are addressed medically as indicated.

NURSING INTERVENTIONS

In 1999, the *Report of the Surgeon General* noted there will never be enough mental health clinicians to treat the vast numbers with a mental illness. Thus, it proves essential that mental health become an integral part of primary care and of other specialties. Nurses can be instrumental in arranging for comprehensive and more effective treatment of depression. In addition to pharmacotherapy and psychotherapy, psychosocial interventions need to be considered and included in the treatment plan as appropriate. Psychosocial interventions, such as psychoeducation, family counseling, visiting nursing services, bereavement groups, and senior citizen center activities, are all strongly recommended as first-line intervention options (Alexopoulos et al., 2001). Kurlowicz and NICHE faculty (1997) provides a comprehensive list of nursing interventions for the management of depression (Box 7-3).

Depressed older adults need an advocate and someone to provide ongoing supportive counseling that reinforces what they have been taught about the illness. They also need assistance in combating the stigma of the illness, problem solving and setting goals, and ongoing reassurance. Just knowing that there is someone to talk to who understands his or her illness and is available to answer questions and provide reassurance is extremely therapeutic for both the patient and caregiver.

BOX 7-3 NURSING CARE PARAMETERS

For all levels of depression, develop an individualized plan integrating the following nursing interventions:

1. Institute safety precautions for suicide risk as per institutional policy (in outpatient settings, ensure continuous surveillance of the patient while obtaining an emergency psychiatric evaluation and disposition).

2. Remove or control etiologic agents.

   a. Avoid, remove, or change depressogenic medications.

   b. Correct or treat metabolic and systemic disturbances.

3. Monitor and promote nutrition, elimination, sleep–rest patterns, physical comfort (especially pain control).

4. Enhance physical function (i.e., structure regular exercise or activity, refer to physical, occupational, recreational therapies); develop a daily activity schedule.

5. Enhance social support (i.e., identify or mobilize support persons [e.g., family, confidante, friends, hospital resources, support groups, patient visitors]); ascertain need for spiritual support and contact appropriate clergy.

6. Maximize autonomy or personal control and self-efficacy (e.g., include patient in active participation in making daily schedules, short-term goals).

7. Identify and reinforce strengths and capabilities.

8. Structure and encourage daily participation in relaxation therapies, pleasant activities.

9. Monitor and document response to medication and other therapies; readminister depression screening tool.

10. Provide practical assistance; assist with problem solving.

11. Provide emotional support (i.e., empathic, supportive listening, encourage expression of feelings, instill hope), support adaptive coping, encourage pleasant reminiscences but do not "force" happiness.

12. Provide information about the physical illness and treatments and about depression (i.e., that depression is common, treatable, and not the person's fault).

13. Educate about the importance of adherence to prescribed treatment regimen for depression (especially medication) to prevent recurrence; educate about specific antidepressant side effects and any dietary restrictions.

14. Ensure mental health community link-up; consider psychiatric nursing home care intervention.

Source: Kurlowicz, L. H., & NICHE Faculty. (1997). Nursing standard of practice protocol: Depression in older adult patients. *Geriatric Nursing, 18*(5), 192–199. Reprinted with permission from Elsevier.

EVIDENCE-BASED MODELS OF CARE DELIVERY

There are many evidence-based programs on mental health promotion recognized by the U.S. Substance Abuse Mental Health Services Administration's National Registry of Evidence-based Programs and Practices (http://nrepp. samhsa.gov) and the National Council on Aging's Center for Healthy Aging (http://healthy agingprograms.org) that can be implemented in primary care clinics and other settings where older adults live and congregate. Numerous efforts, including the recommendation that all primary care providers screen for depression and the advent of antidepressant medications with fewer side effects, have increased the number of older adults receiving treatment for depression. However, the "expertise gap" (primary clinicians are unable to be experts in all areas) has been cited as the primary reason for older adults not receiving adequate treatment for depression (Bartels et al., 2002). Studies have shown that older adults whose primary care practitioners collaborate with a specialist, as opposed to simply consulting a specialist, such as a psychiatrist, psychologist, psychiatric clinical nurse specialist, or other mental health provider, are more adequately treated (Katon et al., 1995; Unutzer, 2002). This growing need for mental health specialists in primary care and medical specialties provides great opportunity for the registered nurse and advanced practice nurse who have developed expertise in treating persons, particularly older adults, with mental illness.

Studies have shown that it is cost-effective to have a depression care manager on an ongoing basis in primary care settings to help persons with depression receive the care they need. Wang and colleagues (2006) noted that "how service sectors share responsibility for people's mental health is changing . . ." (p. 1187). One study found that hiring a care manager may initially be costly but has been shown to be cost-effective in the long-term compared to usual care (Rost, Pyne, Dickinson, & LoSasso, 2005). This study by Rost et al. found that implementing depression case management resulted in an incremental cost-effective ratio ranging from $9,592 to $14,306 per quality-adjusted life–year. Furthermore, adding a depression care manager significantly decreases the number of days with depression. Collaborative models of care, such as Prevention of Suicide in the Primary Care Older Adults: Collaborative Trial (PROSPECT), Improving Mood: Promoting Access to Collaborative Treatment for Late-Life Depression (IMPACT), and Healthy IDEAS: Identifying Depression, Empowering Activities for Seniors, have been effective by using specially trained nurses and other social service providers within primary care or aging service programs (Bruce & Pearson, 1999; Quijano et al., 2007; Unutzer et al., 2002). Important components of these models of care are screening persons for depression, patient education regarding the illness and treatment options and education regarding support services, collaboration with or referral to a mental health specialist in more severe cases, and ongoing supportive counseling or therapy that focuses on problem-solving therapy and behavioral activation. Similar models of care that use specially trained nurses to assess for depression, provide care management, provide liaison with primary care and mental health specialists, and train residential community staff to recognize depression have been shown to be effective in decreasing depressive symptoms among older adults in older adult residential communities (Blanchard, 1995; Llewellyn-Jones et al., 1999; Rabins et al., 2000). "Question, persuade, refer" is a gatekeeper training designed to train non–mental health professionals on how to prevent suicide by asking patients if they are thinking of harming themselves, persuading them to get help, and referring them to appropriate resources (Quinnett, 1995).

An important component of nursing care of older adults with depression that should not be overlooked is the care of the primary caregiver of the depressed person. Caregivers, particularly those caring for a person with a mental illness, are themselves at risk for depression (Horton-Deutsch, Farran, Choi, & Fogg, 2002). Caregivers must be included in the treatment plan and assessed for symptoms of depression. The PLUS intervention, which provides education, assistance in identification, and strengthening of resources and supportive counseling for caregivers, was shown to benefit the depressed patient by improving personal activities of daily living while decreasing the amount of time the caregiver spent in direct caregiving activities (Horton-Deutsch et al.). By decreasing caregiver burden, the nurse has taken steps to prevent disability in both the caregiver and the depressed older adult.

▌ CASE STUDY

Ms. Smith is a 79-year-old black woman. She has lived with her daughter since her husband died 3 years ago. She is a retired school teacher. During an office visit, her daughter says that for approximately 9 months her mother has not been herself. When Ms. Smith is asked how she is doing and why she is here today, she says "my daughter brought me. I am doing just fine—just getting old and don't have the energy I once had." Her daughter says she frequently misses church and would rather be waited on. Ms. Smith's daughter says "My Mom was always busy doing something—she no longer even reads." Ms. Smith denies feeling sad or down. When asked, she does say that she often feels nervous, more so in the morning when she wakes up. She reports waking up at night, worrying, with the inability to get back to sleep. She states, "There is a lot to worry about these days. I worry a lot about my grandchildren. My daughter works too hard. I feel sick and my knees are always hurting. No sense in going to my doctor, nothing he can do for me." When asked, Ms. Smith says her appetite is fair and she has lost a few pounds recently. She denies feelings of worthlessness or thoughts of wanting to die, but does state she has lived a long life and sometimes thinks it would be best if she died in her sleep.

Ms. Smith scores a 9 on the PHQ-9 and a 2 on the PHQ-2 with a normal clock drawing test.

1. Ms. Smith has not been to her primary care provider for 6 months or more. What laboratory testing should she have done and why?

All of Ms. Smith's laboratory work is normal.

2. What are the possible diagnoses for Ms. Smith? Discuss your rationale for choosing her diagnosis.

Ms. Smith's family medical and psychiatric history reveals that Ms. Smith's other daughter has been treated for depression with sertraline and has done very well since being treated.

3. Describe the specific strategies you would use for promoting Ms. Smith's mental health. Describe the treatment plan and follow-up you would recommend.

REFERENCES

Agency for Healthcare Research and Quality. (2002). *Screening for depression: Recommendations and rationale.* Retrieved July 27, 2008, from http://www.ahrq.gov/clinic/uspstf/uspsdepr.htm

Agency for Healthcare Research and Quality. (2007). *Comparative effectiveness of second-generation antidepressants in the pharmacologic treatment of adult depression.* Retrieved July 27, 2008, from http://effectivehealthcare.ahrq.gov/healthInfo.cfm?infotype=rr&ProcessID=7&DocID=61

Agency for Healthcare Research and Quality. (2008). *National Guideline Clearinghouse: Depression clinical practice guidelines.* Retrieved July 27, 2008, from http://www.guideline.gov/summary/summary.aspx?doc_id=9632&nbr=5152&ss=6&xl=999

Alexopoulos, G. S., Abrams, R. C., Young, J. R., & Shamoian, C. A. (1988). Cornell Scale for Depression in Dementia. *Biological Psychiatry, 23*, 271–284.

Alexopoulos, G. S., Borson, S., Cothbert, B. N., Devanand, D. P., Mulsant, B. H., & Olin, J. T., et al. (2002). Assessment of late life depression. *Biological Psychiatry, 52*(3), 164–174.

Alexopoulos, G. S., Katz, I. R., Reynolds, C. F., Carpenter, D., & Docherty, J. P. (2001). The expert consensus guideline series: Pharmacotherapy of depressive disorders in older adults. In *A postgraduate medicine special report.* Minneapolis, MN: McGraw-Hill.

Alexopoulos, G. S., Meyers, B. S., Young, R. C., Campbell, S., Silbersweig, D., & Charlson, M. (1997). Vascular depression hypothesis. *Archives of General Psychiatry, 54*(10), 915–922.

Alexopoulos, G. S., Streim, J. E., & Carpenter, D. (2005). Expert consensus guidelines for using antipsychotic agents in older patients. *Journal of Clinical Psychiatry, 65*(Suppl. 2), 100–102.

American Association of Geriatric Psychiatry. (2001). *Depression fact sheet.* Retrieved November 24, 2004, from http://www.aagponline.org/p_c/depression.asp

American Foundation for Suicide Prevention. (2009). Facts and figures. Retrieved December 27, 2009, from http://www.afsp.org/index.cfm?fuseaction=home.viewpage&page_id=050FEA9F-B064-4092-B1135C3A70DE1FDA

American Psychiatric Association. (2000). *Diagnostic and statistical manual of mental disorders* (4th ed.). Washington, DC: Author.

Arean, P. A., & Cook, B. L. (2002). Psychotherapy and combined psychotherapy/pharmacotherapy for late life depression. *Biological Psychiatry, 52*(3), 293–303.

Bartels, S. J., Dums, A. R., Oxman, T. E., Schneider, L. S., Arean, P. A., Alexopoulos, G. S., et al. (2002). Evidence-based practices in geriatric mental health care psychiatric services. *Psychiatric Services, 53*(11), 1419–1431.

Blanchard, M. R. (1995). The effect of primary care nurse intervention upon older people screened as depressed. *International Journal of Geriatric Psychiatry, 10*, 289–298.

Blazer, D. G. (2003). Depression in late life: Review and commentary. *Journal of Gerontology, 58*(3), 249–265.

Blier, P., & Szabo, S. T. (2005). Potential mechanisms of action of atypical antipsychotic medications in treatment-resistant depression and anxiety. *Journal of Clinical Psychiatry, 66*(Suppl. 8), 30–40.

Brown, M. N., Lapane, K. L., & Luisi, A. F. (2002). The management of depression in older nursing home residents. *Journal of the American Geriatrics Society, 50*, 69–76.

Bruce, M. L., & Pearson, J. L. (1999). Designing an intervention to prevent suicide: PROSPECT (Prevention of Suicide in Primary Care Older Adults: Collaborative Trial). *Dialogues in Clinical Neuroscience, 1*(2), 100–112.

Centers for Disease Control and Prevention. (2005). *MMWR weekly: The role of public health in mental health promotion.* Retrieved December 28, 2009, from http://www.cdc.gov/mmwr/preview/mmwrhtml/mm5434a1.htm

Centers for Disease Control and Prevention. (2008). National Center for Health Statistics. *Fast stats from A to Z.* Retrieved November 3, 2008, from http://www.cdc.gov/nchs/fastats/suicide.htm

Conwell, Y., Duberstein, P. R., & Caine, E. D. (2002). Risk factors for suicide in later life. *Biological Psychiatry, 52*(3), 193–204.

Davidson, J. R., Gadde, K. M., Fairbank, J. A., Krishnan, R. R., Califf, R. M., Binanay, C., et al. (2002). Effect of hypericum perforatum (St. John's wort) in major depressive disorder: A randomized controlled trial. *JAMA, 287*(14), 1807–1814.

Davison, T. E., McCabe, M. P., & Mellor, D. (2009). An examination of the "gold standard" diagnosis of major depression in aged-care settings. *American Journal of Geriatric Psychiatry, 17*(5), 359–367.

Demyttenaere, K., Bruffaerts, R., Posada-Villa, J., Gasquet, I., Kovess, V., Lepine, J. P., et al. (2004). Prevalence, severity, and unmet need for treatment of mental disorders in the World Health Organization World Mental Health Surveys. *JAMA, 291*(2), 2581–2590.

Desai, A. K., & Grossberg, G. T. (2003). Herbals and botanicals in geriatric psychiatry. *American Journal of Geriatric Psychiatry, 11*(15), 498–506.

Evans, D. L., Charney, D. S., Lewis, L., Golden, R. N., Gorman, J. M., Krishnan, R. R., et al. (2003). Depression Bipolar Support Alliance consensus statement on the treatment of mood disorders in the medically ill. Unpublished manuscript.

Fava, G. A., Grandi, S., Zielenzny, M., Canestrari, R., & Morphy, M. A. (1994). Cognitive behavioral treatment of residual symptoms in primary major depressive disorder. *American Journal of Psychiatry, 151*(9), 1295–1299.

France, R., & Robson, M. (1997). The management of depression. *Cognitive behavioral therapy in primary care: A practical guide*. London: Jessica Kingsly.

Gallo, J. J., & Rabins, P. V. (1999). Depression without sadness: Alternative presentations of depression in late life. *American Family Physician, 60*, 820–826.

Goldstein, D. J., Lu, Y., Detke, M. J., Lee, T. C., & Iyengar, S. (2005). Duloxetine versus placebo in patients with painful diabetic neuropathy. *Pain, 116*(1-2), 109–118.

Hedelin, B., & Strandmark, M. (2001). The meaning of depression from the life-world perspective of older adult women. *Issues in Mental Health Nursing, 22*, 401–420.

Horton-Deutsch, S. L., Farran, C. J., Choi, E. E., & Fogg, L. (2002). The PLUS intervention: A pilot test with caregivers of depressed older adults. *Archives of Psychiatric Nursing, 16*(2), 61–71.

Hybels, C. F., & Blazer, D. G. (2003). Epidemiology of late-life mental disorders. *Clinics in Geriatric Medicine, 19*, 663–696.

Katon, W., Korff, M. V., Lin, E., Walker, E., Simon, G. E., Bush, T., et al. (1995). Collaborative management to achieve treatment guidelines: Impact on depression in primary care. *JAMA, 273*(13), 1026–1031.

Kessler, R. C., Berglund, P., Demler, O., Jin, R., Koretz, D., Merikangas, K. R., et al. (2003). The epidemiology of major depressive disorder: Results from the National Cormorbidity Survey Replication (NCS-R). *JAMA, 289*(23), 3095–3105.

Kroenke, K., Spitzer, R. L., & Williams, J. B. W. (2003). The Patient Health Questionnaire-2: Validity of a two item depression screener. *Medical Care, 41*(11), 1284–1292.

Kurlowicz, L. H., & NICHE Faculty. (1997). Nursing standard of practice protocol: Depression in older adult patients. *Geriatric Nursing, 18*(5), 192–199.

Lebowitz, B. D., Pearson, J. L., Schneider, L. S., Reynolds, C. F., Alexopoulos, G. S., Bruce, M. L., et al. (1997). Diagnosis and treatment of depression in late life: Consensus statement update. *JAMA, 278*(14), 1186–1190.

Llewellyn-Jones, R. H., Baikie, A., Smiters, H., Cohen, J., Snowdon, J., & Tennant, C. (1999). Multifaceted shared care intervention for late-life depression in residential care: Randomized controlled trial. *British Medical Journal, 319*, 676–682.

Lyness, J. M., King, D. A., Cox, C., Yoediono, Z., & Caine, E. D. (1999). The importance of subsyndromal depression in older primary care patients: Prevalence and associated functional disability. *Journal of the American Geriatrics Society, 47*, 757–758.

Mayberg, H. S. (2003). Modulating dysfunctional limbic-cortical circuits in depression: Towards development of brain-based algorithms for diagnosis and optimised treatment. *British Medical Bulletin, 65*, 193–207.

McDonald, W. M. (2000). Geriatric psychiatry. In K. R. R. Krishnan (Ed.), *Educational review manual in psychiatry* (pp. 1–44). New York: Castle Connolly Graduate Medical.

Mental Health America. (2006.) *Factsheet: Depression in older adults*. Accessed January 23, 2009, at http://www.nmha.org/index.cfm?objectid=C7DF94FF-1372-4D20-C8E34FC0813A5FF9

Mitchell, A. J., & Coyne, J. C. (2007). Do ultra-short screening instruments accurately detect depression in primary care? *British Journal of General Practice, 57*(535), 144–151.

National Institute of Mental Health. (2008). *Suicide in the U.S.: Statistics and prevention*. Retrieved August 21, 2008, from http://www.nimh.nih.gov/health/publications/suicide-in-the-us-statistics-and-prevention.shtml#CDC-Web-Tool

Nease, D. E., Jr., & Maloin, J. M. (2003). Depression screening: A practical strategy [abstract]. *Journal of Family Practice, 52*(2), 118.

Nelson, J. C. (2001). Diagnosing and treating depression in the elderly. *Journal of Clinical Psychiatry, 62*(Suppl. 24), 18–22.

Nemeroff, C. B., Musselman, D. L., & Evans, D. L. (1998). Depression and cardiac disease. *Depression and Anxiety, 8*(Suppl. 1), 71–79.

Oxman, T. E., Barrett, J., & Gerber, P. (1990). Symptomatology of late-life minor depression among primary care patients. *Psychosomatics, 31*, 174–180.

Parmelee, P. A., Katz, I. R., & Lawton, M. P. (1992). Incidence of depression in long-term care settings. *Journal of Gerontology: Medical Sciences, 47*, 189–196.

Paykel, E. S., Scott, J., Tesdale, J. D., Johnson, A. L., Garland, A., Moore, R., et al. (1999). Prevention in relapse in residual depression by cognitive therapy. *Archives of General Psychiatry, 56*(9), 829–835.

Pearson, S. D., Katelnick, D. J., Simon, G. E., Manning, W. G., Helstad, C. P., & Henk, H. J. (1999). Depression among high utilizers of medical care. *Journal of General Internal Medicine, 14*(8), 461–468.

President's New Freedom Commission on Mental Health. (2003). *Achieving the promise: Transforming mental health care in America.* Retrieved January 18, 2010, from http://www.mentalhealthcommission.gov/reports/Finalreport/FullReport.htm

Quijano, L. M., Stanley, M. A., Petersen, N. J., Casado, B. L., Steinberg, E. H., Cully, J. A., et al. (2007). Healthy IDEAS: A depression intervention delivered by community-based case managers serving older adults. *Journal of Applied Gerontology, 26*, 139–156.

Quinnett, P. (1995). *QPR for suicide prevention.* Spokane, WA: QPR Institute.

Rabins, P. V., Black, B. S., Roca, R., German, P., McGuire, M., Robbins, B., et al. (2000). Effectiveness of a nurse-based outreach program for identifying and treating psychiatric illness in the older adults. *JAMA, 283*(21), 2802–2809.

Raskin, J., Pritchett, Y. L., Wang, F., D'Souza, D. N., Waninger, A. L., Iyengar, S., et al. (2005). A double-blind, randomized multicenter trial comparing duloxetine with placebo in the management of diabetic peripheral neuropathic pain. *Pain Medicine, 6*(5), 346–356.

Rost, K., Pyne, J. M., Dickinson, L. M., & LoSasso, A. T. (2005). Cost-effectiveness of enhancing primary care depression management on an ongoing basis. *Annals of Family Medicine, 3*(1), 7–14. Retrieved July 27, 2008, from http:www.annfammed.org/cgi/content/full/3/1/7

Salzman, C., Wong, E., & Wright, B. C. (2002). Drug and ECT treatment of depression in older adults, 1996–2001: A literature review. *Biological Psychiatry, 52*(3), 265–284.

Scott, J., Tesdale, J. D., Paykel, E. S., Johnson, A. L., Abbott, R., Hayhurst, H., et al. (2000). Effects of cognitive therapy on psychological symptoms and social functioning in residual depression. *British Journal of Psychiatry, 177*, 440–446.

Steffens, D. (2004). Establishing diagnostic criteria for vascular depression. *Journal of the Neurological Sciences, 226*(1-2), 59–62.

Steffens, D. C., & Krishnan, K. R. (1998). Structural neuroimaging and mood disorders: Recent findings, implications for classification, and future directions. *Biological Psychiatry, 43*(10), 705–712.

Styron, W. (1990). *Darkness visible: A memoir of madness.* New York: Random House.

Thase, M. (2002). What role do atypical antipsychotic drugs have in treatment-resistant depression? *Journal of Clinical Psychiatry, 63*(2), 95–103.

Tweedy, K., Morrison, M. F., & DeMichele, S. G. (2002). Depression in older women. *Psychiatric Annals, 327,* 417–429.

Unutzer, J. (2002). Diagnosis and treatment of older adults with depression in primary care. *Biological Psychiatry, 52*(3), 285–292.

Unutzer, J., Katon, W., Callahan, C. M., Williams, J. W., Hunkeler, E., Harpole, L., et al. (2002). Collaborative care management of late-life depression in the primary care setting. *JAMA, 288*(22), 2836–2845.

Unutzer, J., Schoenbaum, M., Katon, W., Fan, M., Pincus, H., Hogan, D., et al. (2009). Health care costs associated with depression in medically ill fee-for-service Medicare participants. *Journal of the American Geriatric Society, 57*(3), 506–510.

U.S. Department of Health and Human Services. (1999). *Mental health: A report of the Surgeon General.* Rockville, MD: U.S. Department of Health and Human Services, Substance Abuse and Mental Health

Services Administration, Center for Mental Health Services, National Institute of Mental Health.

U.S. Department of Health and Human Services. (2000). *Healthy people 2010*. Washington, DC: Author.

Vaishnavi, T., & Taylor, W. D. (2006). Neuroimaging in late-life depression. *International Review of Psychiatry, 18*(5), 443–451.

Wang, P. S., Demler, O., Olfson, M., Pincus, H. A., Wells, K. B., & Kessler, R. C. (2006). Changing profiles of service sectors used for mental health care in the United States [abstract]. *American Journal of Psychiatry, 163*(7), 1187.

Wang, P. S., Lane, M., Olfson, M., Pincus, H. A., Wells, K. B., & Kessler, R. C. (2005). Twelve-month use of mental health services in the United States: Results from the National Comorbidity Survey Replication. *Archives of General Psychiatry, 62*(6), 590–592.

World Health Organization. (2003). *Investing in mental health*. Geneva: Author. Accessed December 28, 2009, at http://www.who.int/mental_health/en/investing_in_mnh_final.pdf

World Health Organization. (2005). *United States of America: Mental health atlas 2005*. Retrieved January 30, 2006, from http://www.who.int./mental_health/evidence/atlas/

World Health Organization. (2006). *Preamble to the Constitution of the World Health Organization*. Retrieved December 28, 2009, from http://www.who.int/governance/eb/who_constitution_en.pdf

World Health Organization. (2006). *Working together for health: World health report 2006*. Geneva: Author.

World Health Organization. (2007). Mental health policy, planning, and service development information sheet, sheet 4. Retrieved December 28, 2009, from http://www.who.int/mental_health/policy/services/4_Humanresource&training_Infosheet.pdf

World Health Organization. (2009). Depression. Accessed December 28, 2009, at http://www.who.int/mental_health/management/depression/definition/en/

Yesavage, J. A., & Brink, T. L. (1983). Development and validation of a geriatric depression scale: A preliminary report. *Journal of Psychiatric Research, 17*, 37–49.

Zielinski, R. J., Roose, S. P., Devanand, D. P., Woodring, S., & Sackeim, H. A. (1993). Cardiovascular complications of ECT in depressed patients with cardiac disease. *American Journal of Psychiatry, 150*(6), 904–908.

8

Nursing Assessment and Treatment of Anxiety in Late Life

Marianne Smith

The experience of anxiety symptoms is often a complex phenomenon in older adults. Anxiety is a diffuse, unpleasant, and vague feeling of apprehensive expectation and worry that is accompanied by a range of behavioral symptoms, such as restlessness, fatigue, difficulty concentrating, irritability, muscle tension, and sleep disturbance (American Psychiatric Association [APA], 2000). Anxiety is the primary symptom in a diverse array of anxiety disorders; regularly occurs as a comorbid condition or symptom in both late-life depression and dementia; is the direct consequence of a wide variety of physical health conditions that are common among aging individuals; and is aroused in response to a wide variety of social, environmental, personal, and health-related stressors that tend to cluster in later life (Bryant, Jackson, & Ames, 2008; Cairney, Corna, Veldhuizen, Herrmann, & Streiner, 2008; Sareen et al., 2006; Seignourel, Kunik, Snow, Wilson, & Stanley, 2008). Irrespective of causal factors, the increased disability, reduced health-related quality of life, and greater healthcare use among older adults with anxiety disorders (Hoffman, Dukes, & Wittchen, 2008; Porensky et al., 2009) demands that nurses and allied health providers pay thoughtful attention to diverse symptoms that may represent late-life anxiety.

Understanding and managing anxiety symptoms and disorders in late life are challenging for a number of reasons. Of perhaps most importance, anxiety symptoms exist on a continuum from "normal" reactions to life experiences to "pathological" levels that impair function and create substantial suffering. All people experience anxiety symptoms, to a greater or lesser extent, throughout their lives. Use of diagnostic hierarchies and arbitrary "caseness" criteria that reflect problems of young adults is questionable given how little is known about "normal" anxiety in older adults, and in turn, how much anxiety constitutes a "case" (Bryant et al., 2008).

Distinguishing appropriate anxiety and worry from excessive anxiety and worry is often difficult for older adults themselves, and for mental health providers and primary care providers (PCP) who provide treatment for diverse health complaints (Bartels et al., 2004; Lecrubier, 2007). In addition, the literature is inconsistent regarding the characteristics of anxiety disorders in older adults; its prevalence in late life (particularly new-onset anxiety disorders); and the extent to which comorbid psychiatric and medical illness account for the observed frequency of anxiety symptoms (Bryant et al., 2008). Unlike depression and dementia, considerably less research has been conducted specifically with older adults who experience anxiety symptoms and disorders (Lenze & Wetherell, 2009; Vink, Aartsen, & Schoevers, 2008). Although older adults are increasingly the focus of assessment and intervention research, the transfer of knowledge into practice lags behind (Wetherell, Maser, & van Balkom, 2005b). In turn, accurate identification of late-life anxiety disorders and provision of evidence-based treatments in "routine care" are goals that have yet to be achieved (Ayers, Sorrell, Thorp, & Wetherell, 2007; Lenze & Wetherell, 2009; Mohlman, 2004).

Despite the slow progression of anxiety-related research, anxiety symptoms are commonly observed among older adults, often have profound and negative effects, and regularly result in both increased use of health services and diminished quality of life for both the person who experiences the distress and his or her caregivers. Nurses and other allied health providers are challenged to recognize and understand the wide array of problems and health conditions that serve as antecedents to anxiety-related symptoms; to conduct comprehensive, interdisciplinary assessments that use a biopsychosocial framework and examine complex interactions between physical, mental, personal, social, and environmental factors; and to devise effective and lasting interventions that maximize function and comfort.

This chapter emphasizes the often unique problems and issues that may arise in the identification and treatment of late-life anxiety symptoms and disorders, and assumes that the reader has a basic understanding of both anxiety disorders and treatment strategies used with younger age groups. Anxiety symptoms, which are defined here as distressing physical and emotional experiences that often occur as a cluster but do not meet criteria for diagnosis as a disorder, are an important focus of nursing care and are considered throughout the chapter. Commonly occurring comorbid conditions, including depression, cognitive impairment, physical health conditions, and life stressors, are described. Assessment methods, including factors to consider in the diagnostic workup, presentation of anxiety symptoms in late life, interviewing considerations, and scales that may assist in quantifying symptoms, are considered. Finally, treatment considerations, including nonpharmacological and pharmacological interventions that target late-life anxiety disorders, are reviewed.

ANXIETY DISORDERS IN LATE LIFE

A number of important issues are essential to consider if nurses and allied healthcare providers hope to identify, assess, and treat anxiety symptoms and disorders accurately in older adults. Frequently quoted statistics noting that the prevalence of anxiety disorders is lower in older adults compared to younger age groups may inadvertently reduce clinicians' attention to important symptom clusters that are representative of diagnosable disorders, and more importantly, distressing experiences that warrant intervention (Bryant et al., 2008; Wetherell et al., 2005b). Phobias, particularly agoraphobia associated with a specific event, such as falling, generalized anxiety disorders (GAD), and posttraumatic stress disorders associated with trauma earlier in life are all increasingly recognized as emerging for the first time in late life (Gagnon, Flint, Naglie, & Devins, 2005; Karlsson et al., 2009; Rucci et al., 2009; Yehuda et al., 2009).

Moreover, anxiety disorders are the most common psychiatric disorders among people of all ages and affect a substantial number of older adults (Kessler, Berglund, Demler, Jin, & Walters, 2005). Variations in the rates of anxiety reported often reflect the type of anxiety (e.g., symptom clusters, specific disorders, all anxiety disorders) and the setting in which the research occurs (e.g., clinical versus community setting). A review of studies conducted between 1980 and 2007 found that the prevalence of anxiety disorders among community-dwelling older adults ranged from 1.2% to 15%, whereas anxiety symptoms ranged from 15% to 52.3% (Bryant et al., 2008). Notably, rates for both anxiety disorders and symptoms were systematically higher when research was conducted in clinical settings (Bryant et al., 2008), a finding that has important implications for treating anxiety and other mental disorders in primary care settings (Katon & Roy-Byrne, 2007).

The importance of detecting and treating mental distress and disorders among older adults in primary care settings, as highlighted in *Mental Health: A Report of the Surgeon General* (U.S. Department of Health and Human Services, 1999), has been underscored in hundreds of studies on depression (Blasinsky, Goldman, & Unutzer, 2006); depression and comorbid pain (Kroenke, Shen, Oxman, Williams, & Dietrich, 2008); and dementia care (Callahan et al., 2006). Assessment and treatment of anxiety disorders in primary care has received considerably less attention (Katon, Lin, & Kroenke, 2007). However, findings to date provide considerable support that anxiety disorders are common among primary care patients (14.5% to 19.5%), but are widely underrecognized and undertreated (Kroenke, Spitzer, Williams, Monahan, & Lowe, 2007; Lecrubier, 2007), and that use of brief screening tools and collaborative approaches that use "stepped care" are effective in treating anxiety (Kroenke et al., 2007; Lowe et al., 2008b; Roy-Byrne et al., 2008; van't Veer-Tazelaar et al., 2009; Wetherell, Birchler, Ramsdell, & Unutzer, 2007).

Resounding themes that emerge from anxiety-related research in primary care settings have important implications for nurses and allied health providers. First, older adults often present with diverse symptoms and complaints as outlined in Box 8-1.

Systematic assessment using a standardized scale is critically important to document and monitor anxiety-related symptoms over time (Katon & Roy-Byrne, 2007; Spitzer, Kroenke, Williams, & Lowe, 2006; Weiss et al., 2009). In addition, concurrent treatment of anxiety and comorbid problems, such as depression, pain, or other medical conditions, is essential (Bair, Wu, Damush, Sutherland, & Kroenke, 2008; Katon et al., 2007; Roy-Byrne et al., 2008; Teh et al., 2009). Finally, effective treatment often relies on collaborative care (CC) by nurse

care managers, PCPs, and mental health specialists, and "stepped care" approaches that combine and systematically adjust pharmacological and psychosocial interventions to achieve optimal outcomes (Bair et al., 2008; Engel et al., 2008; Mittal, Fortney, Pyne, Edlund, & Wetherell, 2006; Teh et al., 2009).

COMORBID CONDITIONS

Perhaps the most important consideration in identifying and treating clinically significant anxiety among older adults is recognition of the wide range of comorbid conditions. Depression, cognitive impairment, physical health problems, pain, and both personal and environmental stress are all widely recognized as complicating the identification and treatment of anxiety disorders in older adults. Each creates similar and yet somewhat different anxiety symptoms that must be distinguished as a separate anxiety disorder, or understood as being the result of the comorbid mental or physical health problem. Treatment approaches are largely guided by underlying causal factors, making this differentiation an important first step in care planning.

Depression and Anxiety

Concurrent anxiety and depression is alternatively labeled as "anxious depression" or "comorbid anxiety and depression" depending on the position taken related to use of diagnostic hierarchies (Jeste, Hays, & Steffens, 2006; Moffitt et al., 2007). Like rates of anxiety disorders overall, estimated prevalence of morbid anxiety and depression tends to vary according to the setting and sample used. Community surveys of older adults indicate that 3.2% to 6.4% report significant anxiety, 11.5% to 12.9% report significant depression, and 1.9% to 4.5% report comorbid anxiety and depression symptoms (Brenes et al., 2008; Holwerda et al., 2007). Considering the problems from a slightly different perspective, from 23% to 47.5% of older adults who meet criteria for major depression also meet criteria for an anxiety disorder (Beekman et al., 2000; Cairney et al., 2008; Campbell et al., 2007), suggesting that assessment of both disorders is often essential to address adequately the spectrum of difficulties experienced.

Comorbid anxiety and depression in older adults produce greater severity of illness and poorer treatment responses than is observed in either condition alone (Andreescu et al., 2007; Campbell et al., 2007; Lenze et al., 2001). Older adults with comorbid anxiety and depression have more severe somatic symptoms, poorer social function, reduced quality of life and well-being,

BOX 8-1 ANXIETY SYMPTOMS IN OLDER ADULTS

Cognitive	Vigilance and scanning	Motor tension	Autonomic arousal and somatic
Anxiety	Hyperattentiveness	Shakiness	Anorexia
Worry	Feeling "on edge"	Jitteriness	Body aches and pains
Apprehensive expectation	Impatience	Jumpiness	Diaphoresis, sweating
Rumination	Irritability	Trembling	Diarrhea
Anticipation that something bad is about to happen	Distractibility	Tension	Dizziness
• Fear of fainting	Difficulty concentrating	Muscle aches	Dry mouth
• Fear of losing control	Insomnia	Fatigability	Dyspnea
• Fear of dying	Difficulty falling asleep	Inability to relax	Headache
• Fear that family members are ill, injured	Interrupted sleep	Eyelid twitch	Faintness
	Fatigue on awakening	Furrowed brow	Fatigability
		Strained face	Flushing
		Fidgeting	Frequent urination
		Restlessness	Insomnia
		Easy startle	Heart pounding
		Sighing	Hot or cold spells
			Light-headedness
			Nausea, upset stomach
			Palpitations
			Pallor
			Parathesias
			Pulse increased at rest
			Tremor
			Vomiting

Source: APA, 1980; Dada, Sethi, & Grossberg, 2001; Rickels & Rynn, 2001; Small, 1997.

greater cognitive and memory impairment, and greater suicidal ideation (Bierman, Comijs, Jonker, & Beekman, 2005; Brenes et al., 2007; Brenes et al., 2008; Katon et al., 2007). In addition, medically ill older patients who experience anxiety and depression have greater disability and poorer outcomes compared to those who do not experience psychiatric symptoms (Lenze et al., 2001).

Furthermore, the association between comorbid anxiety and depression and chronic pain has many implications for nursing assessments and interventions (Mok & Lee, 2008). Although the downward spiraling relationship between depression and pain is well understood (Kroenke et al., 2008; Unutzer et al., 2008), additional research emphasizes the negative associations between anxiety and pain, and comorbid anxiety and depression and pain. Pain that interferes with daily activities is associated with more severe anxiety, worse daily function, higher health service use, and lower likelihood of responding to anxiety treatments (Teh et al., 2009). Comorbid anxiety and depression and chronic pain are similarly associated with more severe pain, greater disability, and poorer health-related quality of life than when pain occurs alone or in association with either anxiety or depression (Bair et al., 2008).

Cognitive Impairment and Anxiety

Anxiety symptoms associated with cognitive impairment, early dementia, or behavioral symptoms in middle to later dementia are another area of concern in the nursing care of older adults. An important and increasing focus in memory research is the frequency with which anxiety symptoms occur in older adults with mild cognitive impairment. Population-based studies indicate that over 46% of older persons with mild cognitive impairment experience anxiety-related symptoms, and 83% of those with anxiety and mild cognitive impairment develop Alzheimer's disease during the 3-year follow-up (Palmer et al., 2007).

Anxiety is also one of several neuropsychiatric symptoms that commonly occur during the course of dementia. Although early reports suggested that as many as 80% of individuals with Alzheimer's disease experience anxiety (Teri et al., 1999), later studies indicate that anxiety occurs in 22% to 25% of older adults with dementia (Smith et al., 2008b; Tatsch et al., 2006). Box 8-2 provides common symptoms of anxiety in dementia. Of importance, anxiety is considered a distinct phenomenon from agitation, one that warrants methodical assessment to ensure that unique aspects of dementia-related apprehension and worry are adequately addressed (Twelftree & Qazi, 2006).

Physical Health Conditions and Anxiety

Another challenging area for nurses and other allied health personnel is the differentiation of anxiety stemming from an anxiety disorder and anxiety related to general medical conditions that tend to cluster in later life. Physical illness and both anxiety symptoms and disorders are connected and interact in several important ways (Roy-Byrne et al., 2008; Sable & Jeste, 2001). An important first consideration is the arousal of apprehension and worry that "logically" accompany late-life health problems and their treatment. Fear of pain, disability, dependency, and a host of other health-related problems associated with physical illness may trigger anxiety-related symptoms, causing considerable emotional distress. Furthermore, physiological activation associated with anxiety often includes somatic symptoms (e.g., fatigue, gastrointestinal symptoms, and headache) that further complicate the clinical picture (Lenze et al., 2005a).

The overlap in physical symptoms that may result from anxiety disorders or medical illnesses regularly confounds accurate diagnosis and treatment. As illustrated in Box 8-3, a wide variety of physical health problems are known to cause anxiety-related symptoms.

Of equal importance, medications that are regularly used to treat physical illness may have side effects that mimic anxiety-related symptoms (Box 8-4), making thorough assessment of both

BOX 8-2 CLINICAL INDICATORS OF ANXIETY IN DEMENTIA

Angry outbursts	Increased muscle tension	Scared
Asking repeated questions	Insomnia	Shadowing caregiver
Changes in eating patterns	Irritability	Shakiness
Crying	Losing control	Tachycardia
Dry mouth	Pacing	Tearfulness
Facial tension	Poor attention span	Trembling
Fidgeting	Poor eye contact	Urinary frequency
Glancing about	Rapid, disconnected speech	Voice changes
Hyperventilation	Repetitive motions	Voice quivering
Inability to sit still	Restlessness	Wariness

Source: Mahoney, E. K., Volicer, L., & Hurley, A. (2000). Anxiety. In E. K. Mahoney, L. Volicer, & A. Hurley (Eds.), *Management of challenging behaviors in dementia* (pp. 109–124). Baltimore: Health Professions Press. Used with permission.

physical illness and its treatment an important focus of nursing care. Medications and substances associated with anxiety symptoms include the following (APA, 2000; Dugue & Neugroschl, 2002; Small, 1997):

Anxiety disorders also exist comorbidly with physical illness, particularly gastrointestinal, respiratory, and cardiovascular diseases; cancer; primary insomnia; and conditions that cause chronic pain (Hidalgo et al., 2007; Katon et al., 2007; Mok & Lee, 2008; Mussell et al., 2008; Roy-Byrne et al., 2008; Teh et al., 2009). Of importance to nurses and allied health providers, comorbid anxiety and physical illness is regularly associated with reduced quality of life, including both greater disability and reduced well-being (Brenes, 2007; Brenes et al., 2005; Roy-Byrne et al.; Sareen et al., 2006) and greater health services use and cost of care (Gurmankin Levy, Maselko, Bauer, Richman, & Kubzansky, 2007).

The importance of interactions between physical health conditions and anxiety is underscored by the potential downward spiral of disability that may occur as anxiety symptoms interfere with daily function in a kind of "self-fulfilling prophecy." For example, the person who has fallen is anxious about falling again and restricts his or her activity. Activity restriction in turn causes disuse atrophy, which increases the risk of falling again, places the person more at risk for problems associated with immobility, and creates an even greater sense of apprehension about his or her abilities. One problem complicates another and so the spiral turns downward.

Late-Life Change and Anxiety

Psychosocial issues and changes that occur in later life, including frailty, social isolation, financial changes, caregiving responsibilities, safety issues, and other age-related changes, may also arouse anxious feelings and behaviors and contribute to diagnostic difficulties. As noted earlier,

BOX 8-3 GENERAL MEDICAL CONDITIONS THAT CAUSE ANXIETY SYMPTOMS

Metabolic	Cardiovascular	Endocrine	Respiratory	Neurological	Other Conditions
Acidosis	Angina pectoris	Cushing syndrome	Chronic obstructive pulmonary disease	Cerebral anoxia	Influenza
Dehydration	Arrhythmia	Hyperthyroidism and hypothyroidism	Pneumonia	Cerebral neoplasm	Hepatitis
Electrolyte imbalance (e.g., hypercalcemia)	Cerebral atherosclerosis	Hyperadrenocorticism	Hyperventilation	Delirium	Constipation
Hyperthermia	Congestive heart failure	Hypoparathyroidism or hyperparathyroidism	Hypoxia	Dementia	Pain
Porphyria	Mitral valve prolapse	Hypoglycemia, hyperinsulinism		Epilepsy	
	Pulmonary embolism	Pheochromocytoma		Parkinson's disease	
		Vitamin B_{12} deficiency		Postconcussion disorders	
				Vestibular dysfunction	
				Encephalitis	

Source: APA, 2000; Dugue & Neugroschl, 2002; Small, 1997.

BOX 8-4 MEDICATIONS AND SUBSTANCES ASSOCIATED WITH ANXIETY SYMPTOMS

Intoxication	**Withdrawal**	**Medications**	**Heavy Metal and Toxins**
Alcohol	Alcohol	Analgesics and anesthetics	Carbon dioxide
Amphetamines	Anxiolytics	Anticholinergics	Carbon monoxide
Cannabis	Barbiturates	Anticonvulsants	Gasoline, paint, other volatile substances
Cocaine	Cocaine	Antidepressants	
Hallucinogens	Hypnotics	Antihistamines	Nerve gases
Inhalants	Narcotics	Antihypertensives	Organophospate insecticides
Phencyclidine	Nicotine	Antiparkinsonian medications	
	Sedatives	Antipsychotics, atypical antipsychotics	
		Bronchodilators (e.g., albuterol, terbutaline)	
		Caffeine	
		Corticosteroids	
		Digoxin	
		Insulin	
		Lithium carbonate	
		Meclizine HCL	
		Nonsteroidal anti-inflammatory agents	
		Over-the-counter cough and cold preparations (e.g., pseudoephedrine, caffeine)	
		Over-the-counter hypnotics	
		Tobacco	
		Theophylline	
		Thyroid preparations (e.g., thyroxine)	

Source: APA, 2000; Dugue & Neugroschl, 2002; Small, 1997.

determining what is "excessive" worry is sometimes difficult when the older person faces a number of real-life problems and stressors.

Because anxiety disorders are widely recognized as having an onset in adolescence and early adulthood, thoughtful examination of long-standing patterns of behavior is essential. For a variety of historical and social reasons, many older adults who experienced mental illness during their lifetime were not identified, diagnosed, or treated. As a result, a life review that includes assessment of long-standing patterns of coping, social history, and both treated and untreated physical health problems is often essential to establishing a diagnosis of anxiety disorder.

ASSESSMENT OF ANXIETY IN LATER LIFE

The array of confounding factors that may mimic, precipitate, and coexist with anxiety disorders in late life emphasizes the importance of comprehensive physical, social, and environmental assessment. Like assessment of other health problems in older people, use of a biopsychosocial framework and attention to both current and historical factors is essential to the accurate identification and treatment of anxiety.

History and Physical

Careful and comprehensive history, physical examination, and routine laboratory studies are recommended as part of the diagnostic workup for anxiety disorder in later life (Swinson et al., 2006). Collaborative approaches between primary care and mental health providers are often essential to identify, diagnose, and treat anxiety symptoms and disorders accurately in tandem with other medical illness (Mittal et al., 2006; Roy-Byrne & Wagner, 2004). Similarly, collateral history from a family member or caregiver who knows the person well can provide important information about current symptoms and past

history (Swinson et al.). Components of the diagnostic workup are as follows:

Medical history
- Current and past medical disorders
- Drug and alcohol use; caffeine intake
- Prescribed and over-the-counter medications; use of herbal or home remedies
- Recent changes in health conditions and their treatment (e.g., change in medications)

Psychiatric history and assessment
- Past psychiatric history, including "nervous breakdowns" or other nontreated mental illness
- Rule out mood disorders, psychotic disorders, delirium, and dementia
- Consider changes that may represent subsyndromal conditions or early impairment

Laboratory
- Complete blood count, electrolytes, serum glucose, hepatic and renal function tests, thyroid function tests, vitamin B_{12} and folate levels, urinalysis, urine toxicology

Other tests
- Electrocardiogram, chest radiograph
- Brain imaging and neuropsychologic testing if cognitive impairment is suspected

Collateral history
- Substantiation of symptom onset, range, duration, intensity by family or close friends
- Long-standing personality, coping, life history
- Recent events that may contribute

As with assessment of other psychiatric and mental health conditions in late life, avoiding the use of medical jargon and adopting terms and descriptions used by the patient to describe the problem (including exploration of somatic symptoms) may be particularly useful. History of anxiety symptoms that existed earlier in life and are now exacerbated because of social or personal changes (e.g., symptoms were "managed" through family or work habits) is important to consider. Likewise, the presence of traumatic life events (e.g., combat, holocaust survivor, prisoner of war) that may serve as antecedents to late-life onset of posttraumatic stress disorder (Yehuda et al., 2009), or history of anxiety disorder in a first-degree relative (Swinson et al., 2006), may also contribute to understanding the current clinical picture.

Phrasing of questions is an important consideration when interviewing older adults who may not consider their distress as the result of anxiety (Flint, 2005; Smith, Ingram, & Brighton, 2008a; Swinson et al., 2006). For example, "Have you been concerned about or fretted over a number of things?" or "Do you have a hard time putting things out of your mind?" may be more fruitful than traditional questions about worry, rumination, or obsessive thoughts. Likewise, assistance may be needed to place distressing experiences in a temporal framework to understand the duration of problems. In this instance, offering the person a significant date or event to cue memories is often helpful (e.g., "Were you having this experience before [Christmas]?" vs. "When did this first happen?"). Adjusting questions that target possible antecedents to symptoms (e.g., "What were you doing when you noticed the chest pain?") or associated features (e.g., "When you can't sleep, what is usually going through your head?") may also produce meaningful clinical data.

Anxiety Symptoms

The wide range of anxiety symptoms that may occur as the result of an anxiety disorder, anxious depression, cognitive impairment, physical illness, or psychosocial stress emphasizes the importance of being inclusive until the nature of the person's distress is better understood. Refer again to Box 8-1 to review anxiety-related symptoms that may emerge in clinical practice.

The context of worries is often used to differentiate pathological anxiety (which is excessive) from "normal" worries. As in other age groups, apprehension, anxiety, or worry may be associated with a variety of stressors (e.g., financial changes, health conditions, family changes or problems). Unlike chronic worry that is excessive and disabling, "adaptive worry" is situational and temporary, and may even contribute to effective coping by anticipating future needs (Montorio, Wetherell, & Nuevo, 2006). Clinicians regularly have difficulty deciding what is justified given the nature and extent of problems an older adult has experienced. For example, the rationale offered for an older person's fear of leaving home may be related to crime rates and fear of mugging. Whether that fear is reasonable or excessive largely depends on rates of crime in the older person's community, a question that may only be answered with collateral information from family or caregivers.

Assessment Scales

Detection of clinically significant anxiety regularly relies on the use of a standardized scale to ensure that diverse symptoms are documented (Smith et al., 2008a). Several scales have demonstrated effectiveness with older adults and may be easily used by nurses and other providers to assess symptom clusters and monitor outcomes over time. Three scales that may be self-administered or clinician scored and used in a variety of settings with older adults are briefly reviewed next, along with two scales that are effective for addressing comorbid conditions.

The Geriatric Anxiety Inventory (Pachana et al., 2007) is composed of 20 statements that are scored Yes = 1 and No = 0 for a total score of 0 to 20. A score of 8 or greater correctly classified 78% of older adults with anxiety disorders, and is recommended as a cut-point. The GAD-7 (Spitzer et al., 2006) rates the seven symptoms that comprise the diagnostic criteria for GAD on a scale from 0 to 3, for a total score of 0 to 21. Scores from 5 to 9 indicate mild anxiety, scores from 10 to 14 reflect moderate anxiety, and scores greater than or equal to 15 indicate severe anxiety. Increasing evidence supports the use of the GAD-7 as a general screening tool in primary care and other settings (Kroenke et al., 2007; Lowe et al., 2008a; Swinson, 2006). The Generalized Anxiety Disorder Severity Scale (GADSS) was developed to assess GAD symptoms in primary care patients by telephone interviews (Shear, Belnap, Mazumdar, Houck, & Rollman, 2006). Six items that assess the worry frequency, severity, and related distress and impairment are scored from 0 to 4 for a total score of 0 to 24. Preliminary evidence supports the use of the GADSS with older adults (Andreescu et al., 2008; Weiss et al., 2009), although cut-points for clinically significant anxiety are not reported.

Two additional scales are valuable when comorbid conditions are suspected. The Hospital Anxiety and Depression Scale is widely used to assess late-life anxiety and depression (Kenn, Wood, Kucyj, Attis, & Cunane, 1987; Schroder et al., 2007; Spinhoven, Ormel, Sloekers, Speckens, & Van Hemert, 1997). The Hospital Anxiety and Depression Scale is a self-report measure that consists of two subscales (anxiety and depression) that each have seven items. Each item is rated 0 to 3 using narrative anchors, with total subscale scores of 0 to 21. Scores of less than 7 indicate a disorder (anxiety or depression) is likely not present, scores of 8 to 10 suggest a disorder is possible, and scores of 11 or greater indicate a disorder is probable.

The Rating Anxiety in Dementia scale is valuable when cognitive impairment is believed to impair the older person's ability to self-report anxiety-related emotions and behaviors (Shankar, Walker, Frost, & Orrell, 1999). The Rating Anxiety in Dementia scale is clinician-scored on the basis of observation and interview with the older adult, collateral interview with a person who knows the patient well, and review of behavioral symptoms noted in the medical or facility record. Twenty

items are rated from 0 to 3 for a total score of 0 to 60. Scores of 11 and above are considered clinically significant anxiety.

▪ TREATMENT OF ANXIETY IN LATE LIFE

The treatment methods used with late-life anxiety disorders fall into the two general classes of pharmacological and nonpharmacological interventions. As in the treatment of younger age groups, the selection of interventions depends largely on the specific anxiety diagnosis, individualized symptom presentation, and concomitant medical conditions and medications being taken by the patient. No matter what type of intervention is used, the relationship between the older person and the therapist or health provider is often critically important in treatment effectiveness.

The value of the therapeutic alliance is a particularly salient issue in treatment of late-life anxiety disorders. The nature of anxiety, which includes apprehensive expectations, worry, fearfulness, and often the feeling that one is either dying or going crazy, creates a special need for reassurance and psychological comfort measures (e.g., encouragement, support, reality testing), particularly among older people who often have seemingly valid competing explanations for their experiences. Additional time is often needed to discuss problems and experiences, explore possible alternative explanations for symptoms, and provide support for "staying the course" in treatment when relief is slow to develop.

Nonpharmacological Interventions

Nonpharmacological interventions are often preferred by older adults who may be concerned about medication side effects, costs, or the addition of more medication to an already extensive medication regimen (Thorp et al., 2009; Wetherell et al., 2004). Although a growing number of studies investigate psychosocial treatments for late-life anxiety, and the perceived value of nonpharmacological interventions to treat late anxiety disorders is quite high, the number of published studies is still disproportionately low (Lenze & Wetherell, 2009).

Systematic reviews and critiques of research that target psychosocial treatment of late-life anxiety disorders support the use of cognitive–behavioral therapy (CBT), relaxation training (RT), and supportive therapy (Ayers et al., 2007; Hendriks, Oude Voshaar, Keijsers, Hoogduin, & van Balkom, 2008; Thorp et al., 2009; Wetherell, Lenze, & Stanley, 2005a). General conclusions related to the state of science on this topic include the important observations that differences exist in treatment response based on the specific type of therapy; overall outcomes with older adults tend not to be as strong as in younger adults; and augmenting traditional approaches with methods to enhance learning (e.g., telephone calls, homework prompts, retention-building exercises) may be a strategic approach with older people (Ayers et al.; Mohlman & Price, 2006).

Cognitive–Behavioral Therapy

CBT takes many forms and generally includes structured therapy to identify, evaluate, control, and modify negative thoughts and cognitive distortions and attributions combined with behavioral strategies to confront fears and promote habituation. Various strategies are used to link thoughts, behaviors, and physical symptoms, with an aim of promoting more adaptive coping and reducing anxious arousal. Traditional CBT strategies include education about symptoms and self-monitoring techniques (e.g., thought monitoring, physiological arousal), cognitive restructuring, exposure methods and response prevention, behavioral activation, and problem solving (Kraus, Kunik, & Stanley, 2007).

A recent meta-analysis of behavioral treatments for late-life anxiety identified 19 clinical trials that met identified inclusion criteria (e.g., age of subjects, type of therapy, and size of trial) (Thorp et al., 2009). The analysis examined five conditions that emerged within the 19 studies: (1) wait list or no-treatment control conditions; (2) CBT with RT;

(3) CBT alone; (4) RT alone; and (5) active control conditions, such as psychoeducation, supportive counseling, group discussion, or other time spent with participants that served as an attention placebo. Notable outcomes include the following: (1) spontaneous remission during a wait-list period is unlikely; (2) active control conditions have moderate effects on anxiety reduction; (3) CBT and RT both have a large effect on depression, and an even larger effect on anxiety symptoms; and (4) combined RT and CBT does not seem to be more effective than either alone, suggesting that "more may not be better" for older adults (Thorp et al.).

In spite of identified methodological issues that may limit the generalizability of CBT trial results (Lenze & Wetherell, 2009; Mohlman, 2004; Thorp et al., 2009), the many positive outcomes associated with CBT provide a considerable impetus to refine, expand, and develop new methods for use with anxious older adults. Several variations are noted in the literature, including the translation of CBT principles to primary care, nursing home, and home healthcare settings. Each of these variations provides considerable opportunities for nurses to participate in the provision or support of therapeutic interventions to reduce anxiety and promote positive coping.

CBT in Primary Care

Most older adults seek treatment for mental disorders and distress in their primary care setting, not specialty mental health clinics, making this setting an important focus for nursing care, consultation, and collaborative services (Roy-Byrne & Wagner, 2004). Providing CBT in primary care settings often involves specialized training to facilitate the delivery of interventions that may be formally or informally delivered, creating many opportunities for nurses to participate. For example, one approach is to educate PCPs to use key principles of CBT (e.g., assessment of symptoms; education; self-monitoring; behavioral activation; access of resources; or changing responses to thoughts, feelings, and sensations) in their clinical practice with patients (Kraus et al., 2007). Many interventions add only minutes to the time spent with older patients and overall benefits may be further enhanced by involving nursing personnel to best use time in the waiting room (e.g., completing self-report items), or discussing concerns before or after seeing the PCP.

CC models provide another important opportunity for nurse involvement in providing CBT strategies in primary care settings. CC approaches are designed to improve outcomes by promoting education, engagement, and self-care by patients in collaboration with a specially trained "nonspecialist" therapist or care manager (often a nurse), psychiatrist, and the PCP (Roy-Byrne et al., 2005).

Use of an interactive computer-assisted CBT program, CALM Tools for Living, in primary care settings provides another opportunity for nurse involvement (Craske et al., 2009). Nurses and social workers are trained to facilitate the patient's use of structured educational modules about anxiety disorders; self-monitoring; breathing retraining; cognitive restructuring; exposure to external cues, images, memories; and relapse prevention. Diverse educational approaches (text, videos, list-making, homework assignments, reviews, or quizzes) are used to personalize and reinforce program concepts. Study outcomes indicate that patients with each of the four primary anxiety disorders included in the study sample (GAD, posttraumatic stress disorder, social anxiety disorder, and phobic disorder) report significant and substantial reductions in anxiety and depression symptoms, and significant increases in their expectation for positive outcomes and self-efficacy (Craske et al.).

Applications of CBT that involve individual sessions provided by trained clinicians in primary care settings also provide promising results (Stanley et al., 2009; Wetherell et al., 2009). A pilot study of "modular psychotherapy" in primary care examined the potential of tailoring 12 weekly sessions to the specific symptoms and needs of older participants using 14 possible standardized CBT-related modules (Wetherell et al.). Module topics addressed customary CBT approaches, such as education about anxiety and symptom monitoring, relaxation training, cognitive restructuring, thought-stopping, exposure, and behavioral activation, and less traditional topics, such as sleep hygiene, pain management, life review, acceptance, and relapse prevention. Substantial improvement in anxiety symptoms, worry, depression symptoms, and mental health–related quality of life were observed for subjects in both the intervention and active control group, suggesting that even modest changes in approach may positively influence outcomes. A study investigating CBT for GAD among older adults in primary care provided 10 individual sessions over 12 weeks that included education and awareness, motivational interviewing, relaxation training, cognitive therapy, exposure, problem-solving skills training, and behavioral sleep management (Stanley et al.) resulted in greater improvement in worry severity, depression symptoms, and general mental health, and produced meaningful, but not statistically significant, changes in GAD severity (Stanley et al.). In sum, various forms of CBT hold promise for treating late-life anxiety in primary care settings.

CBT in Home Care

Cognitive–behavioral approaches are also being translated for use in home health care, a setting in which nurses play a predominant and influential role. The importance of providing CBT in home care is underscored by both the frequency of anxiety disorders (31%) among home care patients, and the regularity with which cognitive, psychosocial, medical, or functional disabilities occur (Diefenbach, Tolin, Gilliam, & Meunier, 2008; Preville, Cote, Boyer, & Hebert, 2004).

Preliminary work in providing CBT to treat late-life anxiety in home care builds on work in other settings (Wetherell, Sorrell, Thorp, & Patterson, 2005c) and includes eight sessions using traditional approaches (e.g., psychoeducation, symptom review, relaxation training, problem solving, behavioral activation) and expanded reviews, self-monitoring work sheets, and booster telephone calls (Diefenbach et al., 2008; Mohlman et al., 2003). Outcomes of the feasibility study point to the importance of increasing attention to problem-solving to cope with stress, and improving collaboration between therapists (who provide CBT) and home health providers (e.g., care managers and nurses) who are often pivotal in facilitating needed social services to promote function and activity involvement (Diefenbach et al.). As with other applications of CBT, these findings have important implications for nurses who may work in the home health setting or provide specialized mental health treatment to elders in their own homes. The combined emphasis on problem-solving and cooperation between care providers is also consistent with CC models.

CC: IMPACT as a Model

An important and increasingly discussed approach in primary care settings is the use of CC models. The highly successful depression care study, Improving Mood Promoting Access to Collaborative Treatment (IMPACT) (Unutzer et al., 2002; Unutzer, Powers, Katon, & Langston, 2005), provides considerable support for using supportive counseling, patient education, self-monitoring, behavioral activation, and problem-solving therapy (PST) by a specially trained care manager (often a nurse) who works collaboratively with a consulting psychiatrist and the older person's PCP. Important features of the IMPACT model include the involvement of the older adult in choosing medication and/or PST, systematic monitoring of depression symptoms over time by the care manager, use of "stepped care" guidelines that recommend changing treatments to ensure that patients achieve optimal outcomes, and ongoing communication between care partners. Compared to usual care, the CC interventions reduced levels of depression, pain, and functional impairment and improved satisfaction and quality of life (Lin et al., 2003; Saur et al., 2007; Unutzer et al., 2002).

Notably, IMPACT patients with comorbid panic disorder (PD) and comorbid posttraumatic stress disorder reported higher levels of psychiatric and medical illness, greater functional impairment, and lower quality of life at baseline than participants without anxiety disorders (Hegel et al., 2005). However, older patients with comorbid anxiety disorders receiving CC achieved outcomes similar to those without anxiety disorders, both in terms of overall depression severity and clinically significant improvement (Hegel et al.). Although the IMPACT trial did not specifically address anxiety disorders (or measure anxiety symptoms as an outcome), results of the multisite, 5-year study provide an important standard against which anxiety-focused studies may gauge results.

CC for Anxiety

A small number of studies have examined the use of CC models to treat anxiety disorders in adults in primary care, military primary care, and nursing home settings (Engel et al., 2008; Katon, Roy-Byrne, Russo, & Cowley, 2002; Rollman et al., 2005; Roy-Byrne et al., 2005). All have demonstrated positive outcomes, and all have important implications for nursing practice and research.

Like the IMPACT study, an anxiety care manager (called by different names in each study) is pivotal in the provision of systematic treatment that involves patient choice, symptom monitoring, use of nonpharmacological and pharmacological treatments, and stepped care following treatment algorithms to ensure optimal outcomes. Although approaches to date primarily focus on the needs of adults 18 to 70 years of age, rather than older adults per se ($\geq$ 65 years), the approaches used and resultant findings have many important implications for nursing practice, research, and education. Two studies are described in depth to provide perspective related to key mechanisms, differences, and opportunities for nurses.

A CC model targeting treatment of PD and GAD among primary care patients combined many of the same elements used in IMPACT, including screening patients for PD and GAD, collaborating with PCPs, using specially trained anxiety care managers who were supervised by study physicians, encouraging patient choices related to nonpharmacological and pharmacological interventions, carefully monitoring symptoms and adjusting treatment to optimize outcomes, and systematic communication among care partners (Rollman et al., 2005). In this trial, however, nonpharmacological interventions included specially designed PD and GAD workbooks with lesson plans aimed at self-care. Lesson plans were reviewed and discussed during telephone visits with anxiety care managers who were centrally located (versus being onsite in primary care clinics). In addition, electronic medical records were used to communicate among collaborators. Significantly greater reductions in anxiety and depression symptoms, and improvement in mental health–related quality of life, were observed in CC patients compared to usual care recipients (Rollman et al.).

A somewhat different CC program targeting PD in primary care patients used specially trained behavioral health specialists to provide a shortened version of CBT (six individual sessions over 12 weeks plus six follow-up telephone contacts over 9 months) (Roy-Byrne et al., 2005). Like other CC models, patient education about PD and its treatment was provided by video; behavioral health specialists were supervised weekly by psychiatrists and an experienced CBT psychologist; medication changes were guided by an established algorithm and recommended to the PCP; and communication was optimized using telephone, fax, and email. Unique aspects of this CC intervention included the use of a patient workbook about medication benefits and limitations, and a 1-hour educational program for PCPs on recognition and treatment of PD and use of the anxiety medication algorithm. The CC intervention resulted in significantly greater reductions in panic attacks and depression symptoms and improved function and mental health–related quality of life, and was considered a cost-effective alternative to usual care (Katon et al., 2006; Roy-Byrne et al., 2005).

The many positive outcomes associated with CC models targeting depression in older adults and anxiety disorders in mid- to late-life adults have important implications for nurses. Many opportunities exist for nurses to serve as specially trained "care managers," and the older person's PCP or the consulting psychiatric specialist on the CC team.

Relaxation Training

A solid base of evidence supports the use of RT to treat late-life anxiety disorders (Ayers et al., 2007; Stanley et al., 2009; Thorp et al., 2009). Commonly reported RT methods include progressive muscle relaxation, deep breathing, meditation, and education about tension and stress. These methods are used in combination with one another, and with CBT.

The meta-analysis conducted by Thorp and colleagues (2009) suggests that RT is as effective as CBT, and in some ways may be superior because training providers to implement RT is relatively easier than training them to use CBT. Moreover, evidence indicates that older adults report high satisfaction with RT (Thorp et al.). Nurses often use RT principles in a diverse array of care situations and settings, making its use with late-life anxiety a natural extension of existing skills.

Supportive Therapy

No research targeting supportive methods as an intervention with late-life anxiety disorders is reported in the literature. However, 8 of 19 CBT clinical trials reviewed by Thorpe and colleagues (2009) included active control conditions that used supportive methods including group discussion, supportive counseling, "nonformal training in CBT or RT," psychoeducation, time for quiet reflections, and weekly medication management. Although used as "attention placeboes" in clinical trials, these active control conditions demonstrated moderate effects in reducing both depression and anxiety among older adult participants. Thus, interventions that encourage sharing problems, discussion, problem solving, informal learning, self-monitoring, and reflection, in the absence of structured methods characteristic of CBT, may be viable options for treating late-life anxiety.

Use of supportive therapy is consistent with both provision of care to individuals with chronic mental disorders and use of the therapeutic alliance as a curative factor. In some situations, nondirective talking therapy in which the therapist takes a more active role by providing encouragement, support, gentle direction or guidance, education, and reassurance may be beneficial in the treatment of older people. The addition of follow-up or "booster" telephone calls as an adjunct to CBT, and as a primary focus in CC models, underscores the importance of combining supportive approaches with other therapeutic methods to achieve optimal outcomes with older adults.

Psychoeducational Strategies

Education about symptoms and symptom management is often a component of anxiety management and is regularly provided as part of both CBT and CC models. The aim of educational approaches often has a dual focus of helping the person to understand distressing symptoms within the context of having an identified disorder (i.e., physical, psychological, and behavioral symptoms of the anxiety disorder) and assisting the person to reframe or restructure those experiences to relieve distress and increase comfort. Psychoeducational approaches may be particularly useful with older adults who are not familiar with psychological concepts; tend to present with somatic complaints and symptoms; and attribute their distress and discomfort to medical, not mental health, problems.

In addition to teaching older adults about symptoms of their illness, another important focus of psychoeducation with older adults is problem solving. Helping older adults develop and use problem-solving methods is often essential

for adaptive coping and restoring wellness. PST is increasingly advanced as a specific and structured intervention that involves training personnel, as was undertaken in IMPACT and other CC models (Arean, Hegel, Vannoy, Fan, & Unuzter, 2008; van't Veer-Tazelaar et al., 2009). Given the nonspecific focus of PST (e.g., the approach can be applied to any topic), these skills are an important component of the nurses' therapeutic repertoire.

Alternative Therapies and Interventions

Many supportive and alternative therapies are reviewed in the literature and may be valuable in treating older adults with anxiety symptoms or disorders. A variety of therapies are described in the context of treating anxiety-provoking medical conditions (e.g., cancer, myocardial infarction), or anxiety that is associated with medical settings (e.g., critical care) or procedures (e.g., presurgery, perisurgery, or postsurgery). In this context, nursing interventions to reduce anxiety states include music therapy; aromatherapy; massage (e.g., foot, back); therapeutic touch; light therapy; pet therapy; exercise therapy; self-hypnosis; distraction or redirection (e.g., reminiscence, life review, current events, television viewing); activity involvement; acupuncture; acupressure and auricular acupressure; and cognitive–behavioral strategies, such as guided imagery, relaxation exercises and therapy, and other stress reduction methods.

Despite the common sense appeal of many of these interventions, there is no empirical research to support their use for treatment of late-life anxiety disorders. However, several have demonstrated effectiveness with older individuals who experience anxiety (and agitation) as a consequence of dementia (Kolanowski & Buettner, 2008; Kolanowski, Litaker, & Buettner, 2005). Likewise, treatment of anxiety symptoms, whether or not they are representative of a true threshold-level anxiety disorder, is often a nursing challenge. These supportive, therapeutic, hands-on interventions may be particularly salient to nurses working in day-to-day caregiving settings, and as such make an important contribution to the care and treatment of frail older people.

Preventive Methods

The prevalence of anxiety symptoms among older adults suggests that preventive approaches are needed to reduce the risk that symptom clusters progress to a full-blown anxiety disorder that causes even greater levels of distress and impairment (van't Veer-Tazelaar et al., 2006). A program implemented in the Netherlands targets older adults with subthreshold anxiety (and depression) using "stepped care" to reduce the risk of new-onset depression and anxiety disorders (van't Veer-Tazelaar et al., 2009).

The intervention combines bibliotherapy and PST to help older patients understand their symptoms and engage in more active self-management. The approach consists of four steps, each of which lasts 3 months: (1) watchful waiting monitors elders with clinically significant anxiety for change in their symptoms; (2) CBT-based bibliotherapy provides telephone calls and home visits by a trained nurse who delivers a self-help course; (3) brief CBT-based PST provides seven sessions on problem solving by a trained nurse aimed at helping patients regain control of their lives; and (4) referral to primary care offers patients with continuously elevated symptoms pharmacotherapy by their PCP. Compared to usual care, the stepped care intervention is effective in reducing the onset of depression and anxiety disorders (van't Veer-Tazelaar et al., 2009). As emphasized in the section on CC models, many opportunities exist for nurses to monitor symptoms, provide educational interventions, facilitate problem solving using guided or informal methods, and collaborate with other providers to help older patients cope more effectively with anxiety and worry.

Pharmacological Interventions

Medication interventions continue to be the mainstay of treatment for anxiety disorders in both younger and older adults. Regrettably, many medications used with younger people have adverse consequences when used with older adults (e.g., benzodiazepines). A wide variety of normal aging changes influence drug actions in older people: cardiovascular changes contribute to pharmacokinetic alterations; respiratory system changes increase sensitivity to sedative effects; sensitivity to both peripheral and central anticholinergic effects is more likely with advancing age; glomerular filtration rate declines and affects renal clearance; and perhaps most important, volume of drug distribution (e.g., the ratio of total drug in the body to the amount circulating in the plasma) is altered by decreased total body water, reduced lean body mass, and increased body fat, which in turn increases the drug's half life and extends the time needed for drugs to reach steady state. If liver disease is present, reduced hepatic blood flow and metabolism further compound problems, particularly with benzodiazepines that undergo hydroxylation (e.g., diazepam).

Additional problems are often created by the presence of multiple comorbid medical conditions and medications used to treat them. Potential drug–drug interactions that worsen side effects, alter plasma concentrations, and otherwise negatively influence medication performance or create toxicity are all important factors to consider with older people. Furthermore, as the sheer number of medications increases, the complexity of the regimen often also increases (e.g., number of times per day medications are taken, number and type of medications taken at different times of day), creating additional risks for misunderstanding, confusion, and mismanagement of the medication regimen. Because medications have both benefits and associated hazards, geriatric-conscious providers strive to reduce the number of medications used by older people, simplify medication regimens, educate patients regarding the purpose and side-effect profiles of medications prescribed, and provide alternative nonpharmacological interventions whenever possible.

Rational treatment of anxiety disorders in late life demands use of a biopsychosocial framework that blends supportive, assistive, nonpharmacological interventions with prudent use of psychoactive medications that are carefully prescribed and systematically monitored. Cognitive–behavioral and other psychotherapies should be combined with education and support for patients and family members. Interventions should address significant life stressors and optimize both mental health and physical function, including attention to sleep, exercise, and nutrition needs, to facilitate best response to medication interventions.

As in the treatment of other late-life mental disorders, medication interventions are often specifically selected for the type of disorder the person experiences, taking into consideration unique symptom presentations and other conditions and medications currently in use. General principles related to the selection and use of psychotropic medications in older adults clearly apply to anxiolytic medications. Although use of nonpharmacological interventions as the first line of intervention is always desirable, use of medications is guided by the individual's level of distress and the presence of specific indications, such as anxious depression. Development of clear therapeutic goals and outcome criteria facilitates decision making as doses are titrated, medications are changed, and decisions are made to augment therapy. Clinicians must be confident that a maximum trial with a specific agent is completed without adequate response before making changes. The adage "start low and go slow" applies but should include additional recommendations to monitor symptom improvement carefully, watch for untoward side effects, offer encouragement to patients and families because symptom reduction may take time, and persist in treatment to achieve optimal therapeutic outcomes. The last point is underscored by research that reports older patients receive "some" but not appropriate levels of treatment (Jackson, Passamonti, & Kroenke, 2007; Lecrubier, 2007).

Evidence for Pharmacotherapy

As with psychosocial interventions, research targeting pharmacological treatment of late-life anxiety is slowly accumulating. Most treatment recommendations continue to rely on research conducted with younger age groups and are further guided by the experiences of a growing group of geriatric psychiatrists and nurse practitioners. Although several practice guidelines for the treatment of anxiety disorders now exist (Baldwin et al., 2005; Bandelow et al., 2008; McIntosh et al., 2004; Swinson et al., 2006), none specifically address the unique problems of aging persons.

General cautions related to treating older adults include the need to pay attention to comorbid medical conditions, psychosocial stressors, comorbid anxiety and depression, and observations that poorer treatment outcomes, including delayed or diminished responses and increased likelihood of dropping out of treatment, are common (Swinson et al., 2006). The sage advice offered in the Canadian Clinical Practice Guideline (Swinson et al.), that "a strong doctor–patient relationship is essential [when treating older patients], and interventions should include environmental, social, recreational, supportive, and spiritual programs, as well as psychoeducational programs that include the patient's family" (p. 70S), also applies to nurses.

Other general recommendations from treatment guidelines (Baldwin et al., 2005; McIntosh et al., 2004; Swinson et al., 2006) that are salient to the treatment of late-life anxiety include the following:

■ Shared decision making between the individual and healthcare provider should be foremost in all aspects of treatment, starting with diagnosis.
■ Patients, families, and caregivers (when appropriate) should be provided with information about the nature, course, and treatment options for the identified anxiety disorder, including risks and benefits of specific drug treatments.

- Information about self-help and support groups, and online sources of information, should be provided.
- Selective serotonin reuptake inhibitors are effective across the range of anxiety disorders and are generally suitable as first-line treatment.
- Benzodiazepines are effective for many anxiety disorders, but use should only be short-term (2–4 weeks) because of side effects and dependence.
- Use of tricyclic antidepressants, monoamine oxidase inhibitors, antipsychotics, and anticonvulsants should be considered in light of the evidence to support their use in specific anxiety disorders and individualized risks and benefits.
- Monitoring outcomes using short, self-report measures to document symptom change is essential.
- Regular review and adjustment of treatment is needed to ensure optimal therapeutic outcomes are achieved.
- PCPs may effectively treat anxiety disorders, but referral to a specialty mental health provider is recommended if two treatments have been tried and the person continues to have significant symptoms.

Antidepressants for Late-Life Anxiety

Selective serotonin reuptake inhibitors are considered the first line of intervention for treating anxiety disorders in adults (Baldwin et al., 2005; Sheehan & Sheehan, 2007), and a small body of evidence supports their use with older adults (Swinson et al., 2006). Clinical trials support the use of citalopram and escitalopram for treating older adults with GAD and other anxiety disorders (Blank et al., 2006; Lenze et al., 2005b; Lenze et al., 2009). In addition, sertraline (Schuurmans et al., 2006; Sheikh, Lauderdale, & Cassidy, 2004), paroxetine (Flint, 2005; Stocchi et al., 2003), and venlafaxine, a serotonin and norepinephrine reuptake inhibitor (Boyer, Mahe, & Hackett, 2004;

Flint, 2005), have all shown promise for treating late-life GAD (Table 8-1).

Benzodiazepines Although positive outcomes are often possible with newer antidepressant medications, the time needed to achieve optimal symptom reduction may warrant short-term adjunctive use of short-acting benzodiazepines. However, use of benzodiazepines for more than a few weeks is generally not recommended for older adults, and thoughtful monitoring is required because of the associated risks of adverse side effects. Most risks stem from normal aging changes that alter pharmacokinetics and potentiate negative side effects, such as cognitive impairment, gait instability and increased risk of falls and hip fractures, psychomotor impairment, sedation, disinhibition, and dependency. Physical dependency may result in rebound symptoms, suggesting that any elderly patient who has taken benzodiazepines continuously for more than 6 weeks be gradually tapered over several weeks (Lauderdale & Sheikh, 2003). Short-life benzodiazepines, such as lorazepam (Ativan) or oxazepam (Serax), are preferred because they are inactivated by direct conjugation in the liver and are less likely than older drugs like diazepam (Valium) or chlordiazepoxide (Librium) to accumulate and create toxicity.

Azapirones Clinical trials also support the use of buspirone (Buspar) to treat anxiety disorders among older adults (Flint, 2005; Lauderdale & Sheikh, 2003; Swinson et al., 2006). Although studies in geriatric samples suggest that buspirone is well tolerated, has few adverse effects, and reduces chronic anxiety, experience in clinical practice settings suggests an inconsistent therapeutic benefit (Lauderdale & Sheikh).

In summary, as the evidence needed to guide best practices in the treatment of late-life anxiety continues to grow, the best medication and psychosocial interventions are devised by individual

TABLE 8-1

Antianxiety Medications

Generic Name	Trade Name	Class	Starting Dose	Step-Up Dose	Target Dose	Top Dose	Food and Drug Administration Approval	Comments
First Line								
Citalopram	Celexa	SSRI	10 mg/d	10 mg/d	20 mg/d	40 mg/d	PD	Possibly fewer cytochrome P-450 drug interactions
Paroxetine	Paxil	SSRI	10 mg/d	10 mg/d	20 mg/d	40 mg/d	GAD, PD, OCD, PTSD, social phobia	Slightly sedating; has cytochrome interactions
Sertraline	Zoloft	SSRI	25 mg/d	25 mg/d	100 mg/d	200 mg/d	PD, OCD, PTSD	Has minimal P-450 interactions
Venlafaxine XR	Effexor XR	SNRI	37.5 mg/d	37.5 mg/d	75–100 mg/d	225 mg/d	GAD	May increase blood pressure at higher doses
Buspirone	Buspar	SA	5 mg bid	10 mg bid	10 mg bid-tid	30 mg	GAD	Does not induce dependence or withdrawal symptoms
Second Line								
Alprazolam	Xanax	BZD	0.125 mg bid	0.125 mg bid	0.25 mg prn	1 mg/d		Short onset and duration of action; difficult to taper
Lorazepam	Ativan	BZD	0.5 mg tid-qid	0.5 mg/d	1 mg tid	4 mg/d		Moderate duration of action; no active metabolites
Mirtazapine	Remeron	ATA	15 mg/d	15 mg/d	30–45 mg/d	45 mg/d		Sedation and weight gain may be prominent

Abbreviations: SSRI, serotonin reuptake inhibitor; SNRI, serotonin norepinephrine reuptake inhibitor; SA, serotonin agonist; BZD, benzodiazepine; ATA, atypical tetracyclic antidepressant; PD, panic disorder; GAD, generalized anxiety disorders; OCD, obsessive-compulsive disorder; PTSD, posttraumatic stress disorder.

Source: Adapted by Schultz (2009) from Rollman, B. L., Belnap, B. H., Reynolds, C. F., 3rd, Schulberg, H. C., & Shear, M. K. (2003). A contemporary protocol to assist primary care physicians in the treatment of panic and generalized anxiety disorders. *General Hospital Psychiatry, 25,* 74–82. Used with permission.

interdisciplinary teams composed of nurses, social workers, psychologists, psychiatrists, and other ancillary personnel who have expertise in geriatric psychiatry, and who work together to assess and treat older adults using a biopsychosocial framework.

Community and Family Resources

A final consideration in the identification and treatment of late-life anxiety symptoms and disorders relates to accessing sources of assistance. At present, the blended specialization of geriatric–psychiatric care, in nursing, psychology, social work, and psychiatry, is limited to a small group of specialists and services. Although geropsychiatric specializations are growing, day-to-day care and treatment of late-life anxiety disorders are more often provided by generalist health providers in primary care settings, by psychiatric specialists who lack geriatric expertise, or geriatric specialists who lack psychiatric expertise. As a result, access to more specialized information may be needed to promote quality of care.

Several national resources are worthy of mention. Perhaps most important is the Anxiety Disorder Association of America, which offers a wide variety of resources that target education and advocacy, including informational materials (including those that are specific to late-life anxiety), an online bookstore, self-help tools, and assistance to find treatment in accessible locations. The Anxiety Disorder Association of America sponsors an annual conference, offers full- and half-day professional workshops, and maintains an easy-to-use Web site at http://www.adaa.org/.

Although not specific to late-life anxiety disorders, several other national organizations offer assistance related to anxiety disorders. The National Institute of Mental Health provides a wide variety of educational products, including books, fact sheets, and summaries that can be accessed from its Web site (http://www.nimh.nih.gov/anxiety/anxietymenu.cfm). The free publication, *Anxiety Disorders*, provides a brief overview of various anxiety disorders and lists organizations to contact for further information. The APA provides an informational page about anxiety (http://www.psych.org/public_info/anxiety.cfm), the American Psychological Association (http://apa.org/therapy/anxiety.html) offers assistance to find a psychologist and information on how therapy may help individuals with anxiety disorder, and the American Association of Geriatric Psychiatry (http://www.aagponline.org/links.asp) provides a comprehensive list of links to diverse aging and mental health organizations, advocacy groups, governmental programs, and professional organizations.

Collectively, these resources provide a wide variety of educational materials that may be used directly or adapted for use with older adults and their families, healthcare professionals, and community service providers who may be unfamiliar with anxiety disorders. A common theme throughout the literature is underidentification of anxiety disorders that result in unnecessary suffering for older individuals and their families or caregivers. Use of educational resources such as these may be essential to promote appropriate referral and treatment.

SUMMARY AND CONCLUSIONS

Nurses are in a key position to identify anxiety-related symptoms and initiate assessment that leads to appropriate management and treatment. Although some older adults have long-standing experiences with anxiety disorders that have persisted throughout their lives, many others experience these symptoms for the first time in later life. Whether that symptom represents a diagnosable anxiety disorder is perhaps less important than the fact that the individual will suffer needlessly if assessment and treatment are not undertaken. Comprehensive assessment using a biopsychosocial framework, and maximizing the benefits of the therapeutic alliance with the apprehensive, uncomfortable, and often frightened older person, offers the opportunity to understand complex problems and issues, and then devise appropriate interventions.

Joan Wellbrook, an otherwise healthy woman, experienced her first cardiac event at age 82 years. After a brief hospitalization and stent placements, Joan was discharged to return to her rural home where she had lived alone since her husband's death 20 years ago. Discharge orders included no driving, only light housekeeping, and cardiac rehabilitation three times per week for 12 weeks. Her return home relied on the agreement that her son and daughter would provide in-home assistance until follow-up assessments with her cardiologist and internist suggested that she could return to her usual level of independence, which included paid employment as a nurse, volunteer work, and transporting her 93-year-old sister to appointments.

Although her cardiac status remained stable following discharge, Joan experienced a diverse array of uncomfortable and frustrating gastrointestinal symptoms (GI), including upset stomach, loss of appetite, gas, belching, and diarrhea. She blamed her newly prescribed cardiac medications for her discomforts, stating that the effects were nearly "worse than being dead." Apprehension and worry about her GI distress resulted in irritable, angry, and demanding interactions with her adult children, who encouraged their mother to record and discuss the distressing symptoms with her medical providers. Difficulties concentrating, chronic fatigue, new-onset sleep disturbance, and weight loss further complicated her sense of well-being, but were considered "normal reactions" to a life-altering experience by her health providers.

After 4 weeks, Joan was allowed to resume driving, work, and other usual activities of living on a gradual basis. However, new apprehensions about driving alone, bad weather, and having another heart attack interfered with her willingness to leave home. At the same time, she began to worry about being a burden to her adult children, in spite of their regular assurances to the contrary. Her GI-related symptoms and associated worries, irritability,

and physical symptoms persisted despite the positive feedback about her progress in cardiac therapy, and became increasingly out of context given her long-standing patterns of autonomy and medical assurances that her cardiac condition was stable. After 8 weeks of medication adjustments attempting to reduce her GI-related distress, Joan's internist offered her a choice between taking more medication or a trial of problem-solving treatment aimed at improving her mood and outlook on life. Joan responded that there was "nothing wrong with her problem solving," noting "I'm a BS-prepared nurse you know! I'm not stupid! And if I want to talk, I'll talk to my daughter and my son." In turn, a trial of sertraline, 12.5 mg daily, was initiated, supplemented with lorazepam, 0.25 mg three times per day. Lorazepam provided immediate relief for distressing GI symptoms, as Joan reported "I feel like myself for the first time since this happened." Over 4 weeks, sertraline was titrated to 37.7 mg and lorazepam was reduced to an "as needed" basis. Joan's distressing symptoms all slowly resolved over the following 6-month period, and she returned to her usual roles working, volunteering, and taking an active role in helping others. After a year, sertraline therapy was titrated down and discontinued without reoccurrence of anxiety-related symptoms, although Joan maintains a "relapse prevention plan" in the drawer with her checkbook to remind her of bothersome symptoms that might signal a return.

Questions:

1. What diagnosis did Joan's internist likely record in the medical record? What symptoms support or refute that diagnosis?

2. What guiding principles for late-life anxiety detection and treatment were observed or neglected in Joan's case?

3. What nursing roles, besides the offer of PST, may have facilitated Joan's management of distressing symptoms?

REFERENCES

American Psychiatric Association. (1980). *Diagnostic and Statistic Manual of Mental Disorders (DSM-III)* (3rd ed.). Washington, DC: American Psychiatric Press.

American Psychiatric Association. (2000). *Diagnostic and Statistical Manual of Mental Disorders (DSM-IV-TR)* (4th ed.). Washington, DC: Author.

Andreescu, C., Belnap, B. H., Rollman, B. L., Houck, P., Ciliberti, C., Mazumdar, S., et al. (2008). Generalized anxiety disorder severity scale validation in older adults. *American Journal of Geriatric Psychiatry, 16*(10), 813–818.

Andreescu, C., Lenze, E. J., Dew, M. A., Begley, A. E., Mulsant, B. H., Dombrovski, A. Y., et al. (2007). Effect of comorbid anxiety on treatment response and relapse risk in late life depression: Controlled study. *British Journal of Psychiatry, 190,* 344–349.

Arean, P., Hegel, M., Vannoy, S., Fan, M.-Y., & Unuzter, J. (2008). Effectiveness of problem-solving therapy for older, primary care patients with depression: Results from the IMPACT project. *Gerontologist, 48*(3), 311–323.

Ayers, C. R., Sorrell, J. T., Thorp, S. R., & Wetherell, J. L. (2007). Evidence-based psychological treatments for late-life anxiety. *Psychology and Aging, 22*(1), 8–17.

Bair, M. J., Wu, J., Damush, T. M., Sutherland, J. M., & Kroenke, K. (2008). Association of depression and anxiety alone and in combination with chronic musculoskeletal pain in primary care patients. *Psychosomatic Medicine, 70*(8), 890–897.

Baldwin, D. S., Anderson, I. M., Nutt, D. J., Bandelow, B., Bond, A., Davidson, J. R., et al. (2005). Evidence-based guidelines for the pharmacological treatment of anxiety disorders: Recommendations from the British Association for Psychopharmacology. *Journal of Psychopharmacology, 19*(6), 567–596.

Bandelow, B., Zohar, J., Hollander, E., Kasper, S., Moller, H. J., Zohar, J., et al. (2008). World Federation of Societies of Biological Psychiatry (WFSBP) guidelines for the pharmacological treatment of anxiety, obsessive-compulsive and post-traumatic stress disorders: First revision. *World Journal of Biological Psychiatry, 9*(4), 248–312.

Bartels, S. J., Coakley, E. H., Zubritsky, C., Ware, J. H., Miles, K. M., Arean, P. A., et al. (2004). Improving access to geriatric mental health services: A randomized trial comparing treatment engagement with integrated versus enhanced referral care for depression, anxiety, and at-risk alcohol use. *American Journal of Psychiatry, 161*(8), 1455–1462.

Beekman, A. T., de Beurs, E., van Balkom, A. J., Deeg, D. J., van Dyck, R., & van Tilburg, W. (2000). Anxiety and depression in later life: Co-occurrence and communality of risk factors. *American Journal of Psychiatry, 157*(1), 89–95.

Bierman, E. J., Comijs, H. C., Jonker, C., & Beekman, A. T. (2005). Effects of anxiety versus depression on cognition in later life. *American Journal of Geriatric Psychiatry, 13*(8), 686–693.

Blank, S., Lenze, E. J., Mulsant, B. H., Dew, M. A., Karp, J. F., Shear, M. K., et al. (2006). Outcomes of late-life anxiety disorders during 32 weeks of citalopram treatment. *Journal of Clinical Psychiatry, 67*(3), 468–472.

Blasinsky, M., Goldman, H., & Unutzer, J. (2006). Project IMPACT: A report on barriers and facilitators to sustainability. *Administrative Policy in Mental Health & Mental Health Services Research, 33,* 718–729.

Boyer, P., Mahe, V., & Hackett, D. (2004). Social adjustment in generalised anxiety disorder: A long-term placebo-controlled study of venlafaxine extended release. *European Psychiatry: the Journal of the Association of European Psychiatrists, 19*(5), 272–279.

Brenes, G. A. (2007). Anxiety, depression, and quality of life in primary care patients. *Primary Care Companion Journal of Clinical Psychiatry, 9*(6), 437–443.

Brenes, G. A., Guralnik, J. M., Williamson, J. D., Fried, L. P., Simpson, C., Simonsick, E. M., et al. (2005). The influence of anxiety on the progression of disability. *Journal of the American Geriatric Society, 53*(1), 34–39.

Brenes, G. A., Kritchevsky, S. B., Mehta, K. M., Yaffe, K., Simonsick, E. M., Ayonayon, H. N., et al. (2007). Scared to death: Results from the Health, Aging, and Body Composition study. *American Journal of Geriatric Psychiatry, 15*(3), 262–265.

Brenes, G. A., Penninx, B. W., Judd, P. H., Rockwell, E., Sewell, D. D., & Wetherell, J. L. (2008). Anxiety, depression and disability across the lifespan. *Aging & Mental Health, 12*(1), 158–163.

Bryant, C., Jackson, H., & Ames, D. (2008). The prevalence of anxiety in older adults: Methodological issues and a review of the literature. *Journal of Affective Disorders, 109*(3), 233–250.

Cairney, J., Corna, L. M., Veldhuizen, S., Herrmann, N., & Streiner, D. L. (2008). Comorbid depression and anxiety in later life: Patterns of association, subjective well-being, and impairment. *American Journal of Geriatric Psychiatry, 16*(3), 201–208.

Callahan, C. M., Boustani, M. A., Unverzagt, F. W., Austrom, M. G., Damush, T. M., Perkins, A. J., et al. (2006). Effectiveness of collaborative care for older adults with Alzheimer disease in primary care: A randomized controlled trial. *Journal of the American Geriatrics Association, 295*(18), 2148–2157.

Campbell, D. G., Felker, B. L., Liu, C. F., Yano, E. M., Kirchner, J. E., Chan, D., et al. (2007). Prevalence of depression-PTSD comorbidity: Implications for clinical practice guidelines and primary care-based interventions. *Journal of General Internal Medicine, 22*(6), 711–718.

Craske, M. G., Rose, R. D., Lang, A., Welch, S. S., Campbell-Sills, L., Sullivan, G., et al. (2009). Computer-assisted delivery of cognitive behavioral therapy for anxiety disorders in primary-care settings. *Depression & Anxiety, 26*(3), 235–242.

Dada, F., Sethi, S., & Grossberg, G. T. (2001). Generalized anxiety disorder in the elderly. *Psychiatric Clinics of North America, 24*(1), 155–164.

Diefenbach, G. J., Tolin, D. F., Gilliam, C. M., & Meunier, S. A. (2008). Extending cognitive-behavioral therapy for late-life anxiety to home care: Program development and case examples. *Behavior Modification, 32*(5), 595–610.

Dugue, M., & Neugroschl, J. (2002). Anxiety disorders. Helping patients regain stability and calm. *Geriatrics, 57*(8), 27–31.

Engel, C. C., Oxman, T., Yamamoto, C., Gould, D., Barry, S., Stewart, P., et al. (2008). RESPECT-Mil: Feasibility of a systems-level collaborative care approach to depression and post-traumatic stress disorder in military primary care. *Military Medicine, 173*(10), 935–940.

Flint, A. J. (2005). Generalised anxiety disorder in elderly patients: Epidemiology, diagnosis and treatment options. *Drugs & Aging, 22*(2), 101–114.

Gagnon, N., Flint, A. J., Naglie, G., & Devins, G. M. (2005). Affective correlates of fear of falling in elderly persons. *American Journal of Geriatric Psychiatry, 13*(1), 7–14.

Gurmankin Levy, A., Maselko, J., Bauer, M., Richman, L., & Kubzansky, L. (2007). Why do people with an anxiety disorder utilize more nonmental health care than those without? *Health Psychology, 26*(5), 545–553.

Hegel, M. T., Unutzer, J., Tang, L., Arean, P. A., Katon, W., Noel, P. H., et al. (2005). Impact of comorbid panic and posttraumatic stress disorder on outcomes of collaborative care for late-life depression in primary care. *American Journal of Geriatric Psychiatry, 13*(1), 48–58.

Hendriks, G. J., Oude Voshaar, R. C., Keijsers, G. P., Hoogduin, C. A., & van Balkom, A. J. (2008). Cognitive-behavioural therapy for late-life anxiety disorders: A systematic review and meta-analysis. *Acta Psychiatrica Scandinanvia, 117*(6), 403–411.

Hidalgo, J. L., Gras, C. B., Garcia, Y. D., Lapeira, J. T., del Campo del Campo, J. M., & Verdejo, M. A. (2007). Functional status in the elderly with insomnia. *Quality of Life Research, 16*(2), 279–286.

Hoffman, D. L., Dukes, E. M., & Wittchen, H. U. (2008). Human and economic burden of generalized anxiety disorder. *Depression & Anxiety, 25*(1), 72–90.

Holwerda, T. J., Schoevers, R. A., Dekker, J., Deeg, D. J., Jonker, C., & Beekman, A. T. (2007). The relationship between generalized anxiety disorder, depression and mortality in old age. *International Journal of Geriatric Psychiatry, 22*(3), 241–249.

Jackson, J. L., Passamonti, M., & Kroenke, K. (2007). Outcome and impact of mental disorders in primary care at 5 years. *Psychosomatic Medicine, 69*(3), 270–276.

Jeste, N. D., Hays, J. C., & Steffens, D. C. (2006). Clinical correlates of anxious depression among elderly patients with depression. *Journal of Affective Disorders, 90*(1), 37–41.

Karlsson, B., Klenfeldt, I. F., Sigstrom, R., Waern, M., Ostling, S., Gustafson, D., et al. (2009). Prevalence of social phobia in non-demented elderly from a Swedish population study. *American Journal of Geriatric Psychiatry, 17*(2), 127–135.

Katon, W., Lin, E. H., & Kroenke, K. (2007). The association of depression and anxiety with medical symptom burden in patients with chronic medical illness. *General Hospital Psychiatry, 29*(2), 147–155.

Katon, W., & Roy-Byrne, P. (2007). Anxiety disorders: Efficient screening is the first step in improving outcomes. *Annals of Internal Medicine, 146*(5), 390–392.

Katon, W., Roy-Byrne, P., Russo, J., & Cowley, D. (2002). Cost-effectiveness and cost offset of a collaborative care intervention for primary care patients with panic disorder. *Archives of General Psychiatry, 59*(12), 1098–1104.

Katon, W., Russo, J., Sherbourne, C., Stein, M. B., Craske, M., Fan, M. Y., et al. (2006). Incremental cost-effectiveness of a collaborative care intervention for panic disorder. *Psychological Medicine, 36*(3), 353–363.

Kenn, C., Wood, H., Kucyj, M., Attis, J., & Cunane, J. (1987). Validation of the Hospital Anxiety and Depression Rating Scale (HADS) in an elderly psychiatric population. *International Journal of Geriatric Psychiatry, 2*(3), 189–193.

Kessler, R. C., Berglund, P., Demler, O., Jin, R., & Walters, E. (2005). Lifetime prevalence and age-of-onset distributions of DSM-IV disorders in the National Co-Morbidity Survey replication. *Archives of General Psychiatry, 62*, 593–602.

Kolanowski, A., & Buettner, L. (2008). Prescribing activities that engage passive residents. An innovative method. *Journal of Gerontological Nursing, 34*(1), 13–18.

Kolanowski, A. M., Litaker, M., & Buettner, L. (2005). Efficacy of theory-based activities for behavioral symptoms of dementia. *Nursing Research, 54*(4), 219–228.

Kraus, C. A., Kunik, M. E., & Stanley, M. A. (2007). Use of cognitive behavioral therapy in late-life psychiatric disorders. *Geriatrics, 62*(6), 21–26.

Kroenke, K., Shen, J., Oxman, T. E., Williams, J. W., Jr., & Dietrich, A. J. (2008). Impact of pain on the outcomes of depression treatment: Results from the RESPECT trial. *Pain, 134*(1-2), 209–215.

Kroenke, K., Spitzer, R. L., Williams, J. B., Monahan, P. O., & Lowe, B. (2007). Anxiety disorders in primary care: Prevalence, impairment, comorbidity, and detection. *Annals of Internal Medicine, 146*(5), 317–325.

Lauderdale, S. A., & Sheikh, J. I. (2003). Anxiety disorders in older adults. *Clinical Geriatric Medicine, 19*(4), 721–741.

Lecrubier, Y. (2007). Widespread underrecognition and undertreatment of anxiety and mood disorders: Results from 3 European studies. *Journal of Clinical Psychiatry, 68*(Suppl. 2), 36–41.

Lenze, E. J., Karp, J. F., Mulsant, B. H., Blank, S., Shear, M. K., Houck, P. R., et al. (2005a). Somatic symptoms in late-life anxiety: Treatment issues. *Journal of Geriatric Psychiatry and Neurology, 18*(2), 89–96.

Lenze, E. J., Mulsant, B. H., Shear, M. K., Alexopoulos, G. S., Frank, E., & Reynolds, C. F., 3rd. (2001). Comorbidity of depression and anxiety disorders in later life. *Depression & Anxiety, 14*(2), 86–93.

Lenze, E. J., Mulsant, B. H., Shear, M. K., Dew, M. A., Miller, M. D., Pollock, B. G., et al. (2005b). Efficacy and tolerability of citalopram in the treatment of late-life anxiety disorders: Results from an 8-week randomized, placebo-controlled trial. *American Journal of Psychiatry, 162*(1), 146–150.

Lenze, E. J., Rollman, B. L., Shear, M. K., Dew, M. A., Pollock, B. G., Ciliberti, C., et al. (2009). Escitalopram for older adults with generalized anxiety disorder: A randomized controlled trial. *Journal of the American Geriatrics Association, 301*(3), 295–303.

Lenze, E. J., & Wetherell, J. L. (2009). Bringing the bedside to the bench, and then to the community: A prospectus for intervention research in late-life anxiety disorders. *International Journal of Geriatric Psychiatry, 24*(1), 1–14.

Lin, E. H., Katon, W., Von Korff, M., Tang, L., Williams, J. W., Jr., Kroenke, K., et al. (2003). Effect of improving depression care on pain and functional outcomes among older adults with arthritis: A randomized controlled trial. *JAMA, 290*(18), 2428–2429.

Lowe, B., Decker, O., Muller, S., Brahler, E., Schellberg, D., Herzog, W., et al. (2008a). Validation and standardization of the Generalized Anxiety Disorder Screener (GAD-7) in the general population. *Medical Care, 46*(3), 266–274.

Lowe, B., Spitzer, R. L., Williams, J. B., Mussell, M., Schellberg, D., & Kroenke, K. (2008b). Depression, anxiety and somatization in primary care: Syndrome overlap and functional impairment. *General Hospital Psychiatry, 30*(3), 191–199.

Mahoney, E. K., Volicer, L., & Hurley, A. (2000). Anxiety. In E. K. Mahoney, L. Volicer, & A. Hurley (Eds.), *Management of challenging behaviors in dementia* (pp. 109–124). Baltimore: Health Professions Press.

McIntosh, A., Cohen, A., Turnbull, N., Esmonde, L., Dennis, P., Eatock, J., et al. (2004). *Clinical guidelines* and evidence review for panic disorder and generalised anxiety disorder. Sheffield: University of Sheffield/London National Collaborating Centre for Primary Care.

Mittal, D., Fortney, J. C., Pyne, J. M., Edlund, M. J., & Wetherell, J. L. (2006). Impact of comorbid anxiety disorders on health-related quality of life among patients with major depressive disorder. *Psychiatric Services, 57*(12), 1731–1737.

Moffitt, T. E., Harrington, H., Caspi, A., Kim-Cohen, J., Goldberg, D., Gregory, A. M., et al. (2007). Depression and generalized anxiety disorder: Cumulative and sequential comorbidity in a birth cohort followed prospectively to age 32 years. *Archives of General Psychiatry, 64*(6), 651–660.

Mohlman, J. (2004). Psychosocial treatment of late-life generalized anxiety disorder: Current status and future directions. *Clinical Psychology Review, 24*(2), 149–169.

Mohlman, J., Gorenstien, E. E., Kleber, M., de Jesus, M., Gorman, J. M., & Papp, L. A. (2003). Standard and enhanced cognitive-behavior therapy for late-life generalized anxiety disorder: Two pilot investigations. *American Journal of Geriatric Psychiatry, 11*(1), 24–31.

Mohlman, J., & Price, R. (2006). Recognizing and treating late-life generalized anxiety disorder: Distinguishing features and psychosocial treatment. *Expert Reviews in Neurotherapy, 6*(10), 1439–1445.

Mok, L. C., & Lee, I. F. (2008). Anxiety, depression and pain intensity in patients with low back pain who are admitted to acute care hospitals. *Journal of Clinical Nursing, 17*(11), 1471–1480.

Montorio, I., Wetherell, J. L., & Nuevo, R. (2006). Beliefs about worry in community-dwelling older adults. *Depression & Anxiety, 23*(8), 466–473.

Mussell, M., Kroenke, K., Spitzer, R. L., Williams, J. B., Herzog, W., & Lowe, B. (2008). Gastrointestinal symptoms in primary care: Prevalence and association with depression and anxiety. *Journal of Psychosomatic Research, 64*(6), 605–612.

Pachana, N., Byrne, G., Siddle, H., Koloski, N., Harley, E., & Arnold, E. (2007). Development and validation of the Geriatric Anxiety Inventory. *International Psychogeriatrics, 19*(1), 103–114.

Palmer, K., Berger, A. K., Monastero, R., Winblad, B., Backman, L., & Fratiglioni, L. (2007). Predictors of progression from mild cognitive impairment to Alzheimer disease. *Neurology, 68*(19), 1596–1602.

Porensky, E. K., Dew, M. A., Karp, J. F., Skidmore, E., Rollman, B. L., Shear, M. K., et al. (2009). The burden of late-life generalized anxiety disorder: Effects on disability, health-related quality of life, and healthcare utilization. *American Journal of Geriatric Psychiatry, 17*(6), 473–482.

Preville, M., Cote, G., Boyer, R., & Hebert, R. (2004). Detection of depression and anxiety disorders by home care nurses. *Aging and Mental Health, 8*(5), 400–409.

Rickels, K., & Rynn, M. (2001). Overview and clinical presentation of generalized anxiety disorder. *Psychiatric Clinics of North America, 24*(1), 1–17.

Rollman, B. L., Belnap, B. H., Mazumdar, S., Houck, P. R., Zhu, F., Gardner, W., et al. (2005). A randomized trial to improve the quality of treatment for panic and generalized anxiety disorders in primary care. *Archives of General Psychiatry, 62*(12), 1332–1341.

Roy-Byrne, P. P., Craske, M. G., Stein, M. B., Sullivan, G., Bystritsky, A., Katon, W., et al. (2005). A randomized effectiveness trial of cognitive-behavioral therapy and medication for primary care panic disorder. *Archives of General Psychiatry, 62*(3), 290–298.

Roy-Byrne, P. P., Davidson, K. W., Kessler, R. C., Asmundson, G. J., Goodwin, R. D., Kubzansky, L., et al. (2008). Anxiety disorders and comorbid medical illness. *General Hospital Psychiatry, 30*(3), 208–225.

Roy-Byrne, P. P., & Wagner, A. (2004). Primary care perspectives on generalized anxiety disorder. *Journal of Clinical Psychiatry, 65*(Suppl. 13), 20–26.

Rucci, P., Miniati, M., Oppo, A., Mula, M., Calugi, S., Frank, E., et al. (2009). The structure of lifetime panic-agoraphobic spectrum. *Journal of Psychiatric Research, 43*(4), 366–379.

Sable, J. A., & Jeste, D. V. (2001). Anxiety disorders in older adults. *Current Psychiatry Reports, 3*(4), 302–307.

Sareen, J., Jacobi, F., Cox, B. J., Belik, S. L., Clara, I., & Stein, M. B. (2006). Disability and poor quality of life associated with comorbid anxiety disorders and physical conditions. *Archives of Internal Medicine, 166*(19), 2109–2116.

Saur, C. D., Steffens, D. C., Harpole, L., Fan, M. Y., Oddone, E., & Unutzer, J. (2007). Satisfaction and outcomes of depressed older adults with psychiatric clinical nurse specialists in primary care. *Journal of the American Psychiatric Nurses Association, 13*(1), 62–70.

Schroder, C., Johnson, M., Morrison, V., Teunissen, L., Notermans, N., & van Meeteren, N. (2007). Health condition, impairment, activity limitations: Relationships with emotions and control cognitions in people with disabling conditions. *Rehabilitation Psychology, 52*(3), 280–289.

Schuurmans, J., Comijs, H., Emmelkamp, P. M., Gundy, C. M., Weijnen, I., van den Hout, M., et al. (2006). A randomized, controlled trial of the effectiveness of cognitive-behavioral therapy and sertraline versus a waitlist control group for anxiety disorders in older adults. *American Journal of Geriatric Psychiatry, 14*(3), 255–263.

Seignourel, P. J., Kunik, M. E., Snow, L., Wilson, N., & Stanley, M. (2008). Anxiety in dementia: A critical review. *Clinical Psychology Review, 28*(7), 1071–1082.

Shankar, K. K., Walker, M., Frost, D., & Orrell, M. (1999). The development of a valid and reliable scale for rating anxiety in dementia (RAID). *Aging & Mental Health, 3*(1), 39–49.

Shear, K., Belnap, B. H., Mazumdar, S., Houck, P., & Rollman, B. L. (2006). Generalized anxiety disorder severity scale (GADSS): A preliminary validation study. *Depression & Anxiety, 23*(2), 77–82.

Sheehan, D. V., & Sheehan, K. H. (2007). Current approaches to the pharmacologic treatment of anxiety disorders. *Psychopharmacology Bulletin, 40*(1), 98–109.

Sheikh, J. I., Lauderdale, S. A., & Cassidy, E. L. (2004). Efficacy of sertraline for panic disorder in older adults: A preliminary open-label trial. *American Journal of Geriatric Psychiatry, 12*(2), 230.

Small, G. W. (1997). Recognizing and treating anxiety in the elderly. *Journal of Clinical Psychiatry, 58*(Suppl. 3), 41–47; discussion 48–50.

Smith, M., Ingram, T., & Brighton, V. (Eds.). (2008a). *Detection and assessment of late life anxiety evidence-based guideline.* Iowa City, Iowa: The University of Iowa College of Nursing Gerontological Nursing Interventions Research Center, Research Translation and Dissemination Core.

Smith, M., Rosenblatt, A., Samus, Q., Steele, C., Baker, A., Harper, M., et al. (2008b). Anxiety symptoms among assisted living residents: Implications of the "no difference" finding for subjects with and without dementia. *Research in Gerontological Nursing, 1*(2), 1–9.

Spinhoven, P., Ormel, J., Sloekers, P. P., Speckens, A. E., & Van Hemert, A. M. (1997). A validation study of the Hospital Anxiety and Depression Scale (HADS) in different groups of Dutch subjects. *Psychological Medicine, 27*, 363–370.

Spitzer, R. L., Kroenke, K., Williams, J. B., & Lowe, B. (2006). A brief measure for assessing generalized anxiety disorder: The GAD-7. *Archives of Internal Medicine, 166*(10), 1092–1097.

Stanley, M. A., Wilson, N. L., Novy, D. M., Rhoades, H. M., Wagener, P. D., Greisinger, A. J., et al. (2009). Cognitive behavior therapy for generalized anxiety disorder among older adults in primary care: A randomized clinical trial. *Journal of the American Geriatric Society, 301*(14), 1460–1467.

Stocchi, F., Nordera, G., Jokinen, R. H., Lepola, U. M., Hewett, K., Bryson, H., et al. (2003). Efficacy and tolerability of paroxetine for the long-term treatment of generalized anxiety disorder. *Journal of Clinical Psychiatry, 64*(3), 250–258.

Swinson, R. P. (2006). The GAD-7 scale was accurate for diagnosing generalised anxiety disorder. *Evidence Based Medicine, 11*(6), 184.

Swinson, R. P., Antony, M. M., Bleau, P., Chokka, P., Craven, M., Fallu, A., et al. (2006). Clinical Practice Guidelines: Management of anxiety disorders. *Canadian Journal of Psychiatry, 51*(Suppl. 2), 1S–91S.

Tatsch, M. F., Bottino, C. M. d. C., Azevedo, D., Hototian, S. R., Moscoso, M. A., Folquitto, J. C., et al. (2006). Neuropsychiatric symptoms in Alzheimer disease and cognitively impaired, nondemented elderly from a community-based sample in Brazil: Prevalence and relationship with dementia severity. *American Journal of Geriatric Psychiatry, 14*(5), 438–445.

Teh, C. F., Morone, N. E., Karp, J. F., Belnap, B. H., Zhu, F., Weiner, D. K., et al. (2009). Pain interference impacts response to treatment for anxiety disorders. *Depression & Anxiety, 26*(3), 222–228.

Teri, L., Ferretti, L. E., Gibbons, L. E., Logsdon, R. G., McCurry, S. M., Kukull, W. A., et al. (1999). Anxiety in Alzheimer's disease: Prevalence, and comorbidity. *Journal of Gerontology: Medical Sciences, 54A*(7), M348–352.

Thorp, S. R., Ayers, C. R., Nuevo, R., Stoddard, J. A., Sorrell, J. T., & Wetherell, J. L. (2009). Meta-analysis comparing different behavioral treatments for late-life anxiety. *American Journal of Geriatric Psychiatry, 17*(2), 105–115.

Twelftree, H., & Qazi, A. (2006). Relationship between anxiety and agitation in dementia. *Aging & Mental Health, 10*(4), 362–367.

Unutzer, J., Hantke, M., Powers, D., Higa, L., Lin, E., Vannoy, S., et al. (2008). Care management for depression and osteoarthritis pain in older primary care patients: A pilot study. *International Journal of Geriatric Psychiatry, 23*(11), 1166–1171.

Unutzer, J., Katon, W., Callahan, C. M., Williams, J. W., Jr., Hunkeler, E., Harpole, L., et al. (2002). Collaborative care management of late-life depression in the primary care setting: A randomized controlled trial. *JAMA, 288*(22), 2836–2845.

Unutzer, J., Powers, D., Katon, W., & Langston, C. (2005). From establishing an evidence-based practice to implementation in real-world settings: IMPACT as a case study. *Psychiatric Clinics of North America, 28*(4), 1079–1092.

U.S. Department of Health and Human Services (DHHS). (1999). *Mental Health: A Report of the Surgeon General*. Rockville, MD: Substance Abuse and Mental Health Services Administration, Center for Mental Health Services, National Institutes of Health, National Institute of Mental Health.

van't Veer-Tazelaar, N., van Marwijk, H., van Oppen, P., Nijpels, G., van Hout, H., Cuijpers, P., et al. (2006). Prevention of anxiety and depression in the age group of 75 years and over: A randomised controlled trial testing the feasibility and effectiveness of a generic stepped care programme among elderly community residents at high risk of developing anxiety and depression versus usual care. *BMC Public Health, 6*, 186.

van't Veer-Tazelaar, P. J., van Marwijk, H. W., van Oppen, P., van Hout, H. P., van der Horst, H. E., & Cuijpers, P., et al. (2009). Stepped-care prevention of anxiety and depression in late life: A randomized controlled trial. *Archives of General Psychiatry, 66*(3), 297–304.

Vink, D., Aartsen, M. J., & Schoevers, R. A. (2008). Risk factors for anxiety and depression in the elderly: A review. *Journal of Affective Disorders, 106*(1-2), 29–44.

Weiss, B. J., Calleo, J., Rhoades, H. M., Novy, D. M., Kunik, M. E., Lenze, E. J., et al. (2009). The utility of the Generalized Anxiety Disorder Severity Scale (GADSS) with older adults in primary care. *Depression & Anxiety, 26*(1), E10–15.

Wetherell, J. L., Ayers, C. R., Sorrell, J. T., Thorp, S. R., Nuevo, R., Belding, W., et al. (2009). Modular psychotherapy for anxiety in older primary care patients. *American Journal of Geriatric Psychiatry, 17*(6), 483–492.

Wetherell, J. L., Birchler, G. D., Ramsdell, J., & Unutzer, J. (2007). Screening for generalized anxiety disorder in geriatric primary care patients. *International Journal of Geriatric Psychiatry, 22*, 115–123.

Wetherell, J. L., Kaplan, R. M., Kallenberg, G., Dresselhaus, T. R., Sieber, W. J., & Lang, A. J. (2004). Mental health treatment preferences of older and younger primary care patients. *International Journal of Psychiatry & Medicine, 34*(3), 219–233.

Wetherell, J. L., Lenze, E. J., & Stanley, M. A. (2005a). Evidence-based treatment of geriatric anxiety disorders. *Psychiatric Clinics of North America, 28*(4), 871–896, ix.

Wetherell, J. L., Maser, J. D., & van Balkom, A. (2005b). Anxiety disorders in the elderly: Outdated beliefs and a research agenda. *Acta Psychiatrica Scandinavia, 111*(6), 401–402.

Wetherell, J. L., Sorrell, J. T., Thorp, S. R., & Patterson, T. L. (2005c). Psychological interventions for late-life anxiety: A review and early lessons from the CALM study. *Journal of Geriatric Psychiatry & Neurology, 18*(2), 72–82.

Yehuda, R., Schmeidler, J., Labinsky, E., Bell, A., Morris, A., Zemelman, S., et al. (2009). Ten-year follow-up study of PTSD diagnosis, symptom severity and psychosocial indices in aging holocaust survivors. *Acta Psychiatrica Scandinavia, 119*(1), 25–34.

9

Psychosis in Older Adults

Janet C. Mentes
Julia K. Bail

Mr. B., 65 years old, sits quietly smoking a cigarette in the corner of the waiting room. Occasionally he rocks back and forth in his seat as if he is restless. When you ask him how he is doing, he tells you in a soft voice about how he is controlled by "people from outer space," who read his thoughts and want him to behave in certain ways.

Mr. J., 79 years old, sits at the side of his bed in a local nursing home, eating his dinner. Suddenly, he becomes agitated and shouts out, "Nigel—please don't feed the elephant . . . . Nigel! Nigel!"

Both of these older men are exhibiting psychoses, caused by different etiologies. From an extensive history, we find that Mr. B. has been experiencing his symptoms since he was a young adult. His symptoms are attributable to chronic schizophrenia, paranoid type. On the other hand, Mr. J.'s history reveals that he had an abrupt change in mental status, indicative of a delirium with psychotic symptoms. On further evaluation, his delirium was found to be secondary to decreased cerebral oxygenation caused by internal bleeding.

BACKGROUND

Historically, "psychosis" was an expansive term referring to a state of being cut off from reality. Psychotic behavior, or psychosis, signified that a person was unable to determine if what he or she was thinking and feeling about the real world was really true (Merriam-Webster, 1997). Currently, psychosis is recognized as a syndrome or constellation of psychiatric symptoms, which occurs in a number of physical and mental disease states. The predominant symptoms of psychosis include hallucinations, which are false sensory impressions affecting any of the five senses, and delusions, which are simply false beliefs (American Psychiatric Association [APA], 2000).

There are two distinct presentations of psychosis in older persons: chronic psychosis in older individuals who have had a lifelong schizophrenia, major depression, or bipolar disorder with psychosis; and older persons who develop psychotic symptoms for the first time in old age. Table 9-1 provides a comparison of psychotic features of various disease states. Psychosis that develops in older individuals can be the result of a primary psychiatric disorder or a secondary psychosis, which can be caused by a number of disease states and can often herald underlying neurological disorders. Disease states associated with psychosis and psychotic symptoms in older persons include:

1. Schizophrenia, early-onset, late-onset, and very late-onset schizophrenic-like psychosis

203

TABLE 9-1

Comparison of Signs and Symptoms Among Psychotic Disorders of Elders

Psychotic Disorder	Delusions	Hallucinations	Other
Alzheimer's disease	Simple; theft, infidelity, abandonment, house is not one's real house	Visual > auditory; people from past, animals	Misidentification[a], Capgras syndrome[b]
Vascular dementia	Complex, persecutory; fear of infidelity	Visual	Capgras syndrome[b], presence of HTN, CAD, CVD
Lewy body disease	Not as evident	Visual; early in course of disease	Mild parkinsonism
Frontal lobe dementia	Bizarre, grandiose	Not as evident	Occurs in persons > 65 years
Parkinson's disease	Paranoid	Visual, small people, animals	Related to dopaminergic medications
Delirium	If present, simple	Visual, tactile, or olfactory	Abrupt onset; person appears physically ill
Substance abuse/use	Paranoid	Visual with illusions, tactile with withdrawal	
Delusional disorder	Nonbizarre, persecutory; focuses on one aspect of life—marital, occupational, interpersonal	Usually absent	Social function intact
Major depression with psychosis	Somatic; body parts missing or diseased, or guilt	Usually absent	Mood disturbance
Bipolar disorder	Grandiose; e.g., believe they are a celebrity	Auditory	Mood disturbance, mania
Early-onset schizophrenia	Bizarre, systematized persecutory	Auditory; e.g., persons making derogatory comments or commenting on behavior	Usual onset before 45 years
Late-onset schizophrenia	Persecutory; e.g., people spying on them or trying to poison them	Visual > auditory	Onset after 45 years
Charles Bonnet syndrome	None	Elaborate visual of people, animals, or geometric patterns	Person has visual deficits

[a] Misidentification syndrome is when the person with dementia cannot recognize family members or even himself or herself.

[b] Capgras syndrome is when the person with dementia believes that familiar people have been replaced by an identical imposter.

Source: Desai, A., & Grossberg, G. (2003). Differential diagnosis of psychotic disorders in the elderly. In C. Cohen (Ed.), *Schizophrenia into later life. treatment, research, and policy* (pp. 55–75). Washington, DC: American Psychiatric Association; Thorpe, L. (1997). The treatment of psychotic disorders in late life. *Canadian Journal of Psychiatry, 42*(Suppl. 1), 19s–27s.

2. Delusional disorder
3. Mood disorders with psychotic features, both major depression and bipolar disorder
4. Delirium
5. Psychosis manifested with other diseases: Parkinson's disease (PD), Alzheimer's disease (AD), and other dementias
6. Psychoses related to substance use, abuse, or polypharmacy
7. Benign hallucinatory state, Charles Bonnet syndrome

Schizophrenia

Schizophrenia is a severe mental disorder characterized by two or more of the following symptoms: delusions; hallucinations; disorganized thinking; disorganized behavior; or negative symptoms (i.e., affective flattening, poverty of speech, or apathy that cannot be attributed to other medical or psychiatric causes). These symptoms cause occupational and personal impairment (APA, 2000). Schizophrenia has been studied within three age groupings: early onset (EOS) before age 40 years, late onset (LOS) between 40 and 60 years of age, and very LOS schizophrenic-like psychosis over 60 years of age (Howard, Rabbins, Seeman, & Jeste, 2000). Some mental health professionals have hotly contested the validity of a diagnosis of LOS because they believe LOS to be pathophysiologically different from EOS (Tune & Salzman, 2003). In relation to EOS, individuals with LOS have a greater prevalence of visual hallucinations (Howard, Castle, Wessely, & Murray, 1993), less prevalence of a formal thought disorder, and fewer negative symptoms, such as flat affect, apathy, and poverty of speech; less family history of schizophrenia; a greater risk for developing tardive dyskinesia; and significant gender differences, with women more likely to have LOS than men (Tune & Salzman). Persons with LOS tend to live in the community and have been able to hold a job, maintain personal relationships, and marry (Castle, Wessely, Howard, & Murray, 1997).

Individuals with EOS who have entered old age present a slightly different picture. Schultze et al. (1997) conducted a cross-sectional study of persons aged 14 to 73 years with EOS. Older participants in the study had decreased hallucinations, delusions, and bizarre behavior and decreased inappropriate affect. In persons with EOS, positive symptoms waned and negative symptoms tended to persist into old age, unlike persons who have LOS. Further, persons with EOS are less likely to have had a successful career and to have married and had a family. Table 9-2 provides comparisons of characteristics of EOS, LOS, and very LOS schizophrenia (Reeves & Brister, 2008).

Delusional Disorder

Generally, delusional disorder increases in middle to old age (Thorpe, 1997) and is manifested by the presence of one or more nonbizarre delusions (APA, 2000). Delusional content is not pervasive and is related to everyday life, such as the belief that one's spouse is having an affair. Often, overall functioning is not impaired or impairment is limited to the area of life that is the focus of the delusion. As in the previous example, the individual may have family problems but be able to function in an occupational setting.

Mood Disorder with Psychotic Features

Major depression and bipolar disorder can be accompanied by psychotic symptoms, both delusions and hallucinations. Mood symptoms are pervasive, and psychotic symptoms can be mood congruent or mood incongruent (APA, 2000). "Mood congruent" means that an individual who is depressed manifests delusions that reinforce this depression, such as delusions of guilt or self-nihilism, and an individual who is manic manifests grandiose delusions. "Mood incongruent" means that the psychotic symptoms are not related to the person's mood. Various sources report that psychotic symptoms are more prevalent in older individuals experiencing their first episode of depression, specifically in older women (Kessing, 2006). Late-onset bipolar disorder is likely to be

TABLE 9-2

Comparison of Some Characteristics of Early-Onset Schizophrenia, Late-Onset Schizophrenia, and Very Late-Onset Schizophrenia-Like Psychosis

Characteristic	Early-Onset Schizophrenia	Late-Onset Schizophrenia	Very Late-Onset Schizophrenia-Like Psychosis
Age	Younger than 40	40 to 59	60 or older
Female preponderance	Absent	Present	Strongly present
Positive symptoms	Usually strongly present	Usually strongly present	Usually strongly present
Negative symptoms	Strongly present	Rare	Usually absent
Thought disorder	Strongly present	Rare	Usually absent
Family history of schizophrenia	Present	Sometimes present	Rare
Early life maladjustment	Present	Unlikely	Rare
Brain structural abnormalities	Absent	Usually absent	Often present
Cognitive deterioration	Absent	Usually absent	Often present
Required antipsychotic agent dosage	Higher	Lower	Lower
Risk of tardive dyskinesia	Present	Present	Higher

Source: Reeves & Brister (2008).

accompanied by psychotic features and complicated with greater medical and neurological comorbidity. Some mania can be related to certain medical diseases and drugs. Right-sided cerebrovascular disease has been implicated in late-onset mania (Desai & Grossberg, 2003). The presence of psychotic symptoms in mood disorders makes treatment more challenging.

Delirium

Delirium is a syndrome of brain dysfunction that primarily affects one's ability to attend to meaningful stimuli and usually is accompanied by hallucinations and misinterpretation of environmental cues (Mentes, Culp, Maas, & Rantz, 1999; Thorpe, 1997). Hallucinations in delirium are typically visual and accompanied by illusions. Illusions are different than hallucinations in that an illusion is a misperception of a real sensory stimulus and a hallucination is a sensory experience with no real stimulus. Paranoid delusions may also be present. Studies show that delirium is present in 10–15% of older adults who enter the hospital and that an additional 5–30% become delirious during the hospital stay (Francis, 2000). Common causes of delirium include infection, medication toxicity, recent hospitalization, recent surgery under general anesthesia, recent falls, trauma or pain, alcohol or drug abuse, recent stroke or seizure, and nutritional deficiencies (Francis, 2000). Delirium is often misdiagnosed or undiagnosed in older persons by nurses and other care providers (Inouye, Foreman, Mion, Katz, & Cooney, 2001), leading to improper treatment and poor health outcomes, such as longer hospitalizations and decline in functional and cognitive abilities resulting in nursing home placement (Francis). The hallmark signs of delirium are its acute onset (hours to days) and fluctuating levels of consciousness.

Psychosis Manifested with Other Diseases

Many diseases may be accompanied by psychotic symptoms. An estimated 15% of individuals with untreated endocrine disorders, 20% of persons with systemic lupus erythematosus, and as many as 40% of persons with temporal lobe epilepsy have psychotic symptomatology (APA, 2000). In addition, many elderly persons with AD or other dementias (e.g., vascular dementia, Lewy body dementia, frontotemporal dementia) and PD also manifest psychotic symptoms at some time in the course of the disease.

Psychotic symptoms manifested in persons with dementia vary. Delusions manifested in persons with AD include persecutory delusions ("Someone has stolen my possessions") and auditory or visual hallucinations that are not usually frightening to the individual (Soares & Gershon, 1997). As the person becomes more cognitively impaired, the delusions become less elaborate. Hallucinations are reported to affect 21–41% of patients, with visual hallucinations being the most common (Paulsen et al., 2000). Visual hallucinations usually involve people from the past, intruders, or animals. Auditory hallucinations commonly accompany delusions and are usually persecutory (Desai & Grossberg, 2003).

Patients with vascular dementia may also present with psychotic features. Delusions affect 9–40% of patients with vascular dementia and are similar to those in AD patients. Hallucinations are usually visual and occur concurrently with delusions (Desai & Grossberg, 2003). Lewy body dementia is characterized by fluctuations in cognitive impairment, intermittent parkinsonism, and recurrent visual hallucinations (Dodel et al., 2008). The clinician should be suspicious about the possibility of Lewy body dementia in a patient who presents with visual hallucinations early in the course of a dementia. Frontotemporal dementia is a disorder that is much less common than AD, Lewy body dementia, or vascular dementia, and is frequently misdiagnosed. It is characterized by language impairment, personality changes, and behavioral disturbances sometimes occurring for years before a diagnosis is made. The patient exhibits bizarre and grandiose delusions caused by loss of frontal lobe function (Desai & Grossberg).

In PD, psychotic symptoms are most likely related to medications that are used to treat the PD or neuropathology that accompanies the progression of the disease. Common psychiatric symptoms in PD include visual and auditory hallucinations, delusions, agitation, delirium, sleep disturbances, and nightmares. Psychotic symptoms occur more commonly in the later stages of the disease and in PD patients with dementia. Approximately 20% of persons taking dopaminergic agents report visual hallucinations of people or animals (Thorpe, 1997).

It is important to remember that psychosis manifests primarily as delusions or hallucinations. Often, a whole range of problem behaviors in persons with dementia, such as wandering, escape behaviors, or excessive vocalizations, are misidentified and treated as psychotic behavior (Kidder, 2003). This can be problematic because these individuals are then medicated with powerful antipsychotic medications that do nothing to improve the problematic behaviors but can cause serious side effects.

Psychosis Related to Substance Use, Abuse, or Polypharmacy

Older individuals take many medications that can cause alterations in mental state, including psychotic symptoms. The biggest offenders are those drugs with anticholinergic properties, antiarrhythmics, H_2 blockers, benzodiazepines, tricyclic antidepressants, and antiparkinsonian drugs (Desai & Grossberg, 2003).

Abuse of alcohol or other drugs can occur in elderly individuals. Intoxication from or withdrawal of substances of abuse can trigger psychotic symptoms in older individuals. Psychotic symptoms are often very intense, accompanied by agitation and a fluctuating physical status. Therefore, it is important not to overlook substance abuse as a cause of psychotic behaviors in older persons.

Benign Hallucinatory State: Charles Bonnet Syndrome

Isolated visual hallucinations in individuals with significant visual impairment suggest Charles Bonnet syndrome (Shiraishi, Terao, Ibi, Nakamura, & Tawara, 2004). Charles Bonnet syndrome has been strongly linked to low vision, where 10–13% of individuals with bilateral visual acuity worse than 20/60 are reported to have such visual hallucinations. The visual hallucinations are sophisticated and consist of small children, animals, or a vivid movie-like scene. To be diagnosed with Charles Bonnet syndrome, the patient must meet the following criteria: visual hallucinations, partially intact sight, visual impairment, and lack of evidence of brain disease or other psychiatric disorder. The treatment of choice for Charles Bonnet syndrome is information and support, and in a recent study, Crumbliss, Taussig, and Jay (2008) reported that a program of vision rehabilitation may be helpful for patients with Charles Bonnet syndrome.

Epidemiology of Psychotic Symptoms in Older Adults

The number of elderly persons with psychotic symptoms is not precise and has focused primarily on the presence of paranoid ideas. It is difficult to assess the presence of psychotic symptoms by self-report, because older individuals may have comorbid illnesses that prevent disclosure, and

generally individuals of all ages are less likely to report such symptoms. The prevalence of paranoid ideation in the general elderly population has been reported at 4–6%, and this estimate may include persons with dementia (Henderson et al., 1998). One epidemiological study of psychotic symptoms in nondemented elderly persons older than age 85 years reported the prevalence of any one psychotic symptom at 10%. Specific psychotic symptoms reported were 7% exhibiting hallucinations, 5.5% exhibiting delusions, and 7% exhibiting paranoid ideation (Ostling & Skoog, 2002). This investigation is most likely more accurate because data were collected through multiple sources including physical and psychiatric examinations, family interviews, and chart review. In a recent study comparing delusion proneness in a community sample of older and younger adults, 11% of the older participants reported that they felt as if there was a conspiracy against them and 44% stated that they felt they were being persecuted (Laroi, Van der Linden, DeFruyt, van Os, & Aleman, 2006). This finding is supported in another recent study that found that younger older adults (70–82 years) had a lower prevalence of psychotic symptoms (1%) than adults older than 85 years (10%) (Sigstrom et al., 2009).

When considering older nursing home residents, the increased prevalence of psychotic symptoms is related to the increased prevalence of dementia in this population. In an earlier study of psychiatric disorders in nursing home residents, Rovner et al. (1990) documented that 16% of 454 new admissions to a nursing home had either dementia (AD, vascular, or other dementias) with psychotic features or schizophrenia. In a study of 329 nursing home residents with AD who were followed for 4 years, over 50% exhibited psychotic symptoms (Paulsen et al., 2000).

Estimates of schizophrenia in the elderly population include those persons who have EOS schizophrenia who have lived to old age, which comprise about 85% of older persons with schizophrenia, and those persons who develop schizophrenia in old age. The prevalence of LOS schizophrenia (occurring after age 40) is estimated to be 23.5% (Harris & Jeste, 1998), and approximately 4% of persons diagnosed with schizophrenia have very LOS after the age of 60 (Howard et al., 2000).

Psychotic symptoms are not uncommon in older people living in the community, with 1 in 10 community-dwelling persons without dementia having some psychotic symptom and as many as one in two persons with dementia exhibiting psychotic behaviors. These estimates are expected to increase over the next 20 years in tandem with the increasing aged population.

Risk Factors for Psychosis

Psychosis increases with age and is more prevalent in females than in males (Giblin, Clare, Livingston, & Howard, 2004). Further, there is evidence that sensory impairments, both visual and auditory deficits, are more common in older persons with psychotic symptoms. It has not been determined whether sensory impairment is a cause or a result of psychosis (Castle et al., 1997). Social isolation, lack of intimate contacts, such as a spouse or close friends, and premorbid paranoid personality traits have also been cited as risk factors for psychosis in old age (Thorpe, 1997). In addition, Giblin and colleagues (2004) found that older persons with late-onset psychosis were more likely to report significantly higher rates of adverse life events and a higher degree of isolation, loneliness, and impaired function. Cognitive impairment may be a contributing or risk factor for delirium that is associated with psychotic symptoms, and likewise for the psychosis that often accompanies dementia.

ASSESSMENT

Most nurses find it challenging to identify, evaluate, and manage psychosis in older patients. Psychotic symptoms can occur as components of either medical or psychiatric illnesses. Medications are the most common cause of psychosis in the elderly patient with effects that are often reversible (Katz, Jeste, & Tariot, 2002). The clinician should approach the assessment and differential diagnosis of psychosis using a systematic approach (Figure 9-1). Ostling and Skoog (2002) found psychotic symptoms to be associated with a poorer prognosis in patients; they should be identified and treated as expeditiously as possible.

Determine Type of Psychosis

Psychotic disorders can be classified into either primary or secondary psychoses. Primary psychotic disorders include schizophrenia and related disorders, bipolar disorders, psychotic depression, and delusional disorder. The primary disorders comprise the bulk of chronic mental illness in geriatric patients. Secondary psychotic disorders include delirium; psychotic symptoms associated with dementia; and psychotic symptoms secondary to an identifiable medical condition or chemical agent (e.g., drug or alcohol toxicity) (Desai & Grossberg, 2003). It is important to distinguish between these two types to determine prognosis and formulate an appropriate plan of care. The evaluation of a geriatric patient who presents with psychotic symptoms (hallucinations or delusions) should focus on determining whether the psychosis is primary or secondary, and then on eliminating any medical, toxic, or metabolic causes for the symptoms.

Onset of Psychosis

When evaluating psychosis, it is also of the utmost importance to determine when the psychotic symptoms began. An onset earlier in the patient's life, following a chronic course, suggests a primary psychosis, whereas a more sudden onset in a patient without a previous psychiatric history suggests a secondary psychosis (Desai & Grossberg, 2003).

Obtain Accurate and Detailed Medical and Medication History

When assessing elderly patients for psychosis, it is crucial for the clinician to obtain a detailed and accurate history using information collected from

FIGURE 9-1

Assessment Algorithm for Psychosis in Elders.

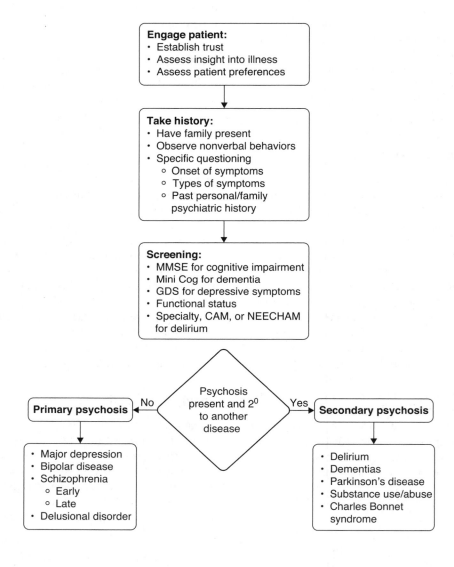

the patient and from collateral sources (i.e., caregiver report, staff reports, and medical records). A good history and medication evaluation is crucial for differential diagnosis.

The Interview

The assessment of psychosis in geriatric patients ideally should begin with the interview. It is essential for the nurse to establish a therapeutic bond with the patient to ensure a positive interview. Patience and active listening help to facilitate this bond and put the patient at ease. Informing the patient about the amount of time for, and content of, the interview is also important. Older patients may respond more slowly to questions, and it is vital to give them ample time to answer before assuming there may be cognitive deficits. The interviewer should avoid any jargon, slang, or medical terminology and should speak slowly and in a low pitched voice. The best time for the interview depends on the patient and his or her needs and preferences. It is helpful to interview the patient when he or she is most awake and alert. Sensory deficits should be accounted for and corrected when possible. It is extremely worthwhile to have a family member or regular caregiver at the interview who is able to clarify responses given by the patient or when there is a question of reliability. The collateral informant becomes especially important when dealing with a psychotic patient who has previously been diagnosed with dementia. Multiple studies of demented patients have shown that caregiver reports yield higher rates of psychopathology than examination and evaluation by the clinician (Ostling & Skoog, 2002).

The nurse may use formal questions and screening tools, and behavioral observation, during the interview to help confirm a diagnosis of psychosis and begin to determine its etiology. Specific questions regarding psychotic symptoms should be used once the older patient is comfortable in the interview setting. The nurse can ask about hallucinations and delusional thinking directly (e.g., "Do you see things that others do not see?" or "Do you hear voices when no one else is around?"). Once

the presence of psychotic symptoms is ascertained, a mental status assessment should be conducted, preferably toward the beginning of the interview. The determination of mental status helps guide the interview, because some of the necessary screening tools to determine the underlying etiology of the psychotic symptoms may be unreliable in patients with cognitive, attention, or orientation impairments. The most well-known and common screening tool is the Mini-Mental State Examination (Folstein, Folstein, & McHugh, 1975). This is a relatively short, 30-item, reliable tool used to screen for cognitive and memory deficits (Kaye & Camicioli, 2000). If time does not permit, the interviewer may use components from the Mini-Mental State Examination, such as the three-item recall and orientation questions. Additionally, there are a variety of brief screening tools for the evaluation of depression, dementia, and delirium that are easy to use during the interview process. The Geriatric Depression Scale (Yesavage et al., 1983) is an example of a useful screening tool because depression in old age is widespread and affects one in six patients in general medical practice and an even higher percentage in nursing homes and hospitals (Bosworth, Hays, George, & Steffens, 2002). The Mini Cog is a simple screening instrument that consists of a three-word recall and clock drawing test that can be used to screen for dementia (Borson, Scanlan, Vitallano, & Dokmak, 2000). The Lippincott's Nursing Center's "How to Try This" series has both printed copies of the Geriatric Depression Scale and the Mini Cog and online videos showing nurses administering these instruments. They can be found at http://www.nursingcenter.com/library/static.asp?pageid=730390. Nurses are encouraged to establish a screening regimen (Figure 9-1) for psychotic patients that includes screening for dementia, delirium, and depression.

Behavioral observation may be the most effective way to assess the acutely psychotic patient because he or she most likely would not be able to sit through and complete an entire interview because of anxiety caused by delusions or hallucinations during the interview. A particularly helpful

212 Chapter 9: Psychosis in Older Adults

technique is to observe the patient at home or in his or her regular living environment to reduce the patient's anxiety level and to allow the nurse to observe for possible triggers of the psychotic behavior. If the psychotic patient is hospitalized, an in-room behavioral assessment may also be very useful. Assessment of functional status should also be included in the complete assessment of psychosis when possible. Mobility should be assessed along with functional level determined by an activities of daily living and instrumental activities of daily living score because this information aids the nurse in determining the patient's potential for independent living after treatment. The interview and behavioral assessment often provide the nurse with enough valuable information to identify the patient's psychotic symptoms and can be a guide as to what the cause of the psychosis may be and how to proceed with evaluation and treatment.

TREATMENT

Treatment of older adults with psychotic symptoms should be based on a thorough assessment that has determined whether the psychosis is primary or secondary and the time of onset of first symptoms (early or late). In secondary psychosis (i.e., psychosis caused by medical illness, dementia, substance use or abuse, or delirium) the most important intervention is to treat the underlying cause. In primary psychotic disorders, specifically schizophrenia, it is important to know the time of onset of first symptoms to plan appropriate care.

Establishing an Environment of Trust

Regardless of the treatment setting, a safe environment and trusting relationship must be established before further interventions are undertaken with older adults with psychosis (Lehman, Lieberman, et al., 2004). These older adults are often isolated, lonely, and have sensory impairments that make negotiation of unfamiliar treatment environments difficult. In outpatient settings, consistency in care providers is essential for the development of a therapeutic alliance.

Strategies for developing a therapeutic alliance include interpersonal presence, effective listening skills, a nonjudgmental attitude, and shared problem solving. Initially, the nurse should listen to the older person's complaints without reinforcing the psychotic symptoms. It is important to understand the delusional or hallucinatory experience from the individual's perspective to better understand his or her level of distress and coping abilities. Often serious medical symptoms or side effects of medications are embedded in a person's delusional system, and if new or different delusions are dismissed as irrelevant, the person is subject to unnecessary suffering. The nurse can provide a safe, nonjudgmental environment where the older individual experiencing psychosis can consistently know that someone will attempt to understand his or her distress and help solve problems. Problem solving with the older individual returns personal control; minimizes paranoid ideas; and promotes adherence to other treatments, such as pharmacotherapeutic and psychosocial interventions (Fung, Tsang, & Corrigan, 2008). If the individual is incapacitated by psychosis, then the first effort should be to control the psychotic symptoms with pharmacotherapy. After stabilization of psychotic symptoms, a therapeutic alliance and a comprehensive treatment plan should be developed that includes the therapeutic strategies discussed in this section.

Pharmacotherapy

Although there are other drugs that may be helpful in the treatment of psychosis, for the purposes of this chapter the focus is on the typical and atypical antipsychotic agents. Major uses for the antipsychotic drugs are in the treatment of schizophrenia and delusional disorder. They may be used on a short-term basis in treating depression with psychotic features, mania, substance abuse–induced psychosis, and aggression and behavioral problems common in older patients with delirium (Stuart & Laraia, 2005). Antipsychotic agents should be used with extreme caution in older persons with psychosis and disruptive behavior related to dementia because of the risk of increased cerebrovascular adverse events and overall mortality (Reeves & Brister, 2008). The development of a pharmacotherapeutic treatment plan should include identification of target symptoms to be treated; drug selection and dose; observed side effects and their treatment; and patient safety, education, and reassurance (Stuart & Laraia). When considering pharmacological treatment of psychotic disorders in older adults, it is important to remember that approximately 80% of older patients have at least one chronic serious physical illness and may be taking multiple medications. It is essential to try to minimize polypharmacy in these individuals for many reasons. Older adults also commonly have sensory deficits and cognitive impairment that can lead to nonadherence to complex medication regimens. The nurse's role in pharmacotherapy is to understand the action of antipsychotic agents, monitor the individual for treatment effectiveness and side effects, and provide information and support for continued adherence to the medication regimen.

Typical Agents

The original drugs used to treat psychosis are known as the "typical" antipsychotics and are predominantly dopamine antagonists. Typical agents, such as haloperidol or fluphenazine, are rarely used as first-line agents today because of numerous shortcomings, such as providing only partial relief of positive symptoms (hallucinations, delusions) with little to no effect on negative symptoms (flat affect, apathy); little effect or worsening of cognitive impairment; increased likelihood of uncomfortable side effects; and increased likelihood of noncompliance. The typical antipsychotics can be considered when a patient has not responded to treatment with atypical antipsychotics.

Atypical Agents

Atypical antipsychotics block dopamine receptor subtype 2 (D2) and serotonin receptor subtype 2 (5HT2) action by inhibiting the reception of the neurotransmitters, dopamine and serotonin, at specific postsynaptic sites. They are useful in treating the positive and negative symptoms of schizophrenia without causing significant extrapyramidal symptoms (EPS). They have also been reported to help treat mood symptoms, hostility, violence, suicidality, and the cognitive impairment that is sometimes seen in schizophrenia.

The atypical agents offer a different pharmacological mechanism of action, an expanded spectrum of therapeutic efficacy, and less severe side effects. For these reasons, they are usually considered as first-line therapy for the treatment of elderly patients with psychosis.

Six agents are available in this class of drugs: (1) aripiprazole, (2) clozapine, (3) risperidone, (4) olanzapine, (5) quetiapine, and (6) ziprasidone. Cloza-pine was the first atypical agent approved for use in the treatment of schizophrenia and has been shown to have good efficacy but has major side-effect issues in the elderly population including agranulocytosis, which is considered a medical emergency, and limits the usability in a population of older adults. First-line choices for older adults are risperidone, olanzapine, or quetiapine. Each agent has special indications; for example, risperidone is a good first choice because of good efficacy with aggressive behavior associated with psychosis and a better side-effect profile including less EPS and fewer falls and injuries (Weiden, Preskorn, Fahnestock, Carpenter, Ross, & Docherty, 2007). Low doses of clozapine or quetiapine are recommended for treating psychosis associated with PD or Lewy body dementia (Dodel et al., 2008). It is important to note that there have been several studies suggesting that either typical or atypical antipsychotic use in older patients is linked with cardiovascular mortality, and so the agents should be carefully monitored (Ray, Chung, Murray, Hall, & Stein, 2009). Refer to Chapter 6 for doses, adverse effects, drug interactions, and geriatric considerations of atypical antipsychotic medications.

Promoting Adherence

Psychotropic medications historically have a relatively poor rate of patient adherence. A review of research has shown that in persons receiving antipsychotics, only half took the medication as prescribed (Lacro, Dunn, Dolder, Leckband, & Jeste, 2002). Risk factors for nonadherence in individuals with schizophrenia include a previous history of nonadherence, recent illicit drug or alcohol use, prior treatment with antidepressants, and patient-reported medication-related cognitive impairment (Ascher-Svanum, Zhu, Faries, Lacro, & Dolder, 2006). In addition, troubling side effects of some types of antipsychotic medications may contribute to nonadherence to the prescribed treatment. In fact, older persons with schizophrenia and other psychoses are at increased risk for such serious side effects as EPS and tardive dyskinesia. Persons with pre-existing cognitive impairment are at high risk for tardive dyskinesia (Katz et al., 2002). Further threats to medication adherence in older persons include the increased prevalence of cognitive and sensory problems that can severely impair the ability to take medications correctly and regularly, and the likelihood that the older person is already on a complex medication regimen to manage other health problems. The addition of even one more medication can confuse the person and expose him or her to further drug-to-drug interactions. Another barrier for medication adherence in older persons living on a fixed income is the cost of the atypical agents, which can be considerable.

Nurses can promote medication adherence in older persons by helping individuals develop routines to promote medication adherence, by carefully monitoring side effects, and by providing medications in a long-acting injectable form (fluphenazine, haloperidol, and risperidone) when an older individual demonstrates difficulty remembering or managing his or her medication regimen (Weiden et al., 2007). Side effects can be assessed by observation and specific questions. Several instruments may be used to assess side effects including the Abnormal Involuntary Movement Scale (Guy, 1976), which assesses for the presence of tardive dyskinesia, and the Simpson-Angus Scale (Simpson & Angus, 1970), which assesses for the presence of EPS, such as akinesias, dyskinesias, and pseudo-Parkinson's syndrome. Use

of depot administration of antipsychotic medications (every 2–4 weeks) in memory-impaired older individuals eliminates the need for the person to remember to take medications on a daily basis.

Nurses can also plan a medication regimen with the older person using simple, descriptive medication instructional materials describing the medication and the time it should be taken or using a pill sorter, which can be prefilled weekly for the older individual by the nurse or family members. In a systematic review of the literature, structured medication groups were shown to increase an individual's knowledge of psychotropic medication and medication adherence (Fernandez, Evans, Griffiths, & Mostacchi, 2006).

Primary Preventive Care

Older individuals with mental disorders are often not advised of preventive health screening options. Individuals with LOS dementia and other diseases with paranoid symptoms have an increased prevalence of sensory deficits, both visual and auditory, which if corrected could improve their response to psychiatric treatment. In addition, as persons with EOS age, they are likely to develop conditions associated with aging, such as sensory deficits, arthritis, heart disease, diabetes, and respiratory disease. Older adults with schizophrenia should be offered preventive services, such as an annual influenza vaccine and a pneumonoccal vaccine, and screenings for hypertension and colorectal, prostate, breast, cervical, and skin cancer. Support and education about the necessity of these examinations are crucial because older persons with schizophrenia may be paranoid about the examination and the intrusiveness of some examinations may make the individual uncomfortable. In addition, older individuals with schizophrenia should be taught health maintenance skills. The importance of diet and exercise to prevent medical problems, alleviate stress, and enhance coping skills is invaluable. Smoking cessation and moderate alcohol intake are other areas for consideration. All older persons with schizophrenia should have a primary care provider whom they trust, and the nurse can help identify a provider who is skilled in caring for persons with chronic mental illness and can reinforce preventive health care practices with the older individual.

Crisis Intervention

During the course of interviewing an older adult with psychosis, it may become evident to the nurse that there is a need for crisis intervention. Given the high prevalence of depression among older adults, and especially those with schizophrenia, it is imperative for the nurse to routinely inquire about suicide. This helps to properly identify older patients who are at risk of committing suicide. An older adult who is depressed with psychotic features may be at even higher risk for self-harm or suicide. Suicide rates in the United States are higher among older adults than any other age group. The highest rate occurs in people older than 75 years, with men older than 85 years of age having the highest rate overall (Menghini & Evans, 2000). More than 90% of adults who end their lives by suicide have an associated psychiatric condition. There are certain disorders that place individuals at higher risk for suicide. These include mood disorders, substance abuse, and schizophrenia. Patients with depression, in addition to their schizophrenia, were at even higher risk for suicide (Kasckow et al., 2007). Suicide is the leading cause of premature death among patients with schizophrenia, and the lifetime prevalence has been estimated at 10% (Meltzer, 1998). Among patients with schizophrenia, 40% report suicidal thoughts, 20–40% make unsuccessful suicide attempts, and 9–13% ultimately end their lives with suicide (Meltzer). The highest priority for nurses treating patients who are suicidal is the maintenance of patient safety. In cases of psychotic patients who are suicidal, hospitalization is clearly indicated.

Several studies have found that persons with schizophrenia are at higher risk for homicide than the general population and psychosis has been linked with increased violence. Schwartz, Reynold, Austin, and Petersen (2003) found that manic symptoms and psychotic symptoms had a significant correlation with homicidal ideation and intent. The investigators recommend that clinicians assess a male schizophrenic patient's overall lethality (homicidal ideation and intent) and evaluate it thoroughly in order to formulate an appropriate plan of care. It is clear that in the case of a psychotic homicidal patient, hospitalization is warranted.

Psychosocial Interventions

Evidenced-based practice for best psychosocial interventions for schizophrenia is in its infancy and few are developed specifically for older adults, but some recommendations do exist based on the Schizophrenia Patient Outcomes Research Team updated treatment recommendations (Lehman, Kreyenbuhl et al., 2004). The most significant finding from the Schizophrenia Patient Outcomes Research Team work is that the individual with schizophrenia needs comprehensive services at the individual, family, and community level plus pharmacotherapy. This is further supported in a recent review of psychosocial therapies for the treatment of schizophrenia by Patterson and Leeuwenkamp (2008). They report that psychosocial treatments can improve adherence, promote symptom reduction, prevent relapse and hospitalizations, and improve patient function and family relationships. Further, multiple integrated services often work best. The characteristics of successful services in each of these areas are discussed and specific therapeutic modalities addressed. It is important to note that although most persons have to be medicated with antipsychotics indefinitely, it is equally important for the nurse to establish a therapeutic relationship with the psychotic individual to engage him or her in the necessary array of therapies.

Individual-Focused Intervention

Individual-focused interventions are those interventions that enhance or improve an individual's function, whether delivered individually or in a group format. Components of successful modalities include a combination of support, education, and cognitive-behavioral strategies to improve the individual's function and ability to self-manage his or her disease (Lehman, Kreyenbuhl, et al., 2004).

Disease management skill training is ideally accomplished in a group format where individuals can share their experiences. The content is broken into smaller learning modules including areas of medication management, communicating with the healthcare provider about symptoms, and how to deal with an increase in symptoms. The disease management modules are designed as a highly interactive learning activity where participants can use psychomotor skills, and coaching is available from the group leaders to master these skills (Liberman, 2003). Liberman strongly advocates for the use of a highly structured modular format for this educational intervention because of the age-related and disease-mediated cognitive changes seen in older persons. Psychoeducational groups that rely more on verbal memory and traditional methods of learning may not be successful with older persons with schizophrenia. Other open-ended formats, such as a weekly medication group that provides support combined with concrete problem-solving strategies around disease symptoms and medication side effects, are also effective (Zygmunt, Olfson, Boyer, & Mechanic, 2002).

Community management skills focus on the successful adaptation of the individual to community living. Many older individuals who have life-long schizophrenia may have spent long periods of time in state psychiatric hospitals and therefore require help to readjust to community living. Use of modular learning as described previously can also be adapted to teaching community living skills. It is important to incorporate "hands on" learning experiences to teach home management skills, such as cooking and cleaning, and social skills, such as making conversation (Liberman, 2003).

Social skills training in combination with other individual modalities discussed here has the potential to improve the ability of an older adult with schizophrenia to live independently

(Kopelowicz, Liberman, & Zarate, 2006). The focus of the skills training is to promote interpersonal competence and coping ability through role playing, feedback, and positive reinforcement.

Cognitive–behavioral therapy (CBT) is a therapeutic approach widely used across a variety of disorders including those individuals with schizophrenia who have refractory positive symptoms, specifically hallucinations and delusions, as well as negative symptoms (Patterson & Leeuwenkamp, 2008). CBT techniques encourage the individual to reevaluate strongly held beliefs through "disputing and challenging, creating dissonance, using coping statements, generating alternative explanations for symptoms, cognitive restructuring of the meaning of symptoms, and behavioral experiments" (Liberman, 2003, pp. 27–28). Older persons with schizophrenia can be coached to question their long-held delusions and reformulate another more reality-based explanation for the symptom. This is done in a supportive environment, encouraging the use of coping self-talk, opportunities to role-play new behaviors, and homework assignments. Liberman describes an easy mnemonic of the Three Cs—Catch the thought (identify irrational cognitions), Check it (assess any thought distortions), and Change it (develop alternative thoughts), to guide the initial sessions.

Family Intervention

Psychoeducation interventions designed to educate and support family members about schizophrenia and its treatment have a strong evidence base including reduction in relapses and rehospitalizations (Lehman, Kreyenbuhl, et al., 2004; Patterson & Leeuwenkamp, 2008). However, traditional psychoeducation programs are designed for individuals who live with their families. Many older persons with schizophrenia live alone but maintain contact with their families (Lefley, 2003). Further, most older persons with schizophrenia have lived with the disease for decades and family members have acquiesced or adapted to the notion of having a chronically ill member. Therefore, it is important to adapt the educational endeavors to include more age-appropriate content, such as the effect of age on schizophrenic symptoms and treatment, and helping aging family members plan for the care of their relative with schizophrenia after they die (Lefley). Culturally sensitive family patterns of caregiving must be addressed. For example, in African-American families, it may be likely that a sibling or younger family member will take responsibility for the individual with schizophrenia (Lefley), and in Chinese and other Eastern Asian cultures parents are cared for by their children in old age.

It is important with older adults who have no family contact, but are living in assisted housing or long-term care facilities, to offer an adapted psychoeducation program to the formal caregivers. The program would focus on educating caregivers about the disease process, how to help the resident cope, and the importance of maintaining pharmacotherapy.

Community Interventions

Community interventions can be an array of services that provide the individual with safe, appropriate housing and support in navigating the healthcare and social welfare systems (Lehman, Kreyenbuhl, et al., 2004). Community services augment the therapeutic modalities discussed previously. Although research conducted in the area of community interventions demonstrates effectiveness, no study has been conducted solely with older individuals. Several of the studies demonstrating positive outcomes included persons older than 50 years of age and may therefore hold promise for elderly persons with schizophrenia (Mohamed, Kasckow, Granholm, & Jeste, 2003).

Case management programs provide support for persons negotiating for services. Case managers do not provide direct service but contract with other providers for services and then oversee the integration of services. Clients come to the case manager, usually a member of the mental health team, who helps to link the client with needed

services and may advocate for service improvements when gaps or deficiencies are identified. Case management programs have primarily demonstrated effectiveness in improving psychological well-being of participants, through the integration of social skills training. Cost-effectiveness in the form of decreased hospitalization and use of emergency services is less well demonstrated (Mohamed et al., 2003).

Supported housing is noninstitutional, permanent housing that offers supportive services based on the individual's functional ability and preference. Supported housing facilities often have a paraprofessional provider on site to provide for general housing needs of the tenants and to help provide the stable housing environment that a person with schizophrenia requires. Previously, the only community housing options available were transitional housing arrangements, and individuals were ultimately expected to live independently. It is now recognized that older, isolated persons with schizophrenia have relatively few options for living arrangements: family, nursing home, public housing, or some form of supported housing. Supported housing for older persons has not been well studied, although program evaluations demonstrate that supported housing helps decrease days of hospitalization, decrease psychiatric symptoms, improve clients' homemaking skills, and increase satisfaction (Leff et al., 2009).

Day treatment programs or partial hospital programs provide an alternative to extended hospitalization through comprehensive services offered on an outpatient basis by a multidisciplinary team of psychiatric nurses, psychiatrists, social workers, and occupational therapists (Mohamed et al., 2003). Programs are scheduled 5 days per week, with some programs having structured, planned participation several days a week and other programs allowing the individual to build his or her own program, based on individual need. Many of the previously described modalities may be used in a day treatment center, such as medication management, group therapies focusing on disease management and social skills, and family education. Although it seems that persons with schizophrenia in day pro-grams demonstrate better community adjustment at a cost-effective price, few studies using this treat-ment option have included persons older than 50 years of age (Mohamed et al).

Clubhouses are participant-run self-help clubs open 7 days a week with supporting paraprofessional staff members. Persons who join the club are called "members," not "patients," to reinforce a healthy social role for members. In addition, members are expected to take an active role in the operation of the clubhouse and may transition from working at the clubhouse to outside employment. Social and supportive services are also available, particularly on evenings and weekends when members may feel most isolated. Again, it is unclear that this service has age-related benefits, because few studies have been conducted with older persons.

Assertive community programs are recom-mended for persons who are at high risk for repeated hospitalization, who have difficulty remaining in traditional treatment settings, and who are home-less (Lehman, Kreyenbuhl, et al., 2004). These programs provide close and personal monitoring of patients through the use of a multidisciplinary team that provides outreach to these patients in their community environment and have been shown to decrease the length of hospitalizations and improve living conditions (Lehman, Kreyen-buhl, et al.).

Community and Family Resources

Families of older persons with schizophrenia have the compounded difficulties of caring for a mem-ber who has a chronic disability while dealing with their own personal aging. Caregiver burden in these families is chronic and fluctuates depend-ing on the symptoms and life stresses that their family member with schizophrenia is experienc-ing. Although many older persons with schizo-phrenia live apart from their families, they still maintain contact with elderly parents, specifically their mothers (Lefley, 2003). In addition, there is evidence that families who are living apart from

their relative with schizophrenia have some of the same stresses as families living with their relative (Laidlaw, Coverdale, Falloon, & Kydd, 2002). Two of the concerns expressed by parents of older per-sons with schizophrenia are unmet service needs for their family member, specifically for perma-nent supported housing and recreation services; and services that help families plan for the future of their relative with schizophrenia (Smith, 2003).

Unfortunately, there are relatively few ser-vices explicitly for older persons with schizophre-nia (Table 9-3). The National Alliance on Mental Illness (NAMI, www.nami.org) is the organization that provides the most comprehensive informa-tion about services for families and persons with schizophrenia and other mental illnesses. Most states have a local chapter of NAMI. The NAMI Web site provides educational resources and infor-mation about support groups, respite care, and maintaining a healthy lifestyle. One of the initia-tives of this organization is to help older family members plan for the legal, financial, housing, and healthcare needs of their relative with schizo-phrenia (Thompson, 2003). The Planned Lifetime Assistance Network programs were developed expressly to meet the needs of aging family mem-bers who want to plan for the future of their rela-tive with schizophrenia or other disabling mental illnesses. These nonprofit programs affiliated with NAMI help families develop a future care plan, establish the resources for payment, and identify the persons or programs responsible for carrying out the plan (NAMI, n.d.).

ETHICAL AND LEGAL ISSUES

Psychiatric Advance Directives

One of the prevailing ethical–legal concerns for persons with schizophrenia and other psychotic disorders is that of self-determination in psychi-atric care decisions. Similar to advance directives for medical care, psychiatric advance directives (PAD) have been proposed to help persons with schizophrenia and other psychiatric disorders to

TABLE 9-3

Resources for Persons with Schizophrenia and Their Families

Organization	Contact Information	Mission/Purpose
National Alliance on Mental Illness	Colonial Place Three 3803 N. Fairfax Drive, Suite 100 Arlington, VA 22203 (703) 524-7600—Main (800) 950-NAMI (6264)—Helpline www.nami.org	Education, advocacy, support, and preventive care for persons with mental illness
Mental Health America	2000 N. Beauregard St., 6th floor Alexandria, VA 22311 (800) 969-6642 www.nmha.org	Education, advocacy, and support for persons with mental illness
Schizophrenia.com	Web community—no address www.schizophrenia.com	Education, support for persons with schizophrenia
Compeer	259 Monroe Ave. Rochester, NY 14607 (800) 836-0475 www.compeer.org	Matches community volunteers in supportive friendship relationships with persons who have mental illness
Judge David L. Bazelon Center for Mental Health Law	1101 15th St. NW, Suite 1212 Washington, DC 20005 (202) 467-5730 www.Bazelon.org	Legal advocacy to advance and serve the rights of persons with mental illness and developmental disabilities
National Alliance for Research on Schizophrenia and Depression	60 Cutter Mill Rd., Suite 404 Great Neck, NY 11021 (800) 829-8289 www.narsad.org	Fundraising for psychiatric brain research worldwide

predetermine the psychiatric care that they want should they become unable to make such decisions when they have a psychotic crisis (Srebnik, Russo, Sage, Peto, & Zick, 2003). PADs promote individual autonomy, enhance communication between families and mental health caregivers about treatment issues, decrease ineffective or unwanted treatments, and prevent crises that may result in involuntary commitment or use of seclusion or restraints. Several studies have indicated that between 40% and 75% of individuals with severe mental illness, such as schizophrenia, are interested in creating PADs (Srebnik et al.). Further, a trusted caseworker or nurse may be the

impetus for this interest. Although there are difficult implementation issues with PADs, patient advocacy groups and mental health professionals support the appropriate use of PADs for persons with severe mental illness. Materials to help with the preparation of a PAD can be obtained from the National Mental Health Association Web site or from the Bazelon Center for Mental Health Law Web site.

Social Stigmatization

Social stigma may be doubly damaging to older persons with chronic psychotic disorders, such as schizophrenia. Ageism plus stigma from having a chronic mental illness can be overwhelming. Levy, Slade, and Kasl (2002) have shown that ageism can affect cognition, physical abilities, and gait in older adults. When the stigma of mental illness is added, the individual feels dehumanized. Schulze and Angermeyer (2003) conducted focus groups of persons with schizophrenia, their relatives, and mental health workers to better understand stigmatizing experiences from the individual's perspective. Stigma was reported at many levels including at the interpersonal and social levels (Schulze & Angermeyer). For example, interpersonal stigma was experienced as derogatory comments about people with mental illness, and social stigma was experienced as stereotyped public images characterizing all people with schizophrenia as violent and dangerous. When individuals with schizophrenia internalize this stigma, they often isolate themselves and distance themselves from society, resulting in nonadherence with treatment, underemployment, and few significant relationships with others, which significantly reduces quality of life. In a recent study Yanos, Roe, Markus, and Lysaker (2008) suggest that therapies that identify and minimize internal negative self-messages, such as CBT, can be helpful in alleviating this internalized stigma. In addition, societal misperceptions about diseases, such as schizophrenia, must be addressed. Programs to combat stigma associated with schizophrenia should have multiple foci, including encouraging the media to represent persons with schizophrenia in a more balanced manner, lobbying for better services for the mentally ill, and providing the individual with support to combat interpersonal stigma. The National Alliance on Mental Illness has several programs for combating stigma associated with mental illness. Their program entitled, "In Our Own Voice: Living with Mental Illness," helps individuals develop confidence through sharing their experience with mental illness with audiences of mental health professionals, students, and lay persons. NAMI also sponsors a monthly Stigmabuster newsletter, available on its Web site (see Table 9-2).

Role of the Geropsychiatric Nurse

Nurses are often the first healthcare professionals to identify psychosis in an older adult, primarily because of the close therapeutic relationship that is engendered between nurse and older patient. Nurses have an integral role in the assessment and treatment of older adults with psychoses resulting from the multiple etiologies discussed in this chapter. They may serve as case managers, coordinating all of the various aspects of treatment, both psychosocial and community services (Lancashire et al., 1997). Nurses who have been trained in CBT techniques may assist in helping persons with schizophrenia manage their symptoms and maintain their treatment regimen (Chan, 2003). Nurses conduct medication groups and other disease management, community skills, and family psychoeducational groups and are an essential member of a multidisciplinary team (Lehman, Kreyenbuhl, et al., 2004). Further, nurses are often the first providers to identify medication nonadherence or uncomfortable side effects, and can intervene before the individual becomes actively psychotic. Medication clinics, which are often a part of an integrated community program and provide supervision of medications and provision of the long-acting injectable form of antipsychotic agents, are often managed by nurses.

Advanced practice nurses with specialty education in adult psychiatric mental health nursing and additional training in care of older adults provide essential mental health services to older adults with acute and chronic mental illness (Algase, Souder, Roberts, & Beattie, 2006). Some advanced practice nurses who are prepared as adult psychiatric mental health nursing nurse practitioners may provide holistic care to older adults with persistent mental illness by prescribing psychoactive medications and providing primary care for older adults.

CASE STUDY

Ms. Mary Graves is a 61-year-old single woman with a history of early onset schizophrenia, paranoid type. She has a 30-year history of smoking cigarettes and has developed chronic obstructive pulmonary disease (COPD) and hypertension. Although she reports chronic auditory hallucinations and has a restricted affect, she does not evidence delusions or thought disorder. The voice that she hears is supportive and encouraging to her and she has not been hospitalized for exacerbation of her mental illness in the past 5 years. She has fair insight into her illness.

Her current treatment consists of depot fluphenazine deconoate (Prolixin) every 2 weeks; inhalers for COPD (albuterol and Advair); and an antihypertensive (hydrochlorothiazide and lisinopril). She attends an outpatient clinic where she receives her medication every 2 weeks and sees a psychiatrist on a monthly and as-needed basis.

Ms. Graves receives social security disability and Medicaid insurance and she works 8 hours per week in a supported work program—"I get too nervous at work, I'm afraid I will make a mistake." She lives in an apartment with another woman who also is an outpatient. They split the cost of rent, but each purchases her own food. Although there is no overt animosity between them, one senses that they interact very little and live "parallel" lives. Ms. Graves has a brother and his family but sees them infrequently. Her mother died several years ago at age 75 and was reported to have been an alcoholic.

Recently, Ms. Graves has begun a relationship with a younger man, John, whom she met at the outpatient clinic. She spends much of her free time with him. She has had few relationships with men so she is obsessed with maintaining this relationship. She reports being sexually active.

In the past 2 weeks she has not been able to sleep; she stays awake because she is convinced that her roommate and next door neighbors are spying on her. In addition, the voices are loudly yelling at her that she is a "dirty slut" for sleeping with John and that she must "cleanse herself" or die. She believes that when she goes outside that people can see that she is unclean. All of these psychotic symptoms began after she was evaluated and diagnosed with cervical cancer in situ.

Questions

1. What would your first psychiatric priority be in caring for Ms. Graves?
   Ms. Graves should be assessed for suicidal ideation and monitored closely, given the presence of positive symptoms, personal shame, and prospect of a life-threatening disease—all of which increase the risk for suicide.

2. Would you recommend that her medications be changed or increased to better manage her symptoms?
   Her depot medication should be augmented with oral antipsychotics—most preferably a small dose of an atypical antipsychotic, such as risperidone or olanzapine (if she is not overweight or at risk for type 2 diabetes) until her psychotic symptoms remit.

3. What type of follow-up care would you recommend?
   Until she is stable, it is proposed that she attend a day hospital program for

(continues)

CASE STUDY *(continued)*

older persons with persistent mental illness on a weekly basis, where she has an advanced practice psychiatric nurse practitioner who manages her care. The day program provides her with an array of person-centered care options including case management services, cognitive behavioral therapy, social skills training, and home and medication management skills. In addition, her advanced practice psychiatric nurse practitioner visits her in her apartment and meets with Ms. Graves and her roommate to assess Ms. Graves' relationship with her roommate.

4. How should the treatment of her cervical cancer be initiated?

   After referral to the day hospital program, she receives a RN case manager who will accompany her to her cancer treatment appointments and who will serve as a liaison between the oncology department and the day hospital program. The RN case manager will ensure that Ms. Graves receives the information she needs to make decisions about her cancer treatment, and provide continuity of care and the support that Ms. Graves needs.

Ms. Graves responds well to her mental health treatment, exhibiting a decrease in her psychotic symptoms; specifically, she feels less paranoid about her roommate and her

neighbors. Concerning her cancer treatment, she consents to and undergoes a hysterectomy and receives one round of chemotherapy for her cervical cancer. A follow-up pap smear indicates that she should have another round of chemotherapy. She refuses the chemotherapy because she lost her hair, felt very sick, and could not spend as much time with John during the first treatments. She is aware that this may mean that her cancer will reoccur, but she is adamant about refusing the follow-up treatments.

5. How would you handle Ms. Graves' refusal of follow-up cancer treatment?

   It is important to assess if Ms. Graves has the capacity to understand the ramifications of her refusal of follow-up care. Decisional capacity assessment includes the following components: understanding, appreciation, reasoning, and expression of a choice and is closely correlated with performance on cognitive tests, such as the Mini-Mental State Examination (Jeste & Saks, 2006). If it is determined that she has made an informed decision, regardless of the nurse's personal beliefs about treatment, it may be more beneficial to support her right to make an informed decision and maintain the therapeutic alliance between Ms. Graves and the nurse (Schlechter, 2008).

SUMMARY

Nurses are in a pivotal position to help dispel misconceptions about psychotic disorders, specifically schizophrenia. Providing accurate public information about these disorders helps to decrease stigma, promotes an older individual's self-esteem, and improves his or her quality of life.

REFERENCES

Algase, D., Souder, E., Roberts, B., & Beattie, E. (2006). Enriching geropsychiatric nursing in advanced practice nursing programs. *Journal of Professional Nursing, 22*, 129–136.

American Psychiatric Association. (2000). *Diagnostic and statistical manual of mental disorders* (4th ed. Text Revision). Washington, DC: American Psychiatric Association.

Ascher-Svanum, H., Zhu, B., Faries, D., Lacro, J., & Dolder, C. R. (2006). A prospective study of risk factors for nonadherence with antipsychotic medication in the treatment of schizophrenia. *Journal of Clinical Psychiatry, 67*, 1114–1123.

Borson, S., Scanlan, J. M., Vitallano, P., & Dokmak, A. (2000). The Mini Cog. A cognitive "vital signs" measure for dementia screening in multi-lingual elderly. *International Journal of Geriatric Psychiatry, 15*, 1021–1027.

Bosworth, H., Hays, J., George, L. K., & Steffens, D. C. (2002). Psychosocial and clinical predictors of unipolar depression outcomes in older adults. *International Journal of Geriatric Psychiatry, 17*, 238–246.

Castle, D., Wessely, S., Howard, R., & Murray, R. (1997). Schizophrenia with onset at the extremes of adult life. *International Journal of Geriatric Psychiatry, 12*, 712–717.

Chan, S. (2003). Brief cognitive behavioral intervention delivered by nurses reduces overall symptoms in schizophrenia. *Evidence-based Mental Health, 6*, 26.

Crumbliss, K., Taussig, M., & Jay, W. (2008). Vision rehabilitation and Charles Bonnet syndrome. *Seminars in Ophthalmology, 23*, 121–126.

Desai, A., & Grossberg, G. (2003). Differential diagnosis of psychotic disorders in the elderly. In C. Cohen (Ed.), *Schizophrenia into later life. Treatment, research, and policy* (pp. 55–75). Washington, DC: American Psychiatric Association.

Dodel, R., Csoti, I., Ebersbach, G., Fuchs, G., Hahne, M., Kuhn, W., et al. (2008). Lewy body dementia and Parkinson's disease with dementia. *Journal of Neurology, 25*(Suppl. 5), 39–47.

Fernandez, R. S., Evans, V., Griffiths, R. D., & Mostacchi, M. S. (2006). Educational interventions for mental health consumers receiving psychotropic medication: A review of evidence. *International Journal of Mental Health, 15*, 70–80.

Folstein, M. F., Folstein, S., & McHugh, P. R. (1975). Mini-Mental State: A practical method for grading the cognitive state of the patients for the clinician. *Journal of Psychiatric Research, 12*(3), 189–198.

Francis, J. (2000). Delirium. In D. Osterweil, K. Brummel-Smith, & J. Morley (Eds.), *Comprehensive geriatric assessment* (pp. 489–506). New York: McGraw-Hill.

Fung, K., Tsang, H., & Corrigan, P. (2008). Self-stigma of people with schizophrenia as a predictor of their adherence to psychosocial treatment. *Psychiatric Rehabilitation Journal, 32*, 95–104.

Giblin, S., Clare, L., Livingston, G., & Howard, R. (2004). Psychosocial correlates of late-onset psychosis: life experiences, cognitive schemas and attitudes to ageing. *International Journal of Geriatric Psychiatry, 19*, 611–623.

Guy, W. (1976). *ECDEU Assessment manual for pharmacology* (Rev. ed.). Washington, DC: U.S. Department of Health, Education and Welfare.

Harris, A., & Jeste, D. (1998). Late-onset schizophrenia: an overview. *Schizophrenia Bulletin, 14*, 39–55.

Henderson, A., Korten, A., Levings, C., Jorm, A., Christensen, H., Jacomb, P., et al. (1998). Psychotic symptoms in the elderly: A prospective study in a population sample. *International Journal of Geriatric Psychiatry, 13*, 484–492.

Howard, R., Castle, D., Wessely, S., & Murray, R. (1993). A comparative study of 470 cases of early- and late-onset schizophrenia. *British Journal of Psychiatry, 163*, 352–357.

Howard, R., Rabins, P., Seeman, M., & Jeste, D. (2000). Late-onset schizophrenia and very-late onset schizophrenia-like psychosis: An international consensus. The International Late-Onset Schizophrenia Group. *American Journal of Psychiatry, 157*, 172–178.

Inouye, S., Foreman, M., Mion, L., Katz, K., & Cooney, L. (2001). Nurses' recognition of delirium and its symptoms: Comparison of nurse and researcher ratings. *Archives of Internal Medicine, 161*, 2467–2473.

Jeste, D., & Saks, E. (2006). Decisional capacity in mental illness and substance use disorders: Empirical database and policy implications. *Behavioral Sciences and the Law, 24*, 607–628.

Kasckow, J., Montross, L., Golshan, S., Hohamed, S., Patterson, T., Sollanzano, E., et al. (2007). Suicidality in middle aged and older patients with schizophrenia and depressive symptoms: relationship to functioning and quality of life. *International Journal of Geriatric Psychiatry, 22*, 1223–1228.

Katz, P. R., Jeste, D. V., & Tariot, P. N. (2002). Pharmacotherapy for the older patient with psychosis. *Journal of the American Medical Directors Association, 3*(Suppl. 4), H34–H41.

Kaye, J., & Camicioli, R. (2000). Dementia. In D. Osterweil, K. Brummel-Smith, & J. Morley (Eds.), *Comprehensive geriatric assessment* (pp. 507–554). New York: McGraw-Hill.

Kessing, L. (2006). Differences in diagnostic subtypes among patients with late and early onset of a single depressive episode. *International Journal of Geriatric Psychiatry, 21*, 1127–1131.

Kidder, S. (2003). Psychosis and the elderly—Whose delusion is it? *Geriatric Times, IV*(2), 25–26.

Kopelowicz, A., Liberman, R., & Zarate, R. (2006). Recent advances in social skills training for schizophrenia. *Schizophrenia Bulletin, 32*(Suppl. 1), S12–S23.

Lacro, J. P., Dunn, L. B., Dolder, C. R., Leckband, S. G., & Jeste, D. V. (2002). Prevalence of and risk factors for medication nonadherence in patients with schizophrenia: A comprehensive review of recent literature. *Journal of Clinical Psychiatry, 63*, 892–909.

Laidlaw, T., Coverdale, J., Falloon, I., & Kydd, R. (2002). Caregivers' stresses when living together or apart from patients with chronic schizophrenia. *Community Mental Health Journal, 38*, 303–310.

Lancashire, S., Haddock, G., Tarrier, N., Baguley, I., Butterworth, C., & Brooker, C. (1997). Effects of training in psychosocial interventions for community psychiatric nurses in England. *Psychiatric Services, 48*, 39–41.

Laroi, F., Van der Linden, M., DeFruyt, F., van Os, J., & Aleman, A. (2006). Associations between delusion proneness and personality structure in nonclinical participants: Comparison between young and elderly samples. *Psychopathology, 39*, 218–226.

Leff, H. S., Chow, C. M., Pepin, R., Conley, J., Allen, I. E., & Seaman, C. A. (2009). Does one size fit all? What we can and can't learn from a meta-analysis of housing models for persons with mental illness. *Psychiatric Services, 60*, 473–482.

Lefley, H. (2003). Changing caregiving needs as persons with schizophrenia grow older. In C. Cohen (Ed.), *Schizophrenia into later life: Treatment, research, and policy* (pp. 251–268). Washington, DC: American Psychiatric Association.

Lehman, A., Kreyenbuhl, J., Buchanan, R., Dickerson, F., Dixon, L., Goldberg, R., et al. (2004). The Schizophrenia Patient Outcomes Research Team (PORT): Updated treatment recommendations 2003. *Schizophrenia Bulletin, 30*, 192–217.

Lehman, A., Lieberman, J., Dixon, L., McGlaslan, T., Miller, A., Perkins, D., et al. (2004). *Practice guideline for the treatment of patients with schizophrenia* (2nd ed.), Washington, DC: American Psychiatric Association.

Levy, B., Slade, M., & Kasl, S. (2002). Longitudinal benefit of positive self-perceptions of aging on functional health. *Journal of Gerontology Psychological and Social Science, 57*, P409–P417.

Liberman, R. (2003). Biobehavioral treatment and rehabilitation for older adults with schizophrenia. In C. Cohen (Ed.), *Schizophrenia into later life: Treatment, research, and policy* (pp. 223–250). Washington, DC: American Psychiatric Association.

Meltzer, H. Y. (1998). Suicide in schizophrenia: Risk factors and clozapine treatment. *Journal of Clinical Psychology, 59*(Suppl. 3), 15–20.

Menghini, V., & Evans, J. (2000). Suicide among nursing home residents: A population based study. *Journal of the American Medical Directors Association, 1*, 47–50.

Mentes, J., Culp, K., Maas, M., & Rantz, M. (1999). Acute confusion indicators: Risk factors and prevalence using MDS data. *Research in Nursing & Health, 22*, 95–105.

Merriam-Webster. (1997). *The Merriam-Webster dictionary*. Springfield, MA: Merriam-Webster.

Mohamed, S., Kasckow, J., Granholm, E., & Jeste, D. (2003). Community-based treatment of schizophrenia and other severe mental illnesses. In C. Cohen (Ed.), *Schizophrenia into later life: Treatment, research, and policy* (pp. 205–222). Washington, DC: American Psychiatric Association.

National Alliance on Mental Illness (n.d.). *PLAN (Planned lifetime assistance network)*. Retrieved August 3, 2009, from http://www.nami.org/Template.cfm?Section=Helpline1&template=/ContentManagement/ContentDisplay.cfm&ContentID=4861

Ostling, S., & Skoog, I. (2002). Psychotic symptoms and paranoid ideation in a nondemented population-based sample of the very old. *Archives of General Psychiatry, 59*, 53–59.

Patterson, T., & Leeuwenkamp, O. (2008). Adjunctive psychosocial therapies for the treatment of schizophrenia. *Schizophrenia Research, 100*, 108–119.

Paulsen, J., Salmon, D., Thal, I., Romero, R., Weisstein-Jenkins, C., Galasko, D., et al. (2000). Incidence of and risk factors for hallucinations and delusions in patients with probable AD. *Neurology, 54,* 1965–1971.

Ray, W., Chung, C., Murray, K., Hall, K., & Stein, M. (2009). Atypical antipsychotic drugs and the risk of sudden cardiac death. *New England Journal of Medicine, 360,* 225–235.

Reeves, R., & Brister, J. (2008). Psychosis in late life: Emerging issues. *Journal of Psychosocial Nursing, 46*(11), 45–52.

Rovner, B., German, P., Broadhead, J., Moriss, R., Brant, L., Blaustein, J., et al. (1990). The prevalence and management of dementia and other psychiatric disorders in nursing homes. *International Psychogeriatrics, 2,* 13–24.

Schlechter, A. (2008). Capacity assessment and intervention in a 56 year old man with schizophrenia. *Mount Sinai Journal of Medicine, 75,* 153–155.

Schultze, S., Miller, D., Oliver, S., Arndt, S., Flaum, M., & Andreasen, N. (1997). The life course of schizophrenia: Age and symptom dimensions. *Schizophrenia Research, 23,* 15–23.

Schulze, B., & Angermeyer, M. C. (2003). Subjective experiences of stigma. A focus group study of schizophrenic patients, their relatives and mental health professionals [Electronic version]. *Social Science & Medicine, 56,* 299–312.

Schwartz, R. C., Reynold, C. A., Austin, J. F., & Petersen, S. (2003). Homicidality in schizophrenia: A replication study. *American Journal of Orthopsychiatry, 73,* 74–77.

Shiraishi, Y., Terao, T., Ibi, K., Nakamura, J., & Tawara, A. (2004). The rarity of Charles Bonnet syndrome. *Journal of Psychiatric Research, 38,* 207–213.

Sigstrom, S., Skoog, I., Sacuiu, S., Karlsson, B., Klenfeldt, I., Waern, M., et al. (2009). The prevalence of psychotic symptoms and paranoid ideation in non-demented population samples aged 70-82 years. *International Journal of Geriatric Psychiatry, 24*(12), 1413–1419.

Simpson, G. M., & Angus, J. W. (1970). A rating scale for extrapyramidal side effects. *Acta Psychiatrica Scandanavica, 212,* 11–18.

Smith, G. (2003). Patterns and predictors of service use and unmet needs among aging families of adults with severe mental illness. *Psychiatric Services, 54,* 871–877.

Soares, J., & Gershon, S. (1997). Therapeutic targets in late-life psychoses: A review of concepts and critical issues. *Schizophrenia Research, 27,* 227–239.

Srebnik, D., Russo, J., Sage, J., Peto, T., & Zick, E. (2003). Interest in psychiatric advance directives among high users of crisis services and hospitalization [Electronic version]. *Psychiatric Services, 52,* 981–986.

Stuart, G., & Laraia, M. (2005). *Principles and practice of psychiatric nursing* (8th ed.). St. Louis, MO: Mosby.

Thompson, K. (2003). Stigma and public health policy for schizophrenia [Electronic version]. *Psychiatric Clinics of North America, 26,* 273–294.

Thorpe, L. (1997). The treatment of psychotic disorders in late life. *Canadian Journal of Psychiatry, 42*(Suppl. 1), 19s–27s.

Tune, L., & Salzman, C. (2003). Schizophrenia in late life [Electronic version]. *Psychiatric Clinics of North America, 26,* 103–113.

Weiden, P., Preskorn, S., Fahnestock, P., Carpenter, D., Ross, R., & Docherty, J. (2007). Translating the psychopharmacology of antipsychotics to individualized treatment for severe mental illness: A roadmap. *The Journal of Clinical Psychiatry, 68*(Suppl. 7), 6–46.

Yanos, P., Roe, D., Markus, K., & Lysaker, P. (2008). Pathways between internalized stigma and outcomes related to recovery in schizophrenia spectrum disorders. *Psychiatric Services, 59,* 1437–1442.

Yesavage, J., Brink, T., Rose, T., Lum, O., Huang, V., Adey, M., et al. (1982–83). Development and validation of a geriatric depression screening scale. *Journal of Psychiatric Research, 17*(1), 37–49.

Zygmunt, A., Olfson, M., Boyer, C., & Mechanic, D. (2002). Interventions to improve medication adherence in schizophrenia [Electronic version]. *American Journal of Psychiatry, 159,* 1653–1664.

10

Substance Abuse in Older Adults

Betty D. Morgan
Donna M. White
Ann X. Wallace

Despite recent research, the extent of substance abuse in older adults in the United States is not clearly known. Studies have shown that substance abuse occurs often in this population. Alcohol is the most commonly abused drug, but abuse of marijuana and prescribed medications, such as opioids and sedatives, also occurs (Fingerhood, 2000). Misdiagnosis is common, caused in part by complicated medical and psychosocial issues that are problematic in older adults.

This chapter provides information on what is known about substance abuse in older adults, definition of terms, commonly used drugs, and a review of the literature on substance abuse in the older adult population. Information about assessment and screening tools that are appropriate for use in an older adult population is also included. Interviewing techniques and substance abuse treatment guidelines, along with special issues related to overall health care for older adults, is provided. Finally, caregiver stress is addressed as it relates to family involvement with older adult substance abusers and as it relates to healthcare professionals caring for this population.

PREVALENCE OF SUBSTANCE ABUSE IN OLDER ADULTS

Since 1990, the National Survey on Drug Use and Health (formerly the National Household Survey on Drug Abuse), sponsored by the Substance Abuse and Mental Health Services Administration (SAMHSA), has conducted an annual survey of people in the United States over the age of 12 who are noninstitutionalized civilians. The 2007 survey included 2426 adults age 65 or older (SAMHSA, 2007). However, the age categories in relation to specific substance abuse provide little explanation of older adult substance abuse, because the categories used most frequently were ages 12 to 17, 18 to 25, and 26 years and older. Two tables in the survey provide some detail on substance abuse in the age 65 and older category: 10.7% of the sample reported lifetime illicit drug use, 1% reported illicit drug use in the past year, and 0.7% reported illicit drug use in the past month. Of those age 65 or older, 38.1% indicated some alcohol use in the past month, 7.6% indicated binge alcohol use in the past month, and 1.4% heavy alcohol use in the past month.

Using 1999 data, SAMHSA researchers attempted to project the number of substance abusers in 2020 among older adults, using current prevalence rates and population projections. This projection estimated that in the population of persons aged 50 and older, the number of those who are alcohol or drug dependent will increase from 500,000 to 700,000 by the year 2020. The number of those who use illicit drugs or drink heavily is also expected to increase during this time period, from 930,000 to 1.1 million.

These projections present several potential problems. There is no universally held definition of substance abuse, there is misdiagnosis and lack of reporting of substance abuse problems, and there is a lack of information on recovery or death caused by substance use or misuse. Perhaps most importantly, there is an expected increase in substance abuse in older adults because of the aging of the "baby boom" generation (those born between 1946 and 1964), who in their adolescence and early adulthood experimented and used substances in greater numbers than previous generations (SAMHSA, 2007).

The lack of clarity about the magnitude of the problem of substance abuse in older adults continues to be a public health issue. When money for public health issues is low and other illnesses have higher prevalence rates, this lack of detailed information about elder substance abuse results in fewer dollars for treatment or research.

DEFINITIONS

Substance Abuse

The terms "substance abuse" or "chemical dependency" are defined as "the use of a substance or substances in an uncontrolled, compulsive, and potentially harmful manner" (Savage, 1993, p. 265). Criteria for diagnosis of substance abuse include a maladaptive pattern of use of a substance during a 12-month period that results in impairment indicated by at least one of the following: (1) lack of fulfillment of role obligations, such as job, school, or home; (2) risk of physical danger because of use, such as use while operating machinery or a car; (3) legal problems; and (4) ongoing interpersonal problems as a result of or exacerbated by use of a substance (American Psychiatric Association [APA], 2000).

Dependency

Dependency can be physical and psychological. "Physical dependency" refers to the development of a withdrawal syndrome following abrupt cessation of a drug (Savage, 1993). Physical dependence may be accompanied by tolerance to the substance, which is a pharmacological property of opioid drugs and occurs when increased dosage is required to sustain the same effects of the drug (APA, 2000). Criteria for the diagnosis of substance dependence include a maladaptive pattern of use over a 12-month period that results in (1) tolerance; (2) a withdrawal syndrome or use of a related substance to avoid withdrawal; (3) use of larger amounts of the substance or for a longer period of time than was planned; (4) attempts to cut down or control use; (5) spending a lot of time obtaining, using, or recovering from the substance; (6) change in social, occupational, or recreational activities because of substance use; and (7) continued use despite physical and psychological problems (APA).

Addiction

Addiction is characterized by the psychological dependence and "preoccupation with obtaining or using a substance, loss of control over the use of the substance, and continued use despite adverse consequences" (Savage, 1993, p. 266). The American Society of Pain Management Nurses defines addiction based on definitions by the American Academy of Pain Management, American Pain Society, and the American Society of Addiction Medicine as "A primary, chronic, neurobiological disease with genetic, psychosocial, and environmental factors influencing its development and manifestations. It is characterized by behaviors that include one or more of the following: impaired control over drug use, compulsive use, continued use despite harm and craving" (American Society of Pain Management Nurses, 2003, p. 1).

COMORBID CONDITIONS

The National Institute on Drug Abuse (NIDA) estimates that 6 out of 10 people with a substance abuse problem also have other mental health problems. Stress and trauma, including physical and sexual abuse, are some of the common issues that can increase the risk of developing mental illness or substance abuse. Patients with mood disorders or anxiety disorders are twice as likely to have a substance abuse problem and vice versa, and present with more severe symptoms of both disorders (National Institute on Drug Abuse, 2009a).

DRUGS OF ABUSE

Alcohol

In terms of numbers affected and costs to society, alcohol abuse is the number one problem in North America. Ethanol, the chemical name for alcohol, is metabolized primarily in the liver and in the stomach. Alcohol affects the central nervous system and initially acts as an anxiolytic; cognitive and motor skills are affected as alcohol concentrations increase. "Cellular damage and loss of brain tissue have been documented as a result of alcohol use" (Armstrong, 2008, p. 317). People can experience anxiety, psychoses, depression, paranoia, or auditory hallucinations following ingestion of alcohol. Most show a clearing of the clouded consciousness within hours, but those with previous serious alcohol abuse, brain damage or trauma, and some older adults may remain confused for days or weeks (Armstrong).

Cannabis or Marijuana

Cannabis is the most commonly used illicit drug in the United States. The active ingredient,

tetrahydrocannabinol, produces a calm, mildly euphoric state that may be accompanied by heightened sensations, distorted time perception, psychomotor retardation, and increased appetite. Marijuana is made from the leaves and flowers of the cannabis plant and is usually smoked. Data about the long-term effects of marijuana use are conflicting, with development of pulmonary problems as the clearest consequence of prolonged use and possible effects on memory, attention, and information processing (Armstrong, 2008). Marijuana is often used with other drugs to extend or potentiate a high, prevent a crash, or lessen the anxiety associated with cocaine or other stimulants (D'Avonso, 2001).

Stimulants

This category includes amphetamines (Benzedrine), dextroamphetamines (Dexedrine), cocaine, methamphetamines (Desoxyn), and methylphenidates (Ritalin). Amphetamines were used in the 1950s and 1960s for depression, fatigue, weight problems, and as bronchodilators (D'Avonzo, 2001). Today they are used in the treatment of narcolepsy, attention deficit disorder, and attention-deficit hyperactivity disorder (D'Avonzo). Stimulants are also used to treat depression in the medically ill, particularly geriatric patients and people with HIV/AIDS (Keltner & Folks, 2001).

Stimulant drugs are used illicitly by the oral, intranasal, or intravenous routes. Stimulants produce heightened sensations including feelings of euphoria, increased energy, and decreased social inhibitions. Pleasurable activities, such as sex, seem more intense and are often accompanied by increased feelings of mastery, power, and self-confidence. Impairment in decision making and psychotic reactions can occur that can lead to hostile and violent behavior, especially when combined with alcohol (D'Avonzo, 2001).

Cocaine was introduced as an anesthetic in 1858. Cocaine is extracted from the coca plant and is available in several forms: white powder for intranasal use (snorting), dissolved and injected intravenously, smoked, or freebased in the form of "crack" (rocks of cocaine base). Freebasing involves removal of the water-soluble adulterants from the cocaine, producing a purified substance more palatable for smoking that also has better absorption and produces euphoria within seconds (Kosten & Sofuoglu, 2004). Cocaine can also be used orally in any of these forms. Intravenous, smoking, or freebasing provides an immediate high or rush.

Prescription Drugs

Adults older than 65 years of age consume more prescription medications than any other age group. Prescription drug misuse or abuse among older adults usually involves benzodiazepines and other sedative hypnotics. Benzodiazepines represent 17–23% of drugs prescribed to older adults (Center for Substance Abuse Treatment [CSAT], SAMHSA, 1998). Benzodiazepine use in older adults is correlated with female gender, increased number of drugs used, college education, white ethnicity, and a history of depression (Finlayson, 1995; Lisanti & Gomberg, 2004).

Sedatives and Hypnotics

Many of the drugs in this class are commonly prescribed drugs that are used for a variety of medical problems. Barbiturates (Seconal, Nembutal, Amytal, Tuinal, and Phenobarbital), barbiturate-like drugs (Quaaludes), and benzodiazepines (Valium, Librium, Xanax, Klonopin, Halcion, and Ativan) are all widely abused drugs (D'Avonzo, 2001). Barbiturates are used in headache preparations (Fiorinal, Fiorocet) and as anticonvulsants. Benzodiazepines are used to treat anxiety, panic disorders, and sleep disorders and are indicated as muscle relaxants and anticonvulsants. They cause significant central nervous system depression and reduced anxiety, a loss of inhibition, drowsiness, emotional instability, ataxia, and decreased aggressiveness; on occasion they cause a paradoxical effect of increased aggression, memory loss, and lowered seizure threshold. In high

doses, benzodiazepines can disturb sleep patterns and cause changes in mood or affect (Armstrong, 2008). Barbiturates can be lethal if taken in an overdose and, like benzodiazepines, produce physical and psychological dependence that has a severe, life-threatening withdrawal syndrome (D'Avonzo, 2001).

This group of drugs produces effects similar to alcohol and other sedative hypnotics. The withdrawal syndrome associated with sedative hypnotics is also consistent with the signs and symptoms seen in alcohol withdrawal. In particular, withdrawal from benzodiazepines produces autonomic and anxiety rebound, sensory excitement, and motor and cognitive excitation. These symptoms can be dependent on the amount of the drug ingested and duration of time used. Withdrawal from benzodiazepines is lengthy, and rapid withdrawal can cause seizures (Armstrong, 2008).

Opioids

Opioid refers to opiates and their derivatives, both natural and synthetic. This class of drugs includes legal and illicit drugs. Natural opiates include opium and morphine. Heroin is a semisynthetic narcotic and is an illicit drug in the United States. Synthetic opioids include such drugs as codeine sulfate, propoxyphene, meperidine, hydromorphone, fentanyl, dolophine, oxycodone, and morphine sulfate contin; these drugs are illegal except by prescription. Many of these drugs have short- and long-acting formulations. They can be taken orally, smoked, snorted, injected into soft tissue (skin-popping), or used intravenously (Armstrong, 2008).

These drugs have both sedative hypnotic and analgesic effects. They can produce physical and psychological dependence. Use of these substances by older adults is often related to the management of chronic pain. Two to three percent of older adults use opioids by prescription. Opioids are ranked second only to benzodiazepines among abused prescription drugs in the older adult population and represent the second most commonly cited reason for admission for chemical dependence treatment by adults age 55 and older (SAMHSA, 2007). Aside from the legitimate use of opioids for pain, these drugs can be abused by people seeking the euphoric mood that may result from their use or abuse. Other common effects are relaxation, drowsiness ("nodding"), and sleep.

Nicotine

Nicotine is one of 4000 chemicals found in the smoke from tobacco in cigarettes, cigars, and pipes and is the component of tobacco that acts on the brain (NIDA, 2003). It is a highly addictive substance, and most smokers use tobacco regularly because of addiction to nicotine. The use of tobacco products and smoking tobacco continues to be a primary healthcare concern in the United States. This is a lifelong issue, and prevention means cessation of tobacco use in a younger age group. All the major causes of death among older adults are associated with smoking or secondhand smoke (cancer, heart disease, and stroke). Each of these diseases may be associated with months and years of disabling pain and suffering. Research has shown that smoking cessation results in improvement in health status at any age, including those aged 65 and older. Some health benefits are almost immediate, and the longer one refrains from smoking, the more health improves (Center for Social Gerontology, 2001).

Caffeine

Although caffeine is abused or misused by all age groups, caffeine abuse is not considered substance abuse for the sake of this chapter. Caffeine misuse or overuse may have an effect on the physical condition of older adults, but it does not result in the same negative consequences encompassing all spheres of life as the other substances described in this section.

Other Substances of Abuse

Hallucinogens, inhalants, anabolic steroids, and laxatives are abused in other age groups. Currently, there are few data describing use of these drugs in older adults. However, as the baby boom generation

ages, there may be increased abuse of these substances and more data may become available.

REVIEW OF THE LITERATURE

Research related to substance abuse in older adults has been developed in several areas: (1) definition and prevalence of the problem in the elder population, (2) identification of risk factors associated with substance abuse in elders, (3) morbidity and mortality rates with substance abuse in elders, (4) assessment and screening issues particular to the elder population, and (5) development of new techniques for treatment of substance abuse in elders (Fingerhood, 2000). Additionally, several studies have examined the issue of substance abuse in older women (CASA Report, 1998; Eliason, 2001; Fingeld-Connett, 2004).

Most of the literature and research in the area of substance abuse in the older population has focused on the abuse of alcohol; therefore, the main focus of this chapter is on alcohol abuse and treatment. With the aging of the baby boomer cohort, studies looking at the abuse of other substances, alcohol, and polysubstance abuse need to be undertaken. Although a thorough review of the literature is beyond the scope of this chapter, several research studies are highlighted.

SCREENING TOOLS FOR IDENTIFICATION OF SUBSTANCE ABUSE IN THE OLDER ADULT

There are a number of problems related to identifying substance abuse in the older adult. The use of screening instruments cannot be routinely generalized to older adults who have variant life issues and consequences from drug use and abuse. Most of the literature relies on measures of alcohol and its impact. Other screening tools have been adjusted for applicability for the elderly individual. Although it is generally believed that the patient history and medical record provide a clear picture of substance use, too often patterns of use are overlooked by healthcare professionals or well-intended family members. Interviews and history taking are subject to inaccurate history of substance use and possible signs of dementia. Finlayson, Hurt, Davis, and Morse (1988) found that self-report methods are unreliable because of the aging person's memory deficits. The following are the primary screening tools used when assessing the older adult for potential substance abuse and related life issues.

CAGE Questionnaire

The CAGE questionnaire was developed in the early 1970s by Ewing (1984) of the University of North Carolina at Chapel Hill. It is considered one of the most reliable and nonincriminating sets of questions to gauge an individual's use of a substance, primarily alcohol, and life effects. It consists of four questions that indicate covert problem drinking. It meets the requirements for brevity, ease of administration, sensitivity, and validity (Mayfield, McLeod, & Hall, 1973). It is a screening technique that has become the gold standard for rapid assessment and usability. Because it has only four questions, it has long been considered the best screening tool for assessment of potential substance use and abuse.

Use of the tool, however reliable, continues to limit the scope of potential consequences of an older adult with an entrenched denial system. It offers a window through which a clinician can view the older adult's life concerns, but can also shortsight the person's life consequences that relate to drug use and drinking patterns, loneliness, isolation, loss of family and friends, and health destruction. Another drawback to this tool is that the primary focus is on alcohol. Prescription drugs are not included as part of the screen, although this area of substance use and dependence can be significant for the older adult. Clinicians have attempted to make the tool more comprehensive by adapting the tool by replacing the word "alcohol" with the word "drugs" when asking the questions.

Fingerhood (2000, p. 987) suggests additional questions be asked before the use of the CAGE questionnaire. He advocates the use of general assessment questions in an open-ended frame,

and that one integrates alcohol use inquiry into the interview so that it follows inquiry about less sensitive habits ("We have talked about your usual diet and your smoking. Can you tell me how you use alcoholic beverages?"). For patients who report present or past use of alcohol, screen for evidence of alcoholism; ask "Has your use of alcohol caused any kinds of problems for you?" or "Have you ever been concerned about your drinking?" By the use of these two lead questions, the nurse is now poised to use the CAGE questionnaire, which can build on the information already provided: (1) "Have you ever felt you should **C**ut down on your drinking?; (2) Have people **A**nnoyed you by criticizing your drinking?; (3) Have you ever felt bad or **G**uilty about your drinking?; and (4) Have you ever had an **E**ye opener (drink) first thing in the morning, to steady your nerves?" (Ewing, 1984, p. 1906).

In general, a score of two or more in response to these four questions is considered a positive response and requires further assessment for substance use. A score of one or more on a CAGE questionnaire has a sensitivity and specificity of about 80% in adults older than 60 years and is considered a positive screen for substance use and potential abuse requiring further assessment (Dekker, 2002). A CAGE-T, which has a question that involves trauma ("Have you ever been injured after drinking?") may increase sensitivity in equivocal CAGE screenings of older adults. It is also considered less effective for screening of female problem drinkers.

Michigan Alcoholism Screening Test—Geriatric

The Geriatric Michigan Alcoholism Screening Test (MAST-G) is an adaptation of the original MAST series of 24 questions developed at the University of Michigan (Blow, Schulenber, Demo-Dananburg, Young & Beresford, 1992). Respondents provide a yes or no answer to the questions. Five or more yes answers are considered a positive response to the screening tool and require further assessment for alcohol use or dependence. The sensitivity is 91–93% with a specificity of 65–84% (Blow et al.). The list that follows is the MAST-G series of questions:

1. After drinking, have you ever noticed an increase in your heart rate or beating in your chest?
2. When talking with others, do you ever underestimate how much you actually drink?
3. Does alcohol make you sleepy so often that you fall asleep in your chair?
4. After a few drinks, have you sometimes not eaten or been able to skip a meal because you didn't feel hungry?
5. Does having a few drinks help decrease your shakiness or tremors?
6. Does alcohol sometimes make it hard for you to remember parts of the day or night?
7. Do you have rules for yourself that you won't drink before a certain time of the day?
8. Have you lost interest in hobbies or activities you used to enjoy?
9. When you wake up in the morning, do you ever have trouble remembering part of the night before?
10. Does having a drink help you sleep?
11. Do you hide your alcohol bottles from family members?
12. After a social gathering, have you ever felt embarrassed because you drank too much?
13. Have you ever been concerned that drinking might be harmful to your health?
14. Do you like to end an evening with a nightcap?
15. Did you find your drinking increased after someone close to you died?
16. In general, would you prefer to have a few drinks at home rather than go out to social events?
17. Are you drinking more now than in the past?
18. Do you usually take a drink to relax or calm your nerves?
19. Do you drink to take your mind off your problems?
20. Have you ever increased your drinking after experiencing a loss in your life?
21. Do you sometimes drive when you have had too much to drink?
22. Has a doctor or nurse ever said he or she was worried or concerned about your drinking?
23. Have you ever made rules to manage your drinking?
24. When you feel lonely, does having a drink help?

A shortened version of the MAST-G encompasses a series of 10 selected questions from the full MAST-G. Questions number 2, 4, 5, 6, 18, 19, 20, 22, 23, and 24 comprise the shortened version of the MAST-G. A scoring of two or more yes responses is indicative of an alcohol problem and requires further detailed assessment. The primary focus of this screening tool is alcohol; prescription (medication) drug abuse is not addressed in the screen.

Impressions of Medication, Alcohol, and Drug Use in Seniors

This tool was developed by Gerald Shulman (2003), a noted addiction specialist in the field of elderly substance abuse, to address the limitations of the CAGE and MAST-G. This tool screens for problems with alcohol, prescription drugs, and over-the-counter medication and has a specific aim to reduce feelings of shame in the older adult being evaluated (Box 10-1). Three or more positive answers indicate the need for further assessment.

Screening for substance abuse is a recommended part of a regular examination. Screening should also be considered if the older adult is going through a life transition, such as retirement, taking on a caregiver role, or the death of a spouse (CSAT, 1998). Physical signs that should prompt screening include sleep complaints, memory issues, depression, anxiety, and persistent irritability. Unexplained physical complaints, gait disturbance, frequent falls, bruising, and neglect of hygiene have all been identified as clues to substance abuse in the older adult. Substance abuse should be considered in the older adult who presents as noncompliant

BOX 10-1 IMPRESSIONS OF MEDICATION, ALCOHOL, AND DRUG USE IN OLDER ADULTS

1. Does your use of medication or alcohol make you feel so sleepy that you fall asleep in your chair?

2. Do you find yourself using alcohol to help you sleep?

3. Have you occasionally spent more time drinking or using other drugs than you intended?

4. Have you found yourself thinking a lot about taking your medication or drinking?

5. Do your social and recreational activities often involve drinking?

6. Have you given up activities because they did not involve drinking?

7. Does using medication or alcohol sometimes make it difficult for you to remember what you said or did?

8. Have you ever neglected doing something you should have done because of medications or drinking?

9. Have you ever used medication or alcohol to relieve emotional discomfort, such as sadness, anger, loneliness, or boredom?

10. Have you ever felt you needed medication or alcohol just to keep going?

11. Have you ever told anyone that you drank less than you actually did?

12. In the past 12 months, have you at any time used more medications or drunk more alcohol than you meant to?

13. Have you ever had an injury while drinking that required medical attention?

14. Have you used alcohol with prescribed or over-the-counter medications even after being instructed not to do so?

15. Have you ever found yourself short of money because of what you spent on alcohol?

16. Did your drinking change or increase after some event such as death of a loved one or retirement?

17. Has a relative, or friend, or doctor ever suggested changing the way you use your medications or cutting down on your drinking?

18. Have you ever felt that your medication use or drinking was a problem?

19. Do you ever wonder whether the use of medication or alcohol may be bad for your health, finances, or independence?

20. Has anyone (family, friends, or doctor) raised questions about or objected to your use of medications or alcohol?

Source: Shulman, G. (2003). Senior moments: Assessing older adults. *Addiction Today, 15*(82), 7–19. Reprinted with permission.

or with one or more refractory medical conditions (American Geriatrics Society, 2003; CSAT; Widlitz & Marin, 2002).

If the screening is negative, then healthy lifestyle choices can be reinforced including the guidelines for age-appropriate alcohol consumption. For adults older than 65 years of age, no more than one drink per day and a maximum of two drinks on any drinking occasion is recommended. The limits for women should be somewhat lower.

In selected individuals with multiple comorbidities and medications, abstinence may be the most appropriate recommendation (CSAT, 1998; National Institute on Alcohol Abuse and Alcoholism [NIAAA], 2008).

If the screening is positive, then further assessment is warranted. Determination of the need for treatment and the appropriate setting is critical. The least intensive treatment is recommended (CSAT, 1998).

▍CASE STUDY

Mrs. C. is a 69-year-old white woman who has had a recent fall in her home. Her daughter brings her in to see her primary care provider, where you work as a registered nurse. As you are getting Mrs. C. ready to see the nurse practitioner in the office, you notice several bruises on her arms and legs that do not look like the result of the recent fall. You find out that the daughter (who lives out of state) has been visiting her mother once a month for the 4 months since Mrs. C.'s husband died. How would you proceed with your discussion with Mrs. C.? How would you proceed with the daughter?

Use of the CAGE or one of the other screening tools described may or may not result in an acknowledgment of problem drinking. A discussion about the bruising and concern you have about the bruises can be brought up in a nonjudgmental way before and during the examination by the nurse practitioner. Questions about whether or not there is someone who is hurting Mrs. C. could rule out the possibility of physical abuse. Other issues to include in the evaluation that would heighten the concern about alcohol use are family history of alcohol or other drug use, recent losses, cognitive changes, irritability, anxiety or depression, change in eating and sleeping habits, increased isolation, and medical issues as described later in this chapter. Expressing concern and possible reasons for the falls may allow the daughter to provide some additional information. Raising the issue of alcohol or other drug use as a possible cause of the falls and bruises simply introduces the topic and may raise the daughter's awareness of a potential problem. Offering home healthcare nursing evaluation might be an intervention helpful for further assessment and assistance to Mrs. C.

▍ALCOHOL ABUSE AND THE OLDER ADULT

In a study as far back as 1982, Brody asserted that about 10–15% of elderly patients seeking medical help for any reason has an alcohol-related problem. The older adult who is using or abusing substances in any form poses a difficult challenge for geropsychiatric nurses. Only recently have primary care providers begun to look at this emerging crisis. A review of current literature and methodology to examine this topic reflects a paucity of information. The underidentification of drug use in this particular age group is in response to many variables and societal attitudes.

Discussion and review of the problem require a frank conversation among healthcare providers at the national public policy level, the academic setting, and the clinical level.

Too often, attitudinal stereotyping of aging can influence a healthcare provider from assessing an aging person. The older adult can present a wide range of responses to questions about use of alcohol or other chemicals and too often the abuse potential can be overlooked. In addition, standardized screening tools do not differentiate between early and late-onset elderly alcohol abuse, making treatment of this population more difficult. Close observation that comprehensively assesses the person's needs and issues identifies symptoms that may be subclinical or attributed to a comorbid diagnosis or another etiology.

Fingerhood (2000) describes older adults with two categories of alcoholism: early onset and late onset. In early onset alcohol abuse, the individual had alcoholism present earlier in life. According to studies (Adams & Waskel, 1991; Atkinson, Tolson, & Turner, 1990), two thirds of older alcohol abusers fall into the early onset group. This group is more likely to drink to intoxication; more likely to have been in alcohol treatment in the past; more likely to have legal, financial, or occupational problems; and less likely to have social supports. Often they are undiagnosed or have been diagnosed with substance abuse in various forms, but their long-standing substance use has been treated without success. In addition, untreated substance use in their lifetime may induce a chronic state of health problems with impaired cognition.

Late-onset alcohol abuse occurs after the age of 60. This group is more likely to enter treatment as a result of a crisis (e.g., driving under the influence), more likely to report feelings of depression or loneliness, more likely to deny an alcohol problem, and more likely to have identifiable supportive family or friends (Adams & Waskel, 1991; Atkinson et al., 1990; Fingerhood, 2000). Shulman (2003) states that those individuals who develop late-onset alcoholism generally do so in response to the stress of aging. He defines situations that

increase the likelihood of late-onset alcoholism as the following (p. 18):

- Retirement with the loss of structure, support, and self-esteem provided by employment
- Loneliness and isolation that may be a result of widowhood
- Loss of sensory capabilities and/or reduced mobility exacerbating isolation and loneliness
- Geographical and emotional separation from family and friends with resultant loss of social and emotional support
- Reactive depression
- Combined use of multiple prescribed medications, over-the-counter drugs, and drinking, even in modest amounts
- Increased financial and health problems or concerns about these problems and the individual's ability to remain independent.
- Reduced ability of the aging body to handle alcohol

Older adults should be screened annually for alcohol use and any other time that a major life transition has occurred.

GENDER ISSUES, ALCOHOL, AND THE OLDER ADULT

Women make up a larger percentage of the older population and outnumber men in all decades after the age of 60 (U.S. Bureau of the Census, 2000). More often women fall into the late-onset category of alcohol abuse and are often widowed, lonely, and isolated, with depressive symptomatology. Additionally, women are more vulnerable to the negative effects of alcohol with less alcohol intake than men (Stevenson, 2005). Women are not likely to seek treatment or be identified as being in need of treatment. However, when identified and referred for alcohol treatment, women have been shown to have long-term positive outcomes (Schutte, Byrne, Brennan, & Moos, 2001).

As women age, drug metabolism slows down, and changes in body mass and water content tend to enhance the effects of medications, such as benzodiazepines and alcohol. Less of the drug or alcohol is needed and the effects last longer. This can result in drug or alcohol dependence, although it may not be at all apparent to the person, family, or providers of care (Fingeld-Connett, 2004). This can result in withdrawal symptoms if use is stopped abruptly.

Stevenson (2005) commented that because it is known that women experience more biological damage with shorter drinking histories and less drinks per drinking episode than men, the recommendations for safe levels of alcohol for women are half those for men in young and middle adulthood (NIAAA, 2008). The recommendations for older adults are the same for both men and women, and it is believed that older men become as sensitive to alcohol as women as they age. The NIAAA has recommended no more than one drink per day for older adults, with a maximum of two drinks on any drinking occasion, such as New Years Eve, with somewhat lower limits for women.

HEALTH ASSESSMENT

Historically, substance abuse in older adults has been an underdiagnosed and undertreated problem. Not unlike many other disorders seen in the older adult population, the presentation of substance abuse is often nonspecific and atypical in nature. It can easily be mistaken for other geriatric illnesses or aging changes (DeHart & Hoffman, 1995; Gambert & Albrecht, 2005; Lichtenberg, Gibbons, Nanna, & Blumenthal, 1993; Solomon, Manepalli, Ireland, & Mahon, 1993). Symptoms of substance abuse may appear as psychiatric or physical disorders. Assumptions regarding the prevalence of abuse, and the potential for recovery among older adults, may interfere with the provider's ability to correctly assess and plan for these individuals. Contrary to these assumptions, elders have a 75% recovery rate, the highest of any age group (CSAT, 1998).

The use of health assessment and review of standard laboratory tests supplement standardized screens. Health assessment, performed by a skilled clinician–practitioner, can elicit much information regarding use of substances, even before review of laboratory data and clinical indices. A review of systems approach offers a comprehensive view of overall health and the interplay of substances within the person's life patterns. In addition, a biopsychosocial review of the individual's life can illuminate substance use as it interfaces with the maturational changes of the aging adult. Very often, a person can have decades of substance use or abuse that can be confounded by the clinical presentation of dementia. In this case, it may be helpful to use a combination of tests and screening tools to make a more accurate clinical diagnosis. The geropsychiatric nurse is able to obtain an accurate assessment of the older adult with substance abuse, and complicated maturational issues may be defined. Nurses can play a "vital role in identifying the range of alcohol-related problems" (Eliason, 1998, p. 23) in the older adults with whom they work.

Masters (2003) asserts that "the increases in affluence, education, and life expectancy achieved in the twentieth century have produced an aging population that has not only increased in numbers but also has more leisure time and disposable income, a more positive attitude toward alcohol, and higher rates of alcohol consumption than in previous generations" (p. 155). She further states that "longer life expectancy is associated with greater exposure to health risks and a concomitant increase in chronic disease and polypharmacy" (p. 155). Thus, a specific screening instrument for the older adult, combined with structured health assessment questions, elicits the broadest base of information on which to base a comprehensive plan of care.

Strategies that may assist geropsychiatric nurses in assessment of this unique population include (1) health assessment techniques and tools geared toward the older adult, (2) strong knowledge base of alcohol and other substances and the physiological effects on the older adult, (3) routine use of geriatric standardized screening tools to examine for substance use or abuse in this population,

(4) cultural awareness of substance use or abuse within a family or culture, (5) team approach for all providers to address the older adult's use of a substance, (6) humane planning for substance abuse education and treatment, and (7) awareness of substance abuse programs that use a geriatric track or case manager skilled in the care of this particular population.

MEDICATION ASSESSMENT

A key role in geropsychiatric clinical nursing practice is the assessment of prescribed medications and active or suspected concomitant use of alcohol by the older adult. It is important to understand how the older adult conceptually values his or her prescribed medication. The individual's use of medication and understanding of the therapeutic effect can provide a clue as to the potential for substance use and misuse. A comprehensive review of all over-the-counter and prescription medication is recommended. How the medications are taken can indicate the priority the aging adult places on a particular medication or practice. For example, a person may be unable to obtain antihypertensive medication but may view it as less important than having his prescribed benzodiazepine available, which he uses for a sleep aid. The intended use of the benzodiazepine was as an antianxiety medication, but the older adult begins the practice of self-medication for sleep, leading to misuse of the drug. Development of tolerance to the therapeutic effect can ensue.

In addition, older adults can also believe particular medications assist them in their independence, which they value highly. Use of alcohol may steady their nerves; prescribed narcotics control painful conditions, such as arthritis; mood stabilizers and antidepressants help to battle depression and loneliness; and sleeping pills assist with the common complaint of insomnia. The interplay among these drugs, compounded by the potentiation of additional medications, can wreak havoc in an aging body. In addition, older adults may not fully comprehend the criteria for use of the medication and the clinical reasoning as to why it was prescribed.

MEDICAL CONSEQUENCES OF SUBSTANCE ABUSE

Alcohol is the most commonly abused substance in any age group. Alcohol, or ethanol, is a central nervous system depressant, and is classified as a sedative–hypnotic. At lower doses, the effect is psychologically calming, whereas at higher doses it produces sleep induction. Central nervous system depression is not the only neuronal response. Some neurons, rather than decreasing their rate of firing, actually increase firing. This produces a removal of inhibitory response and may contribute to the disinhibition seen at lower doses, evidenced by excitement and aggression (Grilly, 2002). Alcohol causes a multiplicity of physical and psychological effects. When combined with other central nervous system depressants, alcohol can have a significant synergistic effect. Alcohol is capable of causing physical and psychological dependence. Physically, no body system is unaffected by alcohol, resulting in significant neurological, gastrointestinal, and cardiovascular effects. Psychologically, alcohol affects complex cognitive skills, fine and gross motor skills, visual accommodation, and unconditioned reflexes (Grilly).

Alcohol intake produces slowed mental functions, decreased coordination, slurred speech, ataxia, euphoric or labile mood, and decreased blood pressure and pulse. Withdrawal symptoms usually develop within 6 to 8 hours after cessation of alcohol ingestion. Withdrawal symptoms include increased blood pressure and pulse, nausea, vomiting, anxiety, tremor, and diaphoresis. Severe withdrawal signs and symptoms include hallucinations, seizures, and delirium tremens (Lisanti, 2001; Mayo-Smith, 2009). The severity of withdrawal is highly individualized and can cover a wide range of clinical presentations. Varying opinions exist as to the effect of age on the severity of withdrawal. Kraemer, Mayo-Smith, and Calkins (1997) concluded that age did not significantly change the severity of withdrawal scores when quantitative self-report measures or instruments were used. However, the study cohort, age 60 and older, did demonstrate an increased risk for delirium and functional impairment. Despite these findings, other sources include older age as a risk factor for increased severity of withdrawal. Additional risk factors for severity of withdrawal include past history of alcohol dependence and withdrawal, history of alcohol-related seizures, or delirium tremens (Mayo-Smith).

REVIEW OF SYSTEMS

The assessment includes a careful review of systems, validation of information from family and friends when appropriate, and a complete physical examination and diagnostics. Changes that occur in gastrointestinal, cardiovascular, neurological, renal, musculoskeletal, and hematological systems are of particular significance when assessing the older adult with substance abuse (Edlund & Spain, 2003; Holbert & Tueth, 2004).

Gastrointestinal

Various gastrointestinal disorders are related to the abuse of alcohol. Alcohol is toxic to the gastric mucosa and can subsequently cause stomatitis, esophagitis, gastritis, and exacerbation of gastroesophageal reflux and ulcer disease. These disorders may be further complicated by the concurrent use of aspirin or nonsteroidal anti-inflammatory agents. Alcohol delays gastric emptying and lowers esophageal sphincter tone. The effect of alcohol on the small intestine produces a decrease in the absorption of nutrients, including folic acid and vitamin B_{12}. These effects, coupled with delayed gastric motility, can prompt the use of laxatives that may further interfere with the absorption of nutrients (Katzung, 2001).

In older adults there is a decrease in gastric alcohol dehydrogenase, the enzyme that converts alcohol to acetaldehyde, in the first step of alcohol metabolism. This contributes to higher blood alcohol levels and increases the hepatic burden in older adults. Gastric alcohol dehydrogenase levels are lower for women regardless of age (CSAT, 1998). There is an age-related decrease in hepatic size and blood flow, which can be further affected by alcohol and drug use. This can produce a slowed metabolic rate of certain drugs with an increased risk of toxicity. Older adults also demonstrate a decreased ability to recover from hepatic damage (Beers & Berkow, 2000).

Alcohol-related pancreatitis is usually caused by ingestion of five to six drinks per day for an extended period of time. Clinically, individuals with pancreatitis have upper abdominal pain, nausea, vomiting, weight loss, and diarrhea (Nace, 2005). Biliary tract diseases, such as gallstones and heavy alcohol consumption, are responsible for most cases of acute pancreatitis in the United States (Costello, 2008; Friedman, L., 2009). A return to drinking after a period of abstinence can produce recurrent pancreatitis. Recurrent episodes can lead to chronic pancreatitis.

Effects on the liver include fatty infiltration, hepatitis, and cirrhosis. Alcohol-related liver disease is correlated to the level of alcohol consumption. Additional risk factors include genetic profile, female gender, concomitant viral hepatitis, and duration of drinking history. Fatty infiltration is usually asymptomatic and may be produced by several days of heavy drinking.

Alcoholic hepatitis, an inflammatory process, can produce a presentation similar to gallbladder disease, with hepatomegaly, fever, jaundice, leukocytosis, and pain. Elevations of hepatic enzymes aspartate aminotransferase and alanine aminotransferase, with aspartate aminotransferase higher than alanine aminotransferase, are often part of the clinical presentation of alcohol-induced hepatic disease (Saitz, 2009). Alcohol-induced cirrhosis remains a common cause of morbidity and mortality and is the second most common cause for liver transplantation. Currently, hepatitis C is the primary cause for liver transplantation. Because many of the hepatitis C patients requiring transplantation also have alcohol abuse histories, the full impact of alcohol-induced cirrhosis may be underestimated (Haber & Batey, 2009).

Cirrhosis, a process of fibrosis, can cause portal hypertension, esophageal varices, edema, and ascites. Initial clinical presentation may include anorexia, fatigue, weakness, and weight loss. Jaundice, ascites, and edema are seen later in the course of the disease. Hepatic encephalopathy may develop secondary to an accumulation of toxic substances, including ammonia (Saitz, 2009).

Cardiac

Cardiovascular age-related changes include decreased myocardial contractility and cardiac reserve, vascular resistance, and increased risk of atrial fibrillation and other arrhythmias (Smith & Cotter, 2008). These changes are all exacerbated by alcohol abuse. Alcohol abuse can cause decreased myocardial contractility and left-ventricular ejection fraction, and has cardiac muscle depressant actions that are not fully understood (Friedman, H. S., 2009). Alcohol can also contribute to an increase in blood pressure frequently observed in older adults. Hypertension can persist for days to weeks after acute alcohol withdrawal. This effect is more predominant in white men; however, after menopause the effect intensifies in women (Friedman, H. S.).

In most studies, alcohol, a vasodilator, increases coronary blood flow secondary to increased myocardial oxygen demand. This can worsen myocardial ischemia and is more likely to be seen in the setting of coronary artery disease. Alcohol is related to functional and conduction abnormalities. These abnormalities are seen in cardiomyopathy (Friedman, H.S., 2009). This may produce a clinical presentation of heart failure and arrhythmia with decreased exercise tolerance, tachycardia, dyspnea, edema, palpitations, and cough. Although treatment choices for cardiomyopathy are limited and the course is variable, the cessation of alcohol use can produce an improvement in cardiac function (Friedman, H. S.; Massie & Amidon, 2003). Arrhythmias, particularly including atrial fibrillation, can be seen after episodes of heavy alcohol ingestion. Older adults with a history of cardiac disease are at increased risk.

Neurological

Neurological age-related changes include slowed reaction time, forgetfulness, decreased short-term memory, slowed time for task completion, and altered kinesthetic sense (Beers & Berkow, 2000; Edlund & Spain, 2003). Alcohol and other sedative hypnotics can exacerbate all age-related neurological changes. Intoxication, withdrawal, seizures, and delirium are all neurological effects of alcohol. Alcohol abuse coupled with age-related changes in balance and coordination place the older adult at increased risk for trauma secondary to falls (Brust, 2009).

A common neurological effect of alcohol, particularly long-term drinking, is polyneuropathy. Deficiencies of thiamine and other B vitamins, which may be a toxic effect of alcohol, or nerve compression can cause this neuropathy. This type of neuropathy begins distally, usually noted in the feet before the hands, and progresses proximally. Pain, burning, tingling, and numbness are reported. This may progress to muscle weakness and wasting, producing a foot-drop gait (Brust, 2009; Nace, 2005).

Functional brain changes that result from alcohol include impaired learning and a decrease in concentration, abstract thinking, judgment, short-term memory, and problem solving. These changes contribute to the behavioral manifestations noted with substance abuse. Advancing age is considered a risk factor for dementia related to alcohol (CSAT, 1998; Grilly, 2002). One review discussed the need to understand further the effects of alcohol on Alzheimer's disease, which is the most common cause of dementia. This review suggests that the use of alcohol can worsen the impairments produced by this form of dementia (Wiscott, Kopera-Frye, & Seifert, 2001).

Thiamine deficiency is also responsible for Wernicke's encephalopathy. This condition presents with confusion, ataxia and lateral gaze abnormalities, and nystagmus. The symptoms can develop over days to weeks. Early treatment with intravenous thiamine before glucose administration can produce partial to full recovery (Brust, 2009). However, without early treatment the encephalopathy can develop into Korsakoff's syndrome, an irreversible condition. This condition is primarily one of memory loss and confabulation. Unlike other forms of dementia, memory impairment is the predominant feature with sparing of other cognitive functions (Masters, 2001; Saitz, 2009).

Risk of stroke is also increased with abuse of alcohol. The effect of alcohol on cerebral blood flow is not entirely clear. Ethanol acts as a vasoconstrictor, whereas the metabolite of ethanol, acetate, acts as a vasodilator. Older adults are more sensitive to the vasoconstrictive effects. This sensitivity along with other risk factors for vascular disease increases the risk for ischemic stroke. The increased risk for hemorrhagic stroke is related to the antithrombotic effects of alcohol (Friedman, H. S., 2009).

Renal and Pharmacokinetics

Normal age-related renal changes include decreased renal blood flow producing a reduction in the glomerular filtration rate, measured by creatinine clearance. Excretion of drugs is predominantly a function of renal clearance. As function declines, drugs have a prolonged half-life. Distribution of drugs is affected by the decrease in muscle mass, total body water, and albumin, all of which accompany aging. This results in higher alcohol levels with less alcohol ingested and higher levels of protein-bound drugs (CSAT, 1998; Katsung, 2001). Age-related physiological changes, coupled with the significant consumption of prescription medications and drug interactions with alcohol, produce considerable risk to this population (Culberson, 2006).

Musculoskeletal

Alcohol contributes to decreased bone density, accelerated bone loss, and skeletal muscle atrophy (Edlund & Spain, 2003; Nakahara et al., 2003). These effects in conjunction with the age-related changes of decreased muscle mass and strength and accelerated bone loss contribute to poor mobility and falls. Alcohol abuse can cause acute myopathy (rhabdomyolysis) that presents with pain, tenderness, and edema in proximal muscle groups after excessive ingestion of alcohol. This acute process can elevate creatine phosphokinase, lactic acid dehydrogenase, aspartate aminotransaminase, and myoglobinuria. Acute myopathy can be significant enough to cause myoglobulinemia and acute tubular necrosis. Chronic myopathy is characterized by painless, proximal muscle wasting and weakness that increase the risk of falls (Nace, 2005). Alcohol has also been associated with hyperuricemia, gout, and osteoporosis (Saitz, 2009).

Hematological

Many older adults have chronic illnesses that may put them at increased risk for anemia; however, anemia is not a normal part of aging (Toy, 2004). Anemia in the setting of alcohol abuse can be related to acute or chronic gastrointestinal bleeding and present as iron deficiency anemia or a pancytopenia related to the direct bone marrow toxicity of alcohol. All aspects of cell development are affected by alcohol. Erythropoietin production can be affected by hepatic and pancreatic disease, producing hypoproliferative disorders. Red blood cell maturation and survival are affected by alcohol and the decreased availability of folic acid. Additionally, hypersplenism seen in severe liver disease contributes to red blood cell destruction.

Gastrointestinal bleeding can cause iron deficiency anemia, whereas alcohol-related bone marrow toxicity can cause pancytopenia. Folate and vitamin B_{12} deficiency can cause a macrocytic anemia characterized by a decreased red blood cell count and an elevated mean corpuscular volume (Saitz, 2009). Diagnosis can be challenging if the anemia is related to concurrent etiologies (Nace, 2005; Saitz).

Immune

Frequent serious infections are often seen with alcohol abuse. Various aspects of the immune system are affected by alcohol, including lower polymorphonuclear leukocyte counts, contributing to decreased ability to fight infection. Decreased lymphocytes also contribute to impaired cell-mediated immunity. Alcohol abuse may decrease total white blood cell and platelet counts. The ability of white blood cells to fight infection may also be diminished. The risk of cancer is increased by the abuse of alcohol. Cancers of the esophagus, larynx, oral cavity, and pharynx are among the cancers increased by alcohol abuse. The effects of alcohol and smoking, behaviors that commonly coexist, contribute to oropharyngeal cancers (Dani, Kosten & Benowitz, 2009). Significant increases in liver, stomach, colon, breast, and ovarian cancers are also noted with alcohol abuse (Nace, 2005).

TREATMENT ISSUES

NIDA has set forth principles of drug addiction treatment. Although these principles guide treatment for all ages, the principles are important for treatment of older adults (NIDA, 2009b, pp. 2–5):

- Addiction is a complex but treatable disease that affects brain function and behavior.
- No single treatment is appropriate for everyone.
- Treatment needs to be readily available.
- Effective treatment attends to multiple needs of the individual, not just his or her drug abuse.
- Remaining in treatment for an adequate period of time is critical.
- Counseling (individual or group) and other behavioral therapies are the most commonly used forms of drug abuse treatment.
- Medications are an important element of treatment for many patients, especially when combined with counseling and other behavioral therapies.
- An individual's treatment and services plan must be assessed continually and modified as necessary to ensure that it meets his or her changing needs.
- Many drug-addicted individuals also have other mental disorders.

- Medically assisted detoxification is only the first stage of addiction treatment and by itself does little to change long-term drug abuse.
- Treatment does not need to be voluntary to be effective.
- Drug use during treatment must be monitored continuously, because lapses during treatment do occur.

Treatment programs should assess for the presence of HIV/AIDS, hepatitis B and C, tuberculosis, and other infectious diseases, and provide targeted risk-reduction counseling to help patients modify or change behaviors that place them at risk of contracting or spreading infectious diseases.

TREATMENT PHILOSOPHIES

Most primary care providers are familiar with the acute treatment or detoxification programs and protocols to prevent sudden withdrawal states. As stated in the *Principles of Drug Abuse Treatment* (NIDA, 2009b), medical detoxification is only the beginning step in treatment and does little to alter the more complex behavioral changes needed to occur in long-term cessation of drugs. Despite this clear statement and principle, most of the available treatment in the United States is focused on this first step of treatment with referral to self-help groups, such as Alcoholics Anonymous or Narcotics Anonymous, as the only follow-up on discharge from detoxification units.

Several different philosophies of long-term drug and alcohol treatment exist, and a brief review of the philosophies that have shown evidence of positive outcomes for older adults is provided. Studies have indicated that older adults, both men and women, respond better to programs that are tailored to the older adult, including one-to-one counseling, nonconfrontational approaches, with a slower pace and attention to comorbid medical and psychiatric problems (Atkinson, 1995; Blow, 2000). A supportive model with low level of stimulation in the environment may assist in minimizing any confusion that might be present in older adults. Cognitive–behavioral therapy that addresses negative affect and improves social support may also be helpful (Loukissa, 2007). Relatively little formal research has been conducted comparing the various treatment approaches to addiction in older adults. Oslin, Pettinati, and Volpicelli (2002) reported that older adults are more adherent with treatment as measured by attendance than are younger adults.

Harm reduction is one approach that may be helpful in treating substance abuse in older adults. Harm reduction meets the patient at his or her own level in terms of desire for change in his or her harmful behavior. The techniques used in harm reduction assist in helping the person decrease exposure to risky behaviors, which leads to a healthier lifestyle. Fingeld-Connett (2004) described a brief intervention for older women with substance abuse called A-FRAMES. The model includes assessment, feedback, responsibility, advice, menu, empathy, and self-efficacy. The model was an adaptation of the model developed by Bien, Miller, and Tonigan (1993) and has been shown to be effective in older adults in one study (Fleming, Manwell, Barry, Adams, & Stauffacher, 1999). An example of use of harm reduction is included in the following brief case discussion.

CASE STUDY

Mr. P. is a 74-year-old widower who is very connected with his oldest daughter and her children who live nearby. He had a long history of drug and alcohol use in his younger years but stopped his use totally when his wife threatened to leave him over two decades ago. His wife died a year and a half ago and Mr. P. is fairly isolated, other than his contact with this daughter and her children. He acknowledges that he has had a few drinks since her death, but this is "nothing to worry about." His daughter has been increasingly concerned with his drinking and says that he has fallen several times, and has been obviously "drunk," according to her children who have been very upset by this. He reports that his daughter is concerned about allowing her 15-year-old to continue to visit, and he is distraught by this possibility.

The fact that this is of concern to him makes it an appropriate place to focus an intervention using harm reduction strategy. The first step might include planning how he will not drink on days that the grandchildren or his daughter will visit, so that he may continue his contact with them, therefore decreasing the harm to him of further isolation. Success with this step in treatment may help him plan for future strategies, such as strategies to decrease the falls associated with his drinking. If he is unsuccessful in not drinking on days that the daughter or grandchildren visit, then this information can be used to highlight the fact that he may not be as in control of the drinking as he thought he was, and may be in need of additional treatment.

Specific Alcoholics Anonymous or Narcotics Anonymous meetings for older adults are offered in some senior citizen centers and offer additional support networks and a form of socialization for older adults. This addition of support and socialization, which decreases isolation and loneliness, has been shown to increase significantly the chance for treatment adherence for substance abuse (Barrick & Connors, 2002).

CASE STUDY

Frank is a 67-year-old African-American man who was admitted to the hospital for treatment of osteomyelitis of the left foot with gangrenous ulcerations on the heel. He has a history of hypertension and now is presenting with shortness of breath and wheezing. He previously worked as a truck driver but is now on disability. He was married, but his wife died 2 years ago from cancer of the esophagus. Frank is estranged from his only daughter, who is a nurse. He now lives alone in a small apartment. He has few if any supports in his life, does not drive, receives health care from emergency rooms, and does not regularly seek health care unless severely ill or in need of a prescription refill.

Frank has a long history of alcohol use and dependence. In addition, he has a three-decade use of narcotics and intravenous heroin use and dependence. His initial use of opioids was for pain management after a motor vehicle accident with resultant crushing injuries to both legs 30 years ago. Subsequent surgeries improved mobility and ambulation, but pain management has remained problematic. Throughout these years, increasing amounts of Percocet, Vicodan, and Dilaudid provided limited relief. Seven years ago, Oxycontin was prescribed and pain relief was improved. Frank began supplementing use of opioids with snorting heroin when he was in his early thirties, and he progressed to intravenous heroin as the pain continued. He has continued to drink alcohol and has been in treatment for alcohol dependence four times with minimal sustained sobriety.

Frank does not see his use of narcotics as problematic, but only as needed for pain relief. He also does not view combining medications as problematic. He has been unwilling to address heroin dependence until this admission. Frank fears amputation of his foot because of repeated infections.

He now combines use of alcohol and narcotics throughout the day. The actual amount of alcohol ingested daily fluctuates based on his financial status, but he states he generally consumes 6 to 12 beers per day. Currently, he rates his pain an 8 on a pain scale of 1 to 10 (10 being the worst).

This case presents with the multisystem, complicated medical issues confronting many older adults with substance abuse problems. Lack of a consistent provider, lack of emotional and financial support, and complicated pain and substance abuse lead to the need for a multidisciplinary team approach, which can be initiated by nurses. From a harm reduction point of view, working with Frank around his fear of amputation may assist in development of a therapeutic relationship focused on his needs and concerns. Development of a plan to help him deal with this fear and ways to improve his health can then lead to the role of alcohol and drug abuse in his repeated infections and risk for amputation.

Discussion questions are as follows: (1) Can you identify any areas where you, the nurse, can connect with Frank about his goals, (2) What factors complicate the treatment of Frank's pain, and (3) What other information about Frank's history would be helpful for you in planning for his care?

MEDICATIONS USED IN TREATING ADDICTIVE DISORDERS

Medications are used to detoxify patients from substances. Most primary care providers are familiar with detoxification protocols. Alcohol detoxification is described briefly as it relates to the older adult, because it has life-threatening implications. The rest of the medications described are used in the longer-term treatment of alcoholism and other drugs of abuse. Geriatric and psychiatric nurses should be familiar with these drugs as a foundation for referral to addiction specialty services, and for monitoring drug–drug interactions.

In recent years, the use of pharmacological agents to support abstinence has gained acceptance in both the scientific and recovery community. Traditionally, the model used to support long-term lifestyle changes in a person with an addictive disorder was an abstinence-based approach (Davison, Sweeney, & Bush, 2006).

New research evidence provides the basis for use of a pharmacological strategy to provide neurological stabilization using a variety of medications. An individual seeking recovery may verbalize resistance or ambivalence toward the use of medications as part of their program. It may be related in part to the perpetuated myth that "the use of any medication is contrary to Alcoholics Anonymous (AA) philosophy or just another crutch" (AA Member Medications and Other Drugs, 1984). Although this myth is erroneous, it continues to plague those who seek recovery using a variety of methods. "All approved drugs have been shown to be effective adjuncts to the treatment of alcohol dependence. Thus, consider adding medication whenever you are treating someone with active alcohol dependence or someone who has stopped drinking in the past few months but is experiencing problems such as craving or slips" (NIAAA, 2005, p. 13).

In addition, pharmacological agents are best used in conjunction within an overall program of counseling support, self-help groups, and medical monitoring. Used as part of a comprehensive system to support recovery, medications can specifically assist the person who is experiencing intense craving or a brief return to episodic drinking or drug use, commonly referred to as a "slip." Keeping in mind no one avenue toward recovery is absolute, the following medications provide an adjunctive role to assist and support abstinence and thereby effect a change toward a chemical-free lifestyle.

Medications Used in the Treatment of Alcoholism

Alcohol Detoxification and the Older Adult

Observation and a thorough history and physical examination may lead the nurse to believe that an older adult is at risk for withdrawal from alcohol. Symptoms of minor withdrawal may start as soon as 6 to 12 hours after the last drink and may include nonspecific symptoms, such as tremor, anxiety, nausea, hypervigilance, insomnia, tachycardia, and hypertension. Major withdrawal symptoms begin 10 to 72 hours after the last drink and include vomiting; diaphoresis; and visual, auditory, and tactile hallucinations. Grand mal seizures may occur and a life-threatening situation can ensue. Delirium tremens may occur 24 to 72 hours after the last drink but can occur up to 10 days later. Patients exhibiting signs of delirium tremens appear disoriented and confused, and have tachycardia, hypertension, and hyperthermia (Letizia & Reinbolz, 2005).

Use of rating scales, such as the Clinical Institute Withdrawal Assessment Scale, assists in rating the severity of alcohol-related withdrawal and is helpful in assessing risk for withdrawal and treatment response. Hospitalization may be necessary for safe withdrawal because "detoxification is generally seen as medically riskier for an older adult person" (CSAT, 1998, p. 69). The benzodiazepines are most often used to withdraw people safely from alcohol. The shorter-acting benzodiazepines, such as lorazepam (Ativan) or oxazepam (Serax), are preferred for older adults and doses are adjusted to one half or one third of a dose for a normal adult (Finlayson, 1995).

Long-Term Treatment of Alcohol Abuse

Disulfarim (Antabuse) has been used for treatment of alcoholism for many years. This medication was developed as an aversive technique to promote abstinence from use of alcohol. The principle used with this strategy is that the individual fears the response of their own body to ingestion of alcohol, knowing there is a chemical reaction that will precipitate them feeling extremely ill.

Even small amounts of alcohol, such as is found in vinegar, mouthwash, hand sanitizers, and cologne, when used while taking disulfarim may result in flushing, feelings of heat in the face and upper body, hypotension, dizziness, blurred vision, palpitations, nausea and vomiting, air hunger, and numbness of the upper extremities. The consequences of this kind of reaction make any patients who are not in good health poor candidates for this treatment. It is contraindicated for patients who have cardiac disease, and fulminant hepatotoxicity can occur in one in 50,000 people. Impulsive heavy drinking while taking disulfarim may be fatal (Trigoboff, 2009). There may be limited uses for disulfarim with the younger-old, but the potential for complications does not make this a safe choice for the frail elder.

Acamprosate (Campral) is a medication that decreases the symptoms associated with early abstinence, such as dysphoria, irritability, anxiety, insomnia, and restlessness. It is used following detoxification and improves the patient's ability to remain sober. This medication requires compliance to a regimen of taking medication three times per day. It takes approximately 5 days for acamprosate to reach a therapeutic level in the body and provide efficacy as an intended treatment for alcohol dependence (Combine Monograph, 2004). The side effects are primarily gastrointestinal problems, but these can be minimized by titrating the dosage by 333 mg three times a day once a week (up to 666 mg three times a day). Patients are instructed to take the medication with meals to improve adherence. Acamprosate is contraindicated in patients with abnormal renal function. Renal function and creatinine clearance tests should be evaluated before initiation of treatment.

Medications Used in Treatment of Opiate Dependence

Buprenorphine

This medication has been shown in research to be efficacious in the treatment of opioid dependence. It is approved by the Food and Drug Administration (FDA) for individuals aged 16 to 65 years and not specifically tested with an elderly population (NIDA, 2009a). Buprenorphine is a partial opioid receptor agonist; it has both agonist and antagonist properties. The medication has a short half-life with a long duration of action (NIDA).

Although it is best used as a single tool in a comprehensive program to support recovery, the major advantage to this medication is that it can be provided in an office-based opioid treatment setting. This helps to decrease the stigma so often associated with treatment for an addictive disorder. However, as stated previously, there is currently no FDA approval for use in those older than age 65 years.

Methadone

This medication has long been considered the gold standard for treatment of opioid dependence (Leavitt, 2005). Methadone is an opioid agonist (Addiction Treatment Forum, 2007a). Methadone maintenance therapy (MMT) has provided effective treatment for over four decades to individuals. The goal of MMT is to provide neurological stabilization and assist recovery from the biopsychosocial patterns associated with opioid dependence. MMT is federally regulated and requires close monitoring (Addiction Treatment Forum).

Prescribing methadone for an elderly population can present multiple challenges. As with other use of prescriptive medications to support recovery, use of concomitant depressants is problematic and dangerous, particularly if respiratory status is compromised. Logistically, MMT has challenges that can be difficult for any individual, but for an elderly person it may pose particular problems. A person obtaining methadone for MMT must be present in the early morning at the clinic site for medication administration. In addition, he or she must wait in line. This may be of concern for a population that may have difficulty standing without use of a cane, problems ambulating, a history of syncope, or requiring the use of a wheelchair. In addition, clients in a methadone clinic must be cognizant of the need for transportation and the weather, because often the line for medication administration can be long enough to be outside of the clinic.

Naltrexone

This medication is an opioid antagonist. It helps eliminate opioid craving and was approved for that purpose by the FDA in 1984 (Addiction Treatment Forum, 2007b). This medication can be given in single daily oral doses. Individuals must be completely detoxified from opiates before initiation of naltrexone (Leavitt, 2002). Its primary activity is opioid blockade. It is inexpensive and adverse reactions are rare. It is considered safe but has not been widely used or investigated for use in an elderly population. One study indicated that it was well tolerated in a group of veterans ages 50 to 70 (Oslin, Liberto, O'Brien, Kras, & Norbeck, 1997). Naltrexone should be used with caution in those with impaired liver and kidney function (Oslin et al., 1997).

Antismoking Medications

To assist individuals in the process of smoking cessation, recent developments in pharmacology can support an individual's goal of recovery from nicotine dependence. With the health consequences associated with smoking, clinicians should encourage cessation by the use of two questions during healthcare visits. It is recommended every clinician ask every patient on every visit two key questions: "Do you smoke?" and "Do you want to quit?"

Any of the following pharmacological agents may be used for treating nicotine addiction (Fiore, Bailey, Cohen, & Dorfman, 2008): bupropion SR, nicotine gum, nicotine inhaler, nicotine lozenge, nicotine nasal spray, nicotine patch, or varenicline. These medications have been shown to have a level of efficacy and positive outcome for an individual who seeks to stop the use of tobacco. Nicotine replacement therapies may be the medication treatment of choice for older adults, given the potential for seizures and other side effects from buproprion (McGrath, Crome, & Crome, 2005). The potential adverse side effects and use of these and any medications must be closely monitored, particularly in the elderly population who may be on multiple concomitant medications. Nicotine replacement therapies should be used with caution in patients with cardiovascular disease (Pbert, Ockene, & Reiff-Hekking, 2004). Some of the potential side effects include mouth soreness, hiccups, and ache in the jaw (Pbert et al.).

NURSING INTERVENTIONS TO ADDRESS SUBSTANCE ABUSE IN THE OLDER ADULT

Intervention capability, when working with an older adult who has substance abuse in his or her current lifestyle, requires a particular skill set that includes being adept at recognition, intervention, and referral. The intervention must be negotiated while supporting the integrity of the person and being respectful of their experiences and coping strategies, whether considered harmful or beneficial. Often older adults face discrimination and ageism regarding their own life choices and they may continue to shun healthcare providers or minimize their own use of substances for fear of reprisal, negative responses from family and caregivers, and an unwillingness to cease use altogether of the chemical of choice. Shame-based individuals will continue to remain reclusive about their use of substances (Shulman, 2003). Allowing the older adult a safe arena in which to discuss and respond to routine questions about substance use affords the beginning of a therapeutic relationship in which health promotion can be initiated to improve the quality of life.

Awareness by the nurse that alcohol-use disorders have been found to be a predictor of suicide risk in men and women should prompt an assessment for suicidal thoughts and plans (Waern, 2003). Older adults as a population are at risk for suicide, and this risk is increased with alcohol-use disorders. The deteriorating social function associated with alcohol disorders is thought to play an integral part in the loss of contact, changes in energy for life, and the effort required to sustain a sober lifestyle. Treatment for the older adult with a diagnosed substance-abuse disorder requires a unique blend of compassion and respect from staff who are specifically educated to treat this population. Clearly, the geropsychiatric nurse attuned to the maturational needs and functional changes of the older person has the capacity to address treatment in a humane and respectful manner.

A program of recovery for this population must address quality of life and physical and mental capabilities. In addition, drug use and misuse and amounts of substances used must be clearly addressed in a caring and supportive manner. The confrontational model used in many substance-abuse treatment centers has little impact on a person who views himself or herself at the final stage of life. Shulman (1998) describes traditional intervention strategies to be far less effective with this population. He states that the leverage conditions, such as loss of employment or criminal sanctions, do not have the same importance in this age group. In addition, Shulman further describes that families of the older adult may not respond to standard intervention methods because of the belief that they are being publicly humiliated by the substance abuse of their loved one. Often the goal of initial intervention is to improve the person's health status with the by-product being enjoyment of life. If substance abuse is detected, a brief

intervention can assist the individual to decrease his or her use of substances by using a treatment plan. A series of brief intervention steps facilitate change at this level (Fingerhood, 2000, p. 991).

1. Give feedback on screening
2. Discuss reasons for drinking
3. Discuss consequences of drinking
4. Discuss reasons to cut down or quit
5. Develop strategies for achieving goal
6. Develop an agreement in the form of a written contract
7. Identify obstacles to achieving goal
8. Discuss strategies to overcome obstacles
9. Summarize session

Older adults who abuse substances and become chemically dependent benefit from this structured approach. Using these steps may help to modify heavy use of any substance and may be an effective methodology to create a treatment plan. Older persons who demonstrate mild symptoms of withdrawal may be monitored at home if family members are supportive and present to assist in the overall care. The older adult who exhibits severe withdrawal, who is medically compromised, or who takes a number of prescribed medications requires an inpatient setting for safety and ongoing medical supervision of a potentially dangerous and unpredictable state (Wright, Cluver, & Myrick, 2009).

Medical safety and access to the abused substance are primary considerations in the decision-making process regarding treatment setting. Additional factors to be considered include a history of seizures, delirium tremens, medical comorbidities, co-occurring disorders, suicidality, dependence on more than one substance, lack of support system, and failure of previous treatments (CSAT, 1998).

Use of pharmacological agents to withdraw a person requires a medical and nursing skill set and familiarity with the patterns of any acute abstinence syndrome (withdrawal). A focus on the psychosocial issues with older adults is an essential part of recovery in this age group (Liberto &

Oslin, 1995). The management plan must also address the need for referral to specialists in the field of substance abuse and older adults, and collaborative approaches to the multidisciplinary care plans established.

Families of the older adult with a substance abuse problem may feel humiliated and shamed by the substance abuse. Care provided to families may need to focus on the outcomes of improved health and improved quality of life, rather than focusing on the abuse of substances, as a way to lessen the stigma associated with the substance abuse. Support groups for families, such as Alanon, may be important resources for family members.

Healthcare professionals may also need support in dealing with their own biases about substance abuse by older adults. Nursing psychoeducational meetings or support groups that are focused on case examples, and role-playing with specific techniques for relating to or treating older adults with substance abuse problems in a respectful manner, may provide the needed education and support for nurses who are working with this population.

The ultimate goal is to return older adults to the community with an enriched awareness of personal health in the domains of physical, mental, emotional, and spiritual connectedness in the twilight of their lifetime.

REFERENCES

Adams, S. L., & Waskel, S. A. (1991). Late onset of alcoholism among older mid-western men in treatment. *Psychology Reports, 68,* 432–434.

Addiction Treatment Forum. (2007a). *MAT cycle of recovery from opioid addiction, 16*(2). Retrieved December 12, 2008, from http:/www.atforum.com/SiteRoot/pages/addiction_resources/NTX-Opoid.pdf

Addiction Treatment Forum. (2007b). *Methadone overdoses in MMT, 16*(3). Retrieved December 12, 2008, from http:/www.atforum.com/SiteRoot/pages/addiction_resources/NTX-Opoid.pdf

Alcoholics Anonymous. (1984). *AA member medications and other drugs.* New York: Alcoholic Anonymous World Services.

American Geriatrics Society. (2003). *Clinical guidelines for alcohol use disorders in older adults.* Retrieved September 4, 2008, from www.americangeriatrics.org/products/positionpapers/alcoholPF.shtml

American Psychiatric Association. (2000). *Diagnostic and statistical manual of mental disorders* (4th ed., Text Revision). Washington, DC: Author.

American Society of Pain Management Nurses. (2003). *ASPMN position statement: Pain management in patients with addictive disease.* Pensacola, FL: Author.

Armstrong, M. A. (2008). Substance-related disorders. In K. M. Fortinash & P. A. Holoday Worret (Eds.), *Psychiatric mental health nursing* (4th ed., pp. 304–341). St. Louis, MO: Mosby.

Atkinson, R. M. (1995). Treatment programs for aging alcoholics. In T. P. Beresford & E. S. L. Gomberg (Eds.), *Alcohol and aging.* New York: Oxford University Press.

Atkinson, R. M., Tolson, R. L., & Turner, J. A. (1990). Late versus early onset drinking in older men. *Alcoholism: Clinical and Experimental Research, 14*(4), 574–579.

Barrick, C., & Connors, G. J. (2002). Relapse prevention and maintaining abstinence in older adults with alcohol-use disorders. *Drugs Aging, 19*(8), 583–594.

Beers, M. H., & Berkow, R. (Eds.). (2000). *Merck manual of geriatrics* (3rd ed.). Whitehouse Station, NJ: Merck Research Labs.

Bien, T. H., Miller, W. R., & Tonigan, J. S. (1993). Brief interventions for alcohol problems: A review. *Addiction, 88,* 315–336.

Blow, F. (2000). Treatment of older women with alcohol problems: Meeting the challenge for a special population. *Alcoholism: Clinical and Experimental Research, 24*(8), 1257–1266.

Blow, E. C., Schulenber, K. J., Demo-Dananberg, L. M., Young, J. L., & Beresford, T. I. (1992). The Michigan Alcoholism Screening Test—Geriatric Version (MAST-G): A new elderly specific screening instrument. *Alcoholism: Clinical and Experimental Research, 16,* 372.

Brody, J. A. (1982). Aging and alcohol abuse. *Journal of the American Geriatrics Society, 30,* 123–126.

Brust, J. C. M. (2009). Neurologic disorders related to alcohol and other drug use. In R. K. Ries, D. A.

Fiellin, S. C. Miller, & R. Saitz (Eds.), *Principles of addiction medicine* (4th ed., pp. 1049–1056). Philadelphia: Lippincott Williams and Wilkins.

CASA Report. (1998). *Under the rug: Substance abuse and the mature woman.* New York: National Center on Addiction and Substance Abuse at Columbia University.

Center for Social Gerontology. (2001). *Fact sheets on tobacco and older persons.* Retrieved January 15, 2009, from http://www.tcsg.org/

Center for Substance Abuse Treatment (CSAT), Substance Abuse and Mental Health Services Administration. (1998). *Substance abuse among older adults: Treatment Improvement Protocol (TIP) Series 26.* DHHS Publication No. (SMA) 07-3918. Rockville, MD: U.S. Department of Health and Human Services, Public Health Service.

Combine monograph: Medical management treatment manual. (2004). Rockville, MD: U.S. Department of Health and Human Services.

Costello, M. (2008). Pancreatitis. In T. M. Buttaro, J. Trybulski, P. B. Bailey, & J. Sandberg-Cook (Eds.), *Primary care: A collaborative practice* (3rd ed., pp. 714–722). St. Louis, MO: Mosby Elsevier.

Culberson, J. W. (2006). Alcohol use in the elderly: Beyond the CAGE. *Geriatrics, 61*(11), 20–26.

Dani, J. A., Kosten, T. R., & Benowitz, N. L. (2009). The pharmacology of nicotine and tobacco. In R. K. Ries, D. A. Fiellin, S. C. Miller, & R. Saitz (Eds.), *Principles of addiction medicine* (4th ed., pp. 179–191). Philadelphia: Lippincott Williams and Wilkins.

Davison, J., Sweeney, M., & Bush, K. (2006). Outpatient treatment engagement and abstinence rates following in-patient opioid detoxification. *Journal of Addictive Diseases, 25*(4), 27–35.

D'Avonzo, C. E. (2001). Common drugs of abuse. In M. A. Naegle & C. E. D'Avonzo (Eds.), *Addictions and substance abuse: Strategies for advanced practice nurses* (pp. 333–354). Upper Saddle River, NJ: Prentice Hall Health.

DeHart, S. S., & Hoffman, N. G. (1995). Screening and diagnosis of alcohol abuse and dependence in older adults. *The International Journal of Addictions, 30*(13/14), 1717–1747.

Dekker, A. H. (2002, April). *Alcoholism in the elderly.* Program and abstracts presented at the 33rd Annual Meeting & Medical-Scientific Conference, Atlanta, GA: American Society of Addiction Medicine, April 26, 2002.

Edlund, B. J., & Spain, M. (2003). Geriatric assessment. *Advance for Nurses, 3*, 18–22.

Eliason, M. J. (1998). Identification of alcohol-related problems in older women. *Journal of Gerontological Nursing, 24*(10), 8–15.

Eliason, M. J. (2001). Drug and alcohol intervention for older women: A pilot study. *Journal of Gerontological Nursing, 27*(12), 18–24.

Ewing, J. (1984). Detecting alcoholism: The CAGE questionnaire. *JAMA, 252*(14), 1905–1907.

Fingeld-Connett, D. L. (2004). Treatment of substance abuse in older women: Using a brief intervention model. *Journal of Gerontological Nursing, 30*(8), 30–37.

Fingerhood, M. (2000). Substance abuse in older people. *Journal of the American Geriatrics Society, 48*(8), 985–995.

Finlayson, R. E. (1995). Misuse of prescription drugs. *The International Journal of Addictions, 30*(13/14), 1871–1901.

Finlayson, R. E., Hurt, R. D., Davis, L. J., & Morse, R. M. (1988). Alcoholism in elderly persons: Study of the psychiatric and psychosocial features of 216 inpatients. *Mayo Clinic Proceedings, 63*, 761–768.

Fiore, M. C., Bailey, W. C., Cohen, S. J., & Dorfman, S. F. (2008). *Treating tobacco use and dependence: 2008 Update.* Clinical Practice Guideline. Rockville, MD: U.S. Department of Health and Human Services, Public Health Service.

Fleming, M. F., Manwell, L. B., Barry, K. L., Adams, W., & Stauffacher, E. A. (1999). Brief physician advice for alcohol problems in older adults: A randomized community-based trial. *Journal of Family Practice, 48*, 378–384.

Friedman, H. S. (2009). Cardiovascular consequences of alcohol and other drug use. In R. K. Ries, D. A. Fiellin, S. C. Miller, & R. Saitz (Eds.), *Principles of addiction medicine* (4th ed.). Philadelphia: Lippincott Williams and Wilkins.

Friedman, L. (2009). Liver, biliary tract and pancreas disorders. In S. McPhee & M. Papadakis (Eds.), *Current medical diagnosis and treatment 2009* (48th ed., pp. 582–629). New York: McGraw-Hill.

Gambert, S. R., & Albrecht, C. R. III. (2005). The elderly. In J. H. Lowinson, P. Ruiz, R. B. Millman, & J. G. Langrod (Eds.), *Substance abuse: A comprehensive textbook* (4th ed., pp. 1038–1048). Philadelphia: Lippincott Williams & Wilkins.

Grilly, D. M. (2002). *Drugs and human behavior* (4th ed.). Boston: Allyn & Bacon.

Haber, P. S., & Batey, R. G. (2009). Liver disorders related to alcohol and other drug use. In R. K. Ries, D. A. Fiellin, S. C. Miller, & R. Saitz (Eds.), *Principles of addiction medicine* (4th ed., pp. 989–1008). Philadelphia: Lippincott Williams and Wilkins.

Holbert, K. R., & Tueth, M. J. (2004). Alcohol abuse and dependence: A clinical update on alcoholism in the older population. *Geriatrics, 59*(9), 38–40.

Katzung, B. G. (2001). *Basic and clinical pharmacology* (8th ed.). New York: Lange Medical Books/ McGraw-Hill.

Keltner, N. L., & Folks, D. G. (2001). *Psychotropic drugs* (3rd ed.). St. Louis, MO: Mosby.

Kosten, T. R., & Sofuoglu, M. (2004). Stimulants. In M. Galanter & H. D. Kleber (Eds.), *Textbook of substance abuse treatment* (pp. 189–198). Washington, DC: American Psychiatric Publishing.

Kraemer, K. L., Mayo-Smith, M. F., & Calkins, D. R. (1997). Impact of age, severity, course, and complications of alcohol withdrawal. *Archives of Internal Medicine, 157,* 2234–2240.

Leavitt, S. B. (2002). Naltrexone in the prevention of opioid relapse. *Addiction Treatment Forum.* Retrieved December 12, 2008, from http://www.atforum.com/ SiteRoot/pages/addiction_resources/NTX-Opoid. pdf

Leavitt, S. B. (2005). Addiction recovery: New understandings of an old concept. *Addiction. Treatment Forum, 14*(4). Retrieved December 12, 2008, from http://www.atforum.com/SiteRoot/pages/addiction_ resources/NTX-Opoid.pdf

Letizia, M., & Reinbolz, M. (2005). Identifying and managing acute alcohol withdrawal in the elderly. *Geriatric Nursing, 26*(3), 176–183.

Liberto, J. G., & Oslin, D. W. (1995). Early versus late onset of alcoholism in the elderly. *The International Journal of the Addictions, 30*(13/14), 1799–1818.

Lichtenberg. P. A., Gibbons, T. A., Nanna, M. J., & Blumenthal, F. (1993). The effects of age and gender on the prevalence and detection of alcohol abuse in elderly medical inpatients. *Clinical Gerontologist, 13*(3), 17–27.

Lisanti, E. S., & Gomberg, E. S. L. (2004). Ethnic minorities and the elderly. In M. Galanter & H. D. Kleber (Eds.),

Textbook of substance abuse treatment (3rd ed.). Washington, DC: American Psychiatric Publishing.

Lisanti, P. (2001). Adult health: Acute care. In M. A. Naegle & C. E. D'Avanzo (Eds.), *Addictions and substance abuse: Strategies for advanced practice nursing* (pp. 137–188). Upper Saddle River, NJ: Prentice Hall Health.

Loukissa, D. (2007). Under diagnosis of alcohol misuse in the older adult population. *British Journal of Nursing, 16*(20), 1254–1258.

Massie, B. M., & Amidon, T. M. (2003). Heart. In L. M. Tierney, S. J. McPhee, & M. A. Papadakis (Eds.), *Current medical diagnosis and treatment 2003* (42nd ed., pp. 312–408). New York: Lange Medical Books/McGraw-Hill.

Masters, J. (2003). Moderate alcohol consumption and unappreciated risk for alcohol-related harm among ethnically diverse, urban dwelling elders. *Geriatric Nursing, 24*(3), 155–161.

Masters, S. (2001). The alcohols. In B. G. Katzung (Ed.), *Basic and clinical pharmacology* (8th ed., pp. 382–394). New York: Lange Medical Books/ McGraw-Hill.

Mayfield, D., McLeod, G., & Hall, P. (1973). The CAGE questionnaire: Validation of a new alcoholism and screening instrument. *American Journal of Psychiatry, 131*(10), 1121–1123.

Mayo-Smith, M. F. (2009). Management of alcohol intoxication and withdrawal. In R. K. Ries, D. A. Fiellin, S. C. Miller, & R. Saitz (Eds.), *Principles of addiction medicine* (4th ed., pp. 559–572). Philadelphia: Lippincott Williams and Wilkins.

McGrath, A., Crome, P., & Crome, I. B. (2005). Substance misuse in the older population. *Postgraduate Medical Journal, 81,* 228–231.

Nace, E. P. (2005). Alcohol. In R. J. Frances, S. I. Miller, & A. H. Mack (Eds.), *Clinical textbook of addictive disorders* (3rd ed., pp. 75–104). New York: Guilford Press.

Nakahara, T., Hasimoto, K., Hirano, M., Koll, M., Martin, C. R., & Preedy, V. (2003). Acute and chronic effects of alcohol exposure on skeletal muscle c-myc,p53 and Bcl-2 mRNA expression. *American Journal of Physiological Endocrinology and Metabolism, 285,* E1273–E1281.

National Institute on Alcohol Abuse and Alcoholism. (2005). *Helping patients who drink too much: A clinician's guide.* NIH Publication No. 07-3769. Bethesda, MD: Author.

National Institute on Alcohol Abuse and Alcoholism. (2008). *Alcohol: A Women's Health Issue*. NIH Publication No. 03-4956. Bethesda, MD: Author.

National Institute on Drug Abuse. (2003). *Nicotine addiction*. Retrieved December 14, 2004, from www.nida.nih.gov/researchreports/nicotine

National Institute on Drug Abuse. (NIDA, 2009a). *New innovations in opioid treatment*, NAADAC Knowledge Center Life-Long Learning Series. Alexandria, VA. Retrieved January 28, 2009, from www.nida.nih.gov

National Institute on Drug Abuse (NIDA, 2009b). *Principles of drug abuse treatment: A research based guide* (2nd ed.). Retrieved January 28, 2009, from www.nida.nih.gov

Oslin, D., Liberto, J. G., O'Brien, J., Kras, S., & Norbeck, J. (1997). Naltrexone as an adjunctive treatment for older patients with alcohol dependence. *American Journal of Geriatric Psychiatry, 5*(4), 324–332.

Oslin, D. W., Pettinati, H., & Volpicelli, J. R. (2002). Alcoholism treatment adherence: Older age predicts better adherence and drinking outcomes. *American Journal of Geriatric Psychiatry, 10*, 740–747.

Pbert, L., Ockene, J. K., & Reiff-Hekking, S. (2004). Tobacco. In M. Galanter & H. D. Kleber (Eds.), *Textbook of substance abuse treatment* (3rd ed., pp. 217–234). Washington, DC: American Psychiatric Publishing.

Saitz, R. (2009). Medical and surgical complications of addiction. In R. K. Ries, D. A. Fiellin, S. C. Miller, & R. Saitz (Eds.), *Principles of addiction medicine* (4th ed., pp. 945–967). Philadelphia: Lippincott Williams & Wilkins.

Savage, S. R. (1993). Addiction in the treatment of pain: Significance, recognition and management. *Journal of Pain and Symptom Management, 8*(5), 265–278.

Schutte, K. K, Byrne, F. E., Brennan, P. L., & Moos, R. H. (2001). Successful remission of late-life drinking problems: A 10-year follow-up. *Journal of Studies on Alcohol, 62*(3), 322–344.

Shulman, G. (1998). *The challenge of assessment and treatment of the older alcoholic and substance abuser*. A six-part Web site series—East Carolina University. Retrieved November 10, 2004, from www.counselors@addictioninfo.com

Shulman, G. (2003*)*. Senior moments: Assessing older adults. *Addiction Today, 15*(82), 17–19.

Smith, C. M., & Cotter, V. T. (2008). Normal aging changes, *Nursing standard of practice protocol: Age-related changes in health*. Retrieved December 14, 2008, from: www.consultgerirn.org/topics/normal_aging_changes/want_to_know_more

Solomon, K., Manepalli, J. M., Ireland, G. A., & Mahon, G. M. (1993). Alcoholism and prescription drug abuse in the elderly: St. Louis University grand rounds. *Journal of the American Geriatrics Society, 41*(1), 57–69.

Stevenson, J. S. (2005). Alcohol use, misuse, abuse, and dependence in later adulthood. *Annual Review of Nursing Research, 23*, 245–280.

Substance Abuse and Mental Health Services Administration (SAMHSA). (2007). *Results from the 2006 National Survey on Drug Use and Health: National Findings, 2007*. Rockville, MD: U.S. Department of Health and Human Services, SAMHSA, Office of Applied Studies: NSDUH Series H-32, DHHS Publication N. SMA 07-4293.

Toy, P. (2004). Anemia. In *Current geriatric diagnosis and treatment* (pp. 314–316). New York: Lange Medical Books/McGraw-Hill.

Trigoboff, E. (2009). Substance-related disorders. In C. R. Kneisel & E. Trigoboff (Eds.), *Contemporary psychiatric-mental health nursing* (2nd ed., pp. 323–369). Upper Saddle River, NJ: Prentice Hall.

U.S. Bureau of the Census. (2000). Population projections of the United States by age, sex, race, Hispanic origin and nativity. Washington, DC: Author.

Waern, M. (2003). Alcohol dependence and misuse in elderly suicides. *Alcohol and Alcoholism, 38*, 249–254.

Widlitz, M., & Marin, D. B. (2002). Substance abuse in older adults. *Geriatrics, 57*(12), 29–34.

Wiscott, R., Kopera-Frye, K., & Seifert, L. (2001). Possible consequences of social drinking in the early stages of Alzheimer's disease. *Geriatric Nursing, 22*(2), 100–104.

Wright, T. M., Cluver, J. S., & Myrick, H. (2009). Management of intoxication and withdrawal: General principles. In R. K. Ries, D. A. Fiellin, S. C. Miller, & R. Saitz (Eds.), *Principles of addiction medicine* (4th ed., pp. 551–558). Philadelphia: Lippincott Williams & Wilkins.

III

Issues in Geropsychiatric and Mental Health of Older Adults

11

Delirium

Karen Dick
Catherine R. Morency

CASE STUDY

Mr. V. is a 90-year-old resident of an assisted living facility with a history of gastroesophageal reflux disease, benign prostatic hypertrophy with retention, type 2 diabetes mellitus, pulmonary emboli, and dementia. His medications include moxifloxacin, lisinopril, metoprolol, metformin, dutasteride, tamsulosin hydrochloride, quetiapine fumarate, donepezil hydrochloride, omeprazole, MVI, ASA, and trazodone as needed for sleep. He is independent with his activities of daily living, but requires some help with a chronic indwelling catheter. He is alert and active and participates in activities at his residence. Mr. V. is ambulatory and uses a cane for balance. He wears glasses for vision and hearing aids in both ears. After a recent bout with a URI that affected many residents of his facility, Mr. V. had 2 days of diarrhea and a feeling of needing to void despite his catheter being in place. His temperature was 100.8°F, and he was sent to the local hospital for evaluation.

While in the emergency department in the middle of the night, he continually asked where the elevator was because he needed to go to the dining room. He seemed to think that he was in a restaurant that was closed. He asked if he could please cook himself something to eat. His laboratory values revealed sodium 144, potassium 3.4, blood urea nitrogen 29, creatinine 1.1, glucose 238, white blood cell 11.2, and hematocrit 36.3. A chest radiograph showed a right basilar consolidation. Urinalysis showed white blood cell count greater than 150, positive nitrites, and many bacteria. A subsequent culture of the urine grew *Klebsiella*. Mr. V. was admitted for 3 days to the hospital. The nursing notes described him as "demented" but did not mention that this new behavior was a departure from normal. While hospitalized, visitors who knew him well found him fluctuating between falling asleep during a conversation to being agitated and climbing

(continues)

out of bed to go to the movies. They also noted that his glasses and hearing aids were not sent with him to the hospital for fear of their being lost. On the day of discharge, his attending physician found him oriented to self. Mr. V. thought that the physician was familiar and even guessed that he knew him from the assisted living facility. Despite being afebrile with normal blood work, when he returned the staff believed

that he needed skilled nursing care. Mr. V. now needs help with medications, bathing, and ambulation and is considered a fall risk.

What are the risk factors for delirium in this case? How would you go about evaluating contributing factors? What interventions would be appropriate? This case represents a typical scenario that both acute and long-term care nurses frequently encounter in their daily practice.

INTRODUCTION

Delirium is a serious and significant health problem in the elderly population. It is a syndrome of disturbed consciousness, attention, cognition, and perception. Delirium represents complex interactions between medical conditions, cognitive function, and behavior, and for many elders it is often the first and only indicator of underlying physical illness (Lyness, 1990). Delirium contributes to increased morbidity and mortality, longer hospital stays, functional impairment, and more permanent forms of cognitive impairment if it is not recognized and treated in a timely fashion (Leslie, Marcantonio, Zhang, Leo-Summers, & Inouye, 2008; Levkoff, Besdine, & Wetle, 1986; Levkoff et al., 1992; Lipowski, 1983; Marcantonio et al., 2003; Murray et al., 1993). This syndrome can occur in elders at any point across the care continuum, from community, to long-term care, to acute care settings. Delirium can be present in the emergency department on admission to the hospital, develop while the patient is hospitalized, and persist long after the patient is discharged to home or institutional settings. It is not clear why elders are at such high risk for this syndrome. Some believe that the brain is the "vulnerable" organ in an older adult, and cumulative insults to the body may be

reflected in changes in cognitive functioning from acute brain failure. It is important for clinicians to know that delirium is reversible if it is recognized as an acute change and precipitating causes are removed in a timely fashion.

The incidence estimates for delirium in hospitalized patients vary widely because of both sampling and diagnostic criteria and range from 14 to 56% (Inouye, 1998). Patients who have undergone hip fracture repair are particularly prone to delirium with incidence rates ranging from 35% to 65% (Marcantonio, Flacker, Wright, & Resnick, 2001). Delirium has also been described in patients at the end of life, particularly in patients with advanced cancers. Research has shown that the symptoms of delirium can last from weeks to months (Gruber-Baldini et al., 2003; Murray et al., 1993), and for some a delirium can represent the beginning of a decline trajectory (Levkoff et al., 1992). It has been estimated that the total direct costs of care related to delirium could range from $38 billion to as high as $152 billion annually in the United States (Leslie et al., 2008). Patients with a preexisting dementia are at highest risk for delirium. Because delirium can be life threatening, it must be thought of as a medical emergency that needs prompt recognition, treatment of potentially removable causes, and supportive care. Nurses are in key positions to recognize, identify, and manage patients with delirium in all healthcare settings. Nurses also play a critical role in identifying patients at risk for delirium and instituting measures to limit and even prevent an episode of delirium. The purpose of this chapter is to define delirium, identify individual patient risk factors, review how delirium is diagnosed, and outline treatment and nursing interventions.

TERMINOLOGY

Delirium has been described for thousands of years. Accounts of delirium in the medical literature have consisted primarily of case reports and clinical impressions (Levkoff, Cleary, Liptzin, & Evans, 1991). Even though the epidemiology of delirium has been studied for many decades, one of the greatest barriers to systematically integrating the research and writing to date has been in the lack of a consistent nomenclature. More than 25 terms have been used to describe the confusional state from "acute brain syndrome" to "toxic befuddlement" (Francis & Kapoor, 1990). It has also been described as pseudo-senility, pseudo-dementia, and acute confusional state. This syndrome is labeled in a number of ways depending on the clinical population and the background of the evaluator (Neelon, 1990). Acute confusion is the terminology that is used most commonly. Although delirium and acute confusion are used interchangeably, some do not believe that acute confusion and delirium are the same thing, that delirium is a medical phenomenon. Rasin (1990) states "nurses seem to use the term confusion as an abbreviated means to describe the constellation of clinical manifestations that fall within the medical diagnosis of dementia or delirium" (p. 910). Nurses also tend to identify both cognitive and behavioral manifestations of confusion, as well as a continuum from "slightly confused to highly confused" (Vermeersch, 1991). According to Foreman (1993), the term "acute confusion requires no translation for the bedside practitioners, does not connote etiology, and represents

more closely what is observed clinically by nurses" (p. 6). If confusion is defined as a loss of capacity to think with clarity and coherence, identifying confusion per se is just the labeling of a symptom and can represent different psychiatric syndromes (Johnson, 1990). That is why it is difficult to determine if the terminology and definitions that nurses use represent the same or a different phenomenon as their physician counterparts. For the purpose of this chapter, delirium is used, because it is the terminology most widely used by mental health providers when describing acute cognitive changes in the elderly.

DEFINITION

The description that follows is the generally accepted definition of delirium as stated by the *Diagnostic and Statistical Manual of Mental Disorders Text Revision, 4th edition* (DSM-IV-TR) (American Psychiatric Association, 2000). Again, it is important to remember that it serves as a method for making a clinical diagnosis. These diagnostic criteria for delirium caused by a general medical condition are as follows: (1) a disturbance of consciousness (reduced clarity of awareness of the environment) with reduced ability to focus, sustain, or shift attention; (2) a change in cognition (e.g., memory deficit, disorientation, language disturbance) or the development of a perceptual disturbance that is not better accounted for by a preexisting, established, or evolving dementia; (3) a disturbance that develops over a short period of time (usually hours to days) and tends to fluctuate during the course of the day; and (4) evidence from the history, physical examination, or laboratory findings indicates that the disturbance is caused by the direct physiological consequences of a general medical condition (American Psychiatric Association).

First, regarding the change in cognition that is not accounted for by preexisting dementia, knowledge of the patient's baseline cognitive status needs to be determined. Often this is not immediately known and requires investigation of when the change in mental status actually occurred. This is critical to the diagnosis. In the preceding case study, sending a baseline mental status examination with the patient to the emergency department or providing a description of the changes in behavior that were noted would have been helpful. Second, the DSM-IV-TR also describes other subcategories of delirium including substance-induced delirium, substance-withdrawal delirium, delirium attributed to multiple etiologies, and delirium not otherwise specified, but often the etiology of the delirium is not always known at the time of diagnosis. Third, the question of an incomplete manifestation of the delirium syndrome has been raised. Some believe that it is possible for patients to have some symptoms of delirium but not all; this is referred to as "subsyndromal delirium" (Cole, McCusker, Dendukuri, & Han, 2003). As to how many of the DSM criteria must be met to make the diagnosis of delirium, there remains no clear consensus.

PATHOPHYSIOLOGY

There may be a number of different pathogenic mechanisms that contribute to the development of delirium: the underlying pathophysiology of delirium is not well understood. Mechanisms that have been proposed to explain the physiological precipitants that underlie the development of delirium include acute stress response, drug toxicity, and inflammation, all which can contribute to the disruption of neurotransmission (Fong, Tulebaev, & Inouye, 2009). There remains a lack of agreement as to the exact mechanism, but there is growing evidence to support a role for cholinergic deficiency in delirium (Hshieh, Fong, Marcantonio, & Inouye, 2008). Patients with Alzheimer's dementia have decreased acetylcholine caused by loss of cholinergic neurons and are at high risk of delirium. Anticholinergic drugs are known to precipitate delirium and certain metabolic abnormalities may decrease acetylcholine synthesis in the central nervous system and contribute to the development of delirium.

There is also some evidence that even drugs used commonly in the elderly, such as digoxin, furosemide, prednisone, and theophylline, may have anticholinergic activity (Cole & McCusker, 2002). Finally, increased levels of anticholinergic activity have been shown to correlate with the severity of delirium in some hospitalized elderly patients (Mach et al., 1995).

RISK FACTORS

Although there has been wide variability in reported risk factors associated with delirium, individual, physiological, environmental, and pharmacological risk factors have been identified in Table 11-1 (Foreman, 1986, 1989; Francis, Martin, & Kapoor, 1990; Inouye, Viscoli, Horwitz, Hurst, & Tinetti, 1993; Rockwood, 1993; Schor et al., 1992). It is most likely that predisposing and precipitating factors interact with aggravating factors to influence the course. Research has suggested that between two and six factors may be contributing in any one case of delirium (Rudberg, Pompei, Foreman, Ross, & Cassel, 1997). It is believed that the risk of delirium increases as the number of risk factors increase. Patients with minimal risk factors may have a margin of safety before any dysfunction occurs compared to those who might be near threshold where very little stress may precipitate cognitive dysfunction (Neelon, 1990). It may also be that there are protective or mediating factors that influence the development of delirium. It is important for clinicians not to assume that there is just one single factor and stop in the search for any and all potentially contributing factors when assessing a patient's risk of delirium. Most risk factors may not in most circumstances be modified, but clinicians may be alerted to patients at highest risk and early surveillance and monitoring may allow for more timely interventions (Liptzin, 1995). In regards to pharmacological factors, almost any drug can contribute to delirium with anticholinergics, benzodiazepines, and narcotics being the major offenders. Over-the-counter medications must also be considered.

TABLE 11-1

Risk Factors for Delirium

Individual	Physiological	Pharmacological	Environmental
Advanced age	Postoperative state	Polypharmacy	Stress
Visual impairment	Infection	Withdrawal from alcohol or drugs	New or change in environment
Hearing impairment	Dehydration		Excessive or lack of sensory input, isolation
Preexisting cognitive impairment	Hypoxia		Use of bladder catheters
Preexisting brain disorders: stroke, Parkinson's disease	Anemia		Absence of clock, watch, reading glasses
Previous delirium episodes	Malnutrition		
Severe chronic illnesses	Vitamin B_{12}, folate deficiencies		
Immobility (including restraint use)	Hypovolemia		
Disordered sleep	Hyponatremia, hypernatremia		
Depression	Low perfusion states		

Source: Adapted from Foreman (1986); Foreman (1989); Francis, Martin, & Kapoor (1990); Inouye, Viscoli, Horwitz, Hurst, & Tinetti (1993); Rockwood (1993); and Schor, Levkoff, Lipsitz, Reilly, Cleary, Rowe, et al. (1992).

SUBTYPES AND PATTERNS

Clinical subtypes of delirium have been identified, and these include hyperactive, hypoactive, and mixed variants (Lipowski, 1987; Liptzin & Levkoff, 1992). The hyperactive subtype is the classic picture of the patient who is agitated, restless, combative, and hyperalert. Patients may have fast or loud speech, be distractible, and have quick motor responses. These are the patients who pull out intravenous lines and catheters, try to climb over bedrails, and are at greatest risk for complications from injury and physical or chemical restraints. They also require increased nursing surveillance and care, often straining already depleted staffing resources. Surprisingly, these cases account for less than 25% of all cases but have the worst outcomes, including nursing home placement or death at 1 month (Marcantonio, Ta, Duthie, & Resnick, 2002).

The hypoactive subtype includes patients who have decreased alertness, sparse or slow speech, lethargy, slowed movements, and apathy. These patients may be somnolent or stuporous. Because these patients are quiet and do not present nursing staff with increased demands for care or surveillance, the chance is high that these patients will not be identified as delirious. In one study of hip fracture patients that looked at both delirium severity and psychomotor types, patients with pure hypoactive delirium had better outcomes than patients with hyperactive delirium even after adjusting for severity (Marcantonio et al., 2002). The mixed variant subtype includes symptoms of both hyperactive and hypoactive subtypes with patients cycling between the two and accounts for more than 50% of cases. These patients often are not identified as being delirious until they become agitated and confused with more symptoms of the hyperactive state. Our patient Mr. V. shows features of being in a mixed subtype of delirium: he is described as alternating between falling asleep during a conversation and trying to get out of bed to go to the movies.

Neelon, Frank, Carlson, and Champagne (1989) described three types of patterns of confusion development in hospitalized elderly. In the first pattern, patients with low cognitive reserve, such as dementia, are extremely susceptible to environmentally provoked states, such as sensory deprivation or overload. In the second pattern, patients with low physiological reserve or instability are influenced by physiological factors including pain, hypoxia, and high illness levels. In the third pattern, patients with low biochemical reserve caused by renal and hepatic impairment are vulnerable to toxic agents, such as drugs, which are a key in the development of delirium. The authors postulate that the risk of the development of acute confusion is a cumulative function of the patient's vulnerability, the timing and magnitude of the effect of multiple added stressors, and the support of biopyschosocial integrity (Neelon, 1990). The goal for nursing becomes one of identifying and treating the underlying causes to protect the vulnerable systems that have little reserve (Champagne & Wiese, 1992). Note that in the case study, Mr. V. did not have his glasses or hearing aids, adding to his vulnerability.

RELATIONSHIP BETWEEN DEMENTIA AND DELIRIUM

Patients with an underlying dementia are more susceptible to developing a delirium in the setting of acute illness. This is known as "delirium superimposed on dementia." Many healthcare professionals do not recognize that the patient is delirious and may attribute behavioral or cognitive issues to the patient being demented or sundowning. In one study of registered nurses in an acute care setting done by Fick, Hodo, Lawrence, and Inouye (2007), only 21% were able to identify correctly the hypoactive form of delirium superimposed on dementia. The lack of recognition of delirium in an elderly patient and the labeling of it as dementia may lead to the inappropriate

administration of medications to control behavior and make the problem far worse by delaying appropriate care and treatment.

CLINICAL COURSE

There is no one classic trajectory of delirium, but features that are common to all cases of delirium include sudden onset and fluctuating symptoms. This fluctuation in presentation is problematic, because patients may have periods of lucidity interspersed with inattention and high distractibility. Evaluation of a patient's mental status done once a day (picture morning rounds in the hospital) can totally miss the delirious state. Patients may also have motor restlessness, speech that is difficult to follow, and perceptual disturbances that range from misinterpretations of the environment to frank visual hallucinations. Memory, particularly in relation to recent events, is often impaired and disorientation most commonly to time (day of the week or time of the year) or place is usually present. Patients may also exhibit affective signs of fear, anxiety, or anger. There may be a history of a fragmented and disordered sleep–wake cycle. Symptoms of anxiety, restlessness, and agitation may be worse in the late afternoon or evening, and this presentation has been labeled "sundowning," but it is not clear if sundowning is a component of delirium or a separate clinical entity (Burney-Puckett, 1996; Nowak & Davis, 2007). It is known that institutionalized patients with dementia are at greatest risk of sundowning. The temporal aspects of sundowning allow clinicians to predict vulnerable time periods and to use both pharmacological and nonpharmacological interventions to keep patients calm and safe.

THE PROBLEM OF RECOGNITION

Patients who become confused during the course of their hospitalization, or whose preexisting cognitive impairment worsens, present nursing staff with the challenge of maintaining patient safety, wellbeing, and function (Miller, 1991). Misdiagnosis and subsequent failure to treat can have catastrophic consequences for the patient and have been associated with irreversible brain failure, institutionalization, increased patient care costs, and death (Francis & Kapoor, 1992; Lipowski, 1989; Schor et al., 1992). Nurses and physicians often fail to recognize and diagnose delirium and may attribute any form of cognitive impairment to normal aging (Lipowski, 1987). In hospitalized elderly, a downward decline into acute confusion may be seen as a normal trajectory with no need for intervention (Csokasy, 1999). It has been suggested that between 37 and 72% of patients who become acutely confused are never recognized by physicians and nurses as being in an acute confusional state (Foreman, 1989). Patients may be incorrectly labeled as having a dementia, a psychiatric disorder, or unmanageable behavior (Lipowski, 1983; Wolanin & Phillips, 1981). Other explanations for underdiagnosis by nurses have included lack of knowledge (Brady, 1987), social factors and setting (Morgan, 1985), varied clinical reasoning styles (McCarthy, 1991), the presence of dementia (Fick & Foreman, 2000), degree of cooperation with care (Palmateer & McCartney, 1985), and individual factors in the nurse, patient, and environment that influence patient labeling (Ludwick, 1993). In a study of elderly patients admitted to an acute care hospital, four risk factors for underrecognition of delirium by nurses were identified: (1) the presence of the hypoactive form, (2) age 80 years or older, (3) vision impairment, and (4) dementia (Inouye, Foreman, Mion, Katz, & Cooney, 2001). This study found that nursing staff correctly identified patients with delirium only 31% of the time. When delirium subtypes were examined, patients with hypoactive delirium were seven times less likely to be recognized by the nursing staff. The multidimensional nature of delirium with its fluctuating course, variation in presentation from hyperactive and hypoactive subtypes, and lack of consensus as to its features all contribute to underrecognition. Because nurses have a 24-hour-a-day presence in acute care, intermediate, and long-term care settings, it is critical for nurses caring for elders to identify patients at risk, to assess accurately patients with cognitive and behavioral changes,

and to institute appropriate interventions to support patient safety and recovery. To do this successfully requires ongoing education and training for nurses in all aspects of the delirium syndrome. Likewise, given nursing's role in the delegation or supervision of care by paraprofessionals in home care settings, nurses can provide informal caregivers and paraprofessional staff with education regarding symptom recognition of delirium and action steps to take.

ASSESSMENT AND EVALUATION

Because there is no one single diagnostic test for delirium, the evaluation of the patient should focus first on identifying that the disorder is in fact present, and second that any and all underlying contributing medical conditions and factors are treated or removed. This approach should include the elements discussed next.

Identify the Presence of Delirium

The critical point is to understand the patient's baseline cognitive status and the timing and onset of the symptoms. How is what is being observed different from the patient's baseline? Does the patient have an underlying dementia or other brain diseases, such as Parkinson's disease or history of a stroke? When did the patient first demonstrate a change in cognition or behavior? Clinicians may have to obtain the history from family members, formal caregivers, or staff members if the patient comes from an institutional setting. Because the hallmark of delirium is inattention, using mental status tests that require patient cooperation and attention may prove to be difficult. Standard mental status examinations, such as the Mini-Mental State Examination (Folstein, Folstein, & McHugh, 1975), may be used to question the patient and at least obtain some screening information. It is not uncommon to see patients with acute changes in mental status become more agitated with direct questioning. For patients who may be lethargic and slow to respond, direct questioning may not provide an accurate assessment. Although there are many tests of mental status, only a few are specific to diagnosing delirium:

Delirium Symptom Interview (Albert et al., 1992)

Delirium Rating Scale (Trepacz, Baker, & Greenhouse, 1988)

Confusion Assessment Method (Inouye et al., 1990)

Memorial Delirium Assessment Scale (Breibart et al., 1997)

Delirium Observation Screening (Schuurmans, Shortridge-Baggett, & Duursma, 2003)

NEECHAM Confusion Scale (Neelon, Champagne, Carlson, & Funk, 1996)

Tools that are most useful for nursing practice include those that are brief and easy to use, without being burdensome to the patient. The most commonly used is the Confusion Assessment Method (CAM) developed by Inouye et al. (1990). The CAM is a simple tool that can be used quickly and accurately at the bedside by all clinicians to diagnose delirium. It has a sensitivity of 94–100% and a specificity of 90–95% (Inouye et al., 1990) (Box 11-1). The diagnosis of delirium requires the presence of features 1 and 2 and either 3 and 4. It can also help differentiate between delirium and dementia. The CAM-ICU is a version developed specifically for use in critical care settings and can be used with ventilated patients (Ely et al., 2001).

BOX 11-1 CAM

1. Acute onset and fluctuating course	Usually obtained from a family member or nurse and shown by positive responses to the following questions: "Is there evidence of an acute change in mental status from the baseline?"; "Did the abnormal behavior fluctuate during the day, that is, tend to come and go, or increase and decrease in severity?"
2. Inattention	Shown by a positive response to the following: "Did the patient have difficulty focusing attention, for example, being easily distractible or having difficulty keeping track of what was being said?"
3. Disorganized thinking	Shown by a positive response to the following: "Was the patient's thinking disoriented or incoherent, such as rambling or irrelevant conversation, unclear or illogical flow of ideas, or unpredictable switching from subject to subject?"
4. Altered level of consciousness	Shown by any answer other than "alert" to the following: "Overall, how would you rate this patient's level of consciousness?" Normal = alert Hyperalert = vigilant Drowsy, easily aroused = lethargic Difficult to arouse = stupor Unarousable = coma

Source: Inouye, van Dyck, Alessi, Balkin, Siegal, & Horwitz (1990). Used with permission.

Although CAM is useful for diagnosing the presence of delirium (patients either have it or they do not), another tool is available to quantify the severity or intensity of symptoms. The Memorial Delirium Assessment Scale was originally developed for use with cancer patients with delirium. It scores patients on a scale of 0 to 30 (30 being worst score) using a 10-item inventory that measures arousal, level of consciousness, psychomotor activity memory, attention, orientation, and thinking (Breibart et al., 1997). The Memorial Delirium Assessment Scale can be used in conjunction with CAM for a complete assessment.

It is also important for clinicians to be able to differentiate features of delirium from dementia and depression in elderly patients, because features of all three may coexist in an individual (Table 11-2). It has been estimated that the prevalence of delirium superimposed on dementia ranges from 22 to 89% in both hospitalized and community dwelling elders (Fick, Agostini, & Inouye, 2002). Patients with a hypoactive delirium may be identified as being depressed rather than delirious. When in doubt, always diagnose delirium because patients who go untreated are at greater risk than those patients who simply have a chronic cognitive impairment. Always investigate a change in cognitive or behavioral signs and symptoms in elderly patients, and never assume they are "normal." The family or other caregivers should be asked if the patient had ever experienced previous episodes of delirium and under what circumstances.

Identify and Treat Underlying Medical Conditions

The mnemonic DELIRIUM, outlined next, is a helpful tool for identifying reversible causes of delirium. Rarely is delirium caused by only one factor. It is important to review and treat all possible contributing factors.

Drugs: Review the record for the list of medications, with particular note of anything newly added or omitted that may lend a clue as to the cause of the change in mental status.

Even if a person has been on a medication for years, this does not mean that it is not the cause for a delirium. A drug that was started when a person was 60 years of age is metabolized differently once that same person's liver and kidneys are 80 years old, and the situation may now be compounded by dehydration and sepsis. Is the patient undergoing withdrawal? Is the patient taking any over-the-counter medications? Drug levels may be useful in identifying toxic quantities.

Electrolyte abnormalities, dehydration: The usual evaluation includes blood work to identify imbalances in sodium, potassium, blood urea nitrogen, creatinine, calcium, and glucose. Is the patient dehydrated? A urine-specific gravity and color can indicate hydration status.

Low oxygen states (myocardial infarction [MI], stroke): An oxygenation saturation level quickly rules out a low oxygen state as a contributing factor.

Infection: A urinalysis and culture can rule in a urinary tract infection, which is a common cause of mental status changes. Patients recently discharged from an acute care setting are at risk for developing urinary tract infection as an iatrogenic complication of hospitalization. Auscultate the patient's lungs; pneumonia in an older adult often presents without classic signs of fever and cough, and a change in mental status may be the only indication of an underlying pulmonary process. An elevated white blood count can also indicate an acute infection.

Reduced sensory input: Is the patient without his or her glasses or hearing aids? Is the patient in an understimulating or overstimulating environment? Does that patient have access to orienting devices, such as a watch, clock, or calendar? Has the patient recently undergone multiple transfers across settings (i.e., home to ED, to ICU, to general unit, to a skilled nursing facility)?

Intracranial (cerebrovascular accident, transient ischemic attack, seizure): Does the patient

TABLE 11-2

Comparison of the Clinical Features of Delirium, Dementia, and Depression

Clinical Feature	Delirium	Dementia	Depression
Onset	Acute/subacute, depends on cause, often at twilight or in darkness	Chronic, generally insidious, depends on cause	Coincides with major life changes, often abrupt
Course	Short, diurnal fluctuations in symptoms, worse at night, in darkness, and on awakening	Long, no diurnal effects, symptoms progressive yet relatively stable over time	Diurnal effects, typically worse in the morning, situational fluctuations, but less than with delirium
Progression	Abrupt	Slow but uneven	Variable, rapid or slow but even
Duration	Hours to less than 1 month, seldom longer	Months to years	At least 6 weeks, can be several months to years
Awareness	Reduced	Clear	Clear
Alertness	Fluctuates, lethargic or hypervigilant	Generally normal	Normal
Attention	Impaired, fluctuates	Generally normal	Minimal impairment, but is easily distracted
Orientation	Generally impaired, severity varies	Generally normal	Selective disorientation
Memory	Recent and immediate impaired	Recent and remote impaired	Selective or "patchy" impairment, "islands" of intact memory
Thinking	Disorganized, distorted, fragmented, incoherent speech, either slow or accelerated	Difficulty with abstraction, thoughts impoverished, judgment impaired, words difficult to find	Intact but with themes of hopelessness, helplessness, or self-deprecation
Perception	Distorted, illusions, delusions, and hallucinations, difficulty distinguishing between reality and misperceptions	Misperceptions usually absent	Intact, delusions and hallucinations absent except in severe cases
Psychomotor behavior	Variable, hypokinetic, hyperkinetic, and mixed	Normal, may have apraxia	Variable, psychomotor retardation or agitation
Sleep–wake cycle	Disturbed, cycle reversed	Fragmented	Disturbed, usually early morning awakening
Associated features	Variable affective changes, symptoms of autonomic hyperarousal, exaggeration of personality type, associated with acute physical illness	Affect tends to be superficial, inappropriate and labile, attempts to conceal deficits in intellect, personality changes, aphasia, agnosia may be present, lacks insight	Affect depressed, dysphoric mood, exaggerated and detailed complaints, preoccupied with personal thoughts, insight present, verbal elaboration
Assessment	Distracted from task, numerous errors	Failings highlighted by family, frequent "near miss" answers, struggles with test, great effort to find an appropriate reply, frequent requests for feedback on performance	Failings highlighted by individual, frequently answers "don't know," little effort, frequently gives up, indifferent toward test, does not care or attempt to find answer

Source: Foreman, M., Fletcher, K., Mion, L., & Simon, L. (1996). Assessing cognitive function. *Geriatric Nursing, 17*(5), 229. Copyright 1996 by Elsevier. Reprinted with permission.

have a history of a recent fall, which might indicate a slowly accumulating subdural hematoma? A screening neurological examination might reveal deficits that indicate vascular compromise. Determine if the patient has a history of seizures or other neurological conditions or impairments. Patients may undergo brain imaging, either CT or MRI, to rule out structural abnormalities.

Urinary or fecal retention: An abdominal and rectal examination and review of the intake and output sheet gives a clue as to whether retention of urine or stool is a cause.

Myocardial (congestive heart failure, MI, arrhythmia): Does the patient have a history of heart disease, including MI or arrhythmia? In the older adult, an MI may present with only a change in mental status instead of the classic signs of substernal chest pain. A thorough cardiovascular assessment including an electrocardiogram can help determine cardiac abnormalities.

Applying this mnemonic to Mr. V. reveals the following likely contributing factors to his delirium: urinary tract infection and pneumonia, white blood count of 11.4; no glasses or hearing aids; and dementia. A thorough evaluation of all potentially contributing factors is critical to planning interventions and subsequent care.

SUPPORTING SAFETY AND RECOVERY

The goal of care for patients with a suspected delirium is to support and protect the patient while the underlying causes are identified and treated. There is no question that nursing care of the delirious, older patient can be both challenging and frustrating for even the most experienced nurse. No one thing works; appropriate nursing care of patients with delirium generally includes psychosocial, behavioral, and environmental support. The number of research studies that have tested the effect of specific interventions on patient outcomes is quite limited. The lack of a strong relationship between specific nursing interventions and a change in a patient outcome (i.e., reduction in the delirium state) compels the challenge of assumptions about practices that have been defined as the gold standard. Research has not been able to demonstrate which interventions work best in combination or determine the timing or sequencing of these interventions. Interventions work best when they are tailored to the individual patient. In one study of experienced nursing care of delirious hospitalized elderly, nurses used a range of interventions that were tailored to the patient's degree of confusion (Dick, 1998). For example, reorienting, cueing, and explaining hospital routines were useful strategies when a patient was less confused or agitated. The same cognitive strategies were not useful in patients who were highly confused because they were found to agitate patients further. For these patients, environmental strategies of minimizing stimulation, dimming lights, and minimizing physical presence (i.e., limiting the number of unnecessary interactions) were useful (Figure 11-1). Another finding from this study was that nurses did not always attempt to reorient patients who were disoriented. If the patient was agitated, it made no sense to reply to the hospitalized patient who believes he is in his house and has to go upstairs, "Mr. Smith, you are not at home, you are in the hospital." Sometimes "going to where the patient is" can be very useful and helps to calm the patient, rather than arguing about the patient's perceptions, particularly if they are frightening or worrisome. Examples of an appropriate response might be, "I am here to help you. What is upstairs that you need?" or "Is there something upstairs that you are worried about, Mr. Smith?"

In practice, nurses often learn from trial and error. Most nurses have been taught the standard interventions, such as repeated orientation, promoting proper sleep habits, early mobilization, timely removal of catheters, avoiding restraints, and the use of glasses and hearing aids. These are important components of care for the patient with delirium. The question remains, however, as to what types of interventions work best with what

FIGURE 11-1

Nursing Strategies.

Degree of patient's confusion/agitation

High ◄─────────────────────────────────► Low

Environmental	Physical/sensory	Cognitive
Close observation	Maximizing or minimizing touch	Orienting/reorienting
Dimming lights, noise	Maximizing or minimizing physical presence	Cueing/coaching
Minimizing stimulation/ interventions	Assist with activities of daily living	Explanation/reassurance
Restraints (use as last resort)	Ensuring sensory aids: glasses, hearing aids, watch, clock, calendar	Helping patient "make sense of it"

Source: Dick (1998). Reprinted with permission.

kinds of delirium symptoms and when are they best carried out. For example, a family member may calm patients with a hyperactive delirium by being in constant attendance, and the reduction of environmental stimulation provided by being in a private room may be helpful. A patient with hypoactive delirium may do better with increased stimulation and staff contact. It is important to find out as much as possible about the patient's usual habits and patterns, and if possible recreate them in an attempt to "restore normalcy." This may be hard to do in a busy hospital setting or when no information is available, but attempting to establish familiar routines can be very useful.

In a 1999 publication by Inouye et al., standardized intervention protocols for the management of six risk factors for delirium were used as part of a multicomponent intervention study and later became more formally known as the Hospital Elder Life program. The six standardized protocols were for the management of (1) cognitive impairment, (2) sleep deprivation, (3) immobility,

(4) visual impairment, (5) hearing impairment, and (6) dehydration. This risk factor intervention strategy resulted in significant reductions in the number and duration of episodes of delirium in hospitalized older patients. The intervention had no significant effect, however, on the severity of delirium or on recurrence rates. This finding suggests that primary prevention of delirium is probably the most important treatment strategy.

Physical and chemical restraints should be avoided wherever possible and used only in situations where patients are at risk for injuring themselves or others, or when agitation and restlessness may interfere with necessary medical treatments. A volunteer or "sitter" to stay with the patient during an acute episode reduces the risk of injury and may have a calming effect. Small doses of haloperidol and droperidol may be useful in controlling agitation and psychosis, and dosing should be guided by the patient's initial response and by frequent reassessment. Benzodiazepines are useful in the treatment of alcohol and sedative withdrawal.

It can be very difficult for family members and friends to see their loved one agitated and disoriented. Patients and families need reassurance and explanation that the delirium is related to the medical condition and is not a sign that the patient is "crazy," is "losing his or her mind," or is becoming "senile." A thorough explanation of the condition and short-term course is helpful in allaying fears. Involve family members in the plan of care including providing one-to-one observation, stimulation, support, and bringing in familiar objects from home. Patients also need an opportunity to reflect on the experience and to express their feelings as symptoms subside.

Because it is now known that delirium symptoms can persist for many weeks and months after an acute hospitalization, new models for care of delirious patients in posthospital settings are also needed. One such model is the Delirium Abatement Program, which incorporates assessment of delirium symptoms, evaluation and treatment of reversible causes of delirium, prevention and management of common complications, and restoration of cognitive and self-care function in delirious patients (Bergmann, Murphy, Kiely, Jones, & Marcantonio, 2005). This model has promise for those patients with persistent delirium who cannot be discharged home and who need continued care and support. The goals of treatment for all patients with delirium are to promote recovery, prevent additional complications, maintain the patient's safety, and maximize function.

DOCUMENTATION

Nurses have information that needs to be communicated to the other caregivers who are seeing the patient for only a brief time during the day and not at all at night. Because the nature of delirium is that symptoms wax and wane, and because there are many components of delirium, documentation that is helpful in making an accurate diagnosis is essential. Nurses, however, consistently underdocument cognitive symptoms. In a study

of the medical and nursing records of 55 patients hospitalized with hip fracture who experienced delirium, documentation of essential symptoms including onset and course of the syndrome and disturbances in consciousness, attention, and cognition were seldom or never found in the nursing records (Milisen et al., 2002). Nurses tend to focus on orientation, which is just one marker of mental functioning. In our 1994 study of hospitalized elderly, we found that although nurses' assessment of level of orientation matched an independent rating by a standardized instrument for the detection of delirium symptoms 81% of the time, nurses did less well assessing and documenting alterations in other domains, including fluctuating behavior (56%), perceptual disturbances (41%), and increased or decreased psychomotor behavior (64%) (Morency, Levkoff, & Dick, 1994). Because many delirious patients may do well on the orientation portion of a cognitive status examination, only describing the patient's level of orientation is not useful or complete. In the case of Mr. V., on the day of discharge his attending physician only comments on his orientation, with no mention about his level of functioning, which is radically different from his baseline. This level of functioning and risk for falls changes the amount and type of nursing care that he needs on discharge. Few nursing notes specifically mention fluctuating level of consciousness, which is the hallmark of delirium. Even the terminology used is confusing. For example, what is the difference between mental status and cognitive status? For clarification "mental status" is a broader concept that includes intellectual functioning, and emotional, attitudinal, psychological, and personality aspects of an individual. In contrast, "cognitive status" refers more specifically only to the aspect of intellectual functioning. Nurses should use the term "cognitive status" to refer to what they are evaluating.

Does the lack of documentation about cognitive status mean that it was not assessed or that it was assessed and there was no problem? Does "appears alert and oriented × 3" mean that the nurse actually asked the orientation questions or that there was no discernible problem in general conversation? How many patients with intact social skills are called oriented, but actually are not? There also may be no relationship between level of orientation and patient safety. A patient who is identified as oriented may lack appropriate judgment and attempt to get out of bed while on bedrest, or interfere with medical treatments. Simply put, describing a patient as "oriented" is not particularly useful.

Consider the following nursing documentation of a patient whose admission note says "alert and oriented × 3″ with no other mention of cognitive status. There is nothing about any cognitive problems at home, although the patient was described as a "poor historian." The following day the note says "appears confused" but no clarification. The third day the patient is described as "lethargic" and that night is "agitated." Although the warning signs were there and the patient was at risk for delirium, it is often not until the delirium is a full-blown problem that it is recognized in the nursing documentation. What kind of information in the documentation could have better addressed the issue of delirium? Why is it that if delirium is a medical emergency, nurses continue to be undereducated about its importance in the care of the elderly? Let us reexamine the preceding nursing note. On admission, the patient is accompanied by his wife, who seems to answer most of the history questions. The nurse can take this opportunity to either say to the wife "I'd like him to answer and then I'll ask you to fill in the information," or to ask the wife "Is your husband able to answer the questions?" If, for example, the wife answers, "Well, I handle all the medications," the nurse then can probe as to whether this is because of memory impairment or other cognitive deficit. Asking a simple question such as "Who pays the bills in your home?" gives a wealth of information. Paying the bills correctly and keeping the checkbook in balance requires a high level of cognitive functioning. This would provide good history in the nursing documentation as to whether there might be a preexisting dementia, which puts the person at risk

for delirium. On the first day when the patient "appears confused," an alternative note might have read "patient asked me if he was in a bakery, speech slow and halting, repetitive, awake most of the night, restless but not attempting to get out of bed." This gives information about orientation, speech, sleep, and psychomotor activity. On the following day, instead of "lethargic," the note could read "falling asleep while I was talking to him" or "trouble following directions, appears not to be able to focus." Delirium is not hard to miss in the subtype with psychomotor agitation who is climbing out of bed or verbally loud, but because a person with psychomotor retardation demands less attention from the nursing staff, particularly given the shortage of time, this subtype is more morbid, because it is more difficult to identify. The person may simply appear sleepy or "spacey."

It is also important that nurses accurately describe and document patients' cognitive status during times of transition, because nurses may underestimate the impact of incompletely and inaccurately describing cognitive status. It is easy to label patients as "confused" "disoriented" or "crazy." It does not matter if the patient is being transferred from the intensive care unit to a floor, from a hospital bed to a subacute bed, or from hospital to home: the documentation provided is critical to inform the receiving nursing staff. Often on discharge forms it is common to see such language as "patient is confused." What does that really mean? What does the nurse in the nursing home do with that information? Think about how much more helpful it would be to read something like "Patient with a long history of dementia, previously cared for at home by husband, who became acutely confused during hospital stay but has returned to prehospitalization baseline per husband. She is oriented to place only, is now calm and cooperative, and able to answer some questions." Nurses must be aware of the negative consequences of prematurely labeling patients. This occurs when inaccurate and incomplete information is passed along from setting to setting, and once labeled as "confused," patients may never be identified as having an acute problem. It is much more useful to identify specific patient cognitive abilities and behaviors.

ETHICAL ISSUES

Delirium by its nature impairs the capacity to make decisions. It seems that as long as the person with delirium is making a decision that the healthcare professionals agree with, the person's ability to make decisions is not questioned. However, if a person with delirium is making a decision about treatment that the staff does not agree with or is refusing necessary treatment, it is more likely to see notes stating that the person is not able to make decisions because of impaired cognitive status. In a prospective study of 173 medical and surgical procedures in patients with delirium at a university hospital, investigators found no documented assessments of competency or decision capacity and cognitive assessment in only 4% of cases (Auerswald, Charpentier, & Inouye, 1997). The fluctuating nature of delirium also becomes problematic: decisions involving informed consent are a good example. Are patients really able to make informed decisions with a mental status that waxes and wanes?

Patients who experience delirium may or may not be able to remember a delirious episode. Schofield (1997) found that those patients who had illusions or hallucinations were often able to describe their experiences in detail. The patients were more than willing to talk about their experiences. They ranged from being pleasant and entertaining to horrible and frightening. Patients were also able to remember short verbal commands from nurses. Some reported being reassured by explanations and comforting measures even though they were unable to communicate.

SUMMARY

Although more prevalent in the elderly, delirium is a medical emergency and should not be considered a normal part of aging, or a normal occurrence associated with hospitalization. Confusion is a symptom that something is wrong; it is never normal. Nurses are the key to timely and prompt recognition: there is not treatment without recognition. Now that we have defined delirium, identified individual risk factors, and discussed recognition, diagnosis, and treatment, the questions about the initial case study of Mr. V. can be answered. We now recognize that the risk factors for Mr. V. included advanced age, dementia, visual and hearing impairment, medications, and his chronic medical conditions including an indwelling catheter. Would his hospital course have been different if on admission his delirium were identified and considered to be a medical emergency? Key to proper diagnosis and treatment is the recognition that this may be a delirium in a patient with dementia. One would evaluate the contributing factors by going through the mnemonic of DELIRIUM, identifying contributors, and then working in conjunction with his primary care provider and advanced practice nurse to treat anything that can be treated or removed, remembering not to stop at one factor. Obtaining more information from his assisted living facility would have extremely helpful, asking the following questions: What is his baseline mental and functional status? What is his usual daily routine? Has he ever had similar behavior? If so, what interventions were useful? Appropriate interventions include promoting a more familiar environment by having a family member stay with him, having him wear his glasses and hearing aids, encouraging ambulation to maintain muscle strength and the eating of regular meals, monitoring his blood sugar, and encouraging normal sleep routines and patterns that reduce anxiety and promote familiarity. If one is working in assisted living or long-term care, the most important information that can be sent with the patient to the hospital is information related to baseline functioning and routines. Nurses can make all the difference in patient outcomes, and nowhere is that more true than in a patient with delirium. The following valuable resources are available:

The evidence-based protocol *Acute Confusion/ Delirium* developed by the Gerontological Nursing Intervention Research Center at the

University of Iowa is available at: http://www.nursing.uiowa.edu/products_services/evidence_based.htm

The Nursing Standard of Practice Protocol: Delirium: Prevention, Early Recognition, and Treatment is available through the Hartford Institute for Geriatric Nursing at: http:/consult gerirn.org/topics/delirium/want_to_know_more

The Hartford Institute also has many helpful protocols relating to the hospital care of elders in their *Try This* series available at: http://consultgerirn.org/resources/

More information about the Hospital Elder Life Program is available at: http://www.hospital elderlifeprogram.org

REFERENCES

Albert, M., Levkoff, S., Reilly, C., Liptzin, B., Pilgrim, D., Cleary, P., et al. (1992). The delirium symptom interview: An interview for the detection of delirium symptoms in hospitalized patients. *Journal of Geriatric Psychiatry and Neurology, 5*(1), 14–21.

American Psychiatric Association. (2000). *Diagnostic and statistical manual of mental disorders* (4th ed., Text Revision). Washington, DC: Author.

Auerswald, K., Charpentier, P., & Inouye, S. (1997). The informed consent process in older patients who developed delirium. *The American Journal of Medicine, 103*(5), 410–418.

Bergmann, M., Murphy, K., Kiely, D., Jones, R., & Marcantonio, E. (2005). A model for management of delirious postacute care patients. *Journal of the American Geriatrics Society, 53*(10), 1817–1825.

Brady, P. (1987). Labeling of confusion in the elderly. *Journal of Gerontological Nursing, 13*(6), 29–32.

Breibart, W., Rosenfield, B., Roth, A., Smith, M., Cohen, K., & Passik, S. (1997). The Memorial Delirium Assessment Scale. *Journal of Pain and Symptom Management, 13*(3), 128–137.

Burney-Puckett, M. (1996). Sundown syndrome: Etiology and management. *Journal of Psychosocial Nursing and Mental Health Services, 34*(5), 40–43.

Champagne, M., & Wiese, R. (1992). Research on cognitive impairment: Implications for practice. In S. G. Funk, E. M. Tornquist, M. T. Champagne, & R. A. Wiese (Eds.), *Key aspects of elder care* (pp. 340–346). New York: Springer.

Cole, M., & McCusker, J. (2002). Treatment of delirium in older medical inpatients: A challenge for geriatric specialists. *Journal of the American Geriatrics Society, 50*(12), 2101–2103.

Cole, M., McCusker, J., Dendukuri, N., & Han, L. (2003). The prognostic significance of subsyndromal delirium in elderly medical patients. *Journal of the American Geriatrics Society, 51*(6), 754–760.

Csokasy, J. (1999). Assessment of acute confusion: Use of the NEECHAM Confusion Scale. *Applied Nursing Research, 12*(1), 51–55.

Dick, K. (1998). Acute confusion in the elderly hospitalized patient: An exploration of experienced nursing care. (Doctoral dissertation, University of Rhode Island, 1998), *Dissertation Abstracts International, 59*, 4015.

Ely, E., Margolin, R., Francis, J., May, L., Truman, B., Dittus, R., et al. (2001). Evaluation of delirium in critically ill patients: Validation of the Confusion Assessment Method for the intensive care unit (CAM ICU). *Critical Care Medicine, 29*(7), 1370–1379.

Fick, D., Agostini, J., & Inouye, S. (2002). Delirium superimposed on dementia: A systematic review. *Journal of the American Geriatrics Society, 50*(10), 1723–1732.

Fick, D., & Foreman, M. (2000). Consequences of not recognizing delirium superimposed on dementia in hospitalized elderly patients. *Journal of Gerontological Nursing, 26*(1), 30–40.

Fick, D., Hodo, D., Lawrence, F., & Inouye, S. (2007). Recognizing delirium superimposed on dementia. *Journal of Gerontological Nursing, 33*(2), 40–49.

Folstein, M., Folstein, S., & McHugh, P. (1975). Mini-mental state: A practical method for grading cognitive state of patients for the clinician. *Journal of Psychiatric Research, 12*, 189–198.

Fong, T., Tulebaev, S., & Inouye, S. (2009). Delirium in elderly adults: Diagnosis, prevention and treatment. *Nature Reviews Neurology, 5*, 210–220.

Foreman, M. (1986). Acute confusional states in hospitalized elderly: A research dilemma. *Nursing Research, 35*(1), 34–38.

Foreman, M. (1989). Confusion in the hospitalized elderly. *Research in Nursing & Health, 12,* 21–29.

Foreman, M. (1993). Acute confusion in the elderly. *Annual Review of Nursing Research, 11,* 3–30.

Francis, J., & Kapoor, W. (1990). Delirium in hospitalized elderly. *Journal of General Internal Medicine, 5,* 65–79.

Francis, J., & Kapoor, W. (1992). Prognosis after hospital discharge of older medical patients with delirium. *Journal of the American Geriatrics Society, 40*(6), 601–606.

Francis, J., Martin, D., & Kapoor, W. (1990). A prospective study of delirium in hospitalized elderly. *JAMA, 263*(8), 1097–1101.

Gruber-Baldini, A., Zimmerman, S., Morrison, R., Grattan, L., Hebel, J., Dolan, M., et al. (2003). Cognitive impairment in hip fracture patients: Timing of detection and longitudinal follow-up. *Journal of the American Geriatrics Society, 51*(9), 1227–1236.

Hshieh, T., Fong, T., Marcantonio, E., & Inouye, S. (2008). Cholinergic deficiency hypothesis in delirium: A synthesis of current evidence. *Journal of Gerontology: Biological Sciences, 63*(7), 764–772.

Inouye, S. (1998). Delirium in hospitalized older patients. *Clinics in Geriatric Medicine, 14,* 745–764.

Inouye, S., Bogardus, S., Charpentier, P., Leo-Summers, L., Acampora, D., Holford, T., et al. (1999). A multicomponent intervention to prevent delirium in hospitalized older patients. *New England Journal of Medicine, 340*(9), 669–676.

Inouye, S., Foreman, M., Mion, L., Katz, K., & Cooney, L. (2001). Nurses recognition of delirium and its symptoms: Comparison of nurse and researcher ratings. *Archives of Internal Medicine, 16*(20), 2467–2473.

Inouye, S., van Dyck, C., Alessi, C., Balkin, S., Siegal, A., & Horwitz, R. (1990). Clarifying confusion: The Confusion Assessment Method. *Annals of Internal Medicine, 13*(12), 941–948.

Inouye, S., Viscoli, C., Horwitz, R., Hurst, L., & Tinetti, M. (1993). A predictive model for delirium in hospitalized elderly medical patients based on admission characteristics. *Annals of Internal Medicine, 119,* 474–481.

Johnson, J. (1990). Delirium in the elderly. *Emergency Clinics of North America, 8*(2), 255–264.

Leslie, D., Marcantonio, E., Zhang, Y., Leo-Summers, L., & Inouye, S. (2008). One year health care costs associated with delirium in the elderly population. *Archives of Internal Medicine, 168,* 27–32.

Levkoff, S., Besdine, R., & Wetle, T. (1986). Acute confusional states in the hospitalized elderly. *Annual Review of Gerontology and Geriatrics, 6,* 1–26.

Levkoff, S., Cleary, P., Liptzin, B., & Evans, D. (1991). Epidemiology of delirium: An overview of research issues and findings. *International Psychogeriatrics, 3*(2), 149–167.

Levkoff, S., Evans, D., Liptzin, B., Cleary, P., Lipsitz, L., Wetle, T., et al. (1992). Delirium: The occurrence and persistence of symptoms among elderly hospitalized patients. *Archives of Internal Medicine, 152,* 334–340.

Lipowski, Z. (1983). Transient cognitive disorders in the elderly. *American Journal of Psychiatry, 140*(11), 1426–1436.

Lipowski, Z. (1987). Delirium (acute confusional states). *JAMA, 258,* 1789–1792.

Lipowski, Z. (1989). Delirium in the elderly patient. *The New England Journal of Medicine, 320*(9), 578–582.

Liptzin, B. (1995). Delirium. *Archives of Family Medicine, 4,* 453–458.

Liptzin, B., & Levkoff, S. (1992). An empirical study of delirium subtypes. *British Journal of Psychiatry, 161,* 843–845.

Ludwick, R. (1993). Nurses' response to patient's confusion. (Doctoral dissertation, Kent State University, 1993). *Dissertation Abstracts International, 54,* 1548.

Lyness, J. (1990). Delirium: Masquerades and misdiagnosis in elderly inpatients. *Journal of the American Geriatrics Society, 38*(11), 1235–1238.

Mach, J., Dysken, M., Kuskowski, M., Richelson, E., Holden, L., & Jilk, K. (1995). Serum anticholinergic activity in hospitalized older persons with delirium: A preliminary study. *Journal of the American Geriatrics Society, 43*(5), 491–495.

Marcantonio, E., Flacker, J., Wright, R., & Resnick, N. (2001). Reducing delirium after hip fracture: A randomized trial. *Journal of the American Geriatrics Society, 49*(5), 516–522.

Marcantonio, E., Simon, S., Bergmann, M., Jones, R., Murphy, K., & Morris, J. (2003). Delirium symptoms in post acute care: Prevalent, persistent, and associated with poor functional recovery. *Journal of the American Geriatrics Society, 51*(5), 4–9.

Marcantonio, E., Ta, T., Duthie, E., & Resnick, N. (2002). Reducing delirium after hip fracture: A randomized trial. *Journal of the American Geriatrics Society, 49*(5), 516–522.

McCarthy, M. (1991). Interpretation of confusion in the aged: Conflicting models of clinical reasoning among nurses. (Doctoral dissertation, University of California at San Francisco, 1991). *Dissertation Abstracts International, 53,* 0203.

Milisen, K., Foreman, M., Wouters, B., Driesen, R., Godderis, J., Abraham, I., et al. (2002). Documentation of delirium in elderly patients with hip fracture. *Journal of Gerontological Nursing, 28*(1), 23–29.

Miller, J. (1991). A clinical study to pilot test the environmental optimization interventions protocol. (Doctoral dissertation, Oregon Health Sciences University, 1991.) *Dissertation Abstracts International, 53,* 0772.

Morency, C., Levkoff, S., & Dick, K. (1994). Research considerations: Delirium in hospitalized elders. *Journal of Gerontological Nursing, 20*(8), 24–30.

Morgan, D. (1985). Nurses' perceptions of mental confusion in the elderly: Influence of resident and setting characteristics. *Journal of Health and Social Behavior, 26,* 102–112.

Murray, A., Levkoff, S., Wetle, T., Beckett, L., Cleary, P., Schor, J., et al. (1993). Acute delirium and functional decline in the hospitalized elderly patient. *Journal of Gerontology, 48*(5), M181–M186.

Neelon, V. (1990). Postoperative confusion. *Critical Care Nursing Clinics of North America, 2*(4), 579–587.

Neelon, V., Champagne, M., Carlson, J., & Funk, S. (1996). The NEECHAM Confusion scale: Construction, validation and testing. *Nursing Research, 45*(6), 324–330.

Neelon, V., Funk, S., Carlson, J., & Champagne, M. (1989). The NEECHAM Confusion scale: Relationship to clinical indicators of acute confusion in hospitalized elders. *Gerontologist, 29,* 65A.

Nowak, L., & Davis, J. (2007). A qualitative examination of the phenomenon of sundowning. *Journal of Nursing Scholarship, 39*(3), 256–258.

Palmateer, L., & McCartney, J. (1985). Do nurses know when patients have cognitive impairments? *Journal of Gerontological Nursing, 11*(2), 6–16.

Rasin, J. (1990). Confusion. *Nursing Clinics of North America, 25*(4), 909–918.

Rockwood, K. (1993). The occurrence and duration of symptoms in elderly patients with delirium. *Journal of Gerontology, 48*(4), M162–166.

Rudberg, M., Pompei, P., Foreman, M., Ross, R., & Cassel, C. (1997). The natural history of delirium in older hospitalized patients: A syndrome of heterogeneity. *Age and Ageing, 26*(3), 169–174.

Schofield, I. (1997). A small exploratory study of the reaction of older people to an episode of delirium. *Journal of Advanced Nursing, 25,* 942–952.

Schor, J., Levkoff, S., Lipsitz, L., Reilly, C., Cleary, P., Rowe, J., et al. (1992). Risk factors for delirium in the hospitalized elderly. *JAMA, 267*(6), 827–831.

Schuurmans, M., Shortridge-Baggett, L., & Duursma, S. (2003). The Delirium Observation Scale: A screening instrument for delirium. *Research and Theory for Nursing Practice, 17*(1), 31–50.

Trepacz, P., Baker, R., & Greenhouse, J. (1988). A symptom rating scale for delirium. *Psychiatric Research, 23,* 89–97.

Vermeersch, P. (1991). Response to "The cognitive and behavioral nature of acute confusional states." *Scholarly Inquiry for Nursing Practice, 5*(1), 17–20.

Wolanin, M., & Phillips, L. (1981). *Confusion: Prevention and care.* St. Louis, MO: Mosby.

12

Nursing Assessment of Clients with Dementias of Late Life
Screening, Diagnosis, and Communication

Kathleen Sherrell

Madelyn Iris

Tracy Ann Ramos

As a clinician, teacher, and researcher, I think of myself as somewhat of an expert in the field of dementia. However, when my mother—previously an intellectually brilliant person with a better than average memory—began to show signs of confusion, I denied that she could have dementia. At first, she lost some of her ability to concentrate. She had always been an avid reader, but was now losing her sight, so I sent her books on tape every month. Then I would call her long distance, planning to discuss the book over the phone. When she began to complain that the books were confusing or poorly written, I felt badly because I had not chosen the "right" books. Then Mother began to complain that my sister-in-law was being "mean" to her. This would have been totally out of character for my sister-in-law, but I believed my mother and became upset with my sister-in-law. Eventually, I brought my mother to a medical center near my home for evaluation by a geriatric team. The neuropsychologist invited me to sit in on the examination. At first my mother seemed to pass all the tests with flying colors. She could repeat information back to the examiner, could repeat numbers backward and forward, and showed no signs of impairment. I felt relief. Then she was asked to name as many animals as she could within a short period of time. My mother's vocabulary had always been vast and comprehensive. Yet on this day, she was only able to name three

common barnyard animals. Fluency is a significant factor in assessing the cognitive domain of language, and animal naming is often used as a short test to screen for dementia. That was the only sign of impairment revealed during the neuropsychological examination; nevertheless, she was given a diagnosis of probable Alzheimer's disease. The geriatrician told me that my mother's complaints were likely a sign of paranoia, a behavioral symptom of dementia. She said I should "start preparing for the next stage." Yet I still refused to believe my mother had dementia and that it was becoming worse. When I told my brother the diagnosis, he became angry with me, as if it were my fault because I had initiated the diagnostic process. As time went on, the signs of dementia became more evident. When my mother had to be moved to a nursing home, I finally had to accept the diagnosis. When the day came that she did not know me, I was devastated once more, even though I had known that it was inevitable. This is a brief version of the complex and difficult journey made by my mother, my siblings, and I. In our family as in many others, a diagnosis of dementia has broad repercussions. There is a benefit in knowing the reason for the confusion, but this is often outweighed by the distressing knowledge that the condition is progressive and incurable. This calculation of benefit and cost makes the process of assessment and communicating the diagnosis a complex experience for all concerned. It cannot be adequately described by simple rules and standardized test results.

Kathleen Sherrell

Nurses play an important role in the screening, diagnosing, and communicating of results when working with patients and families of older adults with dementia. This role has not been fully appreciated. The shortfall between the existing role of nursing and a fully realized role depends in large measure on the formalization of nursing knowledge and skills in these areas. This chapter provides a formulation of nursing knowledge and skills needed for assessment of clients with dementias of late life. It encapsulates much of what we have learned working with clients with dementias in a variety of settings, including clinics, nursing homes, research studies, and private practice.

The first section of this chapter deals with nurses' knowledge about dementia. It summarizes the relevant research on the neurobiological characteristics of dementia and more recent research on treatable behavioral and psychological symptoms, and the existential experience of dementia.

The second section of the chapter focuses on the important role of nurses in the assessment process. This section includes a description of selected standardized instruments used in the assessment of dementia. The chapter describes the ideal interdisciplinary practice that is still in the future, but necessary, if nursing practice is to achieve an optimized role in dementia assessment. The role of nurses as a vital part of the assessment team is described.

Professionals need to know how difficult and confusing it is for a person or family members to initiate the search for a diagnosis of dementia. Diagnosis-seeking behavior is a qualitative aspect of assessment and has received less attention in past research than the quantitative use of evaluation tools to establish a diagnosis. Findings from research on diagnosis-seeking behavior in clients with Alzheimer's disease (AD) and their families are presented.

In the final section, the authors discuss techniques of communicating the diagnosis to the person with dementia and to the family. Communication about the dementia diagnosis is complex because of its devastating impact, because it is "incurable," and because up until this point families are often in denial about the possibility of receiving a diagnosis of dementia. We conclude with some recommendations for nursing practice and nursing research into the assessment of clients with AD and other dementias.

ALZHEIMER'S DISEASE AND OTHER DEMENTIAS

In the past 20 years, there has been an exponential increase in knowledge about various kinds of dementia. Although cognitive deficits caused by neurological degeneration remain the principal and most researched features of dementia, the disease is also characterized by clinically important behavioral and psychological symptoms. This section describes recent research advances in the assessment and treatment of behavioral and psychological symptoms and promotes a relatively new focus of research on the existential (or subjective and qualitative) experience of dementia. This recent research contributes to a unique nursing perspective on assessment of dementias.

With the aging of the world's population, research has shown a significant increase in the numbers of older adults with irreversible dementias. It is the most common disease of the aging brain and represents a growing public health problem as the world population expands and ages. According to statistics published by the Administration on Aging (2007), the older population (65 and older) numbered 37.9 million in 2007, an increase of 2.9 million since 2000. The number of Americans aged 45–65 who will reach 65 by the year 2050 is projected to reach 88.5 million. The numbers of persons 85 and older in 2008 were 5.4 million, and these figures are expected to triple to 19 million by 2050. Life expectancy at birth in 2006 was 78.1 years, a 0.3% increase from 2005, with AD surpassing diabetes to become the sixth leading cause of death in 2006. These increases have major implications for the provision of health care generally and for dementia assessment in particular.

THE NEUROBIOLOGY OF DEMENTIA

Dementia has long been recognized as a syndrome of neurobiological etiology. The term "dementia" (from the Latin *demens*, meaning "without mind") has ancient origins. It was used in European vernaculars as early as the 17th and 18th centuries. Cognitive impairment was accepted as the defining feature of dementia by the late 1800s. When Alois Alzheimer published the first paper on the neuropathology of dementia in 1906, his description included the presence of neurofibrils and plaques in the brain. In the 1960s and 1970s, comprehensive neuropathological studies demonstrated that the brain changes described by Alzheimer were a common cause of cognitive decline in older adults. The elucidation of specific diseases under the rubric of dementia has continued into the 21st century.

Dementia, therefore, is not a disease but rather a syndrome, often of a chronic and progressive nature, in which there is a gradual or sometimes rapid decline of cognitive functions accompanied by deterioration in emotional control, language skills, and social behavior. Dementia occurs in AD, cerebrovascular disorders, and other conditions primarily or secondarily affecting the brain. Most frequently, it affects older adults. Usually the course is progressive and irreversible, and despite significant advances present treatments are only minimally effective in slowing the progression. One of the benefits of the diagnosis of dementia is to help distinguish this syndrome from a temporary disturbance in the level of consciousness called "delirium." Dementia can be differentiated from delirium because in the early stages of dementia there is no impairment of perception or consciousness. There is, however, loss of cognitive and intellectual abilities characterized by disorientation, loss of memory, impaired judgment, intellectual and social functioning, personality change, and shallow and labile affect. Along with these progressive cognitive disabilities, there is

also a high prevalence of behavioral and psychological symptoms.

There has been a great deal of controversy regarding the use of the term "dementia" (Sachdev, 2000). Initially, it was used to describe a syndrome that was so general and all-inclusive that it might well be called a "garbage can diagnosis." Research has determined that there are at least 70 possible causes of dementia (Cohen et al., 1993) and that each cause has a unique presentation of symptoms and laboratory results. However, these causes can also have great similarities in presentation, thus making definitive subtype diagnosis very difficult. Even though use of the term is confusing, a proposal to abandon the term is also problematic because the term "dementia" has wide acceptance beyond the medical community in general public health, legislation, community affairs, and lay usage. There is, moreover, a large and growing industry that is dependent on the term. The most commonly used definitions of dementia, from the *Diagnostic and Statistical Manual of Mental Disorders Text Revision* (4th ed.) (American Psychiatric Association, 2000) and International Classification of Diseases and Related Health Problems, 10th revision, emphasize memory impairment along with impairment in other cognitive domains. This "memory impairment" criterion is appropriate for AD, but it is restrictive when applied to dementia from other causes, such as vascular dementia (VaD) or frontotemporal dementia (FTD), in which memory impairment is not the most significant symptom. VaD can produce impairment in several cognitive domains while affecting memory only mildly or not at all, and in FTD, frontal–executive and language disturbance may be quite prominent early in the course of the disease.

Despite the previously mentioned problems with the term, "dementia" is still the most universal term used to describe the cognitive changes affecting intellectual and physical function and occurring mostly in older adults. The major development leading to expanded research on dementia has been the increase in prevalence of AD caused by the aging of our growing population. At present, AD has become the prototypical dementia. Even though more than 70 conditions can cause dementia in older adults (Cohen et al., 1993), AD is by far the most common. AD accounts for more than 50% of dementia cases, followed by VaD (15–20%). Because AD and VaD are the two most common causes of dementia, together accounting for nearly two thirds of all dementia cases, this chapter focuses primarily on assessment of dementia from these two causes. Considerable overlap is present between the two, including progressive cognitive, functional, and behavioral decline; neuronal loss; shared risk factors; and neurochemical deficits (Brashear, 2003; Erkinjuntti et al., 2002; Kalaria & Ballard, 1999). The course of the disease in VaD is said to be more fluctuating, with a more stepwise progression. Also, higher rates of depressive symptoms have been described in VaD compared to AD (Evans, 1990).

BEHAVIORAL AND PSYCHOLOGICAL SYMPTOMS OF DEMENTIA

There are two major groups of symptoms that characterize the dementias: symptoms of cognitive dysfunction, and behavioral and psychological symptoms. In most cases, the two groups of symptoms coexist. For example, in this chapter's introductory vignette, two of the early symptoms were difficulty in concentration, which is a cognitive symptom, and paranoia, which is a behavioral symptom.

A 2005 study of 435 patients with AD found the most prevalent early symptoms included apathy, depression, and irritability, whereas delusional symptoms were the least prevalent. Behaviors to emerge late in the course of the disease were hallucinations and abnormal motor movements (Craig, Mirakhur, Hart, Mcilroy, & Passmore, 2005).

Treatments for cognitive dysfunctions have been limited and not very effective. Instead, the greatest opportunities for intervention and alleviation of patient suffering, family burden, and societal costs lie within the domain of behavioral and psychological symptoms. Before the assessment of behavioral and psychological symptoms,

these symptoms were usually dismissed under the label of agitation. Typically, a patient who was old and "senile" would also be "agitated." Fortunately, times have changed (Tune, 2003). Clinicians now agree that it is often possible to treat dementia-associated symptoms, such as agitation and paranoia, successfully even though it is not possible to reverse or stop the progress of the dementia itself.

In 1996, the International Psychogeriatric Association convened an international consensus conference to develop an operational definition of behavioral and psychological symptoms of dementia. In the past, these symptoms had not received as much attention as had cognitive symptoms. The International Psychogeriatric Association grouped these symptoms into two major clusters: symptoms usually and mainly assessed on the basis of interviews with patients and relatives, which may include anxiety, depressed mood, hallucinations, and delusions; and symptoms usually identified on the basis of observation of patient behavior, which may include aggression, screaming, restlessness, agitation, wandering, culturally inappropriate behaviors, sexual disinhibition, hoarding, cursing, and shadowing (Finkel, Costa e Silva, Cohen, Miller, & Sartorius, 1998). Although there have been many research studies focusing on behavioral and psychological symptoms of dementia, researchers have not been able to differentiate these behaviors and psychological symptoms sufficiently among the different types of dementia. Despite symptoms that are common to individuals with dementia, there is growing awareness that dementias are experienced by each individual in a particularly unique and subjective manner.

Moreover, the uniqueness of each family's experience of coping with the effects of dementia on their loved ones cannot be minimized. Downs (1997) contributed to the nursing perspective on dementia because she built on the profession's historical focus on holistic care. Downs writes of the "emergence of the person in dementia." She describes the need for attention to the person with dementia, especially the individual's sense of self, unique perspective, and individual rights.

In Downs' analysis, it is both possible and necessary to obtain the views of people with dementia. Therefore, research and practice must focus on the sufferer. She distinguishes this approach from the medical model in dementia research, which focuses almost exclusively on the symptoms of the disease. Downs also distinguishes this "emergence of the person" perspective from past research that focused on psychosocial aspects of dementia but concentrated on family caregivers more than on the person with the disease.

Measures of the Behavioral and Psychological Symptoms of Dementia

Several reliable, valid, and clinically useful measures of behavioral and psychological symptoms of dementia are available for nurses to use in the assessment process:

1. The Neuropsychiatric Inventory (Cummings et al., 1994) evaluates a wide range of psychopathology; it records severity and frequency separately. Administration time is 10 minutes. The scoring is from 1 to 144. It has been translated into a number of languages and is widely used in drug trials.

2. The Behavioral Pathologic Rating Scale for Alzheimer's Disease (Reisberg et al., 1987) was designed to be used in prospective studies of symptoms in pharmacological trials and takes 20 minutes to administer.

3. The Cohen-Mansfield Agitation Inventory (Cohen-Mansfield, Marx, & Rosenthal, 1989) rates agitated behaviors in patients with cognitive impairment. It takes between 10 and 15 minutes to complete and can be used by formal caregivers in a clinical setting after training.

4. The Cornell Scale for Depression in Dementia (Alexopoulos, Abrams, Young, & Shamoian, 1988) is a 19-item scale specifically designed for the assessment of depression in dementia and is administered by a clinician, taking 20 minutes with the caregiver and 10 minutes with the patient.

THE ROLE OF NURSES IN THE DEMENTIA ASSESSMENT PROCESS

Nurses are a vital part of the interdisciplinary team needed for the assessment and diagnosis of dementia. This assessment team includes the disciplines of neurology, internal medicine, geriatrics, psychiatry, social work, neuropsychology, and nursing. The importance of nurses in this process is based on (1) the large increase in numbers of people with dementia; (2) the lack of adequate numbers of geriatricians, psychiatrists, and neurologists to address these cases; and (3) the clear demonstration in research that nurses' diagnoses using standardized tools are as accurate as other professional groups (Trapp-Moen, Tyrey, Cook, Heyman, & Fillenbaum, 2001). Another important factor is that the approaches used by other disciplines are frequently less adequate than nursing approaches in assessing the functional, social, and family dimensions of dementia. The medical disciplines involved in the diagnosis of dementia have well-established procedures for assessment and diagnosis, but they are sometimes too narrowly focused to pick up on the true scope of the problems. Nurses have been shown to be very effective in diagnosing dementia.

A study of nurse assessment procedures (Dennis, Furness, Lindesay, & Wright, 1998) showed that nurses performed well in detecting dementia compared to diagnoses made by other medical professionals. Other researchers have provided evidence that community psychiatric nurses are able effectively to differentiate dementia from other psychiatric disorders (Collighan, Macdonald, Herzberg, Philpot, & Lindesay, 1993; Seymour, Saunders, Wattis, & Daly, 1994).

Assessment tools specifically designed for nursing are scarce. Abraham et al. (1990) describe the Psychogeriatric Nursing Assessment Protocol for use in multidisciplinary geriatric–neuropsychiatric outpatient clinics. It was designed to complement other general physical assessments used by nurses and filled a gap in the tool kit for the assessment and diagnosis of behaviorally disordered older adults. This tool was further developed for assessment of patients with AD (Abraham et al., 1994). The complexity of health problems in older adults requires in-depth investigation into each medical problem and its possible relationship to cognitive and behavioral symptoms. Because multiple medical problems are commonly present in the elderly, they are likely to be taking multiple medications, and some of these can affect the central nervous system and cause symptoms of altered cognitive function. The Abraham protocol is accompanied by a rating form that permits quantification of essential data for purposes of clinical summary, epidemiological inquiry, research, and evaluations.

Dementia is a syndrome that, like fever, requires a systematic evaluation to identify its many causes (Mega, 2002). The Consortium to Establish a Registry for Alzheimer's Disease (CERAD) was established in 1986 by the National Institute on Aging to develop standardized assessments for patients with AD (Fillenbaum et al., 1997). Since that time, CERAD has developed and evaluated clinical and neuropsychological test batteries, a neuroimaging protocol, and an assessment of the neuropathological findings at autopsy of the brains of AD patients. The two basic assessments used for evaluating dementia are the CERAD Neuropsychological Battery, which is designed to determine the type and severity of cognitive impairment, and the CERAD Clinical Battery, which assesses the presence, type, and severity of dementia (Morriss, Rovner, Folstein, & German, 1990). The Clinical Battery includes (1) a detailed standardized inquiry using a nonpatient informant to determine changes in the patient's cognitive performance, including memory, orientation, verbal ability, calculation, concentration, judgment, and problem solving; (2) evaluation of activities involving community, home, and hobbies; (3) activities of daily living; (4) instrumental activities of daily living; and (5) the CERAD Clock Drawing Test, which assesses spatial orientation, dysphasia for numbers, and aspects of executive functioning.

Instruments Used for Nursing Assessment

There are many instruments used by nurses for the assessment of dementia, but it should be remembered that most tools do not take race, culture, and educational level into consideration (Wood, Giuliano, Bignell, & Pritham, 2006). These characteristics may be helpful in developing a plan of care that has both socioeconomic and cultural sensitivity. Lack of consideration of these factors in screening has the potential to affect the reliability of screening tools in diverse populations. Screening tools are important because they can assist with early identification of mild to moderate dementia, allowing patients and their families to plan for the future (Boustani, Peterson, Hanson, Harris, & Lohr, 2003).

Dementia Screening Questionnaire for Caregivers

This screening tool was developed for the untrained caregiver and reliably detects dementia (Monnot, Brosey, & Ross, 2005). This tool is somewhat longer than others in the field; however, it is unique in a sense that it allows the caregiver to participate in the process of identifying dementia. The questionnaire is divided into three parts. Part one addresses memory loss and general function. The caregiver is asked to identify all areas that describe the family member. Questions are designed to identify problems in long- and short-term memory, orientation, judgment, insight, and concentration. Part two identifies personality and behavior changes. Questions are designed to illicit changes observed, such as neglect in personal appearance, disorganization, apraxia, irritability, aggression, incontinence, and restlessness. Part three focuses on the caregivers' well-being. Questions are designed to identify caregiver burnout, and it ends with questions from the Yesavage Geriatric Depression scale (Monnot et al., 2005). The questionnaire takes approximately 5 minutes to score by a healthcare professional and determines whether a more in-depth evaluation is warranted.

The Mini-Mental State Examination

The Mini-Mental State Examination (MMSE) is the most widely used screening instrument (Folstein, Folstein, & McHugh, 1975). It was developed as a short, easy-to-administer measure of mental status and as a screening tool for dementia. It has been used extensively in research involving dementia patients and found to be an acceptable measure of mental status. The MMSE yields a total score of 30, with a score of 24 established as the cutoff point for dementia. It consists of 11 questions or commands, such as "What is the year?" or "Write a sentence," and assesses seven categories of cognitive function including orientation to time and place, registration of three words, attention and calculations, recall of three words, language, and visual construction. The MMSE takes 5–10 minutes and does not require extensive training to administer. Folstein determined that a score of 23 points or less with an individual who had more than 8 years of education can be a diagnostic indication of cognitive impairment. There is a need for further evaluation to establish a more definitive diagnosis (Folstein, 1983).

The Cognitive Abilities Screening Instrument (CASI)

The Cognitive Abilities Screening Instrument (CASI) was developed and pilot tested in Japan and the United States to determine cross-cultural applicability and usefulness in screening for dementia, monitoring disease progression, and providing a profile of cognitive impairment (Teng et al., 1994). The CASI contains 25 items that are grouped into cognitive domains according to the items' face validity. The CASI has a total score ranging from 0–100, with a suggested cutoff score of 74 for classifying dementia. It provides quantitative assessment in nine domains: (1) attention, (2) concentration, (3) orientation, (4) long-term memory, (5) short-term memory, (6) language, (7) visual construction, (8) fluency, and (9) abstraction and judgment. Typical administration time is 20–30 minutes. Scores from the MMSE can be estimated from the responses to selected CASI items. In a study by White et al. (1996), the CASI was used to evaluate 4000 men who participated in the Honolulu–Asia Aging Study of Dementia. The CASI scores declined significantly with increasing dementia severity, as measured by family informants and other standardized cognitive tests including the MMSE. Sherrell, Buckwalter, Bode, and Strozdas (1999) conducted a study in which they compared the MMSE and CASI. It was found that the CASI demonstrated greater specificity in determining level of cognitive function than did the MMSE.

Short Portable Mental Status Questionnaire

The Short Portable Mental Status Questionnaire is a short, reliable instrument to detect the presence and degree of intellectual impairment. It is easily administered by a nurse in the office, community, or hospital. It has been standardized and validated (Pfeiffer, 1975).

Older Americans Resources and Services

This methodology was designed to assess functional capacity in five dimensions (social resources, economic resources, mental health, physical health, and activities of daily living) and to measure need for and use of 24 types of generic services (Fillenbaum & Smyer, 1981; George & Fillenbaum, 1985).

The Ten-Point Clock Test

This test is used by many clinicians in the assessment of cognitive impairment and is useful in distinguishing disease process and normal aging. The test is a screen for visuoconstructional difficulties, because constructional apraxia is a common neuropsychological disturbance in dementia and often occurs early in the course of the disease. One system for scoring clock drawing was developed by Manos and Wu (1994) (Figure 12-1). Their research on the ten-point clock test was conducted by nurses on hospital patients and clinic outpatients,

---

FIGURE 12-1

Ten-Point Clock Test.

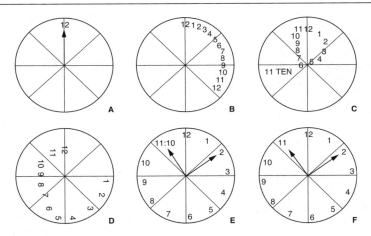

Scoring: **A.** Score = 0. **B.** The number 1 is in the correct position; score = 1. **C.** Numbers 1 and 2 are in the correct positions; score = 2. **D.** Numbers 7, 8, 10, and 11 are in the correct positions; score = 4. **E.** Numbers 1, 2, 4, 5, 7, 8, 10, and 11 are in the correct positions; score = 8. No points for hands of approximately equal length regardless of position. **F.** Numbers 1, 2, 4, 5, 7, 8, 10, and 11 are in correct position for 8 points. The little hand is on the 11 (1 point) and the big hand is on the 2 (1 point); score = 10 points.

Source: Modified from Manos and Wu, 1994.

---

with and without dementia. The purpose was to evaluate the clinical use of the test in screening for and grading cognitive deficits in medical and surgical patients. Clock scores correlated with neuropsychological test scores and with the MMSE. The mean clock score of elderly outpatient controls was 8.5, which was significantly different from the mean of 5.5 scored by patients with dementia. The study, therefore, found the ten-point clock test to be valid in identifying dementia. The results also correlated well with nurses' bedside assessments of observable, functional deficits in their patients. The test was easy to administer, and found to be reliable, valid, and useful as a quick screening and

grading method for cognitive deficits in medical and surgical patients. Moretti, Torre, Antonella, Cozzato, and Bova (2002) used the ten-point clock test and also found it to be reliable and easy to complete. The test detects cognitive impairment even in mild deterioration, which is defined by the MMSE as a score of around 23.

A circle approximately 5 inches in diameter is traced, using a template (see Figure 12-1). The patient is asked to "Put the numbers in the face of the clock," and when the task is completed to "Make the clock say 10 minutes after 11." To score the test, the number 12 is rotated to the top of the page. A line is drawn through the center of the number 12 and the middle of the circle, dividing the circle in half. In the rare instances when the 12 is missing, its expected position is assumed to be counterclockwise from the number 1, at a distance equivalent to the distance between the number 1 and the number 2. A second line is drawn at right angles to the first through the center of the circle, dividing it into quarters. Two more lines are drawn through the center of the circle, dividing it into eighths. One point is given for each of the following numbers that falls in its proper eighth of the circle relative to the 12: 1, 2, 4, 5, 7, 8, 10, and 11. At least half of the spatial volume occupied by the number must be in the correct eighth of the circle. One point is given each to a short hand pointing at the number 11, and a long hand pointing at the number 2. No points are given for the hands if they are approximately equal in length or for a long hand on the 11 and a short hand on the 2, or for hands of any length pointing at other numbers. A short hand on the number 11 and a long hand on the number 3 are worth one point—for the short hand. Numbers drawn outside the circle are scored by simply extending the dividing lines. Marks in place of numbers do not count.

Activities of Daily Living and Instrumental Activities of Daily Living

These are measures of daily function, important in understanding the degree of disability and level of dependence experienced by people with dementia. The Barthel Activities Instrument has had widespread use in research including use with elderly patients. It is easy to use and shows little variation between objective performance of tasks and reports gathered from witnesses. The Barthel Activities Instrument, however, only includes self-care tasks.

Therapeutic Environment

The standardized instruments previously listed are important tools for assessment. However, researchers and clinicians have also described the importance of establishing a therapeutic environment for the assessment process. This has been a forte for nurses over the years. One of the first theoretical nursing models was based on interpersonal relations (Peplau, 1952). Fifty years ago, Peplau described nursing as "a significant, therapeutic, interpersonal process." More recently, Abraham, Smullen, and Thompson-Heisterman (1992) emphasized the need for a "therapeutic climate" as a background for the implementation of the Psychogeriatric Nursing Assessment Protocol. He and his colleagues provide pointers for nurses to follow. Eight of these pointers are particularly relevant in assessing dementia patients:

1. Accommodate physical impairment: This includes being aware of any vision or hearing problems, or any physical symptoms that infringe on the therapeutic effectiveness of the assessment. "An uncomfortable patient is an uncooperative patient" (Abraham et al., 1992, p. 17).

2. Create a warm and inviting atmosphere: The patient needs to feel safe, cared about, and heard. Distractions in the environment and confusing messages do not create this feeling of safety, which is needed for accurate assessment of a dementia patient.

3. Integrate verbal and nonverbal communication: This is particularly important for elderly people who may have lost some of their verbal language abilities. In this case, nonverbal messages take on even more importance than usual. Simple "yes" and "no" questions tend to mask problems when talking to elderly persons and should be avoided. Well-known interviewing skills of active listening, clarifying, and reflecting are also of paramount importance when interviewing elderly persons in general, and particularly those with some dementia.

4. Use all the senses: Listening to the sound of the person's voice and physical presentation (condition of the skin, mobility, and characteristics of speech), and using the sense of

touch to assess strength (e.g., when shaking hands) are all aspects of an intuitive assessment ability that goes beyond the scores of any instrument.

5. Interview several people: Abraham et al. (1992) advises interviewing family members and friends if possible and then following this with a group interview. Obtaining information from others can help clear up any conflicting stories and provide observations of communication patterns within the family and family dynamics.

6. Assess the entire time: Beginning with the initial telephone call, the assessment includes all aspects of each contact (i.e., sitting in the waiting room, walking to the office, and so on).

7. Facilitate storytelling: Stories of the person's past provide a basis to judge what the present dementia symptoms may mean to the patient. Asking them to "tell me a story about a typical day for you" provides information on many levels about their ability to function independently.

8. Clarify, verify, and revisit: Because there are usually language and comprehension problems for persons with dementia, there is a need to clarify confusing or incomplete information.

As they seek to establish a therapeutic environment, nurses need to know the symptoms of dementia that can result from a loss in each cognitive domain and respond with effective strategies for communication. Problems that may hinder communication and some strategies for compensating for them are well described by Weintraub (1998):

1. Attention: This involves the loss of ability to sustain attention and the ability to grasp a normal amount of information from a conversation. Strategies include breaking information down into small portions and repeating instructions as the task is being done.

2. Learning and memory: This involves the loss of ability to learn new information and retain it over time. Strategies include repeating instructions and immediately asking the patient leading questions about the information.

3. Language: This involves the loss of ability to convey messages effectively and to understand what others are saying. Strategies include speaking in simple sentences and devising a system for emergency situations bypassing the need to use the telephone.

4. Visual perception: This involves the loss of ability to look at something and recognize it, find objects in a cluttered array, judge distance and spatial relations, and navigate around the home. Strategies include keeping personal items, objects, and clothing in the same location and simplifying the visual environment.

5. Emotional regulation: This involves loss of the ability to control emotions and even to express emotions (apathy). Strategies include not challenging the patient's responses, but accepting them and using techniques to "defuse" potentially volatile interactions, such as changing the topic.

Principles of communication are important aspects of both assessment and communicating the diagnosis. One of the problems encountered with older adults with dementia is that the need for diagnosis can become more important than the process of assessment. For example, the family of one older adult requested evaluation of the older adult so he could be placed in a drug research program, for which the inclusion criterion was a diagnosis of AD. During the evaluation it became clear that he could relate the story of his past, which included having been orphaned at an early age and placed with several abusive foster parents, coming to a large city, finding work, eventually marrying, buying a home, and raising his children who were now successful adults. However, he could not state what day of the week it was, or the year, or his present address, nor could he count backward from 20 by 2 (serial 2s). The diagnosis seeking in this case was focused more on the criterion for being in the drug study than on the meaning for him of now having his car taken away and of becoming dependent after a life of amazing survival. This is not to dismiss the need for quantitative measures for evaluation. We only urge that professionals be more mindful of the stories that elderly people have to tell about their lives to understand more clearly what the losses caused by dementia may mean to them in the present. In the context of the assessment process, this telling of stories is important in getting to know the person versus the symptoms of his or her disease. Also, telling stories depends on long-term memory, which generally remains intact after other cognitive functions are impaired. Therefore, it is ego saving to focus on that remaining strength as much as or more than on the deficits of short-term memory loss.

THE PROCESS OF DIAGNOSIS SEEKING IN DEMENTIA

This section focuses on the complexity of the entire decision-making process in establishing a diagnosis of dementia. Denial on the part of family members often delays bringing the problem to the attention of a medical professional. Denial can come in many forms. For several reasons, both patients and family members have a difficult time recognizing the changes in memory and behavior that are early signs of developing dementia. First, early changes are similar to changes associated with normal aging or with other preexisting health conditions, such as alcoholism or mental illness or even personal idiosyncrasies. Second, these changes often come and go, and this inconsistency can make it more difficult to take the changes seriously enough to seek evaluation and help. Third, the inconsistency of symptoms in the early stages may not have a significant impact on daily life activities for many months or even years. The recognition and, more importantly, the transformation in interpretation of these changes from usual aging to symptoms of a memory problem are fuzzy and ambiguous. To move from noticing

changes in memory and behavior to labeling such changes as memory loss or cognitive impairment is a complicated process (Berman, Iris, Robinson, & Morhardt, 2002; Iris, Berman, & Morhardt, 2001; Iris et al., 2002). Changes may be recognized, but they are not always seen as problems that need medical intervention. In addition, many physicians see early or mild changes in memory or behavior as part of normal aging and may respond by dismissing them as a concern. Although some family members may reject this conclusion, most feel comforted and reassured and thus the length of time to diagnosis increases.

The process of how families move toward diagnosis has been highlighted in the Pathways study. This study, funded by the Alzheimer's Association, focused on how family members moved from first observing change in their older relative to eventually seeking a medical evaluation (Iris et al., 2002).

In the first phase of this study, the researchers conducted open-ended interviews with 47 family members who played a major role in the process of seeking a diagnosis. Participants were recruited from various sites, including community-based adult day care centers, a geriatrician's private practice, a university-based AD center, and a medical center's geriatric assessment center. Just over 60% of participants were African American and 39% were non-Hispanic whites. Approximately 75% were women, and over half were daughters of the patients (51.5%), followed by wives (15.2%). The remainder was sons, husbands, or other family members, such as siblings or nieces. Areas of inquiry included questions about the circumstances surrounding the diagnosis-seeking behavior, by using key events as triggers for recall. Findings from the first phase showed that there are four critical time points in this process: (1) first notice of change, (2) identification of the change as a problem, (3) first time the problem is brought to the healthcare provider's attention by the family member, and (4) time of diagnosis.

Forty-four family members participated in the second phase, of whom 53% were African American and 45% were non-Hispanic white. Forty-one of these participants were women. The study demonstrated that the time span from first notice of change to the time of diagnosis can be a period of months or even years. Identification of change as a problem warranting medical attention is difficult, because symptoms of cognitive impairment are often seen as natural concomitants of normal aging. In addition, family members are often reluctant to step in and take charge of an older family member's medical care out of respect for the older person's autonomy and independence. Once the changes are seen as a problem, however, families usually act rather quickly to get medical attention and the lag time between points two and three is comparatively short.

When cognitive changes come to the attention of healthcare professionals, however, there are many intervening factors that may delay obtaining a diagnosis. First and foremost, many physicians are not well educated about the dementia process in older people, and they too frequently dismiss the changes as "normal aging." In fact, in the Pathways study, it was unusual for a primary care physician to refer the patient for more specialized assessment, such as neuropsychological testing. Second, changes in health insurance plans frequently led to disruptions in patient–physician relationships. Family members often had to start the process all over again when a new physician was introduced into the picture. The number of physicians involved in the process of obtaining a diagnosis ranged from one or two to as many as six.

COMMUNICATING THE DIAGNOSIS

Informing patients and families about a diagnosis of AD is a complex ethical and practical issue. One challenge for the physician and nurse is deciding how much information to give patients and families about the results of the assessment. Providing too much information can overwhelm some patients and families and give them the impression that the condition is more severe than indicated by test results. Others, in contrast, may want to know

every detail. Providing them with insufficient information could lead them to conclude that the assessment was incomplete and perhaps to doubt the results. Also at issue are the patient's moral and legal rights to receive the diagnosis.

The following are examples of people with dementia and family caregivers describing the manner in which they were given (or not given) information. The verbatim quotes are from patients in an early dementia support group. These quotes show that sensitivity is sometimes missing. The group members frequently describe the kind of "marginalized" position they experience after they have been diagnosed with dementia. "My cardiologist told me I had Alzheimer's disease and therefore shouldn't drive. He painted a vivid picture of little children being mowed down by me. It could have been done in a more helpful way." "Initially my doctor met with me along with my wife and sons. He ignored me and explained everything to them and I was slipping into the background." (A family member) "My father's doctor is an internist and he doesn't really concern himself with his memory."

The most recent American Medical Association guidelines on diagnosis of dementia advise giving the diagnosis directly to the patient if at all possible. Yet researchers suggest that the American Medical Association guidelines do not adequately address the clinical complexities of patient disclosure in dementia. Do patients want to know? Studies of older adult community-based samples revealed that most elderly persons would want to be told that they had dementia (Erde, Nadal, & Scholl, 1988; Holroyd, Turnbull, & Wolf, 2002). Turnbull, Wolf, and Holroyd (2003) found that of 200 subjects older than 65, those with prior involvement with persons with AD were less likely to state that the diagnosis should be given to the patient. In a study by Marzanski (2000), patients already diagnosed with dementia were asked about their preferences regarding "knowing the truth" about their diagnosis of dementia. Of the 50% of participants with satisfactory insight, 70% clearly declared they would like to know more about their illness.

Do families want patients to know? Interestingly, in some studies, most dementia sufferers' relatives (57–83%) did not want the patient to be told of his or her diagnosis, but 70% of the relatives would want to be told the truth if they had the disorder themselves (Barnes, 1997; Maguire et al., 1996). In Marzanski's (2000) study, three families believed the patient suffered as a result of the assessment. Some family members described the patient as someone with AD to other relatives but did not want the patient informed. In Holroyd et al.'s (2002) study, 60 family members of dementia patients attending support groups were asked to answer a questionnaire regarding their experience and attitudes regarding patients being told their dementia diagnosis. Ninety-three percent of family caregivers reported that they had been told the patient's diagnosis by a physician. Only 49% of patients had been told their diagnosis. Only 23% of patients had been told of any symptoms to expect with the illness, whereas 77% of family members were told.

At the moment, the most prominent advocates of truth-telling seem to believe that the nature and degree of the disease may limit the right to information. Johnson, Bouman, and Pinner (2000) studied a group of geriatricians and psychiatrists working with older adults with dementia in the United Kingdom and found that only 40% disclosed the diagnosis to their patients. Although aware of the benefits, they hesitated because of the uncertainty of the diagnosis, the patient's lack of insight, and the potential detrimental effects. The Alzheimer Association of Canada has published an information sheet, available online at http://www.Alzheimer.ca, that recommends establishing a plan for disclosure that takes into account patients' and family members' expectations of what the assessment will reveal. A study by Smith and Beattie (2001) underlines the need to investigate further the psychosocial factors that are involved in the lay interpretation of diagnostic information and the uncertainty associated with the assessment of dementia disorders.

A knowledgeable understanding of cultural norms and health practices within different ethnic groups is important for effective delivery of care. In particular, it is important for the clinician to understand how different ethnic groups view dementia and its associated cluster of behaviors. The American Indians believe that hallucinations are a gift and when the individual hallucinates he or she is communicating with the afterlife (Henderson & Traphagon, 2005). Chinese caregivers, however, interpret memory loss as a natural part of aging and view dementia as a normal phenomenon. Caregivers in Puerto Rico believe that dementia is probably a direct result of a long past misfortune within the family (Janevic & Connell, 2001). The different ethnic explanatory models make communicating the diagnosis even more difficult and treatment of the associated symptoms a challenge. Understanding the family dynamics and extended family relations are both important when communicating the diagnosis. African-American caregivers report stronger support networks, higher levels of life satisfaction, and less depressive symptoms and burnout than white family caregivers (Clay, Roth, Wadley, & Haley, 2008).

Just as with most issues surrounding dementia, the question of whether to report the diagnosis to the patient does not have a clear and definitive answer. It must be a decision based on clinical wisdom that has the best interest of the patient as its core value. Many patients in early stages of dementia not only want to know their diagnosis, but want to know as much as possible about prognosis, research, and advocacy. To quote a member of an early stage AD support group, "I want the information firsthand. I don't want someone else giving me 'trickle-down' facts." However, many patients maintain their denial of the diagnosis into the middle stages of the disease and up to the time when they no longer are capable of having insight. It seems to be their wish to translate symptoms into "What do you expect from a person my age?" or "Why should I know the date? I don't have to go to work anymore!"

Hannah Jane is a 77-year-old white widowed woman; she has two daughters and a son. She grew up and lived most of her life in the New York area and was a college professor by profession. Although Hannah's children Rebecca, Rachael, and Alan did not live nearby, she had a large circle of friends both in the community and academia with whom she loved to socialize. Hannah's children were first alerted to problems 5 years earlier when visiting their mother in New York. Hannah's friend Dora alerted Rebecca to the problem saying "something is not quite right with your mother." Dora had noticed that Hannah seemed to have trouble meeting deadlines in school and had begun forgetting appointments. Hannah's house, which was never neat, seemed in more disarray on this particular visit. Rebecca found bills that had not been paid on time and her mother seemed more "scattered" than usual. Hannah at this point agreed to move closer to her children and into a smaller apartment that would be more manageable. It was not until Hannah moved closer to her daughters that they realized how impaired her short-term memory had become. Rachael filled her pill box and noted there were many days she had not taken her medications. They also noted her sleeping more and not changing her clothes or she would often wear inappropriate clothes for season and weather. The event that finally propelled the family into a diagnostic workup occurred the following summer when Hannah decided to take a road trip back to her old neighborhood in New York. Hannah lost her way and lost her belongings, money, and credit cards. With nowhere to stay and no money, Hannah slept many nights in her car until finally she was found by the police.

The time from when the family first noticed changes in Hannah's cognition to the neurological workup was approximately 5 years. Hannah was found to have difficulty with memory and recall, poor orientation, calculation, and multistep task performance. Her MMSE was recorded as 19/30, and a diagnosis of dementia of the Alzheimer's type was made.

To this day Hannah has not acknowledged any memory deficit and when confronted by the family she states "it's part of getting old." It has been difficult for the family to persuade Hannah to attend appointments. The family expressed fear in causing their mother anxiety by insisting on the appointments; thus they delayed them as long as possible. Up until the neurological workup, the family had not explored community resources, but once the diagnosis had been made they felt a relief of sorts to explore more options to help them cope.

Quite frequently families are in denial, with such statements as "it's her age" or "ever since my father died, she hasn't been quite right." Families tend to generate their own explanatory model for the behavior and symptoms. Many families believe that memory loss is a normal part of aging, and it becomes quite a task to explain otherwise. It usually takes several visits to discuss and explain the process. Unfortunately, there is usually a crisis point before families recognize the need to seek further evaluation and help.

Questions for Discussion

1. What are some of the possible reasons that prevented the family from seeking a diagnostic workup earlier?

2. What additional information would the nurse need to gather before communicating the diagnosis?

3. How could the nurse assist the family and patient with adjusting to the diagnosis of dementia?

SUMMARY

Nurses, especially those with specialized education in geropsychiatric nursing, can function as brokers or bridges between physicians and families and patients, guiding interaction and facilitating communication, especially in a care manager role. An active nursing role in patient and family education about chronic disease management and care is currently a missing component of a comprehensive and holistic professional response to dementia. The realization of nurses' important role in the screening and diagnosis of dementias of late life relies on a solid base of knowledge about dementias, skills in the nursing assessment of such conditions, and the ability to use communication techniques to process the diagnosis with patients and their families. This chapter has provided an overview of these issues.

Solid background information is available about the neurobiology of AD and other dementias. The epidemiological data show that there is a great increase in the number of elderly persons with dementia. This will continue to rise exponentially as the baby boomer cohort enters the vulnerable age in which dementia is more prevalent. Neurobiological research has demonstrated that dementia can result from as many as 70 different disease entities. Thus, it is not a disease itself but rather a syndrome. Even though each cause brings unique symptoms, the general cognitive decline seen in dementia cuts across diagnostic categories. AD is a prototype of the dementia syndrome, and the increase in AD has given impetus to the increased focus in both the clinical and research arena.

Neuropsychiatric features of dementia include a wide range of behavioral and psychological symptoms. Dementia is incurable and inexorably progressive, but the behavioral and psychological symptoms frequently associated with it are treatable. The chapter lists several instruments that nurses can use to assess cognitive changes in dementia, and instruments to assess behavioral and psychological symptoms.

No task in our experience is as professionally challenging as assessment of elderly persons with dementia. The complexity of dementia identification, assessment, and care points to the need for nurses to play a central role in all of these stages as part of an interdisciplinary team. Research demonstrates that nurses who have been specifically trained can assess and assist in the diagnosis of dementia. Beyond using standardized instruments for assessment and diagnosis, nurses can direct the team's attention to social, cultural, biological, and psychological factors and coordinate appropriate responses. Finally, there are no clear guidelines on communicating the diagnosis and how much information to deliver. Although families need all necessary information, it is important not to barrage them with too much information in one session. Acute clinical judgment and humane sensitivity are required to balance the need for information with the need for maintaining a level of hope. Decisions about when to discuss the diagnosis and with whom must be based on clinical wisdom and commitment to the best interests of the patient.

REFERENCES

Abraham, I. L., Fox, J. M., Harrington, D. P., Snustad, D. G., Steiner, D. A., Abraham, L. H., et al. (1990). A psychogeriatric nursing assessment protocol (PNAP) for use in multidisciplinary practice. *Archives of Psychiatric Nursing, 4*(4), 242–259.

Abraham, I. L., Holroyd, S., Snustad, D. G., Manning, C. A., Brashear, H. R., Diamond, P. T., et al. (1994). Multidisciplinary assessment of patients with Alzheimer's disease. *Nursing Clinics of North America, 29*(1), 113–128.

Abraham, I. L., Smullen, D. E., & Thompson-Heisterman, A. A. (1992). Assessing geropsychiatric patients. *Journal of Psychosocial Nursing, 30*(9), 13–19.

Administration on Aging. (2007). *A profile of older Americans: 2006.* Retrieved August 15, 2009, from http://www.aoa.gov/prof/Statistics/profile/high lights.asp

Alexopoulos, G. S., Abrams, R. C., Young, R. C., & Shamoian, C. A. (1988). Cornell Scale for depression in dementia. *Biological Psychiatry, 23*(3), 271–284.

American Psychiatric Association. (2000). *Diagnostic and statistical manual of mental disorders* (4th ed., Text Revision). Washington, DC: Author.

Barnes, R. C. (1997). Telling the diagnosis to patients with Alzheimer's disease: Relatives should act as proxy for patient. *British Medical Journal, 314*(7077), 375–376.

Berman, R., Iris, M., Robinson, C., & Morhardt, D. (2002, October). *Physician feedback in assessing memory changes in older adults: Implications for early diagnosis of dementia.* Poster session during Best Practices Poster Day at the Cognitive Neurology and Alzheimer's Disease Center, Feinberg School of Medicine, Northwestern University, Chicago.

Boustani, M., Peterson, B., Hanson, L., Harris, R., & Lohr, K. (2003). Screening for dementia in primary care: A summary of the evidence for the U.S. Preventive Task Force. *Annals of Internal Medicine, 138*(11), 927–937.

Brashear, H. R. (2003). Galantamine in the treatment of vascular dementia. *International Psychogeriatrics, 15*(Suppl. 1), 187–194.

Clay, O., Roth, D., Wadley, V., & Haley, W. (2008). Changes in social support and their impact on psychosocial outcome over a five year period for African Americans and White dementia caregivers. *International Journal of Geriatric Psychiatry, 23*, 857–862.

Cohen, D., Eisdorfer, C., Gorelick, P., Pavesa, G., Luchins, D., Freels, S., et al. (1993). Psychopathology associated with Alzheimer's disease and related disorders. *Journal of Gerontology, 48*(6), M255–M260.

Cohen-Mansfield, J., Marx, M. S., & Rosenthal, A. S. (1989). A description of agitation in a nursing home. *Journal of Gerontology, 44*(3), M77–M84.

Collighan, G., Macdonald, A., Herzberg, J., Philpot, M., & Lindesay, J. (1993). An evaluation of the multidisciplinary approach to psychiatric diagnosis in elderly people. *British Medical Journal, 306*(6881), 821–824.

Craig, D., Mirakhur, A., Hart, D. J., Mcilroy, S. P., & Passmore, A. P. (2005). A cross study of neuropsychiatry symptoms in 435 patients with Alzheimers. *American Journal of Geriatric Psychiatry, 13*(6), 460–468.

Cummings, J. L., Mega, M., Gray, K., Rosenberg-Thompson, S., Carusi, D., & Gorbein, J. (1994). The Neuropsychiatric Inventory: Comprehensive assessment of psychopathology in dementia. *Neurology, 44*(12), 2308–2314.

Dennis, M., Furness, L., Lindesay, J., & Wright, N. (1998). Assessment of patients with memory problems using a nurse-administered instrument to detect early dementia and dementia subtypes. *International Journal of Geriatric Psychiatry, 13*(6), 405–409.

Downs, M. (1997). The emergence of the person in dementia research. *Ageing & Society, 17*(5), 597–607.

Erde, E., Nadal, E., & Scholl, T. (1988). On truth-telling the diagnosis of Alzheimer's disease. *Journal of Family Practice, 26*(4), 401–406.

Erkinjuntti, T., Kurz, A., Gauthier, S., Bullock, R., Lilienfeld, S., & Damaraju, C. V. (2002). Efficacy of galantamine in probable vascular dementia and Alzheimer's disease combined with cerebrovascular disease: A randomised trial. *Lancet, 359*(9314), 1283–1290.

Evans, D. A. (1990). Estimated prevalence of Alzheimer's disease in the United States. *Milbank Quarterly, 68*(2), 267–289.

Fillenbaum, G. G., Beekly, D., Edland, S., Hughes, J., Heyman, A., & Van belle, G. (1997). Consortium to Establish a Registry for Alzheimer's Disease (CERAD): Development, database structure, and selected findings. *Topics in Health Information Management, 18*(1), 47–58.

Fillenbaum, G. G., & Smyer, M. A. (1981). The development, validity, and reliability of the OARS multidimensional functional assessment questionnaire. *Journal of Gerontology, 36*(4), 428–434.

Finkel, S. I., Costa e Silva, J., Cohen, G. D., Miller, S., & Sartorius, N. (1998). Behavioral and psychological symptoms of dementia: A consensus statement on current knowledge and implications for research and treatment. *American Journal of Geriatric Psychiatry, 6*(2), 97–100.

Folstein, M. F. (1983). The Mini-Mental State Exam. In T. Crook, S. H. Ferris, & R. Bartus (Eds.), *Assessment in Geriatric Psychopharmacology* (pp. 47–51). New Canaan, CT: Mark Powley.

Folstein, M. F., Folstein, S., & McHugh, P. (1975). Mini-mental state: A practical method for grading the cognitive state of patients for the clinician. *Journal of Psychiatric Research, 12*, 185–198.

George, L. K., & Fillenbaum, G. G. (1985). OARS methodology. A decade of experience in geriatric assessment. *Journal of the American Geriatrics Society, 33*(9), 607–615.

Henderson, J., & Traphagon, J. (2005). Cultural factors in dementia. Perspectives from the anthropology of ageing. *Alzheimer's Disease and Associative Disorders, 19*(4), 272–274.

Holroyd, S., Turnbull, Q., & Wolf, A. M. (2002). What are patients and their families told about the diagnosis of dementia? Results of a family survey. *International Journal of Geriatric Psychiatry, 17*(3), 218–221.

Iris, M., Berman, R., & Morhardt, D. (2001, November). *The centrality of circumstance: Decision-making, diagnosis-seeking, and dementia.* Paper presented at the American Anthropological Association Annual Meeting, Washington, DC.

Iris, M., Berman, R., Robinson, C., Engstrom-Goehry, V., Morhardt, D., & Schrauf, R. (2002, October). *Pathways to Alzheimer's disease: Identifying factors that promote or inhibit early detection.* Poster session during Best Practices Poster Day at the Cognitive Neurology and Alzheimer's Disease Center, Feinberg School of Medicine, Northwestern University, Chicago.

Janevic, M., & Connell, C. (2001). Racial, ethnic and cultural differences in the dementia caregiving experience. *The Gerontologist, 41*, 334–347.

Johnson, H., Bouman, W., & Pinner, G. (2000). On telling the truth in Alzheimer's disease: A pilot study of current practice and attitudes. *International Journal of Psychogeriatrics, 12*(2), 221–229.

Kalaria, R. N., & Ballard, C. (1999). Overlap between pathology of Alzheimer's disease and vascular dementia. *Alzheimer's Disease & Associated Disorders, 13*(Suppl. 3), S115–S123.

Maguire, C. P., Kirby, M., Coen, R., Coakley, D., Lawlor, B. A., & O'Neill, D. (1996). Family members' attitudes towards telling the patient with Alzheimer's disease their diagnosis. *British Medical Journal, 313*, 529–530.

Manos, P., & Wu, R. (1994). The ten point clock test: A quick screen and grading method for cognitive impairment in medical and surgical patients. *International Journal of Psychiatry in Medicine, 24*(3), 229–244.

Marzanski, M. (2000). On telling the truth to patients with dementia. *Western Journal of Medicine, 173*(5), 318–323.

Mega, M. S. (2002). Differential diagnosis of dementia: Clinical examination and laboratory assessment. *Clinical Cornerstone, 4*(6), 53–65.

Monnot, M., Brosey, M., & Ross, E. (2005). Screening for dementia: Family caregiver questionnaires reliably predict dementia. *Journal of American Board of Family Practice, 18*(4), 240–256.

Moretti, R., Torre, P., Antonella, R., Cozzato, G., & Bova, A. (2002). Ten point clock test: A correlation analysis with other neuropsychological tests in dementia. *International Journal of Geriatric Psychiatry, 17*(4), 347–353.

Morriss, R. K., Rovner, B. W., Folstein, M. F., & German, P. S. (1990). Delusions in newly admitted residents of nursing homes. *American Journal of Psychiatry, 147*(3), 299–302.

Peplau, H. (1952). *Interpersonal relations in nursing.* New York: Putnam.

Pfeiffer, E. (1975). A Short Portable Mental Status Questionnaire (SPMSQ) for the assessment of organic brain deficit in elderly patients. *Journal of the American Geriatrics Society, 23*(10), 433–441.

Reisberg, B., Borenstein, J., Salob, S. P., Ferris, S. H., Franssen, E., & Georgotas, A. (1987). Behavioral symptoms in Alzheimer's disease: Phenomenology and treatment. *Journal of Clinical Psychiatry, 48*(Suppl.), 9–15.

Sachdev, P. (2000). Is it time to retire the term "dementia"? *Journal of Neuropsychiatry & Clinical Neuroscience, 12*(2), 276–279.

Seymour, J., Saunders, P., Wattis, J. P., & Daly, L. (1994). Evaluation of early dementia by a trained nurse. *International Journal of Geriatric Psychiatry, 9*(1), 37–42.

Sherrell, K., Buckwalter, K. C., Bode, R., & Strozdas, L. (1999). Use of the Cognitive Abilities Screening Instrument (CASI) to assess elderly persons with schizophrenia in long-term care settings. *Issues in Mental Health Nursing, 20*(6), 541–558.

Smith, A. P., & Beattie, B. L. (2001). Disclosing a diagnosis of Alzheimer's disease: Patient and family experiences. *Canadian Journal of Neurological Sciences, 28*(Suppl. 1), S67–S71.

Teng, E. L., Hasegawa, K., Homma, A., Imai, Y., Larson, E., Graves, A., et al. (1994). The Cognitive Abilities Screening Instrument (CASI): A practical test for cross-cultural epidemiological studies of dementia. *International Psychogeriatrics, 6*(1), 45–58.

Trapp-Moen, B., Tyrey, M., Cook, G., Heyman, A., & Fillenbaum, G. G. (2001). In-home assessment of dementia by nurses: Experience using the CERAD evaluations. *Gerontologist, 41*(3), 406–409.

Tune, L. E. (2003). Great progress in diagnosis and treatment of dementia. *American Journal of Geriatric Psychiatry, 11*(4), 388–390.

Turnbull, Q., Wolf, A., & Holroyd, S. (2003). Attitudes of elderly subjects toward "truth telling" for the diagnosis of Alzheimer's disease. *Journal of Geriatric Psychiatry and Neurology, 16*(2), 90–93.

Weintraub, S. (1998, October). *Individual differences in dementia symptoms: Their causes and management.* Paper presented to the National Association of Professional Geriatric Care Managers, Chicago.

White, L., Petrovitch, H., Ross, G., Masaki, K., Abbott, R., Teng, E., et al. (1996). Prevalence of dementia in older Japanese-American men in Hawaii: The Honolulu–Asia Aging Study. *JAMA, 276,* 955–960.

Wood, R., Giuliano, K., Bignell, C., & Pritham, W. (2006). Assessing cognitive ability in research. Use of the MMSE with minority populations and elderly adults with low education levels. *Journal of Gerontological Nursing, 32*(4), 45–54.

13

Nursing Management of Clients Experiencing Dementias of Late Life
Care Environments, Clients, and Caregivers

Ruth Remington
Linda A. Gerdner
Kathleen C. Buckwalter

As people age, they are at greater risk for developing a dementing illness, which is a pathological condition that impairs cognitive function. Dementia is not a single disease, but rather a group of symptoms that negatively impact the person's functional ability. Among these symptoms, cognitive impairment is one of the most devastating losses faced by older adults and their caregivers. Although memory loss may be the earliest and most common indication, dementia also causes changes in personality, behavior, sensorimotor function, and language. A challenge in working with older adults with dementia is to provide care that maintains physical and functional well-being while upholding dignity.

Nurses practicing in most settings can expect, at some time, to care for older adults with cognitive impairment. This chapter explores different environments where the geropsychiatric nurse plays a pivotal role in the promotion of health for people with dementia and their formal and informal caregivers. Most of the care for these persons is provided by nurses or the nursing assistants they supervise. A goal for nursing care is to promote maximum function, dignity, and quality of life for the person with dementia. This chapter presents an overview of nursing interventions with a focus on care environments, clients, and their caregivers.

As the reader advances through the content of this chapter, it is important to understand that cultural values and beliefs about dementia that are held by older adults and family members affect preferences in care and help-seeking behaviors (Janevic & Connell, 2001; Yeo & Gallagher-Thompson, 2006). There is a broad range of ethnic diversity within the United States and heterogeneity within each ethnic group. The depth and breadth of this topic go beyond the scope of this chapter. The reader is referred to *Ethnicity and Dementias* (Yeo & Gallagher-Thompson) for a detailed discussion.

CARE ENVIRONMENTS

Regardless of the care environment, persons with dementia pose numerous challenges to the caregiver. Family caregivers often face caregiving responsibilities for aging parents and young children simultaneously, while trying to maintain employment and other social roles. Community resources that can enhance and support caregiving roles are discussed next.

Adult Day Care

Many times family caregivers become so consumed with the care recipient's needs that they neglect their own. Respite may provide the caregiver with needed temporary relief. Adult day care centers provide health, social, and recreational services to older adults who need supervision for a portion of the day. Older adults with dementia comprise more than one half of the participants in adult day care centers (Alzheimer's Association, 2008). Meals, rest periods, and therapeutic activities are scheduled to maximize the functional ability of the individual. Nursing services may include health teaching, consultation, assessment, research, and coordination of care. Adult day care programs are sponsored by both public and private organizations, with variable schedules, fees, and program foci (Jett, 2008; Linton & Lach, 2007; Miller, 2009). The National Adult Day Services Association in Washington, DC, can provide information on local programs. See its Web site at http://www.nadsa.org/.

Home Health Care

An estimated 70% of persons with dementia live at home at any one time, receiving care from unpaid relatives, friends, and neighbors. These caregivers assist with personal care and management of medical and financial needs, spending on average 16.6 hours per week. In addition, approximately one fourth of older adults using home care services have dementia (Alzheimer's Association, 2008).

Visiting nurse associations provide multidisciplinary healthcare services for persons who need intermittent skilled care at home. Nonskilled, personal care services are offered but not usually covered by insurance. Individual and environmental assessments, treatment for clients, and education for caregivers provided by these agencies can be instrumental in helping to defer institutionalization (Jett, 2008; Miller, 2009).

Assisted Living

Assisted living facilities are residences in which special services are offered to maximize the functional ability of the individual who needs some help with activities of daily living, but not the intensity of care provided by a long-term care facility. Services can include meals, housecleaning, and personal care. Architectural features are adapted to the older or disabled adult. A growing number of facilities have dedicated units for the care of the adult with dementia (Linton & Lach, 2007). Approximately one half of residents of assisted living facilities have dementia and more than half of those are in moderate to late stages of the disease (Alzheimer's Association, 2008).

Small Community Residences

With the goal to transform nursing homes, small community residences are being developed and are believed to provide a better awareness of resident needs and preferences. Assistance with activities of daily living and clinical care are provided, but these are not the focus of the residence. Examples of these settings are Green House (Bowers & Nolet, 2009), Small House (Malony, 2009), and Wellspring (Hill, Milone-Nuzzo, & Kolanowski, 2009). Research is in progress to evaluate these settings.

Long-Term Care Facilities

Persons are usually cared for in the home by family members until caregiving demands exceed the ability to cope or a caregiver is no longer available because of illness or death. It is at this time that a decision may be made for placement in a long-term care facility. The average length of time and the degree of importance with which the caregiving role is viewed may have a major impact on the family member's response to institutionalization and should be examined (Davis & Buckwalter, 2001). Over time, caregiving may become the dominant role of the family member, who may experience ambivalent or adverse feelings, such as guilt and depression, when these responsibilities are relinquished to paid staff in a long-term care facility.

Forty-six percent of nursing home residents have a diagnosis of dementia. Special care units

(SCUs), devoted to the care of persons with dementia, represent only 5.26% of all nursing home beds (Alzheimer's Association, 2008). The services provided on these units should be distinctly different from "traditional" integrated units in their philosophy and environmental design, leading to an improved quality of life for the persons residing within. However, research has shown that the services on SCUs are not always significantly different from those on an integrated unit (Gerdner & Beck, 2006). Recently, Gruneir, Lapane, Miller, and Mor (2008) compared the care of the person with dementia residing on traditional units to those residing in SCUs. They conclude that the most striking finding of this study was the increased use of antipsychotic medications for persons residing on SCUs. Consequently, the education of caregivers regarding elements of "special" care needs to be increased, and nurses are in an excellent position to undertake this challenge. Although only a few states require disclosure, family consumers should be encouraged to obtain comparison information about the characteristics of the SCUs in their geographic area. It is also important for them to know that their personal preference and values are relevant in selecting a unit. Pertinent issues for family consumers and their advocates to explore can include features that distinguish the SCU from an integrated unit. Architectural features and decor, staff training, and activity programs should be adapted to the physical and cognitive deficits of the older adult with dementia. Family members need to know admission, discharge, and transfer criteria; philosophy of care; how the unit is secured; what plan is in place for fire or other emergency; and whether the resident is permitted off the unit with supervision (Gerdner & Buckwalter, 1996).

Hospice Care

Dementia is the fifth leading cause of death for adults older than 65 years of age. Although guidelines exist for hospice eligibility for persons with dementia, only 11% of hospice decedents had a diagnosis of dementia (Mitchell et al., 2007). Persons with dementia who received hospice services remained at home significantly longer (78.8 versus 55.8 days) and had fewer symptoms during the final 90 days of life than those who did not receive such care (Volicer, Hurley, & Blaise, 2003). Barriers to the provision of hospice services include the challenges of estimating a prognosis of 6 months or less and the lack of recognition of dementia as a terminal illness (Mitchell et al.).

Core nursing responsibilities related to end-of-life care when the client with dementia is dying include being (1) a skilled clinician who understands symptom management and can provide comfort care, (2) an advocate to ensure that all members of the healthcare team are available to the client and his or her family members, and (3) a guide to assist the client and family through the dying experience (Norlander, 2001). Norlander has outlined five principles for comprehensive end-of-life nursing care that are applicable to a wide range of client populations, including those with dementia: (1) client and family treatment preferences are discussed among all team members and respected; (2) undesirable symptoms are relieved; (3) emotional, spiritual, and personal suffering are addressed; (4) clients and families are prepared emotionally for death; and (5) grieving is acknowledged. For many years, persons with dementia were disproportionately excluded from hospice or palliative care because it was difficult for clinicians to determine if death was imminent within the 6-month period covered by insurers. More recently, hospice care has moved into nursing homes and SCUs to better accommodate persons with dementia and their families. For example, palliative care is especially challenging for persons with dementia, who may be unable to articulate their need for additional pain medication. Community-based nurses with advanced education in geropsychiatric nursing can play an important role in encouraging early stage clients with dementia and their families to participate in advance care planning (advance directives) and to make their end-of-life care treatment preferences clearly known while they are still cognitively intact enough to participate in the decision-making process. Sensitivity to the psychological conflicts associated with end-of-life decision making can assist the geropsychiatric nurse in supporting the individual and family through this process.

Advance Directives

Despite widespread professional and public promotion, only approximately 25% of people actually execute advance directives. A number of approaches have been developed to help older adults to develop advance directives. Multiple education sessions offering verbal information about advance directives were shown to be more effective than single sessions or written materials to promote formulating advance directives (Bravo, Dubois, & Wagneur, 2008; Linton & Lach, 2007).

Most persons with dementia benefit from the two types of advance directives that exist: a living will or healthcare directive; and durable healthcare power of attorney, healthcare agent, or healthcare proxy. These are legally binding documents that direct health care and decision making when clients are no longer able to make their own decisions (Norlander, 2001). Norlander and McSteen (2000) have outlined six key elements of advance care planning discussion: (1) client goals and values, (2) client experience with death, (3) client understanding of illness, (4) family support and understanding of client goals and values, (5) communication with primary care provider, and (6) identification of resources. Meaningful client input into advance care planning requires a certain level of cognitive ability. Therefore, it is essential that this process take place early enough in the course of the dementing illness for the person's wishes to be known so that his or her wishes can be honored at the end of life.

FRAMEWORKS FOR INTERVENTIONS

The progressively lowered stress threshold (PLST) model, proposed by Hall and Buckwalter (1987), provides a conceptual framework for care of persons with dementia. The model posits that the ability to tolerate stress declines with the progression of the disease. This includes both internal (i.e., pain and fatigue) and external stressors (i.e., overwhelming environmental stimuli). Maximum function can be maintained through a supportive environment in which stress-producing triggers are identified and reduced or eliminated. A plan of care based on the PLST model encompasses interventions that are client-centered, environment-centered, and caregiver-centered, to support the client in functioning within the limits of the dementing illness.

A source of stress and frustration for the older adult with dementia is the inability to plan. The nurse can assist the individual to compensate by providing a consistent routine and limiting the choices that the client is expected to make. Functional losses are caused by progressive, irreversible cortical deterioration; therefore, the client should not be encouraged or expected to regain lost skills. Asking the client to "try harder" only results in increasing frustration. Providing adequate rest is necessary to prevent increased stress levels because of the lowered tolerance to stress and diminished energy reserves. This can be accomplished by alternating stimulating activities with rest periods. Caregivers and families require ongoing education and support regarding the disease process, care routines, and problem-solving strategies (Hall & Buckwalter, 1987). The PLST model has been used to plan, implement, and evaluate care for persons with dementia across institutional and community-based settings (Smith, Gerdner, Hall, & Buckwalter, 2004; Smith, Hall, Gerdner, & Buckwalter, 2006).

The need-driven dementia-compromised behavior model (Algase et al., 1996) offers another perspective, which essentially reframes disruptive behaviors as an expression of unmet needs of the person with dementia. These unmet needs may be emotional, social, physical, or psychological in nature, but because the person with dementia may have lost language skills necessary to communicate their needs, they do so behaviorally. By assessing and organizing personal and environmental factors, the nurse can identify individuals at risk for dysfunctional behavior and individualized interventions can evolve (Algase et al.).

To extend the original model, Kovach, Noonan, Schlidt, and Wells (2005) explain the consequences of behavioral symptoms for the person with dementia. An unmet need causes a series of events leading to negative outcomes, characterized as primary need-driven dementia-compromised behaviors, personal factors, care factors, and contextual factors. The unmet need can result in worsening of the primary behavior and generation of a secondary behavior. This can negatively influence the affective, physical, and functional status of the person with dementia. The need for care is increased with the potential for caregiver role strain, compromising the ability of the caregiver to provide anticipatory care. The resultant environmental stress can have many outcomes, including jeopardizing the safety in the environment for the person with dementia and the caregivers and an increased use of acute and long-term care services.

The cognitive developmental approach is used to characterize cognitive impairment in dementia. This approach proposes that cognitive skills and functional abilities are lost in reverse order from which they were originally acquired. The stages of dementia, from diagnosis to death, are equated to the reverse order of Piaget's developmental levels of children for the purpose of individualizing assessment and intervention (Matteson, Linton, & Barnes, 1996).

The neurodevelopmental sequencing model recommends that interventions should be chosen to match the functional skills of the older adult with dementia to ensure success. Three levels of functional ability direct interventions. For ambulatory individuals, active sports and games and cognitive stimulation with a motor component are examples of interventions. Activities for the wheelchair-bound individual include exercises and sensory stimulation, and for the nonambulatory individual, range-of-motion exercises, massage, and sensory integration activities are appropriate (Buettner & Kolanowski, 2003).

INTERVENTIONS DIRECTED TOWARD THE PERSON

Community-Based Interventions for Early Stage Dementia

To delay the loss of functional abilities and skills, community-based interventions should begin in the early stage of dementia and include the person with dementia in the planning. Multimodal therapies, or those combining two or more interventions, produce the strongest results. Examples of interventions include aerobic and balance exercise classes; cognitive therapies tailored to the individual's daily problems; and recreational therapies, such as art, social engagement, and hobbies. Nonpharmacological therapies that are continuous have greater potential for long-term benefit than short-term, time-limited interventions. Participation with a family member has been shown to improve outcomes (Burgener et al., 2008; Burgener, Buettner, Beattie, & Rose, 2009).

Group Activity

Structured group activities have been shown to reduce agitation in the nursing home environment. In one study, disruptive residents were taken to a 2-hour supervised session, which included orientation activities; movement therapy; or relaxation activities, such as therapeutic touch and music. In addition to the participants becoming calmer, other residents and staff on the unit reported that respite from the disruptive residents facilitated their relaxation. Nursing staff also reported increased job satisfaction (Smith-Jones & Francis, 1992). In a systematic review of psychosocial interventions in early dementia, Bates, Boote, and Beverly (2004) found that reality orientation was effective in improving cognitive ability in persons in the early stages of dementia. Although there was a small decline in improvement at the end of the intervention period, the effect was sustained up to 3 months. No evidence was found, however, to demonstrate the effectiveness of group counseling sessions on well-being or procedural memory stimulation sessions on functional performance and cognitive ability (Bates, Boote, & Beverly).

Time Slips is a creative group-storytelling technique that does not rely on failing memory, allowing persons with Alzheimer's disease and related disorders to express themselves even after their capacity for traditional, literal expression is gone. A group leader presents a picture or image and encourages the group to create a story using the picture as a trigger. Time Slips provides reinforcement for creative activities in a "failure free" environment, supporting creativity.

An observational study using an experimental design was conducted in 20 nursing homes with dementia SCUs. The facilities using Time Slips were found to have improved resident engagement in interactions with others. Staff had more positive attitudes toward persons with dementia. There was no effect on job satisfaction or burnout (Fritch et al., 2009).

Reminiscence

Reminiscence used as an intervention is not simply recalling the past. It is a structured process of reflection on significant life events (Hsieh & Wang, 2003). The ability to retrieve events from long-term memory can persist long after the capacity to recall newly learned information diminishes (Pittiglio, 2000). Reminiscence was effective in stimulating communication, promoting self-esteem (Woodrow, 1998), and decreasing depression in older adults with and without dementia (Hsieh & Wang; Pittiglio; Okumura, Tanimukai, & Asada, 2008). Hsieh and Wang note that although studies of reminiscence therapy do not consistently produce statistically significant results, any intervention that has the potential to decrease depression has clinical significance and should be considered.

Biographical story telling, a form of reminiscence, resulted in improved staff attitudes toward older adults in their care. Staff reported that they understood the older adults better and were able to form closer relationships. Increased involvement with the residents and their families occurred

while gathering biographical data. The intervention demonstrated the potential for increased job satisfaction (Clark, Hanson, & Ross, 2003). Additionally, activities that elicit pleasant memories may produce a soothing effect on the client who is agitated. This process may be enhanced by stimulation of multiple senses (vision, smell, taste, touch, and hearing). Examples of sensory cues include the introduction and discussion of photo albums, personal memorabilia, providing a favorite food item, playing a musical instrument, or listening to music.

An individual or group reminiscence therapy session can begin with techniques to trigger memory recall, such as the use of pictures, photographs, music, foods, tools, or memorabilia. Open-ended questions help to focus the individual on the past (e.g., "Can you tell me what it was like growing up in Springfield?"). These questions stimulate conversation and build rapport. Family and friends can assist in identifying significant historical events (Pittiglio, 2000).

Art

Enhancing the environment with art can have a positive impact on well-being. Exposure to art has been shown to reduce anxiety and depression (Daykin, 2008), minimizing the negative effects of problem behaviors. Art may be an alternate form of communication for persons with dementia when the disease process makes language difficult or impossible. Creative art activities can also offer the person a sense of control by manipulating art materials and making decisions within a limited sphere (Harlan, 1993). In addition, sensory stimulation is provided through the exploration of various art mediums, colors, and forms. Art forms provide for an expression of self, and incorporating the personal identity of the older adult with dementia links art to reminiscence (Kahn-Denis, 1997).

When using art as an intervention, it is important to identify a medium that the person can manage, but is not childlike or demeaning. If the person is only able to color with crayons, provide realistic animal drawings or landscapes to color, rather than coloring books with pictures of dolls or toys (Remington, Abdallah, Melillo, & Flanagan, 2006). Memories in the Making is an activity program designed by Selly Jenny in 1986 and has been adopted by the Orange County Alzheimer's Association and other chapters as a national program to improve quality of life in persons with Alzheimer's disease and related disorders. The program encourages self-expression in a failure-free context through visual arts (painting and drawing) under the guidance of a trained artistic facilitator. Facilitators provide support while allowing the participants to create their own message.

William Utermohlen, a professional artist, was diagnosed with Alzheimer's disease in 1995 and died in 2007. After his diagnosis he continued his work with a series of self-portraits to chronicle the effects of the disease on his artistic abilities. In his memory, these portraits are being exhibited throughout the country. A slide presentation and video excerpt of this exhibit is available online at http://www.alzheimersnotes. com/william-utermohlen-exhibition-self-portrait-of-alzheimers-disease/

Indications for Pharmacological Therapies

Currently there are no pharmacological agents that can cure or stop the progression of dementia. Several agents have been developed that may temporarily improve cognitive function or slow its decline for many with mild to moderate Alzheimer's disease (Table 13-1). Most of these drugs—donepezil (Aricept), rivastigmine (Exelon), and galantamine (Reminyl)—act to increase the amount of acetylcholine in the central nervous system, by inhibiting the enzyme cholinesterase. Acetylcholine is a memory- and cognition-regulating neurotransmitter. Prolonging the activity of acetylcholine on the cholinergic receptors and in the synapses permits more effective transmission (Aschenbrenner & Venable, 2009). Although currently approved only for Alzheimer's-type dementia, it has been

TABLE 13-1

Selected Drugs for Alzheimer's Disease

Drug (Trade name)	Total Daily Dose	Pharmacokinetics	Adverse Effects
Donepezil (Aricept)	5–10 mg qd	Partially metabolized by the liver and partially excreted by kidneys Half-life, 70 hr	Headache, fatigue, insomnia, diarrhea, nausea, anorexia, weight loss, frequent urination
Galantamine (Reminyl)	4–12 mg bid	Mostly metabolized by the liver Half-life, 7 hr	Fatigue, bradycardia, anorexia, diarrhea, weight loss
Rivastigmine (Exelon)	3–6 mg bid to a maximum of 12 mg/day, orally or transdermally	Metabolized by the liver, excreted by the kidneys Half-life, 1.5 hr	Weakness, dizziness, anorexia, nausea, vomiting, weight loss
Memantine (Namenda)	5–10 mg bid	Excreted in urine Half-life, 60–80 hr	Dizziness, headache, constipation

Source: Adapted from Aschenbrenner, D. S., & Venable, S. J. (2009). *Drug Therapy in Nursing* (3rd ed., pp. 323–327). New York: Lippincott; and Miller, C. A. (2009). *Nursing for Wellness in Older Adults: Theory and Practice* (5th ed., pp. 279–281). New York: Lippincott.

suggested that these drugs may be equally effective for people with vascular or Lewy body dementias. Tacrine, the first of the cholinesterase inhibitors approved, is rarely used today because the other drugs in the class have fewer adverse effects (Miller, 2009). Nausea, vomiting, diarrhea, anorexia, and weight loss are common side effects of these medications. Less frequent cholinergic effects include urinary retention, sleep disturbance, seizures, and bronchospasm. Fewer adverse effects are associated with donepezil (Birks, 2006).

Memantine (Namenda) is the first drug shown to be effective in clients with moderate to severe Alzheimer's disease. Memantine, approved by the Food and Drug Administration in 2003, acts by blocking selective receptors that are stimulated by glutamate. A neurotransmitter involved in memory, glutamate is produced in excessive amounts in people with Alzheimer's disease. It has been proposed that memantine may reduce neuronal cell destruction (Garnett, 2003; Libow, 2003). Because the mechanism of action of Namenda is different than other drugs for Alzheimer's disease, it is often prescribed in combination with a cholinesterase inhibitor (Aschenbrenner & Venable, 2009).

Other drugs that are being investigated to manage symptoms of dementia include antioxidants (e.g., ginkgo biloba, vitamin E); nonsteroidal anti-inflammatory drugs; and statins (Miller, 2009). A systematic review that included 59 randomized controlled trials involving pharmacological therapies for dementia showed improvement of cognitive symptoms and global function with cholinesterase inhibitors and memantine. Outcomes of behavior and quality of life showed inconsistent results with these drugs. Studies that compared different cholinesterase inhibitors showed no variation in effect (Raina et al., 2008).

Monitoring Medication Side Effects

Safe administration and ongoing assessment of the client with a dementing illness who is receiving these drugs is an important nursing function related to pharmacological interventions. It is important that nurses ensure that clients have actually swallowed their medication and closely monitor their response (Buckwalter, Stolley, & Farran, 1999). Clients and families should be instructed to take medications as prescribed, because higher doses may not increase cognitive benefits, but are likely to increase side effects. To maximize absorption of the drug, galantamine and rivastigmine should be administered with food, whereas donepezil and memantine can be administered without regard to food (Deglin & Vallerand, 2003).

Complementary and Alternative Therapies

Medicinal Herbs and Nutritional Supplements

Herbs have been recognized for their healing properties since ancient times. Increasingly, herbal remedies and dietary supplements are being suggested as treatments for Alzheimer's disease and other dementias. Although research is being conducted on the safety and effectiveness of these products, many of the claims are anecdotal. In the United States, medicinal herbs are classified as dietary supplements and are not subject to the rigorous scientific research required by the Food and Drug Administration for sale as a prescription drug. Manufacturers may make claims about the effects of the supplements, but are not permitted, by law, to claim that the herbs can prevent or cure disease.

Some herbal supplements may be effective interventions for managing symptoms related to dementia; however, older persons considering their use should be cautioned that the purity and potency of the supplement are not standardized. The chemical composition of the product may be affected by growing and harvesting conditions and storage. The amount of active ingredient in the product may vary from one brand to another. Most importantly, medicinal herbs can have serious adverse interactions with some prescription medications, or increase the risk for bleeding, and should be taken only with the supervision of a health professional.

Researchers have shown interest in ginkgo biloba. Preliminary reports suggest that it improves memory and cognitive function in older adults with dementia; however, results are not consistent.

Ginkgo biloba has antioxidant, anti-inflammatory, and vasodilating properties. Few side effects are reported, but it does inhibit platelet aggregation and can increase the risk of bleeding, especially if the person is taking anticoagulants. Other herbal and dietary supplements promoted for use in dementia include vitamin E and coenzyme Q$_{10}$, because of their antioxidant properties. Studies of these supplements and B vitamins and folate have shown inconsistent results (Keegan, 2001; Miller, 2009; Spoelhof & Foerst, 2002). Although individual nutrients have shown variable results, early studies of a combination of nutrients seem promising. Community-residing subjects with mild to moderate Alzheimer's disease who received a combination of folic acid, vitamin B$_{12}$, vitamin E, S-adenosylmethionine, N-acetylcysteine, and acetyl-L-carnitine showed improved behavioral and cognitive performance, which was maintained for more than 12 months (Chan, Paskavitz, Remington, Rasmussen, & Shea, 2009). In a subsequent randomized clinical trial in persons with moderate to late Alzheimer's disease, cognitive decline was delayed for 6 months in those who took the formulation compared to those who took placebo (Remington, Chan, Paskavitz, & Shea, 2008).

Therapeutic Use of Touch

Hands-on, touch modalities have been practiced by nurses throughout history. Therapeutic back massage promotes relaxation and stimulates the circulation. Touch, in the form of massage, can be viewed as a form of nonverbal communication for the person with dementia whose ability to communicate verbally is declining. Gentle hand massage has been shown to reduce agitation in nursing home residents with dementia (Remington, 2002; Snyder, Egan, & Burns, 1995). These techniques require little training and can be performed by professional and lay caregivers alike. Ongoing assessment is essential because not all patients welcome touch and may perceive it to violate their personal space (Remington et al., 2006).

The effects of therapeutic touch have been shown to reduce the frequency of agitation (Haw-

ranik, Johnson, & Deatrich, 2008; Woods & Dimond, 2002) and the salivary and urine cortisol levels in persons with dementia (Woods & Dimond). Therapeutic touch is derived from an ancient healing practice and is defined as "a method of using the hands to direct human energies to help or heal" (Krieger, 1979, p. 1).

Activities

To improve activities for nursing home residents with dementia, the Centers for Medicaid and Medicare Services, in 2006, directed facilities to provide residents with a program of ongoing activities that meet their physical, mental, and psychosocial well-being. These activities must reflect the lifestyle and interests of the resident and include one-to-one programming for residents who choose not to leave their rooms, group activities, and self-directed activities offered throughout the day. These activities can include physical activities, such as exercise routines; cognitive activities, such as games; and psychosocial activities, such as club-based activities addressing topics of interest (Smith, Kolanowski, Buettner, & Buckwalter, 2009).

Therapeutic activity kits contain items that can be used to provide diversional activity. Items chosen for the kit are individualized with the help of family members and include articles that can provide cognitive and sensory stimulation. Examples of items that can be placed in the activity kit include audiotapes of family members and familiar music, photo albums, videotapes, art therapy, and textured cloth for tactile stimulation and folding activity (Conedera & Mitchell, 2004).

Buettner (1999) conducted a two-part study to test a multilevel sensorimotor intervention for nursing home residents with dementia called "simple pleasures." During part one, trained families and volunteers created 30 therapeutic sensorimotor recreational items that were age- and stage-appropriate for persons with dementia. In part two, the interventions were tested. For example, an activity apron was created and used for residents with repetitive motor patterns, whereas picture dominos were used for residents who were lethargic and isolated. Family members used these items to interact with their loved ones during visits and reported an increase in the quality of their visits. In addition, residents exhibited less agitation with use of the "simple pleasures" intervention. The original 30 items were subsequently tested in two nursing homes. Use of the simple pleasures resulted in additional social opportunities with a decrease in resident inactivity and less agitation. There was an increase in family and friend visits and improved satisfaction reported with these visits (Colling & Buettner, 2002).

Doll Therapy

The therapeutic use of dolls can elicit pleasure and provide a sensory stimulus, reassurance, and comfort in the older adult with dementia and can stimulate verbal and nonverbal communication, improve intimate-care interactions, and reduce wandering behaviors (Ehrenfeld & Bergman, 1995; Mackenzie, James, Morse, Mukaetova-Ladinska, & Reichelt, 2006). Dolls and stuffed animals used for this purpose should be constructed safely with nontoxic dyes and nondetachable parts that the client could swallow. Caregivers must be careful to avoid speaking to the older adult in a childlike manner when dolls are being used therapeutically.

Video Respite

Carefully selected videotapes can engage the older adult while providing a brief period of respite for the caregiver. Video Respite refers to the creation of videotapes that use music, light, movement, and pleasant memories to maintain the interest of the older adult. There are two methods used for creating these tapes. The first involves taping a family member who articulates scripts with individualized content. However, the time and energy involved in creating these tapes may add to existing caregiver burden. Consequently, generic videotapes have been created to reach a wide audience. Professional actors or actresses appear on the tapes by presenting simple, slow-paced conversation. Messages relate to experiences, people,

and objects that are likely to be ingrained in long-term memory. Early research findings revealed that most persons with dementia can watch and participate with the tapes, and staff on SCUs reported the tapes were calming for residents (Lund, Hill, Caserta, & Wright, 1995). More recent investigations of the intervention have shown that there are more positive verbal and nonverbal responses when the tapes are viewed alone, rather than in a group setting (Caserta & Lund, 2002). Research has shown that there is no relationship between cognitive ability and the ability to participate with and respond to the tapes (Caserta & Lund; Malone-Beach, Royer, & Jenkins, 1999); however, video programs that are less complex tend to be more engaging for the person with dementia (Heller, Dobbs, & Strain, 2009). Hall and Hare (1997) evaluated the effectiveness of one selected videotape ("Remembering When") in the series of 10 Video Respite tapes. Although findings did not reveal a significant reduction in agitated behaviors, there was a significant increase in positive behaviors.

Portable Automated Multisensory Intervention Device

A portable automated multisensory intervention device, resembling a stuffed toy, is designed to detect physiological measures of agitation. This information is wirelessly transmitted to a stimulation unit to provide sensory stimuli, such as music, aroma therapy, and light stimuli, to reduce agitation (Riley-Doucet & Debnath, 2009).

Simulated Presence Therapy

Simulated presence therapy uses a similar concept, by capturing a personalized conversation on audiotape about personal memories and family anecdotes. Soundless spaces are incorporated into the tape to encourage the cognitively impaired person to respond and engage in the conversation. Studies have shown significant improvement in problem behaviors and social isolation following the use of presence therapy (Miller et al., 2001; Woods & Ashley, 1995). A systematic review and meta-analysis of studies of simulated presence therapy conducted between 1997 and 2005 indicated that it is an effective intervention for the management of problem behaviors. The authors stress the importance of assessing and monitoring responses to the intervention, because some subjects experienced an increase in agitation. Patients most likely to benefit from simulated presence therapy have moderate to severe dementia and retain conversational skills (Zettler, 2008).

INTERVENTIONS DIRECTED TOWARD THE ENVIRONMENT

Environmental Modification

Whether the person is living at home or in a long-term care facility, it is often necessary to modify the environment to compensate for the person's impaired functional and cognitive status. Safety becomes a primary concern. Potentially harmful items, such as sharp objects and toxic fluids, should be removed from the client's environment. Misinterpretation of environmental stimuli can be confusing and frightening. Mirrors and photographs may need to be covered or removed and television and radio programming should be monitored for appropriateness. In the living area, clutter, highly polished floors, or scatter rugs can lead to falls in patients who may already suffer from an unsteady gait. To the extent possible, keep belongings, frequently used items, and furniture in the same place, so the person with dementia does not have to relearn their whereabouts and may rely more on habit and routine to negotiate the environment.

Home

Maintaining comfort in the home, while creating a safe environment for the older adult with dementia, is a challenge for caregivers. In addition to removing potentially dangerous objects from the client's environment, some relatively simple alterations to the home can have considerable benefits. Using contrasting colors for the walls and woodwork make it easier for the

older adult to more clearly distinguish doorways. Patterned wallpaper, curtains, and upholstery can cause confusion and should be replaced with solid colors wherever possible. Furniture should be in a contrasting color to the floor to make it easier to distinguish. The older adult with dementia may no longer have the skills to properly use rockers, recliners, and furniture on wheels. These types of furnishings may also present a hazard when leaned against to steady oneself. Carpeting, heavy curtains, and upholstered furniture help to absorb sound and can minimize confusion.

Grab bars installed in the bathtub and beside the toilet provide a measure of safety for all members of the household. A handheld shower can make bathing less frightening. Antiscalding devices installed in bathtub faucets and showers can prevent sudden changes in water temperature and accidental burns. Further, lowering the temperature on the hot water heater can prevent burns. Replacing the bathroom door and glass shower doors with shower curtains will continue to offer privacy but prevent the person from getting stuck or locked in the bathroom. If the color of the toilet and floor are similar, changing the toilet seat to a contrasting color helps the person distinguish the seat.

In the kitchen, removing extra pots, dishes, and utensils helps to minimize an overwhelming number of choices. Childproof locks can be installed on cabinet doors and oven doors to restrict access. Control knobs for the stove and oven should be removed to prevent injury. Labels or pictures of objects can help the older adult to identify correct cabinets or drawers.

Cognitive impairment limits the person's ability to differentiate between safe and unsafe acts. Age-related sensory impairments can further contribute to accidents or injury. Environmental camouflage or visual barriers, such as two-dimensional grid patterns on the floor in front of exits or cloth panels over doorknobs, have been shown to be effective in discouraging entrance into areas that are potentially unsafe (Dickinson, McLain, & Marshal-Baker, 1995). Other strategies that have been used with mixed results include placing stop signs before restricted areas, or painting a dark stripe on the floor in front of the "off limits" areas. Paint and wallpaper can be used to disguise or camouflage exits, closets, thermostats, and other potential architectural hazards.

Modifications made to the living environment are done primarily to maintain the safety of the individual. The challenge in planning modifications is in maintaining the independence and dignity of the older adult. The approach will likely need to be adapted as the disease progresses.

Music

Nursing research on the use of music has used two types of music: calming and individualized. Calming or relaxing music is chosen for the qualities of the music that are soothing, such as slow tempo, soft dynamic levels, and repetitive themes. To reduce the cognitive effort necessary to process the music,

lyrics and well-known tunes are avoided. It has been suggested that calming music mediates the release of stress hormones, altering the stress response, resulting in functionally adaptive behaviors. Calming music can be expected to reduce agitation for several persons simultaneously, such as in a group dining room (Ragneskog, Kihlgren, Karlsson, & Norberg, 1993; Remington, 2002; Tabloski, McKinnon-Howe, & Remington, 1995).

Alternatively, the presentation of carefully selected music, based on personal preference, provides an opportunity to stimulate remote memory. This changes the focus of attention and provides an interpretable stimulus, overriding stimuli in the environment that are meaningless or confusing. The elicitation of memories associated with positive feelings (e.g., happiness or love) has a soothing effect on the person with dementia, which in turn prevents or alleviates agitation (Box 13-1). There is a positive

BOX 13-1 RESEARCH WITH INDIVIDUALIZED MUSIC

Theoretical Basis: Mid-Range Theory of Individualized Music for Agitation (Gerdner, 1997)

Theory Testing Through Research: Gerdner (2000) used an experimental repeated measures pretest–posttest crossover design to compare the immediate and residual effects of individualized music to classical "relaxation" music relative to baseline on the frequency of agitated behaviors in 39 elderly persons with dementia residing in six LTCFs in Iowa. The selection of individualized music was based on information obtained from a close family member. Findings showed a significant reduction in agitation during and following individualized music compared to classical music.

Evidence-Based Protocol: Individualized music (Gerdner, 2007) or access information at http://www.guideline.gov/summary/summary.aspx?doc_id=10777

Feasibility: This intervention is relatively inexpensive and required minimal time expenditure. Following instruction by nursing staff, music may be implemented by nursing assistants and family members.

Translating Research into Practice: Gerdner (2005) evaluates the effectiveness of individualized music when implemented by trained staff and family members. Music was administered daily for 30 minutes at a prescribed time and "as needed" by CNAs. Family members were also encouraged to play music for their loved one during visits. A statistically significant reduction in agitation was found during the presentation of music. Music also promoted meaningful interaction between the residents, staff, family, and others.

correlation between the degree of significance music had in the person's life before the onset of cognitive impairment and the effectiveness of the intervention (Gerdner, 1997). A mid-range theory of individualized music was initially tested and supported through research conducted by Gerdner (2000). Since then, there has been an expanding body of research to support the use of this intervention for the management of agitation (Gerdner, 2005; Janelli, Kanski, & Wu, 2002; Park, 2008; Ragneskog, Asplund, Kihlgren, & Norberg, 2001; Sung, Chang, & Abbey, 2006; Sung, Chang, & Abbey, 2008; Suzuki et al., 2004). An evidence-based guideline was developed and has been refined and expanded based on this growing body of research (Gerdner, 2007).

INTERVENTIONS DIRECTED TOWARD THE CAREGIVER

Family Caregivers

Family members often care for persons with dementia in the home during the early to middle stages of cognitive impairment. Indeed, 70% of persons with dementia are cared for in their own home or a family member's home (Alzheimers Association, 2008) (Box 13-2). Caring for a relative with chronic confusion is among the most difficult of family responsibilities, triggering significant emotional, physical, and financial stress. The stress associated with caring for someone

BOX 13-2 DEMENTIA PORTRAYED IN POPULAR LITERATURE AND FILMS

Personal stories can help to facilitate an understanding of Alzheimer's disease from the perspective of the family member and the afflicted person. Professional and lay caregivers can learn from the experiences of those telling their story. Below are some of the many examples of these accounts that are available at larger bookstores.

- Bob Artley and Yasmin Khan (1993). *Ginny: A love remembered.* Ames, IA: Iowa State Press.
- Daniel A. Pollen (1993). *Hannah's heirs: The quest for the genetic origins of Alzheimer's disease.* Oxford: Oxford University Press.
- Esther Strauss Smoller and Kathleen O'Brien (1997). *I can't remember: Family stories of Alzheimer's disease.* Philadelphia: Temple University Press.
- Joyce Dyer (1996). *In a tangled wood: An Alzheimer's journey.* Dallas, TX: Southern Methodist University Press.
- Diana Friel McGowin (1994). *Living in the labyrinth: A personal journey through the maze of Alzheimer's.* New York: Delta.
- Lisa Genova (2009). *Still Alice.* New York: Simon & Schuster.

Movies, contemporary films, and television programs can depict a lifelike example of living with an older adult with dementia. Examples follow:

- *Iris* (2002), Buena Vista Home Video
- *The Notebook* (2004), New Line Cinema
- *Away from Her* (2007), Lions Gate Films
- *The Alzheimer's Project* (2009), HBO Documentary Films: A four-part documentary series changing the way America thinks about Alzheimer's disease, with funding from the National Institutes of Health, Alzheimer's Association, Fidelity Charitable Gift Fund, and Geoffrey Beene Givers Back Alzheimer's Initiative

with Alzheimer's disease and related disorders has been linked to a number of adverse outcomes, including depression, high psychotropic drug use, decline in physical health, and compromised immune response (Gallagher-Thompson & Powers, 1997; Garand et al., 2002; Meshefedjian, McCusker, Bellavance, & Baumgarten, 1998; Mort, Gaspar, Juffer, & Kovarna, 1996; Schulz, O'Brien, Bookwala, & Fleissner, 1995). Nurses are in an excellent position to provide training to empower family members with the knowledge and skills necessary in handling these problematic behaviors, while maintaining their own well-being.

Education and Support in Caregiving Responsibilities

The PLST model, as previously discussed, was used as the basis for a psychoeducational intervention to train in-home caregivers of family members with dementia. The PLST intervention was individualized for each caregiving dyad and focused on psychological support while providing instruction in behavioral techniques aimed at diminishing dysfunctional behaviors in the care recipient. Instruction focused on reducing environmental stressors, compensating for executive dysfunction and communication deficits, providing unconditional positive regard, and planning care based on a lowered stress threshold (Gerdner, Buckwalter, & Reed, 2002). An ongoing nursing relationship is pivotal in guiding family caregivers to establish a routine that maximizes abilities and minimizes stress for both the care recipient and the caregiver.

Referral to Support Groups for Care and Assistance

Family caregiving can become an all-consuming job for which caregivers often receive inadequate support and training (Kelley, Buckwalter, & Maas, 1999). Support groups provide an avenue to meet other family caregivers to share feelings and concerns, and provide emotional support and decrease the caregiver burden. Many support groups also provide learning opportunities

by formal community experts and the informal expertise of other caregivers. Caregivers frequently identify lack of respite care and geographic location as barriers to attending support group meetings. As a means of overcoming these barriers, nurse researchers are exploring the effectiveness of alternative methods, such as Internet support by computers (Beauchamp, Irvine, Seeley, & Johnson, 2005; White & Dorman, 2000) and telephone support (Davis, 1998; Gluechkauf et al., 2007).

Nursing Home Placement

When the family member is no longer able to care for his or her loved one at home, nursing home placement may be warranted. Many caregivers experience decreased depression and burden at 6 and 12 months after placing a family member in the nursing home; however, spouses demonstrate greater burden than adult children caregivers (Gaugler, Mittelman, Hepburn, & Newcomer, 2009). However, relocation to a nursing home does not necessarily mean an end to the stress experienced by family caregivers (Collins, Stommel, Wang, & Given, 1994). Some family caregivers experience feelings of guilt, betrayal, and inadequacy related to their caregiving role. Nursing home placement necessitates the assumption of a new role for the resident and caregiver (Butcher, Holkup, Park, & Maas, 2001). Most families do not know how to make the transition from direct care tasks to a more indirect, supportive, interpersonal role, nor are they likely to receive assistance from nursing home staff in how to go about making changes in their caregiver role. In some cases, families may encounter resistance and resentment from staff who view them as disruptive "outsiders" or "visitors" when they try to carry out decision making and protective care in the facility, resulting in staff–family role conflict (Maas et al., 1994).

Staff Training and Management

Age, education, experience, and training were shown to be associated with attitudes toward dementia care. Caregivers in nursing homes had generally positive attitudes toward older adults with dementia; however, nursing assistants, staff over 50 years of age, and those with greater than 10 years' work experience demonstrated lower scores on measures of hope (Kada, Nygaard, Mukesh, & Geitung, 2009).

Care of persons with dementia and the accompanying problematic behaviors has been reported as a major stressor to nursing staff (Hallberg & Norberg, 1993; Ragneskog et al., 1993) and can potentially lead to burnout. Certified nursing assistants provide the majority of direct care to residents in long-term care facilities. Inadequate training of nurses and certified nursing assistants in gerontological nursing has been linked to poor quality care in nursing homes, with adverse outcomes including falls, restraint, weight loss, urinary incontinence, pressure ulcers, and social isolation (Maas, Specht, Buckwalter, Gittler, & Bechen, 2008). Training can positively influence confidence in dealing with problem behaviors in dementia (Hughes, Bagley, Reilly, Burns, & Challis, 2008). Research has shown that training alone is not sufficient to ensure the retention of knowledge and skills over time. To address this concern, Stevens and colleagues (1998) developed an integrated in-service and staff management system that resulted in maintenance of skill performance over time. Staff nurses are trained to provide the supervision and mentoring of certified nursing assistants, while certified nursing assistants are trained to self-monitor performance. Staff members support this form of management because it is easy to use.

Researchers in Sweden developed a 2-day training session for staff nurses regarding individualized care of persons with dementia. Nurses were subsequently supervised in the application of this knowledge. In evaluating the effectiveness, nurses were encouraged to express personal feelings regarding the challenges they encountered, and problem-solving measures were undertaken. Following a 1-year period, nurses reported a higher degree of support and trust. They also experienced a significant reduction in the frequency and intensity of burnout, and exhibited a more cooperative interaction with clients (Berg, Hansson, & Hallberg, 1994; Edberg, Hallberg, & Gustafson, 1996; Hallberg & Norberg, 1993).

Staff–Family Partnership in Care

When planning care and developing a training program, it is important to recognize that family caregivers are a rich source of information regarding the resident's personal history, individualized routines, and personal preferences. Family may be able to share personal caregiving tips that they have found to be effective through years of trial and error. This knowledge can serve as a foundation for personalized and individualized care. Consequently, family members should be an important part of the dementia care team. Stressors for both the nursing staff and family can be eased by working together in a team approach. However, the degree of involvement varies depending on the family member's desires and abilities.

The Family Involvement in Care (FIC) protocol was developed by Maas et al. (1994) to diminish these potential conflicts, decrease family and staff stress, and increase satisfaction with caregiving roles. The FIC intervention is a step-by-step method designed to help nursing home staff and family members work together by achieving a negotiated partnership, in which control is shared and the particular expertise of each is used to the best advantage. The partnership emphasizes cooperation between staff and families and includes specific and clearly outlined roles for the family caregiver in the institutional setting (e.g., will co-lead reminiscence group every Wednesday afternoon). Key elements of the FIC protocol include (1) orientation of the family to the facility and the partnership role, (2) negotiation and formation of a partnership contract, (3) education of family members for involvement in care, and (4) follow-up family member and staff evaluation and re-negotiation of the partnership contract as needed. Findings from a major study evaluating the effects of the FIC protocol found improvements in both the caregiving experience of family members in nursing homes and the attitude of nursing home staff toward family members (Maas et al.).

DEMENTIA CARE RESOURCES

Theory can be used as a framework to plan, implement, and evaluate care. As research provides a growing foundation of knowledge, care is increasingly anchored in evidence-based protocols. The Electronic Dementia Guide for Excellence (EDGE) project was developed in 1995 by Ann Marie Bradley, Judah Ronch, and Elizabeth Pohlmann and funded by the New York State Department of Health. The project was developed to identify and disseminate intervention protocols generated from research specific to care of persons with dementia. Guidelines include staff training and evaluation of these interventions. The EDGE project can be accessed by the Internet at http://dementiasolutions.com/edge/ index.htm.

The John A. Hartford Institute for Geriatric Nursing is another resource for nurses that can be accessed through the Internet. Its programs identify and develop best nursing practice for older adults and are updated frequently. Abundant resources related to geriatric nursing practice, education, and research are available at www.hartfordign.org.

The Alzheimer's Association (www.alz.org) is a resource for patients, family, and professional caregivers. Through the national association and local chapters, information is available on care of the patient with dementia, and issues related to health, safety, legal, and financial matters.

The Alzheimer's Project produced a four-part HBO documentary on Alzheimer's disease with the National Institute on Aging at the National Institutes of Health, the Alzheimer's Association, Fidelity Charitable Gift Fund, and Geoffrey Beene Gives Back. Fifteen short supplemental films are available at http://www.hbo.com/alzheimers/. The Web site is a good source of community-based information and outreach.

The University of Iowa College of Nursing Gerontological Nursing Interventions Research Center, Research Translation and Dissemination Core, has 37 evidence-based nursing practice guidelines that are available at http://www.nursing.uiowa.edu/products_services/evidence_based.htm. Those guidelines that specifically related to the care of persons with dementia are Bathing Persons with Dementia, Detection of Depression in Older Adults with Dementia, Family Involvement in Care for Persons with Dementia, Individualized Music for Elders with Dementia, and Wandering.

CASE STUDY

Emma was a wonderful 4-ft, 7-in bundle of happy Italian energy for over 80 years. She lived in the center of the city and had her daily stops at the Square to meet her friends at the coffee shop, then did her shopping. She spent most summers at a family camp on the lake. It was at this camp that she developed her love of music and dance, frequently doing the Hully Gully, Alley Cat, waltz, or foxtrot with anyone who would join in.

Over the past few years, she had begun to forget things, like where she was going, or whether she had taken her pills, even though she could remember past events well. Her family physician diagnosed Alzheimer's disease. Increasingly, her confusion led to failing health. She became afraid and did not always recognize her family and would ask for people who had died years before. This confusion lead to failing health, and a decision was made to place her in a nursing home.

In her final days at the nursing home, she just lay on her bed with her eyes closed,

CASE STUDY *(continued)*

appearing petrified. Her family became frustrated with their inability to reach her and to comfort her. While reminiscing about "Grammy Emma" and her love of music, her granddaughter decided to make a recording of her favorite songs and brought it to the nursing home. When the dance music was played, she smiled and started moving her feet as if dancing in bed. She held her great-granddaughter's hand, swinging it to the music and smiled. When the songs finished, she shook her fist until they were played again, then drifted off to sleep and died.

- What are some qualities of musical selections that might have meaning for a person who is unable to communicate verbally?
- What other nonpharmacological interventions might enhance the therapeutic effect of music?
- What type of music do you think would have a calming effect for a patient for whom you are unable to identify a preferred style of music?

SUMMARY

Dementia is characterized by a progressive cognitive and functional decline, affecting the physical and mental health of the older adult. The geropsychiatric nurse working with the older adult with dementia needs to use knowledge and skills from a variety of nursing specialties. The geropsychiatric nurse must be an expert in gerontological and psychiatric nursing. Understanding issues related to the aging process, complicated by cognitive losses, is a key in formulating effective treatment plans. Knowledge of the community and community resources enables the nurse to help families enhance their caregiving role. Treatment plans that address the person, the environment, and the caregiver have the potential to maintain the dignity and quality of life for the person, family, and caregivers.

REFERENCES

Algase, D. L., Beck, C., Kolanowski, A., Whall, A., Berent, S., Richards, K., et al. (1996). Need-driven dementia-compromised behavior: An alternative view of disruptive behavior. *American Journal of Alzheimer's Disease, 1*(6), 10–19.

Alzheimer's Association. (2008). 2008 Alzheimer's disease facts and figures. *Alzheimer's & Dementia, 4*(2), 110–133.

Aschenbrenner, D. S., & Venable, S. J. (2009). *Drug therapy in nursing* (3rd ed.). New York: Lippincott.

Bates, J., Boote, J., & Beverly, C. (2004). Psychosocial interventions for people with a milder dementing illness: A systematic review. *Journal of Advanced Nursing, 45*, 644–658.

Beauchamp, N., Irvine, A. B., Seeley, J., & Johnson, B. (2005). Worksite-based internet multimedia program for family caregivers of persons with dementia. *Gerontologist, 45*(6), 793–801.

Berg, A., Hansson, U. W., & Hallberg, I. R. (1994). Nurses' creativity, tedium and burnout during 1 year of clinical supervision and implementation of individually planned nursing care: Comparisons between a ward for severely demented patients and a similar control ward. *Journal of Advanced Nursing, 20*, 742–749.

Birks, J. (2006). Cholinesterase inhibitors for Alzheimer's disease. *Cochrane Database of Systematic Reviews, 1*, CD 005593 DOI 10.1002/14651858.CD005593

Bowers, B. J., & Nolet, K. (2009). The role of the nurse in the greenhouse model. *The Gerontologist, 49*(S2), 266.

Bravo, G., Dubois, F. F., & Wagneur, B. (2008). Assessing the effectiveness of interventions to promote advance directives among older adults: A systematic review and multi-level analysis. *Social Science & Medicine, 67*, 1122–1132.

Buckwalter, K. C., Stolley, J. M., & Farran, C. J. (1999). Managing cognitive impairment in the elderly: Conceptual, intervention and methodological issues [Electronic version]. *The Online Journal of Knowledge Synthesis for Nursing, 6*(10), 10.

Buettner, L. L. (1999). Simple pleasures: A multi-level sensorimotor intervention for nursing home residents with dementia. *American Journal of Alzheimer's Disease, 14*(1), 41–52.

Buettner, L., & Kolanowski, A. (2003). Practice guidelines for recreation therapy in the care of people with dementia. *Geriatric Nursing, 24*(1), 18–25.

Burgener, S. C., Buettner, L. L., Beattie, E., & Rose, K. M. (2009). Effectiveness of community-based, nonpharmacological interventions for early-stage dementia: Conclusions and recommendations. *Journal of Gerontological Nursing, 35*(3), 50–57.

Burgener, S. C., Buettner, L., Buckwalter, K. C., Beattie, E., Bossen, A. L., Flick, D., et al. (2008). Review of exemplar programs for adults with early-stage Alzheimer's disease. *Research in Gerontological Nursing, 1*(4), 295–304.

Butcher, H. K., Holkup, P. A., Park, M., & Maas, M. (2001). Thematic analysis of the experience of making a decision to place a family member with Alzheimer's disease in a special care unit. *Research in Nursing & Health, 24*(6), 470–480.

Caserta, M., & Lund, D. (2002). Video respite on an Alzheimer's care center: Group versus solitary viewing. *Activities, Adaptation and Aging, 27*(1), 13–26.

Chan, A., Paskavitz, J., Remington, R., & Shea, T. (2009). Efficacy of a vitamin/nutriceutical formulation for early-stage Alzheimer's disease: A 1-year open label pilot study with a 16 month caregiver extension. *American Journal of Alzheimer's Disease & Other Dementias, 23*, 571–585.

Clark, A., Hanson, E. J., & Ross, H. (2003). Seeing the person behind the patient: Enhancing the care of older people using a biographical approach. *Journal of Clinical Nursing, 12*, 697–706.

Colling, K. B., & Buettner, L. L. (2002). Simple Pleasures: Interventions from the Need-Driven Dementia-Compromised Behavior Model. *Journal of Gerontological Nursing, 28*(10), 16–20.

Collins, C., Stommel, M., Wang, S., & Given, C. W. (1994). Caregiving transitions: Changes in depression among family caregivers of relatives with dementia. *Nursing Research, 43*(4), 220–225.

Conedera, F., & Mitchell, L. (2004). Therapeutic activity kits. *Try This: Best Practices in Nursing Care for Hospitalized Older Adults, 1*(4). Retrieved July 28, 2004, from http://www.hartfordign.org/publication/trythis/theraAct.pdf

Davis, L. L. (1998). Telephone-based interventions with family caregivers: A feasibility study. *Journal of Family Nursing, 4*(3), 255–270.

Davis, L. L., & Buckwalter, K. C. (2001). Family caregiving after nursing home admission. *Journal of Mental Health and Aging, 7*(3), 361–379.

Daykin, N. (2008). Review: The impact of art, design and environment in mental healthcare: A systematic review of the literature. *Perspectives in Public Health, 128*(2), 85–94.

Deglin, J. H., & Vallerand, A. H. (2003). *Davis's drug guide for nurses.* Philadelphia: Davis.

Dickinson, J. I., McLain, J. K., & Marshal-Baker, A. (1995). The effects of visual barriers on existing behavior in a dementia care unit. *Gerontologist, 35*(1), 127–130.

Edberg, A., Hallberg, I. R., & Gustafson, L. (1996). Effects of clinical supervision on nurse-patient cooperation quality. *Clinical Nursing Research, 5*(2), 127–149.

Ehrenfeld, M., & Bergman, R. (1995). The therapeutic use of dolls. *Perspectives in Psychiatric Care, 31*(4), 21–22.

Fritch, T., Kwak, J., Grant, S., Lang, J., Montgomery, R., & Basting, A. D. (2009). Impact of Time Slips, a creative expression intervention program on nursing home residents with dementia and their caregivers. *The Gerontologist, 49*(1), 117–127.

Gallagher-Thompson, D., & Powers, D. V. (1997). Primary stressors and depressive symptoms in caregivers of dementia patients. *Aging & Mental Health, 1*(3), 248–255.

Garand, L., Buckwalter, K. C., Lubaroff, D., Tripp-Reimer, T., Frantz, R. A., & Ansley, T. N. (2002). A pilot study of immune and mood outcomes of a community-based intervention for dementia caregivers: The PLST Intervention. *Archives of Psychiatric Nursing, 16*(4), 156–167.

Garnett, W. E. (2003). Memantine for Alzheimer's disease. *Long-Term Care Interface, 4*(12), 14–15.

Gaugler, J. E., Mittelman, M. S., Hepburn, K., & Newcomer, R. (2009). Predictors of change in caregiver burden and depressive symptoms following nursing home admission. *Psychology and Aging, 24*(2), 385–396.

Gerdner, L. A. (1997). An individualized music intervention for agitation. *Journal of the American Psychiatric Nurses Association, 3*(6), 177–184.

Gerdner, L. A. (2000). Effects of individualized vs. classical "relaxation" music on the frequency of agitation in elderly persons with Alzheimer's disease and related disorders. *International Psychogeriatrics, 12*(1), 49–65.

Gerdner, L. A. (2005). Use of individualized music by trained staff and family: Translating research into practice. *Journal of Gerontological Nursing, 31*(6), 22–30.

Gerdner, L. A. (2007). Evidence-based guideline: Individualized music for elders with dementia. In M. G. Titler (Series Ed.), *Series on Evidence-Based Practice for Older Adults.* Iowa City, IA: The University of Iowa College of Nursing Gerontological Nursing Interventions Research Center, Research Translation and Dissemination Core.

Gerdner, L. A., & Beck, C. K. (2006). Impact of Arkansas state regulations for certification of Alzheimer's special care units. *Alzheimer's Care Quarterly, 7*(4), 251–257.

Gerdner, L. A., & Buckwalter, K. C. (1996). Review of state policies regarding special care units: Implications for family consumers and health care professionals. *American Journal of Alzheimer's Disease and Other Dementias, 11*(2), 16–27.

Gerdner, L.A., Buckwalter, K. C., & Reed, D. (2002). The impact of a psychoeducational nursing intervention on frequency of and response to behavioral problems and functional decline in dementia. *Nursing Research, 51*(6), 607–618.

Gluechkauf, R. L., Sharma, D., Shuford, D. W., Byrd, V., Stine, C., Jeffers, S. B., et al. (2007). Telephone-based cognitive-behavioral intervention for distressed rural dementia caregivers: Initial findings. *Clinical Gerontologist, 31*(1), 21–41.

Gruneir, A., Lapane, K. L., Miller, S. C., & Mor, V. (2008). Is dementia special care really special? A new look at an old question. *Journal of the American Geriatrics Society, 56*, 199–205.

Hall, G. R., & Buckwalter, K. C. (1987). Progressively lowered stress threshold: A conceptual model for care of adults with Alzheimer's disease. *Archives of Psychiatric Nursing, 1*, 399–406.

Hall, L., & Hare, J. (1997). Video respite for cognitively impaired persons in nursing homes. *American Journal of Alzheimer's Disease, 12*(3), 117–121.

Hallberg, I. R., & Norberg, A. (1993). Strain among nurses and their emotional reactions during 1 year of systematic clinical supervision combined with the implementation of individualized care in dementia nursing. *Journal of Advanced Nursing, 18*, 1860–1875.

Harlan, J. E. (1993). The therapeutic value of art for persons with Alzheimer's disease and related disorders. *Loss, Grief, & Care: A Journal of Professional Practice, 6*(4), 99–106.

Hawranik, P., Johnston, J., & Deatrich, J. (2008). Therapeutic touch and agitation in individuals with Alzheimer's disease. *Western Journal of Nursing Research, 30*(4), 417–434.

Heller, R. B., Dobbs, B. M., & Strain, L. A. (2009). Video programming for individuals with dementia: Assessing cognitive congruence. *American Journal of Alzheimer's Disease and Other Dementias, 24*(2), 122–128.

Hill, N., Milone-Nuzzo, P., & Kolanowski, A. (2009). Culture change models and resident-specific outcomes in long-term care. *The Gerontologist, 49*(S2), 266.

Hsieh, H., & Wang, J. (2003). Effect of reminiscence therapy on depression in older adults: A systematic review. *International Journal of Nursing Studies, 40*, 335–345.

Hughes, J., Bagley, H., Reilly S., Burns, A., & Challis, D. (2008). Care staff working with people with dementia: training, knowledge and confidence. *Dementia, 7*(2), 227–238.

Janelli, L., Kanski, G., & Wu, Y. (2002). Individualized music—a different approach to the restraint use. *Rehabilitation Nursing, 27*(6), 221–226.

Janevic, M. R., & Connell, C. M. (2001). Racial, ethnic, and cultural differences in the dementia caregiving experience: Recent findings. *The Gerontologist, 41*(3), 334–347.

Jett, K. (2008). Economic, residential, and legal issues. In P. Ebersole, P. Hess, T. A. Touhy, K. Jet, & A. S. Luggen (Eds.), *Toward healthy aging: Human needs & nursing response* (pp. 428–447). Philadelphia: Mosby.

Kada, S., Nygaard, H. A., Mukesh, B. N., & Geitung, J. T. (2009). Staff attitudes towards institutionalised dementia residents *Journal of Clinical Nursing, 18*(16), 2383–2392.

Kahn-Denis, K. B. (1997). Art therapy with geriatric dementia clients. *Journal of the American Art Therapy Association, 14*, 194–199.

Keegan, L. (2001). *Healing with complementary & alternative therapies*. Albany, NY: Delmar.

Kelley, L. S., Buckwalter, K. C., & Maas, M. L. (1999). Access to health care resources for family caregivers of elderly persons with dementia. *Nursing Outlook, 47*(10), 8–14.

Kovach, C. R., Noonan, P. E., Schlidt, A. M., & Wells, T. (2005). A model of consequences of need-driven, dementia-compromised behavior. *Journal of Nursing Scholarship, 37*(2), 134–140.

Krieger, D. (1979). *The therapeutic touch: How to use your hands to help or to heal*. New York: Prentice Hall.

Libow, L. S. (2003). Memantine: A new hope for treating patients with dementia in nursing homes. *Long-Term Care Interface, 4*(9), 8–9.

Linton, A. D., & Lach, H. W. (2007). *Gerontological nursing: Concepts and practice*. Philadelphia: Saunders Elsevier.

Lund, D. A., Hill, R. D., Caserta, M. S., & Wright, S. D. (1995). Video respite: An innovative resource for family, professional caregivers, and persons with dementia. *The Gerontologist, 35*, 683–687.

Maas, M., Buckwalter, K., Swanson, E., Specht, J., Hardy, M., & Tripp-Reimer, T. (1994). The caring partnership: Staff and families of persons institutionalized with Alzheimer's disease. *American Journal of Alzheimer's Disease and Related Disorders & Research*, Nov/Dec, 21–30.

Maas, M. L., Specht, J. P., Buckwalter, K. C., Gittler, J., & Bechen, K. (2008). Nursing home staffing and training recommendations for promoting older adults' quality of care and life: Part 1. Deficits in the quality of care due to understaffing and undertraining. *Research in Gerontological Nursing, 2*(2), 123–133.

Mackenzie, L., James, I. A., Morse, R., Mukaetova-Ladinska, E., & Reichelt, F. K. (2006). A pilot study on the use of dolls for people with dementia. *Age & Ageing, 35*(4), 441–444.

Malone-Beach, E. E., Royer, M., & Jenkins, C. C. (1999). Is cognitive impairment a guide to use of video respite? Lessons from a special care unit. *Journal of Gerontological Nursing, 25*(5), 17–21.

Malony, S. (2009). Mixed methods study of older adults' experiences in a traditional and small house nursing home. *The Gerontologist, 49*(S2), 249.

Matteson, M. A., Linton, A., & Barnes, S. J. (1996). Cognitive developmental approach to dementia. *Image—The Journal of Nursing Scholarship, 28*, 233–240.

Meshefedjian, G., McCusker, J., Bellavance, F., & Baumgarten, M. (1998). Factors associated with symptoms of depression among informal caregivers of demented elders in the community. *Gerontologist, 38*(2), 247–253.

Miller, C. A. (2009). *Nursing for wellness in older adults: Theory and practice* (5th ed.). New York: Lippincott.

Miller, S., Vermeersch, P., Bohan, K., Renbarger, K., Kruep, A., & Sacre, S. (2001). Audio presence intervention for decreasing agitation in people with dementia. *Geriatric Nursing, 22*(2), 66–70.

Mitchell, S. L., Kiely, D. K., Miller, S. C., Connor, S. R., Spence, C., & Teno, J. M. (2007). Hospice care for patients with dementia. *Journal of Pain and Symptom Management, 34*(1), 7–16.

Mort, J. R., Gaspar, P. M., Juffer, D. I., & Kovarna, M. B. (1996). Comparison of psychotropic agent use among rural elderly caregivers and noncaregivers. *Annals of Pharmacotherapy, 30*(6), 583–585.

Norlander, L. (2001). *To comfort always: A nurse's guide to end of life care*. Washington, DC: American Nurses Association.

Norlander, L., & McSteen, K. (2000). The kitchen table discussion: A creative way to discuss end-of-life issues. *Home Healthcare Nurse, 18*(8), 532–540.

Okumura, Y., Tanimukai, S., & Asada, T. (2008). Effects of short-term reminiscence therapy on elderly with dementia: A comparison with everyday conversation approaches. *Psychogeriatrics, 8*, 124–133.

Park, H. (2008). *The effect of individualized music on agitation in patients with dementia who live at home*. PhD dissertation, University of Iowa, Iowa City, Iowa.

Pittiglio, L. (2000). Use of reminiscence therapy in patients with Alzheimer's disease. *Lippincott's Case Management, 5*, 216–220.

Ragneskog, H., Asplund, K., Kihlgren, M., & Norberg, A. (2001). Individualized music played for agitated patients with dementia: Analysis of video-recorded sessions. *International Journal of Nursing Practice, 7*, 146–155.

Ragneskog, H., Kihlgren, M., Karlsson, I., & Norberg, A. (1993). Nursing home staff opinions of work with demented patients and effects of training in integrity-promoting care. *Vard I Norden Nursing Science & Research in the Nordic Countries, 13*(1), 5–10.

Raina, P., Santaguida, P., Ismaila, A., Patterson, C., Cowan, D., Levine, M., et al. (2008). Effectiveness of cholinesterase inhibitors and memantine for treating dementia: Evidence review for a clinical practice guideline. *Annals of Internal Medicine, 148*(5), 379–397.

Remington, R. (2002). Calming music and hand massage with agitated elderly. *Nursing Research, 51,* 317–323.

Remington, R., Abdallah, L., Melillo, K. D., & Flanagan, J. (2006). Managing problem behaviors associated with dementia. *Rehabilitation Nursing, 31*(5), 186–192.

Remington, R., Chan, A., Paskavitz, J., & Shea, T. (2008). Efficacy of a vitamin/nutriceutical formulation for moderate-stage to later-stage Alzheimer's disease: A placebo-controlled pilot study. *American Journal of Alzheimer's Disease & Other Dementias, 24*(1), 27–33.

Riley-Doucet, C. K., & Debnath, D. (2009). Assessment of a Portable Multisensory Autonomous Intervention Device. *The Gerontologist, 49*(S2), 94.

Schulz, R., O'Brien, A. T., Bookwala, J., & Fleissner, K. (1995). Psychiatric and physical morbidity effects of dementia caregiving: Prevalence, correlates, and causes. *The Gerontologist, 35*(6), 771–791.

Smith, M., Gerdner, L. A., Hall, G., & Buckwalter, K. C. (2004). The history, development, and future of the Progressively Lowered Stress Threshold Model: A conceptual model for dementia care. *Journal of the American Geriatrics Society, 52*(10), 1755–1760.

Smith, M., Hall, G. R., Gerdner, L. A., & Buckwalter, K. C. (2006). Application of the Progressively Lowered Stress Threshold (PLST) Model across the continuum of care. *Nursing Clinics of North America, 41*(1), 57–81.

Smith, M., Kolanowski, A., Buettner, L. L., & Buckwalter, K. C. (2009). Beyond bingo: Meaningful activities for persons with dementia in nursing homes. *Annals of Long-Term Care, 17*(7), 22–30.

Smith-Jones, S. M., & Francis, G. M. (1992). Disruptive institutionalized elderly: A cost effective intervention. *Journal of Psychosocial Nursing and Mental Health Services, 30,* 17–20.

Snyder, M., Egan, E. C., & Burns, K. R. (1995). Efficacy of hand massage in decreasing agitation behaviors associated with care activities in persons with dementia. *Geriatric Nursing, 16*(2), 60–63.

Spoelhof, G. D., & Foerst, L. F. (2002). Herbs to magnets: Managing alternative therapies in the nursing home. *Annals of Long-Term Care, 12*(12), 51–57.

Stevens, A. B., Burgio, L. D., Bailey, E., Burgio, K. L., Paul, P., Capilouto, E., et al. (1998). Teaching and maintaining behavior management skills with nursing assistants in a nursing home. *The Gerontologist, 38*(3), 379–384.

Sung, H., Chang, A. M., & Abbey, J. (2006). The effects of preferred music on agitation of older people with dementia in Taiwan. *International Journal of Geriatric Psychiatry, 21*(10), 999–1000.

Sung, H-C., Chang, A. M., & Abbey, J. (2008). An implementation programme to improve nursing home staff's knowledge of and adherence to an individualized music protocol. *Journal of Clinical Nursing, 17*(19), 2573–2579.

Suzuki, M., Kanamori, M., Watanabe, M., Nagasawa, S., Kojima, E., Ooshiro, H., et al. (2004). Behavioral and endocrinolgcal evaluation of music therapy for elderly patients with dementia. *Nursing and Health Sciences, 6,* 11–18.

Tabloski, P. A., McKinnon-Howe, L., & Remington, R. (1995). Effects of calming music on level of agitation in cognitively impaired nursing home residents. *The American Journal of Alzheimer's Disease and Related Disorders & Research, 10*(1), 10–15.

Volicer, L., Hurley, A. C., & Blaise, Z. V. (2003). Characteristics of end-of-life dementia care across care settings. *American Journal of Hospice and Palliative Care, 20*(3), 191–201.

White, M. H., & Dorman, S. M. (2000). Online support for caregivers: Analysis of an internet Alz-heimer's mailgroup. *Computers in Nursing, 18*(4), 168–179.

Woodrow, P. (1998). Interventions for confusion and dementia: Reminiscence. *British Journal of Nursing, 7*(20), 1145–1149.

Woods, D. L., & Dimond, M. (2002). The effect of therapeutic touch on agitated behavior and cortisol in persons with Alzheimer's disease. *Biological Research for Nursing, 4*(2), 104–114.

Woods, P., & Ashley, J. (1995). Simulated presence therapy: Using selected memories to manage problem behaviors in Alzheimer's disease. *Geriatric Nursing, 16*(1), 9–14.

Yeo, G., & Gallagher-Thomson, D. (Eds.). (2006). *Ethnicity and dementias* (2nd ed.). New York: Taylor and Francis.

Zettler, J. (2008). Effectiveness of simulated presence therapy for individuals with dementia: A systematic review and meta-analysis. *Aging & Mental Health, 12*(6), 779–785.

14

Addressing Problem Behaviors Common to Late-Life Dementias

Ruth Remington
May Futrell

Mary is an 87-year-old nursing home resident with a medical history that includes osteoarthritis, hypertension, and advanced dementia. Her roommate is bedbound and noncommunicative. Over the past few weeks, Mary has refused to leave her room and staff members have been leaving her television on all day to provide some stimulation. She has begun to carry on long conversations in her room and the nurses are requesting a psychiatric consultation, believing that Mary is experiencing hallucinations. As you read this chapter, try to identify some interventions that nursing staff can implement before calling for a psychiatric consult.

Problem behaviors associated with late-life dementias are disturbing for the older person and tax the ability of their caregivers. Such behaviors as agitation, wandering, feeding difficulties, sleep disturbances, and inappropriate sexual advances often hasten nursing home placement. These behaviors can also be an indication of stressors that the person with dementia is not able to communicate to caregivers. The individual becomes less able to tolerate stress because of the progressive loss of brain cells. Physical stressors or environmental stimuli may provoke a stressful response in the individual, resulting in problem behaviors. Ineffective management of these behaviors, by both formal and informal caregivers, subjects the individual to additional stress and escalation of the behaviors.

Identification of antecedents to problem behaviors and prompt intervention can help the individual to continue to communicate and function effectively. Caregivers and families can be taught to recognize behaviors that may indicate increasing stress and respond in a way that preserves the dignity and function of the person with dementia.

AGITATION

Agitation is a common management problem in persons with late-life dementia. Up to 50% of community-dwelling older people (Carlson, Fleming, Smith, & Evans, 1995) and 93% of nursing home residents exhibit agitated behaviors, with the highest percentage being in persons with dementia (Beck & Shue, 1994). The presence of agitated behaviors is distressing to the older person and presents considerable challenges to caregivers. Agitated behaviors, coupled with the loss of communication skills, may put the person with dementia at risk for inadequate assessment and treatment. For example, a hearing impairment may increase the person's disorientation, which results in agitation. Additionally, the agitated person is less likely to be offered, or participate in, audiometric testing to identify hearing loss.

The concept of agitation and its expression has not been consistently described in the literature. "Agitation" has been defined as inappropriate vocal, verbal, or motor activity that is not explained by unmet needs that are apparent to the observer (Cohen-Mansfield & Billig, 1986); an excited condition that persists after interventions are carried out to reduce stimuli and manage resistiveness, physical discomfort, and stress (Hurley et al., 1999); and an excess of one or more behaviors occurring in a state of altered consciousness (Corrigan, Bogner, & Tabloski, 1996). Common among these descriptions is that agitation can be verbal, vocal, or motor, either aggressive or non-aggressive, always inappropriate, but most importantly, agitation negatively affects the individual or others in the environment (Remington, Abdallah, Melillo, & Flanagan, 2006).

There is disparity among researchers as to the behavioral components of agitation. Some consider agitation to be specific behaviors, such as hitting, repetitive movement, and negative vocalizations (Cohen-Mansfield, 1986), whereas others group clusters of behaviors including memory problems, delusions and hallucinations (Teri et al., 1992), and resistance to care (Vance et al., 2003). Still others describe agitation as behavioral excess rather than a specific behavior (Corrigan et al., 1996). Terms associated with agitation include disruptive behavior, problem behavior, troublesome behavior, behavior disturbance, dysfunctional behavior, and behavior symptoms associated with dementia (American Geriatrics Society and American Association for Geriatric Psychiatry, 2003).

Agitated behaviors can be physically aggressive (e.g., hitting, kicking, grabbing, or cursing); physically nonaggressive (e.g., pacing, repetitious mannerisms, or handling things inappropriately); or verbal (e.g., complaining, screaming, or repetitious sentences). These behaviors are inappropriate or performed with excessive frequency. The severity of the behaviors is related to the degree of physical danger the behavior poses to the person or caregiver, or the disruptiveness to the person,

caregiver, and the environment (Cohen-Mansfield & Billig, 1986).

When changes in the brain caused by the dementing illness result in impaired memory, reasoning, and language, behavior becomes a primary means of communication with others in the environment (Remington et al., 2006). The pathophysiological basis for agitation is not well understood. It has been suggested that neurotransmitter dysregulations are implicated in the development of agitation. The restlessness associated with agitation is thought to be the result of abnormalities in the striatum, cortex, and thalamus, and mediated in part by γ-aminobutyric acid. Persons with dementia are reported to have a higher sensitivity to norepinephrine, a reduced serotonergic function, and γ-aminobutyric acid deficits (Lindenmayer, 2000; Neugroschi, 2002). Agitation associated with aggression may be related to an increase in noradrenergic activity and a decrease in serotonergic activity.

The presence of agitated behaviors increases the probability of caregiver burden and is an important predictor of nursing home placement (Spillman & Long, 2009). Once in the nursing home, agitation affects the cost of care by increasing the need for staff and special environmental design (Cohen-Mansfield, 1995). Agitation places the health of the individual at further risk. Agitated nursing home residents are more likely to fall than nonagitated residents, and the physically compromised older person with severe agitation is at higher risk for hip fractures, subdural hematoma, or cardiovascular collapse from exhaustion (Beresin, 1988; Cohen-Mansfield & Werner, 1995). Agitation results in individuals being more likely to be physically or chemically restrained. Research has repeatedly shown that, in addition to loss of dignity and potential for injury, agitated persons who are restrained exhibit the same or more agitation, confusion, incontinence, and falls than those who are not restrained. Reduction in restraint use has actually been shown to result in fewer falls and injuries (Fonad, Emami, Wahlin, Winblad, & Sandmark, 2009; Talerico & Evans, 2001; Weinrich, Egbert, Eleazer, & Haddock, 1995).

Chemical restraint, or use of pharmacological agents, is effective in managing agitated behaviors; however, age-related changes subject the agitated individual to longer duration of action of the drug and increased incidence of adverse drug reactions. These medications introduce the potential for gait impairment, falls, anorexia, sedation, hypotension, diminished cognitive function, and may even paradoxically exacerbate the agitation (Chutka, 1997; Gardner & Garrett, 1997).

Antecedents

Examining events or phenomena that precede the occurrence of agitation is the first step in planning interventions to manage agitated behavior (Gerdner & Buckwalter, 1994). Before the work of Cohen-Mansfield and colleagues, information regarding the antecedents of agitation was mostly anecdotal (Cohen-Mansfield, 1986; Cohen-Mansfield & Billig, 1986). More recently, empirical studies have identified factors that precede the manifestation of agitation.

Four factors have been described as precipitating antecedents: (1) patient factors, (2) environmental factors, (3) interpersonal relation factors, and (4) restraints or medication. These may directly cause agitation, or may mediate the development of agitation. Mediating factors include discomfort, unmet needs, and misinterpretation (Kong, 2005).

Cognitive Impairment

Both acute and chronic cognitive impairment in the older adult may present with agitation. Delirium can cause confusion and agitation that can be difficult to differentiate from dementia. Delirium is an acute, reversible form of cognitive impairment, affecting up to 60% of hospitalized older adults (Ely et al., 2001). Nurses identified delirium in only 31% of hospitalized patients (Inouye, Foreman, Mion, Katz, & Cooney, 2001). When the underlying cause for the delirium is identified and treated, the patient may return to baseline behavior.

Cognitive impairment has been shown to be strongly related to manifestations of agitation.

The type of agitated behavior is influenced by the degree of cognitive impairment. Although all types of agitation can occur at any stage of dementia, verbal agitation is more common in persons with increasing age, female gender, and increased cognitive impairment. Nonaggressive agitated behaviors tend to increase with cognitive decline, but the frequency is not related to impairment of activities of daily living. In general, increases in the frequency of agitation are associated with increasing cognitive impairment (Cohen-Mansfield & Libin, 2005), until the development of profound neurological impairment, when the total number of all behaviors, including agitation, tends to decrease.

Changes in the brain that cause impairments in memory, judgment, language, and impulse control predispose a person with dementia to agitation. As language skills are lost, behavior becomes the main form of communication. It has been suggested that agitation may be the person's attempt to communicate needs or feelings that cannot be verbalized in a way that caregivers can understand (Sutor, Rummans, & Smith, 2001). The loss of functioning brain cells associated with dementia causes the person to become less able to receive and process sensory stimuli. As the level of dementia increases, the threshold between baseline and agitated behavior declines, placing the person at a greater risk for agitated behaviors. Agitated behaviors constitute a greater proportion of the individual's behaviors over the course of the disease (Gerdner, 2005; Hall & Buckwalter, 1987).

Sensory Impairment

Sensory impairment has been implicated in the development of agitation. Hearing and vision impairments are common among older adults; however, most can compensate for the losses. For the person with dementia, this can cause misinterpretation of environmental cues. Hearing and vision impairment were shown to be strong predictors of agitation (Vance et al., 2003). It has been suggested that persons with dementia become disoriented by the lack of clear auditory and visual information and are likely to speak more loudly. This, coupled with communication losses, can cause these vocalizations to be considered noisy and disruptive by others in the environment (Algase et al., 1996; Vance et al.). When asked to identify apparent reasons for agitation, nurses reported deafness as a disability predisposing older persons to agitation (Cohen-Mansfield, 1986). Interventions as simple as providing clean eyeglasses and hearing aids with fresh batteries can reduce the effects of sensory impairment on behavior (Gerdner & Buckwalter, 1994; Remington et al., 2006).

Sensory components of activities of daily living have been linked with agitation in persons with dementia. Increased agitation during bathing was postulated to be caused by frustration and a sense of loss of control (Cohen-Mansfield, 1986; Mahoney et al., 1999; Sutor et al., 2001). During meals, increased agitation was attributed to noise (Goddaer & Abraham, 1994; Thomas & Smith, 2009). Aggressive agitated behaviors increased while nursing home residents were touched, in response to a hypothesized violation of personal space (Marx, Werner, & Cohen-Mansfield, 1989).

Physiological

Agitation may be precipitated by physiological processes, such as infections, cardiovascular insufficiency, hypoxia, alcohol use, dehydration, fatigue, and constipation. Pain is an often-overlooked antecedent to agitated behaviors. The worsening of a chronic medical condition may lead to agitated behaviors, just as an increase in agitation may signify a change in the medical condition. Prompt assessment, careful monitoring, and treatment of underlying conditions can alleviate the behavior problem.

Information processing and circadian rhythm generation have been linked to the hypothalamic suprachiasmatic nucleus. The decrease in function of this center, which occurs with aging, is more pronounced in persons with dementia. The resulting altered circadian rhythm has been associated with an increase in agitation (Voicer, Harper, Manning, Goldstein, & Satlin, 2001). This may

explain an increase in agitation in the late afternoon, called "sundown syndrome" as reported by many (Algase et al., 1996; Dewing, 2003; Volicer, et al.). Others have found that agitation was more frequent during the day shift than evening or night shifts (Cohen-Mansfield, Marx, & Rosenthal, 1989). Another rhythm, the lunar phase, has been associated with increases in agitation. There have been anecdotal accounts from caregivers of increased agitation occurring during the full moon. This has not been supported by research (Cohen-Mansfield, Marx, & Werner, 1989).

Personality and Psychiatric

Agitation is a common manifestation of depression, some psychoses, and anxiety. Unresolved past issues, premorbid personality, and coping style have been proposed as influencing the expression of agitation (Cohen-Mansfield & Billig, 1986; Hall, 1994). Delusions and hallucinations are fairly common as causes of agitated behaviors. Ropacki and Jeste (2005) conducted a review of 55 studies of psychosis in dementia. The mean sample size of these studies was 177 subjects (range, 27–1155). In these studies delusions were reported to be present in 36% of subjects and hallucinations in 18%. Most of the studies were conducted in outpatient settings, such as outpatient clinics or research centers.

Pharmacological Effects

Drug toxicity is one of the most common precipitants of agitation. Both prescription and over-the-counter drugs frequently used among older adults for their therapeutic effect are often implicated. Corticosteroids, anticholinergics, levodopa, sedative–hypnotics, and barbiturates are some of the drugs of concern. Withdrawal from central nervous system depressants also produces agitation. The risks associated with psychotropic medications have come under scrutiny, particularly since Beers et al. (1991) first published a list of potentially inappropriate drugs for the elderly, yet these medications continue to be used to manage agitation.

Psychotropic drugs account for more than 45% of the drugs of concern that are prescribed to older adults (Curtis et al., 2004). Side effects include gait impairment, falls, difficulty swallowing, diminished cognitive function, and paradoxical increases in agitation. The risks associated with the use of these drugs are great and the benefits unpredictable (Gerdner & Buckwalter, 1994; Tabloski, McKinnon-Howe, & Remington, 1995). Benzodiazepines are occasionally needed to treat prominent anxiety but are not recommended for long-term use (American Psychiatric Association [APA], 2007). Despite many research reports of improved cognition on withdrawal of inappropriate medications, especially benzodiazepines, these drugs continue to be prescribed to older adults with dementia. It is important that the use of these drugs be closely monitored and reduced and discontinued as soon as is possible (APA; Barton, Sklenicka, Sayegh, & Yaffe, 2008; Curtis et al., 2004).

Environment

Environmental conditions clearly can influence the specific agitated behaviors manifested. Verbal agitation occurring mainly in the evening and when the person is alone suggests that the agitation may be a response to boredom or loneliness. Aggressive behavior occurs most often at night, when it is cold, and when the person is in close contact with others, and can be viewed as a response to a real or perceived threat. Other environmental conditions associated with an increase in agitation include the use of physical restraints, inactivity, and high levels of noise. An increased number of nursing staff, structured activity, music, and the opportunity for social interaction decreased agitated behaviors (Algase et al., 1996; Cohen-Mansfield & Werner, 1995; Kong, 2005).

PAIN

Pain is a frequently cited antecedent to agitated behavior, which further imperils the quality of life of the individual with dementia (Cohen-Mansfield,

1995). The presence of agitation increases the likelihood that the person will receive medications to control behavior. This becomes particularly problematic if the agitation is related to pain, which is better managed with analgesics or non-pharmacological measures. A negative correlation was found between pain reports and the severity of dementia, suggesting that the more severe the dementia, the less the person was able to verbalize pain as a word or number (Buffum, Miaskowski, Sands, & Brod, 2001).

Pain is a relatively common problem for older adults who often have one or more medical conditions that are likely to be painful, such as degenerative joint disease, back pain, or angina (Buffum et al., 2001). In older adults, and particularly those with dementia, pain is frequently undetected, untreated, or undertreated. Persons with dementia self-report less pain than cognitively intact older adults (Horgas, Elliot, & Marsiske, 2009); however, individuals with dementia have fewer analgesics prescribed and are administered less pain medication by nurses, even though the number of diagnoses of painful conditions is similar in both groups. Inadequate pain management threatens the functional ability and quality of life for these persons (Epps, 2001; Kaasalainen et al., 1998; McCaffery & Pasero, 1999).

Pain Assessment Tools

There is a lack of consensus in the literature with regard to the most effective way to assess for the presence of pain in the cognitively impaired elder. Although self-report is the most accurate indicator of pain, research suggests that it is often not reliable for the individual with dementia. Research results demonstrate that no single assessment tool is uniformly effective in this group and that the measure selected should be matched to the person's cognitive abilities and language skills (Jones, Vojir, Hutt, & Fink, 2007). Continued research is needed to develop adequate measurement tools to measure pain objectively in persons with dementia.

One of the most commonly used pain rating scales is the numerical rating scale. In the verbally administered 0 to 10 scale, the person assigns a number to indicate the amount of pain experienced, from 0, indicating no pain, to 10, indicating the worst pain imaginable. Using the same word anchors as the Numerical Rating Scale, the Visual Analog Scale is a visual representation of the range of pain from "none" to "worst." The person is asked to make a mark along a 10 cm vertical or horizontal line to indicate pain intensity (Jones et al., 2007; McCaffery & Pasero, 1999; Pautex, Herrmann, LeLous, & Fabjan, 2005).

The Faces Pain Rating Scale, originally developed for use with children, is another commonly used pain rating scale. The scale is composed of a series of faces, ranging from a smile, depicting no pain, to a sad face, indicating excruciating pain. The Faces Pain Rating Scale has been translated and validated in several languages (McCaffery & Pasero, 1999). This scale has been found to be a somewhat less sensitive measure in older adults with dementia (Pautex et al., 2005).

Simple line drawings of faces have also been used to assess mood states in older adults with dementia. The Dementia Mood Picture Test consists of a series of six faces depicting different moods: good mood, bad mood, happy, sad, angry, and worried. Word descriptors are presented beneath the picture in two-inch letters. Each mood is scored 0 for "yes," 1 for "no," and 2 for "very much" to represent how positive a mood the person indicated (Tappan & Barry, 1995). When using drawings of faces with older adults with dementia, the evaluator should be alert to interpretations of both pain and mood associated with these instruments.

The Verbal Descriptor Scale consists of a list of easily understood adjectives depicting pain intensity. The Verbal Rating Scale is a five-point scale with "0" indicating no pain and "4" indicating unbearable pain. It was found to be better than the Faces Pain Rating Scale and the Visual Analog Scale as an indicator of the magnitude and intensity of pain in persons with dementia; however, it correlated poorly with nurses ratings of the patient's pain (Pesonen et al., 2009).

The Simple Descriptor Scale uses the terms "no pain," "mild," "moderate," and "severe," and is scored by assigning a number between 0 and 3 (McCaffery & Pasero, 1999). Six descriptors used in the McGill Word Scale are "none," "mild," "discomforting," "distressing," "horrible," and "excruciating" (Wynne, Ling, & Remsburg, 2000). The Pain Intensity Scale is composed of six questions. For five of the questions, the subject is asked to respond with one of the following five answers: "not at all," "a little," "moderately," "quite a bit," or "extremely," and is scored from 1 to 5 for each question. The last question asks for the number of days in the week that pain is present (Krulewitch et al., 2000).

These scales are the most commonly used pain scales in the United States and all have demonstrated validity. They are easily administered, scored, and recorded, and well liked by patients. It is important, however, that one scale is used consistently with each patient to minimize confusion (McCaffery & Pasero, 1999).

Proxy pain ratings should never replace self-report of pain; however, observation of behaviors may help the nurse identify pain in a noncommunicative patient. Both vocal behaviors, such as crying, groaning, and screaming, and motor behaviors, such as facial grimacing, rubbing, and fidgeting, have been associated with painful states. The Discomfort Scale for Patients with Dementia of the Alzheimer's Type is an objective scale, based on observed behaviors, developed to measure discomfort in persons with advanced dementia. The scale consists of nine vocal and motor behaviors indicating discomfort. Each behavior is given a score between 0 and 3 to indicate the frequency, intensity, and duration of the behavior. The total score is determined by summing the scores for each behavior, resulting in a total score of between 0 and 27 (Hurley, Volicer, Hanrahan, Houde, & Volicer, 1992). Psychometric evaluation conducted by nurse experts demonstrated reliability and validity of the instrument.

The Pain Assessment in Advanced Dementia scale is a five-item observational tool developed to measure the frequency, duration, and intensity of behaviors that indicate pain in cognitively impaired older adults. The scale consists of five behaviors indicative of pain that were obtained from existing pain scales and the literature. Each of the five behaviors is scored from 0 to 2 to indicate the frequency, duration, and intensity of the behavior. Total score for the instrument is between 0 and 10 (Warden, Hurley, & Volicer, 2003).

A high correlation was found between pain ratings using the Numerical Rating Scale, Faces Pain Rating Scale, and Verbal Descriptor Scale in persons with dementia (Jones et al., 2007). Pautex et al. (2006) found that 61% of persons with severe dementia were able to comprehend at least one pain rating scale. Comprehension rates were better for the Verbal Rating Scale and Faces Pain Rating Scale. The researchers recommend that behavioral rating scales not be routinely used (Pautex et al., 2006).

Barriers to Effective Pain Management

Accurate assessment of pain is essential to effective pain management. Dementia presents many barriers to effective pain assessment. In a review of the literature, McAuliffe, Nay, O'Donnell, and Fetherstonhaugh (2009) described barriers to adequate pain assessment as those related to the person with dementia and those related to nursing staff. Person-related barriers include sensory impairment and communication impairment making it difficult to convey pain experience. They note that it has been suggested that some persons with dementia may have abnormal experience of pain. Staff-related barriers include lack of recognition of pain, insufficient education in identification of pain, misdiagnosis or misinterpretation of patient presentation, and failure to use standard assessment tools (McAuliffe et al.).

The literature is not clear as to whether individuals with dementia actually experience less pain, or have a decreased ability to express pain or appropriately respond to commonly used assessment instruments. One view is that individuals with dementia experience less pain as a result of the neuropathology of the disease (Miller, Nelson, & Mezey, 2000). Alternatively, because dementia of the Alzheimer's type affects the neocortex, sparing the somatosensory cortex, pain perception is likely to be preserved. The emotional responses to pain may be influenced by the changes in the prefrontal cortex and limbic structures, possibly resulting in disinhibition or indifference to pain. The expression of pain may be further compromised because of expressive aphasia and memory impairment associated with dementia (Farrell, Katz, & Helme, 1996). It has also been proposed that the person with dementia may lack the ability to evaluate the situation and anticipate pain causing each repeated pain experience to be new and surprising, causing greater anxiety and distress (Kunz, Mylius, Scharmann, Schepelman, & Lautenbacher, 2009).

Nursing research suggests that individuals with dementia do experience pain, with between 62% and 80% having at least one pain complaint at any given time (Ferrell, Ferrell, & Rivera, 1995; Parmelee, Smith, & Katz, 1993). Older adults may deny the presence of pain, but may admit to hurt, discomfort, soreness, or aching (American Geriatrics Society, 2009). Studies have shown that cognitively impaired persons complain of pain less frequently than cognitively intact persons; however, their complaints are reliable indicators of pain (Krulewitch et al., 2000). In those who can reliably report the existence of pain, many are unable to initiate a request for pain medication on an "as needed" basis (Miller et al., 2000).

Lack of knowledge and skill on the part of professional caregivers presents an obstacle to pain assessment and management. Exacerbation of the behavioral symptoms associated with dementia has been linked to the presence of pain. Some of the reasons nurses cited for undermedicating demented individuals include fear of respiratory depression, of addiction, or of being associated with attempted euthanasia, and excessive concern about side effects (Miller et al., 2000).

Indicators of Pain

Self-report is the most accurate indicator for assessing pain. Because the cognitively impaired person may be unable to communicate his or her distress in a way that caregivers can understand, it may be necessary to use other measures to determine the presence and intensity of pain (Bowser, 2002; Buffum et al., 2001).

In the noncommunicative adult, inference can be made about the pain associated with procedures and obvious pathological conditions, such as open wounds or inflamed joints. This strategy has limited general use with the older adult with dementia, because many of the chronic conditions that cause pain in this group are not visible.

Unusual, new, or escalating behavior in a person with dementia should indicate the need to assess for evidence of pain. Vocal behaviors that may suggest pain include crying, screaming, negative vocalizations, and moaning. Behavioral indicators of pain have been shown to be similar in both cognitively impaired and cognitively intact older adults (Horgas, et al., 2009). Physical behaviors shown to be associated with pain include aggression (Feldt, Warne, & Ryden, 1998) and resistance to care (Mahoney et al., 1999). Additionally, facial grimacing, guarding, rubbing, frowning, and fidgeting may be a sign of pain in the cognitively impaired older adult (Epps, 2001; Hurley et al., 1992).

Less effective indicators are reports of pain from individuals who are close to the person with dementia, such as family members or professional caregivers (McCaffery & Pasero, 1999). There are times, however, when this is the only information available and must be considered. Studies have indicated that health professionals underestimate the amount and severity of pain in individuals with dementia. However, caregivers can be educated to identify signs that a person may be experiencing pain (Miller et al., 2000). Family members may be a source of historical information about the person's past responses to painful situations. Surrogate reports should be used only if the person is unable to communicate his or her pain to caregivers (American Geriatrics Society, 2009).

The least sensitive indicators of pain in the noncommunicative person are physiological measures, such as changes in temperature, pulse, respiratory rate, or blood pressure. Although an increase in blood pressure and heart rate has been associated with pain, these measures are also associated with many other physical and emotional states (McCaffery & Pasero, 1999).

Interventions to Manage Agitation

Interventions shown to decrease agitation include behavioral approaches, environmental modifications, and pharmacological approaches. None of these approaches are universally successful in reducing agitation, and successful management may necessitate use of more than one strategy. The treatment plan needs to be individualized according to ongoing assessment data.

Behavioral Approach

Behavioral treatment of agitation centers on identifying and modifying the physiological, psychosocial, and environmental factors that are antecedents of the agitated behaviors. Comprehensive assessment is a key to developing an individualized treatment plan. It is important to determine the type of agitated behavior exhibited and its frequency, duration, and severity. Any temporal pattern of agitation should be noted. Certain activities, such as bathing, can precipitate agitation. Intervening before the agitation escalates enhances the efficacy of the plan.

Basic Needs Before behavioral interventions can be effective, it is essential to ensure that the individual's basic needs are met. Causes of physical illness and delirium, such as urinary tract infection, should be identified and treated. Frequently, the only presenting sign of infection in the older adult with dementia is agitation or problem behavior (Remington et al., 2006). Other physiological sources of agitation, including pain or discomfort, needing to use the toilet, and restrictive clothing, should be assessed and managed.

Meeting nutritional needs can be a challenge. Agitated persons may not be able to sit long enough to complete a meal. Additionally, because of the presence of apraxia (inability to perform purposeful acts) and agnosia (inability to recognize familiar objects), which are often associated with dementia, the person may be unable to feed himself or herself adequately. Limiting or eliminating alcohol and caffeine, and offering smaller meals, finger foods, and nutritious snacks between meals, can improve intake. Regular vision and hearing evaluations and ensuring that eyeglasses and hearing aids are in use, especially at mealtimes, can decrease confusion and agitation.

Providing a consistent routine is helpful to minimize agitation, because patients with dementia usually find that change strains their ability to adapt. Whenever possible, schedule personal care and meals at the same time of day, with the same caregiver (Remington et al., 2006).

Communication As dementia progresses, language and reasoning skills deteriorate. The person with dementia experiences trouble expressing thoughts in a manner that can be understood by caregivers. Problem behaviors can be viewed as a way of communicating. For example, aggression may express a response to a perceived threat in the environment, whereas repetitious mannerisms are likely to communicate boredom (Cohen-Mansfield & Werner, 1995). Speaking to the person in a calm manner, using a low tone, and with a slow rate can convey a sense of trust. A conscious effort to use good verbal and nonverbal communication skills is needed. Explaining what you intend to do before approaching the person using simple instructions, rather than commands, is important. The person with dementia has an impaired ability to learn or reason. Reorienting a confused person to the environment or trying to teach new information can be frustrating for the older person and the caregiver. An alternative strategy is to redirect the person to a meaningful, "failure-free" activity that he or she can accomplish.

Autonomy and Sense of Control Memory deficits can impair understanding, making tasks and directions seem too difficult or overwhelming to understand. Dividing tasks into small manageable steps and allowing adequate time for completion increases the likelihood of success. Caregivers should be instructed to be patient and avoid criticism and reprimands. It is important to give the individual opportunities to exercise some control when possible. Offering choices with what to eat or what to wear allows the person control in a supervised setting. Eating dessert before the meal or wearing mismatched clothing is less distressful for both the individual and caregivers than escalating agitation in response to frustration.

The application of physical restraints severely limits the agitated person's autonomy. Restraints restrict mobility, usually increase agitation and distress, and should only be used in rare instances to protect the safety of the individual. An alternative to restraints is to remove potentially dangerous objects from the person's environment and provide space for safe pacing.

Environmental Modifications

Environmental factors can influence the development of agitation. Environmental stimuli can be overwhelming or misinterpreted. Voices coming from radios or overhead pagers can lead to confusion and suspicion. Television can be interpreted as reality and perceived as frightening. Caregivers should be instructed to ensure that the surroundings are consistent, predictable, and familiar to help reduce confusion, fear, and agitation.

Clocks and calendars facilitate orientation to time. Simple cues, such as signs or pictures, can prevent a sense of feeling lost. A picture of a toilet on the bathroom door or a picture of the person in his or her bedroom can help to direct them. Because of the loss of short-term memory, the person may not see himself or herself as an old person, and pictures taken when they were younger tend to be more easily identifiable by older adults with dementia. Similarly, if the image of the person viewed in a mirror is distressing to the older person, mirrors may need to be covered or removed.

Activities for the agitated person should be kept simple. Failure-free activities, such as folding napkins, feeding the birds, or counting a pile of coins, can help the older adult have a sense of accomplishment and self-worth. Agitation may be triggered if the instructions are confusing or the environment is too noisy. Care should be taken to avoid unnecessary competing stimuli that may be overwhelming or difficult for the person to interpret. Equally important is preventing under-stimulation, which can lead to boredom, frustration, and further agitation.

There is a growing body of research on the therapeutic effects of music as an environmental modification to reduce agitation in persons with dementia. Instrumental musical selections that have a slow tempo, soft dynamic levels, and repetitive themes tend to have a calming effect. Calming music can be expected to reduce agitation for several persons simultaneously, such as in a group dining room (Remington, 2002; Tabloski et al., 1995). Lyrics and well-known tunes require cognitive effort to process the musical selection and introduce a memory or emotional response that may either enhance or diminish the effect of the music. Individualized or familiar music is selected based on the individual's preference and is intended to evoke an emotional response. The reduction in agitation shown with individualized music is attributed to the memories associated with the familiar music and lyrics (Gerdner, 2000, 2007).

Simple interventions to modify the environment have been shown to reduce agitation. Caregiver singing during bathing resulted in increased cooperation with care and the need for fewer instructions from caregivers (Gotell, Brown, & Ekman, 2002). Audio presence, or simulated presence therapy, is a personalized tape recording of a family member discussing memories or pleasurable topics. Significant improvement in problem behaviors and social isolation was reported following the use of presence therapy (Miller et al., 2001; Woods & Ashley, 1995). Brief interventions of hand massage or slow-stroke back massage reduced the frequency of agitated behaviors (Remington, 2002; Rowe & Alfred, 1999; Snyder,

Egan, & Burns, 1995). See Box 14-1 for an overview of the Remington (2002) study.

Pharmacological Approach

Pharmacological agents should be used only if the agitated behaviors interfere with daily functioning. Age-related changes in the older adult increase the incidence of adverse drug reactions. Additionally, the use of these pharmacological agents may actually exacerbate the agitation, resulting in even more medication being prescribed. Medications used to treat underlying medical conditions can also increase agitated behavior as a side effect of the medication or the resultant change in the person's health status. If behavioral symptoms are not severe, behavioral interventions should be used first. If pharmacological agents are necessary, the lowest effective dose should be used. Gradual dosage reductions should be attempted several times per year to withdraw the medication. Acetaminophen, 1.3 g every 8 hours, was shown to reduce pain-related behaviors associated with musculoskeletal pain in community-residing persons with dementia (Elliot & Horgas, 2009).

Antipsychotic Medications

Behavioral symptoms of dementia cause distress to patients and pose the risk of injury to patients and caregivers. There is a clear need to treat symptoms, such as agitation, psychosis, and mood disorders; however, there is the potential for serious safety concerns, warranting careful assessment (Ballard & Howard, 2006). Serious adverse effects, including stroke and death, have been reported with risperidone and olanzapine (Howland, 2008). Delusions and hallucinations are common in dementia and often respond well to low doses of antipsychotics. Several studies have reported the effectiveness of haloperidol (Haldol), risperidone (Risperdal), and olanzapine (Zyprexa) in managing physical aggression, verbal outbursts, and difficulty sleeping in patients with dementia. The

BOX 14-1   RESEARCH

This study investigated calming music and hand massage as nonpharmacological interventions to reduce agitation in nursing home residents with dementia. Using a four-group repeated measures experimental design, agitation was measured during four 10-minute observation periods: (1) before the intervention, (2) during the intervention, (3) immediately after the intervention, and (4) at 1 hour. The experimental intervention consisted of a 10-minute exposure to either calming music; hand massage; both calming music and hand massage simultaneously; or no intervention (control group).

Each of the experimental interventions reduced the frequency of agitated behaviors more than no intervention. The benefit was sustained over the hour and actually increased over time. Each of the interventions produced similar results, and there was no additive benefit to the combination of calming music and hand massage.

The findings of this study show that either calming music or hand massage is effective in reducing agitated behaviors. Both of these interventions are easily administered, require little training, and incur little cost. The use of nonpharmacological interventions alone or to supplement an individualized plan of care for the agitated individual has the potential to reduce the use of physical and chemical restraints and to improve quality of life for the older adult with dementia.

Source: Adapted from Remington (2002).

most common side effects with these drugs include extrapyramidal symptoms, orthostatic hypotension, sedation, and tardive dyskinesia. Haloperidol is associated with a higher rate of extrapyramidal symptoms than risperidone and olanzapine (Bower, McCullough, & Pille, 2002; Neugroschi, 2002). Where feasible, caregivers should encourage individuals taking antipsychotics to make slow position changes to minimize postural hypotension. Alcohol should be avoided. Parkinsonian symptoms (difficulty swallowing, tremor, rigidity, and shuffling gait) should be promptly reported to the prescriber so that a dosage adjustment can be made. Signs of tardive dyskinesia include uncontrolled rhythmic movements of face and extremities, lip smacking, and tongue thrusting, and are indications that the drug be discontinued (Abdallah, Remington, Melillo, & Flanagan, 2008).

Antidepressants

In patients with coexisting depression and associated agitation, antidepressants can be used to manage disruptive behaviors. In persons with dementia, the prevalence of depression has been estimated to be up to 96% (Gellis, McClive, & Brown, 2009). Depression often leads to anxiety and an inability to initiate meaningful activity, worsening the behavioral problems of dementia (Gellis et al.). The literature reports that most antidepressants have similar efficacy; however, the selective serotonin reuptake inhibitors have a better side-effect profile in older adults (Gellis et al.). Trazodone, a heterocyclic antidepressant with serotonin reuptake inhibition, can induce sedation and should be considered in persons who have disturbed sleep (Neugroschi, 2002).

Mood Stabilizers

Anticonvulsant medications have been shown to be effective for the treatment of agitation and aggression. Such drugs as carbamazepine (Tegretol), valproic acid (Depakote), and gabapentin (Neurontin) are believed to control aggression by affecting neurohormonal mediators. The most common side effects are sedation and gastrointestinal disturbance. Serum drug levels, hepatic function tests, and a complete blood count should be monitored for carbamazepine and valproic acid (Bower et al., 2002; Gellis et al., 2009). Table 14-1 presents an overview of medications used in the treatment of problem behaviors in older adults with dementia.

OTHER PROBLEM BEHAVIORS

Wandering

Wandering is a behavioral problem associated with Alzheimer's disease. Individuals at risk for this behavior include community-residing or institutionalized older adults with dementia. Wandering is defined by the North American Nursing Diagnosis Association (2007) as "meandering, aimless, or repetitive locomotion that exposes the individual to harm; frequently incongruent with boundaries, limits, or obstacles" (pp. 246–247). According to Peatfield, Futrell, and Cox (2002), "there is no single cause for wandering and no single solution" (p. 45). There are, however, common wandering behaviors

TABLE 14-1

Selected Pharmacological Therapy for Problem Behaviors Common to Late-Life Dementias

Drug	Starting Dose	Total Daily Dose	Adverse Effects
Antipsychotics			
Haloperidol (Haldol)	0.25–0.5 mg qd or bid	1–3 mg	Sedation, extrapyramidal symptoms, akathesia, tardive dyskinesia, acute dystonia
Risperidone (Risperidal)	0.25 mg bid	1–3 mg	Sedation, hypotension, tardive dyskinesia, hyperglycemia, extrapyramidal symptoms
Olanzapine (Zyprexa)	2.5 mg qhs	5–10 mg	Sedation, weight gain, hypotension, tardive dyskinesia, hyperglycemia, extrapyramidal symptoms
Antidepressants			
Trazodone (Desyrel)	25–50 mg hs or bid	50–250 mg	Sedation, hypotension
Mood stabilizers			
Carbamazepine (Tegretol)	200 mg qhs	300–400 mg	Sedation, gastrointestinal distress, agranulocytosis, aplastic anemia
Gabapentin (Neurontin)	100 mg qd or bid	300–2400 mg	Sedation, tremor, ataxia
Valproic acid (Depakote, Depakene)	125 mg qhs	250–1000 mg	Nausea, sedation, tremor, ataxia

Source: Adapted from Aschenbrenner, D. S., & Venable, S. J. (2009). *Drug therapy in nursing* (3rd ed., pp. 309–327). New York: Lippincott.

and situations that can provoke these behaviors described in Box 14-2. Consideration of physiological changes, psychological needs, and the environment is important when planning an intervention to lessen the problem behavior.

The first step in management of wandering includes assessment of the individual and the behavior (Futrell & Melillo, 2002). Further assessment should be conducted to evaluate for cognitive decline, depression, anxiety, agitation, wandering patterns, and neurocognitive deficits, and for premorbid lifestyle (Futrell, Melillo, & Remington, 2008). The frequency with which memory and behavior problems occur and the degree to which the problem upsets the caregiver are of importance. Nursing staff should try to determine whether the wandering is an attempt by the resident to acquire additional attention, sensory stimulation, or access desired items.

Assessment tools and instruments that can be used to assess the risk of wandering include the Mini-Mental State Exam (Folstein, Folstein, & McHugh, 1975), Revised Algase Wandering Scale (Nelson & Algase, 2007), Short Geriatric Depression Scale (Sheikh & Yesavage, 1986), Cohen-Mansfield Agitation Inventory: Long Form (Cohen-Mansfield, 1999; Cohen-Mansfield, Marx, & Rosenthal, 1989), and Memory and Behavior Problems Checklist, 1990R (Roth et al., 2003; Zarit & Zarit, 1990).

Management of wandering behavior is difficult. An individualized approach to the problem is necessary. Music therapy, social interaction, structured physical activity, environmental adaptation, and technological devices are interventions that seem to lessen problem behaviors (Peatfield et al., 2002). The need for formal caregivers to transmit knowledge related to these strategies to families and to offer families psychosocial support is recommended (Peatfield et al.). It is also suggested that staff in institutions and families who are caring for individuals with wandering problems need to learn how to communicate with patients who exhibit this behavior.

BOX 14-2 COMMON WANDERING BEHAVIORS AND SITUATIONS THAT CAN PROVOKE WANDERING

Wandering Behaviors	**Situations That Can Provoke Wandering**
Exit seeking	Cognitive impairment
Purposeless walking	Nocturnal confusion
Pacing	Full bladder
Persistent locomotion	Medication effects
Getting lost	Unfamiliar surroundings
Searching	Emotional frustration
Following caregiver	Hunger or thirst
Hyperactivity	Pain
Repetitive visits to the same place	Constipation
Walking to unauthorized places	Overstimulation or understimulation
Nighttime walking aimlessly	Lifestyle before illness (e.g., night-shift worker)

Interventions to address wandering behavior can be grouped into four categories: (1) environmental modifications, (2) interventions addressing technology and safety, (3) physical and psychosocial interventions, and (4) caregiving support and education (Box 14-3) (Futrell & Melillo, 2002; Futrell et al., 2008). Safety of the individual who wanders requires environmental modifications at home or in the institution. A secure area where wandering can take place is necessary. In the institutional setting, one caregiver can watch problem wanderers in a secured area, allowing other caregivers time for patient care. Technology devices that monitor wandering and locate wanderers are available. These devices may alleviate stress for family caregivers in the home environment. Use of door latches, safety locks, and other environmental modifications may also promote safety. Increasing the visual appeal of environmental surroundings with art gives the bored individual a more stimulating experience. It is not clear what part boredom plays in wandering behavior. On the other hand, overstimulation seems to cause patients to wander as much as boredom. Identifying patterns of wandering may be helpful in care planning.

Social interaction of staff and visitors with individuals who wander during mealtimes can decrease wandering and ensure eating. Structured activities, exercise, and the use of music also decrease wandering. Wandering during the night may also occur. This problem is often caused by medications or too much sleeping during the day. It is useful to ask if the individual's lifestyle was that of a day or night person. For instance, did he or she work the night shift? The type of job or the sleeping patterns that existed before the onset of dementia is information useful for individualized care planning. Observation of the individual alerts the caregiver to specific stressors that trigger the problem behavior. Interventions should be evaluated and discontinued if the problem wandering does not decrease.

The Need-Driven Dementia–Compromised Behavior Model offers caregivers structure for planning care that is individualized (Algase et al., 1996). According to Ann Whall, this is "a middle-range theoretical model that addresses what has been called 'disruptive behavior' or 'disturbed behavior' (DB) in individuals with dementia" (Whall, 2002, p. 5). She further suggests the model "posits that behavior, such as wandering, aggression, and problematic vocalizations, is an attempt to convey some meaning" (p. 5). Knowing that this wandering behavior may represent meaning to the individual prompts the nurse to assess for and address contributing factors.

In summary, wandering becomes a problem when it disrupts the individual's sleep, eating, safety, or the caregiver's ability to provide care. Assessment of premorbid factors, the disease process, behaviors typical of the disease, and medications and their side effects is important when individualizing interventions for wandering behavior. Other factors, such as the environment and the knowledge and skill of the caregiver, should be considered when planning care for older adults with dementia who are at risk for wandering behaviors.

Sleep Disturbances

Sleep–wake cycle disturbances are common in older adults with cognitive impairment. Nighttime awakening and excessive napping often become problems for those caring for older adults with dementia. Medications and their side effects may cause drowsiness and vivid dreams. Too much caffeine and a warm room may prevent the patient from sleeping and may cause night wandering. It may become necessary to assist the patient with bedtime routines and to consider the individual's previous wake cycle when considering interventions related to sleep. Hunger or the need to urinate may cause sleep disturbance. Brief naps, especially in the morning, may refresh the older individual if sleep has been disturbed. Naps longer than 1 hour or naps late in the day may, however, interfere with night sleep.

Eating Difficulties

Eating disorders appear in the ambulatory (early) stage of dementia. They can become acute and need

BOX 14-3 INTERVENTIONS TO ADDRESS WANDERING

Environmental modifications

- Provide a secure place to wander, such as a wandering lounge—a large, safe walking area
- Enhance the environment by increasing visual appeal, such as tactile boards or three-dimensional wall art
- Place or paint a wall mural over doorways to disguise exits
- Place gridlines in front of doors to decrease exit seeking
- Make exits less visible and accessible by covering panic bars with cloth
- Allow walking where doors are not in the path
- Use safety locks, complex and less accessible door latches
- Maintain safety by removing clutter and disabling appliances
- Provide stimulation clues, such as pictures and signs
- Use a combination of large-print signs and portrait-like photographs to aid in way finding
- Use a multifaceted approach to environmental modifications because it is more effective than singular modifications

Technology and safety

- Use technological devices to locate and monitor wandering
- Use a verbal alarm system because it is more effective than an aversive alarm system
- Use mobile locator devices for quickly locating wanderers

Physical and psychosocial interventions

- Assess for and treat depression
- Decrease wandering during structured activities by using social interaction of staff or visitors or music
- Music sessions are more effective than reading sessions in decreasing wandering behavior
- Prevent risky situations by adequate supervision
- Walking should not be unnecessarily limited
- Promote safe walking
- Decrease wandering by eliminating stressors from the environment, such as cold at night, changes in daily routines, and extra people at holidays
- Decrease wandering by providing regular exercise, such as walking after meals
- Systematic behavioral conditioning at mealtime to improve food intake, to sit at the table longer, and to stabilize weight
- Use mattress therapy for treatment of agitated wandering

Caregiving support and education

- Educate caregivers to assist in their ability to care for the wanderer
- A facility-based approach could include identification of the problem, a wandering prevention program, interactions with staff, and staff mobilization around the problem
- Dementia care training for residential care staff using training modules

Sources: Futrell, Melillo, & Remington (2008); and Futrell & Melillo (2002).

immediate attention. Individuals may either lose interest in eating or eat constantly. Eating too little or too much may be a result of boredom, overstimulation, or the disease process. Feeding difficulty of the older adult with dementia is a multidimensional phenomenon that is amenable to nursing intervention. Attention to issues related to feeding not only affects the physical health, but the mental health of the individual and can add to caregiver burden (Chang & Roberts, 2008). Individuals may not be able to feed themselves or prepare the food, or they may forget to eat, which may lead to inadequate food intake and poor nutrition.

Weight changes are common in dementia. As the disease progresses, supervision of eating helps to prevent malnutrition. Visitors, family, and volunteers can assist during mealtime in the home or institutional setting. This assistance may make eating less chaotic, while providing a social dimension. For patients who overeat, restricting access to food and providing structure and supervision may help.

Norberg and Athlin (1989) suggest interventions should target the appropriate eating or feeding problem: (1) problems associated with the ability to eat and drink, (2) problems associated with the social dimension of eating, and (3) problems associated with the environmental aspect. Similarly, Watson and Deary (1994) identified three components of feeding difficulty in individuals with dementia: (1) patient obstinacy or passivity, which reflects the lack of cooperation with feeding; (2) nursing intervention, or the amount of help or supervision required with feeding; and (3) indicators of feeding difficulty, such as food spillage and leaving food on the plate at the end of the meal. Understanding the basis of the eating disorder helps caregivers to select specific interventions that have a high likelihood of success (Chang & Roberts, 2008).

With these suggested components in mind, mealtimes for those with dementia may need to be longer. Older adults with dementia take longer to chew and swallow. Finger foods, proper body positioning, and frequent small meals in the same place and at the same time each day may appeal to some individuals. In late stages, the individual may

need to be reminded to open his or her mouth and chew (Cacchione, 2000). Caregivers should consider the use of music at mealtimes, social interaction with family and other patients, and colorful surroundings. When music was played during meals, nursing home residents with dementia have been shown to spend more time with dinner and eat more. Relaxing music played during the main meal of the day reduced the overall level of agitation among nursing home residents (Goddaer & Abraham, 1994). Soothing music had a more positive effect than rock music or tunes from the 1920s and 1930s (Ragneskog, Kihlgren, Karlsson, & Norberg, 1996).

Kinahan (1999) suggests "persons with dementia often consume more at breakfast or lunch than at the evening meal" (p. 34). She further states, "this coincides with the sundowning phenomenon seen at the end of the day, which is displayed as restlessness, insecurity, and agitation" (p. 245). Caregivers who are aware of this behavior can make an effort to encourage intake earlier in the day.

Providing a consistent caregiver may improve communication between an individual with dementia and the caregiver during feeding. McGillivray and Marland (1999) recommend primary nursing to provide consistency of caregivers to improve communication of an individualized plan of care. Training and supervision of assistive personnel enhances their understanding of the patient's disability by helping them to carry out feeding in a sensitive and therapeutic manner.

Sexual Disturbances

Although uncommon, hypersexuality can cause embarrassment and fear for formal and informal caregivers of persons with dementia (Robinson, 2003). Inappropriate sexual behaviors are reported to occur in 7–25% of persons with dementia. The neurobiology of inappropriate behaviors is not fully understood; however, the frontal lobes, temporolimbic system, striatum, and hypothalamus have been implicated (Ozkan, Wilkins, Muralee, & Tampi, 2008). Dysfunction in these areas can impair mechanisms of self-control and understanding of sexual arousal (Wallace & Safer, 2009). Touching the genitals or undressing is not necessarily sexual. These behaviors should be understood and treated as a problem behavior of dementia, not deliberate. It is often a manifestation of other unmet needs such as boredom, rather than sexual ones (Robinson).

The assessment of the older adult exhibiting hypersexual behaviors should ascertain whether treatable conditions, such as depression, pain, constipation, or medication interactions, are contributing to the behaviors (Wallace & Safer, 2009). Nonpharmacological interventions should be initiated first. A firm but calm response needs to be given if unwanted advances are made. Substituting a more appropriate behavior or activity may reduce or eliminate the behavior. The older adult could be gently redirected with food or conversation (Robinson, 2003). If the person exposes genitals, he or she should be taken back to his or her room for privacy (Ozkan et al., 2008). Cover the lap with a pillow and attempt to distract him or her. Staff development that explores attitudes about sexuality and aging among older adults and societal myths about sexuality can enhance appropriate care of the adult exhibiting hypersexual behavior (Wallace & Safer).

According to Lyketsos, Steele, and Steinberg (1999), "men may develop hypersexuality, manifested by inappropriate propositioning, inappropriate touching, or public displays of masturbation. In women, repeated touching and rubbing of the genital area may be the result of vaginal infection, uterine prolapse, or similar physical problems" (p. 223).

In persons with dangerously hypersexual or aggressive behavior, medication may be used as a last resort. Few research data are available on pharmacotherapy for treatment for inappropriate sexual behaviors; most is from case reports (Ozkan et al., 2008). Antidepressants are commonly used because of their antilibido effect. The selective serotonin reuptake inhibitors have a relatively safe profile in the older adult. Hormonal manipulation using antiandrogens causes a decrease in libido and a reduction of hypersexual behaviors, but has the potential for considerable side effects including cardiovascular side effects, sedation, weight gain, depression, hot flashes, and hyperglycemia. Neuroleptics block dopamine receptors decreasing libido but also have many potential adverse effects including hypotension, arrhythmias, syncope, and extrapyramidal symptoms. Comprehensive and continuous assessment is necessary if medications are used to treat hypersexual behaviors (Wallace & Safer, 2009).

SUMMARY

Problem behaviors of the dementia patient present major challenges to caregivers. The cause or causes of these behavioral disturbances are often not clearly identified. Caregivers need to be alert to a variety of stressors that may precipitate problem behaviors. Physical stressors might be a urinary tract infection or pain. Mental health disturbances, such as depression and anxiety, can also be stressors, leading to problem behaviors. The environment where care is given and the individuals providing care may provoke a stressful response. No single stressor is universally responsible for problem behaviors.

Thorough assessment is a first step in planning interventions for compassionate care. Assessing the individual's behavior and reasons for the onset or continuation of the behavior is accomplished with assistance from the caregiver and the family. Careful attention to the environment, the medical and mental health condition of the individual, and medications being given for this and other conditions is important during the assessment process.

Information regarding the caregiver relationship with the older adult with dementia and knowledge of the physical and mental status of the older person are important before recommending a management plan. Once an individualized plan has been developed, education and support of caregivers are essential. A "fallback" plan should be available for emergencies, and caregivers need to be informed that treatment may take longer and need more than one attempt to be successful. Supporting the caregiver is an important role of the geropsychiatric nurse.

REFERENCES

Abdallah, L. M., Remington, R., Melillo, K. D., & Flanagan, J. (2008). Using antipsychotic drugs safely in older patients. *Nursing 2008, 38*(10), 28–31.

Algase, D. L., Beck, C., Kolanowski, A., Whall, A., Berent, S., Richards, K., et al. (1996). Need-driven dementia-compromised behavior: An alternative view of disruptive behavior. *American Journal of Alzheimer's Disease, 11*(6), 10–19.

American Geriatrics Society Panel on the Pharmacological Management of Persistent Pain in Older Persons (2009). Pharmacological management of persistent pain in older persons. *Journal of the American Geriatrics Society, 57*(8), 1331–1346.

American Geriatrics Society and American Association for Geriatric Psychiatry. (2003). Consensus statement on improving the quality of mental health care in U.S. nursing homes: Management of depression and behavior symptoms associated with dementia. *Journal of the American Geriatrics Society, 51*(9), 1287–1298.

American Psychiatric Association. (2007). *Practice guideline for the treatment of patients with Alzheimer's disease and other dementias.* Arlington, VA: American Psychiatric Association.

Ballard, C., & Howard, R. (2006). Neuroleptic drugs in dementia: Benefits and harm. *Nature Reviews: Neuroscience, 7*, 492–500.

Barton, C., Sklenicka, J., Sayegh, P., & Yaffe, K. (2008). Contraindicated medication use among patients in a memory disorders clinic. *The American Journal of Geriatric Pharmacotherapy, 6*(3), 147–152.

Beck, C. K., & Shue, V. M. (1994). Interventions for treating disruptive behavior in demented elderly people. *Nursing Clinics of North America, 29*(1), 143–155.

Beers, M. H., Ouslander, J. G., Rollingher, I., Reuben, D. B., Brooks, J., & Beck, J. C. (1991). Explicit criteria for determining inappropriate medication use in nursing homes. *Archives of Internal Medicine, 151*, 1825–1832.

Beresin, E. V. (1988). Delirium in the elderly. *Journal of Geriatric Psychiatry and Neurology, 1*, 127–143.

Bower, F. L., McCullough, C. S., & Pille, B. L. (2002). Synthesis of research findings regarding Alzheimer's disease: Part II, care of people with AD. *Online Journal of Knowledge Synthesis for Nursing, 9*(4), 1–38.

Bowser, A. (2002). Management of pain in patients with cognitive impairment requires a thoughtful approach. *Central Nervous System Education for the Long-term Care Professional, 1*(2), 1, 12.

Buffum, M. D., Miaskowski, C., Sands, L., & Brod, M. (2001). A pilot study of the relationship between discomfort and agitation in patients with dementia. *Geriatric Nursing, 22*(2), 80–85.

Cacchione, P. (2000). Cognitive and neurologic function. In A. Lueckenotte (Ed.), *Gerontologic nursing* (pp. 615–654). St. Louis, MO: Mosby.

Carlson, D. L., Fleming, K., Smith, G. E., & Evans, J. M. (1995). Management of dementia-related behavioral disturbances: A non-pharmacologic approach. *Mayo Clinic Proceedings, 70*, 1108–1115.

Chang, C., & Roberts, B. L. (2008). Feeding difficulty in older adults with dementia. *Journal of Clinical Nursing, 17*(17), 2266–2274.

Chutka, D. S. (1997). Medication use in nursing home residents. *Nursing Home Medicine, 5*, 180–187.

Cohen-Mansfield, J. (1986). Agitated behaviors in the elderly II. Preliminary results in the cognitively deteriorated. *Journal of the American Geriatrics Society, 34*(10), 722–727.

Cohen-Mansfield, J. (1995). Assessment of disruptive behavior/agitation in the elderly: Function, methods, and difficulties. *Journal of Geriatric Psychiatry and Neurology, 8*(1), 52–60.

Cohen-Mansfield, J. (1999). Assessment measurement of inappropriate behavior associated with dementia. *Journal of Gerontological Nursing, 25*(2), 42–51.

Cohen-Mansfield, J., & Billig, N. (1986). Agitated behaviors in the elderly I. A conceptual review. *Journal of the American Geriatrics Society, 34*(10), 711–721.

Cohen-Mansfield, J., & Libin, A. (2005). Verbal and physical non-aggressive agitated behaviors in elderly persons with dementia: Robustness of syndromes. *Journal of Psychiatric Research, 39*(3), 325–332.

Cohen-Mansfield, J., Marx, M. S., & Rosenthal, A. S. (1989). A description of agitation in a nursing home. *Journal of Gerontology: Medical Sciences, 44*(3), M77–M84.

Cohen-Mansfield, J., Marx, M. S., & Werner, P. (1989). Full moon: Does it influence agitation in nursing home residents? *Journal of Clinical Psychology, 45*(4), 611–613.

Cohen-Mansfield, J., & Werner, P. (1995). Environmental influences on agitation: An integrative summary of an observational study. *The American Journal of Alzheimer's Care and Related Disorders & Research,* *10*(1), 32–39.

Corrigan, J. D., Bogner, J. A., & Tabloski, P. A. (1996). Comparisons of agitation associated with Alzheimer's disease and acquired brain injury. *American Journal of Alzheimer's disease, 11*(6), 20–24.

Curtis, L. H., Ostbye, R., Sendersky, V., Hutchinson, S., Dans, P. E., Wright, A., et al. (2004). Inappropriate prescribing for elderly Americans in a large outpatient population. *Archives of Internal Medicine, 164*(15), 1621–1625.

Dewing, J. (2003). Sundowning in older people with dementia: evidence base, nursing assessment and interventions. *Nursing Older People, 15*(8), 28–32.

Elliot, A. F., & Horgas, A. L. (2009). Effects of an analgesic trial in reducing pain behaviors in community-dwelling older adults with dementia. *Nursing Research, 58*(2), 140–145.

Ely, E. W., Margolin, R., Francis, J., May, L., Truman, B., Dittus, R., et al. (2001). Evaluation of delirium in critically ill patients: Validation of the Confusion Assessment Method for the Intensive Care Unit (CAM-ICU). *Critical Care Medicine, 29,* 1370–1379.

Epps, C. D. (2001). Recognizing pain in the institutionalized elder with dementia. *Geriatric Nursing, 22*(2), 71–77.

Farrell, M. J., Katz, B., & Helme, R. D. (1996). The impact of dementia on the pain experience. *Pain, 67,* 7–15.

Feldt, K. S., Warne, M. A., & Ryden, M. B. (1998). Examining pain in aggressive cognitively impaired older adults. *Journal of Gerontological Nursing, 24*(11), 14–22.

Ferrell, B. A., Ferrell, B. R., & Rivera, L. (1995). Pain in cognitively impaired nursing home patients. *Journal of Pain and Symptom Management, 10,* 591–598.

Folstein, M., Folstein, S., & McHugh, P. (1975). Mini Mental State Exam: A practical guide for grading the cognitive state of patients for clinicians. *Journal of Psychiatric Research, 12*(3), 189–198.

Fonad, E., Emami, A., Wahlin, T. B., Winblad, B., & Sandmark, H. (2009). Falls in somatic and dementia wards at Community Care Units. *Scandinavian Journal of Caring Sciences, 23*(1), 2–10.

Futrell, M., & Melillo, K. D. (2002). Evidence-based protocol: Wandering. *Journal of Gerontological Nursing, 28*(11), 14–22.

Futrell, M., Melillo, K. D., & Remington, R. (2008). Wandering: Evidence-based guideline. In M. G. Titler (Series Ed.), *Series on evidence based practice for*

older adults. Iowa City IA: The University of Iowa College of Nursing Gerontological Nursing Interventions Research Center, Research Translation and Dissemination Core.

Gardner, M. E., & Garrett, R. W. (1997). Review of drug therapy for aggressive behaviors associated with dementia. *Nursing Home Medicine, 5*(6), 199–208.

Gellis, Z. D., McClive, K. P., & Brown, E. L. (2009). Treatments for depression in older persons with dementia. *Annals of Long-Term Care, 17*(2), 29–37.

Gerdner, L. A. (2000). Effects of individualized versus classical "relaxation" music on the frequency of agitation in elderly persons with Alzheimer's disease and related disorders. *International Psychogeriatrics, 12*(1), 49–65.

Gerdner, L. A. (2005). Temporal patterning of agitation and stressors associated with agitation: Case profiles to illustrate the Progressively Lowered Stress Threshold Model. *Journal of the American Psychiatric Nurses Association, 11*(4), 215–222.

Gerdner, L. A. (2007). Evidence-based guideline: Individualized music. In M. G. Titler (Series Ed.), *Series on evidence-based practice for older adults.* Iowa City, IA: The University of Iowa College of Nursing Gerontological Nursing Interventions Research Center, Research Translation and Dissemination Core.

Gerdner, L. A., & Buckwalter, K. C. (1994). A nursing challenge: Assessment and management of agitation in Alzheimer's patients. *Journal of Gerontological Nursing, 20*(4), 11–20.

Goddaer, J., & Abraham, I. L. (1994). Effects of relaxing music on agitation during meals among nursing home residents with severe cognitive impairment. *Archives of Psychiatric Nursing, 8,* 150–158.

Gotell, E., Brown, S., & Ekman, S. L. (2002). Caregiver singing and background music in dementia care. *Western Journal of Nursing Research, 24*(2), 195–216.

Hall, G. R. (1994). Caring for people with Alzheimer's disease using the conceptual model of Progressively Lowered Stress Threshold in the clinical setting. *Nursing Clinics of North America, 29,* 129–141.

Hall, G. R., & Buckwalter, K. C. (1987). Progressively lowered stress threshold: A conceptual model for care of adults with Alzheimer's disease. *Archives of Psychiatric Nursing, 1,* 399–406.

Horgas, A. L., Elliot, A. F., & Marsiske, M. (2009). Pain assessment in persons with dementia: Relationship between self-report and behavioral observation. *Journal of the American Geriatrics Society, 57*, 126–132.

Howland, R. H. (2008). Risks and benefits of antipsychotic drugs in elderly patients with dementia. *Journal of Psychosocial Nursing, 46*, 19–23.

Hurley, A. C., Volicer, L., Camberg, C., Ashley, J., Woods, P., Odenheimer, G., et al. (1999). Measurement of observed agitation in patients with dementia of the Alzheimer's type. *Journal of Mental Health and Aging, 5*(2), 117–133.

Hurley, A. C., Volicer, B. J., Hanrahan, P. A., Houde, S., & Volicer, L. (1992). Assessment of discomfort in advanced Alzheimer's patients. *Research in Nursing & Health, 15*, 369–377.

Inouye, S. K., Foreman, M. D., Mion, L. C., Katz, K. H., & Cooney, L. M. (2001). Nurses' recognition of delirium and its symptoms. *Archives of Internal Medicine, 161*(20), 2467–2473.

Jones, K. R., Vojir, C. P., Hutt, E., & Fink, R. (2007). Determining mild, moderate, and severe pain equivalency across pain intensity tools in nursing home residents. *Journal of Rehabilitation Research and Development, 44*(2), 305–314.

Kaasalainen, S., Middleton, J., Knezacek, S., Hartley, T., Stewart, N., Ife, C., et al. (1998). Pain and cognitive status in the institutionalized elderly: Perceptions and interventions. *Journal of Gerontological Nursing, 24*(8), 24–31.

Kinahan, M. J. (1999). Nutritional issues. In S. Molony, C. Waszynski, & C. Lyder (Eds.), *Gerontological nursing: An advanced practice approach* (pp. 221–257). Stamford, CT: Appleton & Lange.

Kong, E. (2005). Agitation in dementia: Concept clarification. *Journal of Advanced Nursing, 52*(5), 526–536.

Krulewitch, H., London, M. R., Skakel, V. J., Lundstedt, G. J., Thomason, H., & Brummel-Smith, K. (2000). Assessment of pain in cognitively impaired older adults: A comparison of pain assessment tools and their use by nonprofessional caregivers. *Journal of the American Geriatrics Society, 48*, 1607–1611.

Kunz, M., Mylius, B., Scharmann, S., Schepelman, K., & Lautenbacher, S. (2009). Influence of dementia on multiple components of pain. *European Journal of Pain, 13*, 317–325.

Lindenmayer, J. (2000). The pathophysiology of agitation. *Journal of Clinical Psychiatry, 61*, 5–10.

Lyketsos, C., Steele, C., & Steinberg, M. (1999). Behavioral disturbances in dementia. In J. Gallo, J. Busby-Whitehead, P. Rabins, R. Sillman, J. Murphy, & W. Reichel (Eds.), *Reichel's care of the elderly: Clinical aspects of aging* (pp. 214–228). Philadelphia: Lippincott Williams & Wilkins.

Mahoney, E. K., Hurley, A. C., Volicer, L., Bell, M., Gianotis, P., Hartshorm M., et al. (1999). Development and testing of the resistiveness to care scale. *Research in Nursing & Health, 22*, 27–38.

Marx, M. S., Werner, P., & Cohen-Mansfield, J. (1989). Agitation and touch in the nursing home. *Psychological Reports, 64*, 1019–1026.

McAuliffe, L., Nay, R., O'Donnell, M., & Fetherstonhaugh, D. (2009). Pain assessment in older people with dementia: Literature review. *Journal of Advanced Nursing, 65*(1), 2–10.

McCaffery, M., & Pasero, C. (1999). *Pain: Clinical manual.* St. Louis, MO: Mosby.

McGillivray, T., & Marland, G. R. (1999). Assisting demented patients with feeding: Problems in a ward environment. A review of the literature. *Journal of Advanced Nursing, 29*, 608–614.

Miller, L. L., Nelson, L. L., & Mezey, M. (2000). Comfort and pain relief in dementia: Awakening a new beneficence. *Journal of Gerontological Nursing, 26*(9), 32–40.

Miller, S., Vermeersch, P. E., Bohan, K., Renbarger, K., Kruep, A., & Sacre, S. (2001). Audio presence intervention for decreasing agitation in people with dementia. *Geriatric Nursing, 22*(2), 66–77.

Nelson, A. L., & Algase, D. L. (Eds.). (2007). *Evidence-based protocols for managing wandering behaviors.* New York: Springer.

Neugroschi, J. (2002). Agitation: How to manage behavior disturbances in the older patient with dementia. *Geriatrics, 57*(4), 33–40.

Norberg, A., & Athlin, E. (1989). Eating problems in severely demented patients: Issues and ethical dilemmas. *Nursing Clinics of North America, 24*, 781–789.

North American Nursing Diagnosis Association. (2007). *Nursing diagnosis: Definitions and classifications, 2007–2008.* Philadelphia: Author.

Ozkan, B., Wilkins, K., Muralee, S., & Tampi, R. R. (2008). Pharmacotherapy for inappropriate sexual behaviors in dementia: A systematic review of literature. *American Journal of Alzheimer's Disease & Other Dementias, 23*(4), 344–354.

Parmelee, P. A., Smith, B., & Katz, L. R. (1993). Pain complaints and cognitive status among elderly institution residents. *Journal of the American Geriatrics Society, 41*(5), 517–522.

Pautex, S., Herrmann, F., LeLous, P., & Fabjan, M. (2005). Feasibility and reliability of four pain self-assessment scales and correlation with an observational rating scale in hospitalized elderly demented patients. *Journal of Gerontology: Medical Sciences, 60A*(4), 524–552.

Pautex, S., Michon, A., Guedira, M., Emond, H., Le Lous, P., Samaras, D., et al. (2006). Pain in severe dementia: Self-assessment or observational scales? *Journal of the American Geriatrics Society, 54*(7), 1040–1045.

Peatfield, J., Futrell, M., & Cox, C. (2002). Wandering: An integrative review. *Journal of Gerontological Nursing, 28*(4), 44–50.

Pesonen, A., Kappila, T., Tarkkila, P., Sutela, A., Ninisto, L., & Rosenberg, P. H. (2009). Evaluation of easily applicable pain measurement tools for the assessment of pain in demented patients. *ACTA Anaesthesiologica Scandinavica, 53*, 657–664.

Ragneskog, H., Kihlgren, M., Karlsson, I., & Norberg, A. (1996). Dinner music for demented patients: Analysis of video-recorded observations. *Clinical Nursing Research, 5*, 262–282.

Remington, R. (2002). Calming music and hand massage with agitated elderly. *Nursing Research, 51*(5), 317–323.

Remington, R., Abdallah, L., Melillo, K. D., & Flanagan, J. (2006). Managing problem behaviors associated with dementia. *Rehabilitation Nursing, 31*(5), 186–192.

Robinson, K. M. (2003). Understanding hypersexuality: A behavioral disorder of dementia. *Home Healthcare Nurse, 21*(1), 43–47.

Ropacki, S. A., & Jeste, D. V. (2005). Epidemiology of and risk factors for psychosis of Alzheimer's disease: A review of 55 studies published from 1990 to 2003. *American Journal of Psychiatry, 162*(11), 2022–2030.

Roth, D. L., Gitlin, L. N., Coon, D. W., Stevens, A. B., Burgio, L. D., Gallagher-Thompson, D., et al. (2003). Psychometric analysis of the Revised Memory and Behavior Problems Checklist: Factor structure of occurrence and reaction ratings. *Psychology and Aging, 18*(4), 906–915.

Rowe, M., & Alfred, D. (1999). The effectiveness of slow-stroke massage in diffusing agitated behaviors in individuals with Alzheimer's disease. *Journal of Gerontological Nursing, 25*(6), 22–34.

Sheikh, J. I., & Yesavage, J. A. (1986). Geriatric Depression Scale (GDS): Recent evidence and development of a shorter version. *Clinical Gerontologist, 5*(1-2), 165–173.

Snyder, M., Egan, E. C., & Burns, R. (1995). Efficacy of hand massage in decreasing agitation behaviors associated with care activities in persons with dementia. *Geriatric Nursing, 16*(2), 60–63.

Spillman, B. C., & Long, S. K. (2009). Does high caregiver stress predict nursing home entry? *Inquiry, 46*(2), 140–161.

Sutor, B., Rummans, T. A., & Smith, G. E. (2001). Assessment and management of behavioral disturbances in nursing home patients with dementia. *Mayo Clinic Proceedings, 76*, 540–550.

Tabloski, P. A., McKinnon-Howe, L., & Remington, R. (1995). Effects of calming music on the level of agitation in cognitively impaired nursing home residents. *The American Journal of Alzheimer's Care and Related Disorders & Research, 10*(1), 10–15.

Talerico, K. A., & Evans, L. K. (2001). Responding to safety issues in frontotemporal dementias. *Neurology, 56*(11 Suppl. 4), S52–S55.

Tappan, R. M., & Barry, C. (1995). Assessment of affect in advanced Alzheimer's disease: The Dementia Mood Picture Test. *Journal of Gerontological Nursing, 21*(3), 44–46.

Teri, L., Traux, P., Logsdon, R., Uomoto, J., Zarit, S., & Vitaliano, P. P. (1992). Assessment of behavioral problems in dementia: The Revised Memory and Behavior Problems Checklist. *Psychology and Aging, 7*, 622–631.

Thomas, D. W., & Smith, M. (2009). The effect of music on caloric consumption among nursing home residents with dementia of the Alzheimer's type. *Activities, Adaptation & Aging, 33*(1), 1–16.

Vance, D. E., Burgio, L. D., Roth, D. L., Stevens, A. B., Fairchild, D., & Yurick, A. (2003). Predictors of agitation in nursing home residents. *The Journals of Gerontology: Medical Sciences, 58B*(2), M129–M137.

Volicer, L., Harper, D. G., Manning, B. C., Goldstein, R. B., & Satlin, A. (2001). Sundowning and circadian rhythms in Alzheimer's disease. *The American Journal of Psychiatry, 158*(5), 704–711.

Wallace, M., & Safer, M. (2009). Hypersexuality among cognitively impaired older adults. *Geriatric Nursing, 30*(4), 230–237.

Warden, V., Hurley, A. C., & Volicer, L. (2003). Development and psychometric evaluation of the Pain Assessment in Advanced Dementia (PAINAD) Scale. *Journal of the American Medical Directors Association, 4*(1), 9–15.

Watson, R., & Deary, I. J. (1994). Measuring feeding difficulty in patients with dementia: Multivariate analysis of feeding problems, nursing intervention and indicators of feeding difficulty. *Journal of Advanced Nursing, 20,* 283–287.

Weinrich, S., Egbert, C., Eleazer, G. P., & Haddock, K. S. (1995). Agitation: Measurement, management and intervention research. *Archives of Psychiatric Nursing, 5,* 251–260.

Whall, A. L. (2002). Developing needed interventions for the Need-Driven Dementia-Compromised Be-havior Model. *Journal of Gerontological Nursing, 28*(10), 5.

Woods, P., & Ashley, J. (1995). Simulated presence therapy: Using selected memories to manage problem behaviors in Alzheimer's disease patients. *Geriatric Nursing, 16*(1), 9–14.

Wynne, C. F., Ling, S. M., & Remsburg, R. (2000). Comparison of pain assessment instruments in cognitively intact and cognitively impaired nursing home residents. *Geriatric Nursing, 21*(1), 20–23.

Zarit, S. H., & Zarit, S. M. (1990). Cognitive impairment. In P. M. Lewinsohn & L. Teri (Eds.), *Clinical geropsychology: New directions in assessment and treatment* (pp. 38–80). New York: Pergaman.

15

Family Caregiving

Susan Crocker Houde

"Informal caregiving" refers to the unpaid care provided by family, friends, and other relatives to functionally impaired individuals in the community. It was estimated in 2006 that between 30 and 38 million adult informal caregivers provided care to an adult with functional limitations living in the community. Caregivers were estimated to provide an average of 21 hours of care weekly (AARP, 2007). If informal caregivers were reimbursed for the care they provide, the costs to society would be substantial. The American Association of Retired Persons (AARP) Public Policy Institute estimated the economic value of informal caregiving in the United States for the year 2006 conservatively as $354 billion (AARP, 2007). Most informal care to older adults in the home is provided by family members. Many older adult care recipients have dementia and have difficulty functioning independently in the community. It is estimated that 70% of those with dementia are cared for by family and friends in the home (Alzheimer's Association, 2007). The cost of caring for an older adult with Alzheimer's disease has been estimated to be approximately $43,000, which is more than four times the individual estimated economic value of care considered in the AARP cost estimation (AARP, 2007; MetLife, 2006).

Approximately 14% of caregivers are 65 years and older, and many of the older caregivers are wives providing care to functionally impaired husbands (Alzheimer's Association, 2009). Women are estimated to provide 66% of the informal care in the United States (AARP, 2009). If a wife is not present, a daughter is often the primary caregiver. Other relatives who may provide informal care in the home include daughters-in-law, sons, husbands, siblings, and nieces. If a relative is not available, friends and neighbors may serve as informal caregivers. Many of the daughter caregivers are in their mid-40s, provide care an average of 20 hours or more per week, are in the workforce, and are married (National Alliance for Caregiving & AARP, 2004). Employment may make it difficult for daughters to provide the needed care, and paid work hours frequently may need to be reduced. An average reduction of paid work hours by middle-aged female caregivers of 41% has been found, which may impact caregivers' retirement income, job security, and savings (Johnson & Lo Sasso, 2006).

Female caregivers have been found to spend more time than males providing informal care to functionally impaired older adults (National Alliance for Caregiving & AARP, 2004). There are differences in the type of care provided by male and female caregivers. Females are more likely than males to provide hands-on care, such as assistance with activities of daily living (ADLs), including bathing, dressing, toileting, bowel and bladder care, eating, and ambulation (Cancian & Oliker, 2000). Males are more likely to provide care with instrumental ADLs, including money management, home repairs, and transportation, although they also provide emotional and social support and assistance with ADLs (Kaye, 1997). The responsibilities of caregivers are many and varied, including preventing wandering and falls, providing care related to health problems, incontinence care, and medication management. Providing social support is also an important role of the caregiver.

EMOTIONAL RESPONSES TO CAREGIVING

Well-Being and Positive Responses to Caregiving

Caregiving of functionally impaired older adults with dementia has been reported to result in a variety of emotional responses. Much has been written about the increase in stress and burden that may be experienced by caregivers because of the added responsibility of caring for a family member. For many, however, caregiving is viewed as a positive experience. A number of factors have been identified as being associated with a positive caregiving relationship, including a sense of fulfillment or reward by the caregiver, feelings of caring, and companionship with the care recipient (Cohen, Colantonio, & Vernich, 2002). Caregivers have reported an improved relationship with the family member receiving the care, an increased sense of competence in providing the care, personal growth, and an improved understanding of the aging process (Amirkhanyan & Wolf, 2003). Caregivers who report a higher level of satisfaction with caregiving experiences and those with a high level of mastery or emotional support have been found to report lower levels of depression regardless of the level of caregiving stress (Martire, Parris Stephens, & Atienza, 1997; Yates, Tennstedt,

& Chang, 1999). Negative effects of caregiving, such as burden, have been found to be offset by the positive rewards of caregiving, resulting in fewer symptoms of depression (Amirkhanyan & Wolf; Cohen et al.).

The well-being of caregivers has been explored in the literature. It is considered to be a complex and multidimensional concept (Berg-Weger & Tebb, 1998). The Caregiver Well-Being Scale, has been developed to measure the resources and strengths of caregivers (Figure 15-1) (Tebb, 1995). The scale is useful as a means for the geropsychiatric nurse to identify assets, supports, and resources that may be helpful in counseling of family caregivers with the goal of promoting well-being (Berg-Weger, Rubio, & Tebb, 2001). The instrument may facilitate communication with caregivers about priorities and changes that they can make in their daily life that could increase their sense of well-being. It may be used for both screening and intervention planning, and may assist in the identification of caregiver coping strategies using a strength-based perspective (Berg-Weger et al).

The Caregiver Well-Being Scale consists of 45 items and has two subscales. The scales address basic human needs and activities of living (Tebb, 1995). The basic needs subscale consists of items related to four areas: (1) attendance to physical needs, (2) expression of feelings, (3) self-esteem and esteem for others, and (4) security. The Scale is useful in identifying areas that may be of concern to the caregiver and may assist the geropsychiatric nurse in making plans with the caregiver that may increase the quality of life for the caregiver. The Caregiver Well-Being Scale may be a helpful guide for the nurse in better understanding the daily life of caregivers and determining areas where support and guidance are needed (Tebb). The activities of living subscale includes items related to household maintenance, leisure activities, time for self, family support, and maintenance of functions outside the home (Rubio, Berg-Weger, & Tebb, 1999). The coefficient α of the scale was high at 0.94, and it has demonstrated high criterion and construct validity.

FIGURE 15-1

Caregiver Well-Being Scale.

Below are listed a number of basic needs. For each need listed, think about your life over the past three months. During this period of time, indicate to what extent you think each need has been met by circling the appropriate number on the scale provided below.

1 = Never or almost never   2 = Seldom, occasionally   3 = Sometimes
4 = Often, frequently   5 = Almost always

	1	2	3	4	5
1. Having enough money	1	2	3	4	5
2. Eating a well-balanced diet	1	2	3	4	5
3. Getting enough sleep	1	2	3	4	5
4. Attending to your medical and dental needs	1	2	3	4	5
5. Having time for recreation	1	2	3	4	5
6. Feeling loved	1	2	3	4	5
7. Expressing love	1	2	3	4	5
8. Expressing anger	1	2	3	4	5
9. Expressing laughter and joy	1	2	3	4	5
10. Expressing sadness	1	2	3	4	5
11. Enjoying sexual intimacy	1	2	3	4	5
12. Learning new skills	1	2	3	4	5
13. Feeling worthwhile	1	2	3	4	5
14. Feeling appreciated by others	1	2	3	4	5
15. Feeling good about family	1	2	3	4	5
16. Feeling good about yourself	1	2	3	4	5
17. Feeling secure about the future	1	2	3	4	5
18. Having close friendships	1	2	3	4	5
19. Having a home	1	2	3	4	5
20. Making plans about the future	1	2	3	4	5
21. Having people who think highly of you	1	2	3	4	5
22. Having meaning in your life	1	2	3	4	5

(continues)

FIGURE 15-1

Caregiver Well-Being Scale. *(continued)*

Activities of Living

Below are listed a number of activities of living that each of us do or someone does for us. For each activity listed, think over the past three months. During this period of time, indicate to what extent you think each activity of living has been met by circling the appropriate number on the scale provided below. You do not have to be the one doing the activity. You are being asked to rate the extent to which each activity has been taken care of in a timely way.

1 = Never or almost never   2 = Seldom, occasionally   3 = Sometimes
4 = Often, frequently   5 = Almost always

1. Buying food	1	2	3	4	5
2. Preparing meals	1	2	3	4	5
3. Getting the house clean	1	2	3	4	5
4. Getting the yard work done	1	2	3	4	5
5. Getting home maintenance done	1	2	3	4	5
6. Having adequate transportation	1	2	3	4	5
7. Purchasing clothing	1	2	3	4	5
8. Washing and caring for clothing	1	2	3	4	5
9. Relaxing	1	2	3	4	5
10. Exercising	1	2	3	4	5
11. Enjoying a hobby	1	2	3	4	5
12. Starting a new interest or hobby	1	2	3	4	5
13. Attending social events	1	2	3	4	5
14. Taking time for reflective thinking	1	2	3	4	5
15. Having time for inspirational or spiritual interests	1	2	3	4	5
16. Noticing the wonderment of things around you	1	2	3	4	5
17. Asking for support from your friends and family	1	2	3	4	5
18. Getting support from your friends and family	1	2	3	4	5
19. Laughing	1	2	3	4	5
20. Treating or rewarding yourself	1	2	3	4	5
21. Maintaining employment or career	1	2	3	4	5
22. Taking time for personal hygiene and appearance	1	2	3	4	5
23. Taking time to have fun with family and friends	1	2	3	4	5

Source: S. Tebb, M. Berg-Weger, & D. Rubio. This scale may be used by permission only. For permission please contact Dr. Susan Tebb at (314)977–2730.

Stress and Burden in Caregivers

Caring for a family member with dementia can be a stressful experience for the caregiver (Gaugler, Leitsch, Zarit, & Pearlin, 2000). The emotional response to caregiving may be related to one's relationship with the care recipient, the caregiver's usual response to stress, and other life circumstances and experiences of the caregiver (Bumagin & Hirn, 2001). Competing role responsibilities have also been considered a factor in contributing to stress in the caregiver. Care recipients who are excessively demanding of the caregiver also create stress for the caregiver (Zarit & Zarit, 1998). Factors that have been identified as being associated with vulnerability to stresses among caregivers include being a caregiver at age 65 or older, caregiving of a family member with a high level of need, declining physical health of the caregiver, and a low educational level of the caregiver (Navaie-Waliser et al., 2002). In a comparison of caregivers of family members who had cancer, dementia, diabetes, or were frail elders, Kim and Schulz (2008) found that cancer and dementia caregivers reported the highest levels of emotional stress. Emotional stress was also associated with older age, female gender, and higher levels of caregiver burden.

Caring for a spouse with dementia can be especially difficult emotionally for a caregiver, because of changes in the relationship that occur as a result of the disease process. Intimacy and companionship that previously were important in their relationship may no longer be possible. In advanced stages of the disease, the spouse with dementia may not be able to recognize the spouse who provides the care. A decrease in trust by the spouse with dementia may also result, and this can contribute to great difficulty in the provision of care. This, too, contributes to the emotional stress of the spousal caregiver (Ebersole, 2004). Wives report decreased marital satisfaction, decreased leisure time activity participation, and a decreased perception of the quality of family relationships as a result of caregiving (Seltzer & Li, 2000). Role overload is a risk factor for wife caregivers (Cho, Zarit, & Chiriboga, 2009). It has also been found that wives may be more likely to report negative effects of caregiving than husbands. This variation may be related to gender differences in attention to emotions, coping styles, and caregiving tasks (Rose-Rego, Strauss, & Smyth, 1998).

There is concern that some of the gender differences seen in the reported levels of stress among family caregivers may be the result of male caregivers minimizing the level of stress they are experiencing (Kaye, 1997). There are also differences in the levels of stress reported among adult–child caregivers. Daughters who provide care report higher levels of emotional strain than sons (Mui, 1995). Other gender differences have been reported. Female caregivers report not having as much time for themselves, including less time for doing the things they enjoy, such as hobbies and travel. Females also report feeling more physical strain and physical or mental health problems as a result of caregiving responsibilities (National Academy on an Aging Society, 2000).

The impact of caring for a parent on marital quality has been explored, and it was found that a decline in marital quality accumulates over time. Those caregivers who had been caregiving for several years reported less happiness in their marriage and declines in well-being (Bookwala, 2009).

Social isolation has also been identified as a factor that may contribute to stress and burden in family caregivers of older adults with dementia. Family caregivers often report giving up leisure time activities, taking time off from work, and spending less time with family members as a result of their caregiving activities (Ory, Hoffman, Yee, Tennstedt, & Schulz, 1999). In fact, spousal caregivers often become socially isolated from their family members (Ory, Yee, Tennstedt, & Schulz, 2000). Loneliness may result because of the increased responsibility of caregiving, the social isolation that may occur, and the loss of companionship of the spouse with dementia (Bergman-Evans, 1994). Wife caregivers who report that caregiving has a negative impact on social activities may be likely to place their husbands in nursing homes sooner than those who do not (Cho et al., 2009).

It is not uncommon for caregivers to feel they have a lack of support from others as they provide care (Ory et al., 2000). This lack of support may lead to a sense of burden. Burden has been shown to result in a decrease in life satisfaction, lower energy levels, or depression in caregivers (Bumagin & Hirn, 2001). Emotional response to caregiving may depend on the losses experienced by the caregiver as a result of providing the care. Losses may include the lack of personal time, the need to readjust employment, economic costs, and sleep difficulties. It becomes increasingly difficult for caregivers of older adults with dementia as the patient's functional ability decreases and disruptive behavior increases.

Caregiving and Culture

Cultural differences have been found in the emotional responses to caregiving. White caregivers have reported more stress and fewer rewards from caregiving than African-American caregivers (White, Townsend, & Stephens, 2000). There have been a number of studies completed that explore differences in perceptions of caregiving by caregivers of different ethnic groups. In focus groups of African-American, Chinese American, Hispanic American, and European ethnicities, Vickrey and colleagues (2007) found similarities and differences between ethnic groups. Focus group participants commonly reported the need for more information about dementia and resources for caring for those with dementia, and worry about safety, finances, and the ability to care for the care recipient in the future. The African-American, Chinese American, and Hispanic American groups each reported benefits of caregiving including more spirituality, more tolerance, increased sense of purpose, companionship and more time together, and increased appreciation of health. African Americans and Chinese Americans reported prayer, religion, and meditation as being valuable in the caregiving role. Language differences were seen as barriers to care for Chinese Americans, and African Americans perceived discrimination as a barrier (Vickrey et al.).

Scharlach et al. (2006) also conducted focus groups to explore the underutilization of services with Russian, Chinese, Korean, Filipino, Native American, Vietnamese, Hispanic, and African-American caregivers. Caregivers perceived caregiving positively as a source of personal satisfaction and fulfillment rather than as a source of strain or burden. Caregivers in the focus groups saw their cultural approach to caregiving as different from the overall culture in the United States regarding treatment of older adults. There was concern among some groups about the acculturation of younger people in their culture and how changes in cultural norms may affect care of older adults in the future. The four themes that emerged in relation to limited use of formal services included "(1) reliance on informal support networks rather than formal services; (2) lack of knowledge and available services; (3) mistrust of formal service providers; and (4) unavailability of culturally appropriate services" (Scharlach et al., p. 143). Family well-being and the needs of a care recipient were more a concern than caregiver needs, which may result in lower use of services targeted only for caregivers. There was interest expressed for services that used a family-centered approach and benefited the care recipient. In-home respite was seen as a desirable service, and services that were culturally appropriate were also favored (Scharlach et al.).

In a comparison of whites and African Americans in rural Alabama (Kosberg, Kaufman, Burgio, Leeper, & Sun, 2007), religion was used as a coping mechanism for both ethnicities, but the white caregivers reported more burden in personal and social restrictions and physical and emotional health. African Americans had fewer negative health effects and fewer restrictions. There was no difference between groups in social support, but the African-American caregivers were more likely to be involved in formal religious activities. Both groups had low levels of formal service use (Kosberg et al.). Several reasons have been proposed as to the causes for differences in the responses to caregiving, including differences in cultural meaning, the role of religion in assisting in coping with caregiving stress, and cultural differences in support systems (Hooyman & Kiyak, 2002).

It was concluded in a literature review of caregiving by Hispanic caregivers that little is known about the caregiving experience of Hispanics and the influence of culture and background on the caregiving experience (Mier, 2007). To tailor interventions that support caregivers of different ethnicities in a manner that is culturally appropriate and that fulfills a perceived need, more exploration is needed about the caregiving experience and the success of interventions for caregivers of different cultural backgrounds.

Social Support and the Family Caregiver

Social support in the caregiving role has been shown to alleviate stress of caregivers. African-American caregivers have been found to be more resilient than white caregivers and reported higher levels of satisfaction, fewer depressive symptoms, and more satisfaction with social support than white caregivers (Clay, Roth, Wadley, & Haley, 2008). Lack of support for caregivers has been widely explored. Family caregivers have reported issues related to nonsupport including negative interactions with family members, offers of assistance with poor follow-through by family members, lack of contact with friends because of caregiving demands, poor fit between what assistance is offered and the needs of the caregiver, lack of competence in those offering support, negative interactions with friends, criticism from family members, and long-standing family conflict that interferes with support (Neufeld & Harrison, 2003). The geropsychiatric nurse should be sensitive to the difficulties that caregivers may experience in obtaining the social support needed to help alleviate feelings of burden and overload. A careful assessment of available supports and issues related to obtaining the social support needed to continue caring for the family member with dementia in the community setting may assist the caregiver in problem solving social support issues and prevent feelings of isolation that are so common with family caregivers.

Ambivalence and the Care of Family Members with Dementia

Family members who experience guilt and indecision about care needs may experience ambivalence about seeking help with caregiving (Adams, 2006). Intergenerational ambivalence is an area of interest in the social research community that has implications for family caregiving. Past foci in intergenerational relationships have focused on solidarity, which emphasizes consensus and cohesion in family relationships, or conflict and the weakening of family ties (Lüscher & Pillemer, 1998). The concept of ambivalence in intergenerational relationships considers the complexity of the coexistence of both solidarity and conflict in adult family relationships. When one experiences both positive and negative feelings about something, ambivalence is experienced (Maio, Fincham, Regalia, & Paleari, 2004). Higher levels of intergenerational ambivalence have been associated with poorer mental well-being and more depressive symptoms (Fingerman, Pitzer, Lefkowitz, Birditt, & Mroczek, 2008). Intergenerational ambivalence in relation to family caregiving is an important consideration when providing care to caregiving families. Considering the complexity of the relationship between adult children and their parents can greatly facilitate the understanding of emotional responses to caregiving by family members and can assist nurses in addressing the emotional responses to caregiving by both the family caregiver and the care recipient. The ability for clinicians to measure intergenerational ambivalence may be an important consideration, and more valid and reliable methods of measurement are necessary to advance both research and clinical significance of this important conceptual area (Pillemer & Suitor, 2008).

Coping with Caregiving

Caregivers respond to burden by using emotion-focused, problem-focused, and dysfunctional coping strategies (Cooper, Katona, Orrell, & Livingston, 2008). Emotion-focused strategies include religion, humor, emotional support, acceptance, and trying to look at the positive aspects of caregiving. Problem-focused strategies include seeking help and advice from others, planning, or attempting to improve the caregiving situation. Dysfunctional coping strategies include substance use, venting, self-distraction, self-blame, denial, or giving up (Cooper et al.). In a study conducted by Cooper and colleagues, those caregivers who used more dysfunctional coping strategies were more anxious than other caregivers at baseline and 1 year later. Caregivers who report increased burden responded with all types of coping strategies; however, those who used more problem-focused strategies reported increased levels of anxiety in 1 year compared with those who used more emotion-focused strategies and reported less anxiety in 1 year. It was proposed that perhaps caregivers using more problem-focused strategies became frustrated and anxious because many problems facing the caregiver cannot be resolved.

Geropsychiatric nurses may want to consider the results of this study when assessing learning needs and addressing anxiety in family caregivers. Interventions to reduce dysfunctional coping and emphasize emotion-focused coping may be appropriate for some family caregivers (Cooper et al., 2008).

Research has supported that taking breaks from caregiving may help the caregiver maintain a balance in his or her life, which is reported to be a problem for caregivers (Knussen et al., 2008). Maintaining social contact and feeling that one has time to do what is of personal interest may help to prevent feelings of burden. The cost of respite or companionship for an older adult with dementia in the home may be high if social support is not available to fill these needs. Organizing for coverage for an older family member who cannot stay alone can also be overwhelming for a family caregiver who is consumed by caregiving tasks, family responsibilities, and career responsibilities. A caregiver may delay seeking assistance in the home setting until he or she is in a state of crisis, which may result in psychiatric or physical health problems for the caregiver. An important role for the geropsychiatric nurse is to assess the coping ability of the caregiver and to discuss options that are realistic in relation to assisting the caregiver with maintaining balance in his or her life. Assessing what is realistic from an economic and personal perspective is very important, because if the caregiver is overwhelmed it may not be possible for him or her to consider carefully the options available to prevent burnout, resulting in institutionalization of the cognitively impaired family member. The geropsychiatric nurse can better facilitate this careful analysis of realistic options by exploring the needs of the family caregiver and having a strong knowledge of the availability of resources in the community and costs of using available resources.

Psychiatric Health Effects

In a review of the caregiving literature, Schulz et al. (1995) found that there was a strong link between dementia caregiving and psychiatric health effects. Losses in self-identity and decreasing levels of intimacy may contribute to role overload and depression in the caregiver (Adams, McClendon, & Smyth, 2008). Depression symptoms and the use of psychotropic drugs were higher among caregivers than noncaregivers. Cognitive decline has been shown to be associated with depression in caregivers and may have important implications for a caregiver's long-term ability to provide care in the home setting (Vitaliano et al., 2009). Social isolation resulting from communication difficulties with the care recipient and a less stimulating environment may contribute to a caregiver's cognitive decline (Vitaliano et al.). Providing care to family members who display disturbing behaviors may result in higher levels of burden, which is associated with increased depression (Clyburn, Stones, Hadjistavropoulos, & Tuokko, 2000; Hinton, Haan, Geller, & Mungas, 2003). Higher levels of anxiety have also been found in caregivers (Yee & Schulz, 2000). Problem behaviors, and a decline in the health of a loved one, were found to be factors contributing to the negative psychiatric health effects in caregivers. Self-efficacy in dealing with problem behaviors has been found to have a direct inverse relationship with depression symptoms in family caregivers (Gilliam & Steffen, 2006).

Caregiver readiness to assume the caregiving role can have an impact on the psychiatric effects associated with caregiving. Those family members who are prepared to assume the role and make the decision to provide care based on a choice may have an easier transition to the caregiving role. Many caregivers assume the caregiving role unexpectedly and are not prepared or ready to reorganize the pattern of their life to adjust to the additional responsibilities of caregiving. Support within the caregiver's immediate family also may not be present, so the disruption of not only the life of the caregiver but also of his or her family members may add to stress, burden, and depression of the caregiver and other family members. Pressure from siblings or other family members to assume the caregiving role of a parent, when the caregiver is not ready to assume the role, can lead to depression, anger, and resentment (Carruth, Tate, Moffett, & Hill, 1997). Struggling to know how much care should be provided by the caregiver and when to set limitations or to take over are frequently noted as struggles for new caregivers and continue to be issues as the family member with cognitive impairment changes over time. Determining how much assistance to provide may be a source of continued conflict and indecision for family caregivers (Adams, 2006). The needs of caregivers based on whether they are ready for the caregiving role, transitioning into the caregiving role, or experienced in the role may be different, so a careful assessment by the gerospsychiatric nurse can facilitate assisting the caregiver to meet their caregiving needs and needs for emotional and social support.

There are gender differences in relation to the presence of depression symptoms among family caregivers. Females have been found to report symptoms of depression more frequently than males and should be considered at risk for depression (Yee & Schulz, 2000). Research-based estimates project that 50% of female caregivers are at risk for clinical depression, and this increase seems to be attributable to the caregiving experience (Yee & Schulz). Male caregivers have been found to get assistance with caregiving and be more active in preventive health behaviors (Yee & Schulz). These differences may contribute to the lower levels of depression seen in males. Working was associated with reduced levels of depression in husband caregivers in a study conducted in Japan (Sugiura, Ito, Kutsumi, & Mikami, 2009). This may be related to a positive "spillover" effect from a work role that compensates for a negative effect from a caregiving role (p. 153). Experienced caregiving daughters reported higher levels of depression than experienced caregiving sons, and sons reported a decline in depression over time (Bookwala, 2009). Interventions that are targeted to women may be helpful in decreasing the high incidence of psychiatric symptoms in this population. Specific interventions for caregivers are discussed later in this chapter.

Physical Health Effects

Family caregiving may have a negative impact on the health of those providing the care to their relative. Twenty-two percent of family caregivers of individuals with dementia have been found to experience emotional or physical problems (Ory et al., 1999). Caregiving may also provide an adverse effect on one's physical health, and African-American caregivers have been found to be in poorer health than white caregivers (Wallsten, 2000). However, when controlling for educational level, differences in subjective physical health between whites and African-Americans were no longer evident (Knight, Longmire, Kim, & David, 2007).

Caring for someone with behavior problems has been associated with poorer caregiver self-reported health, less engagement in health-promoting behaviors by the caregiver, and increased healthcare spending by the caregiver. These health outcomes of caregiving were mediated by feelings of overload in that those who were feeling more overloaded by caregiving reported more negative health outcomes (Son et al., 2007). Perceived self-efficacy in being able to obtain respite may be associated with positive health behaviors in family caregivers, and the caregiver's self-efficacy in the ability to control upsetting thoughts has been associated with lower levels of cumulative health risk (Rabinowitz, Mausbach, Thompson, & Gallagher-Thompson, 2007). Interestingly, not all studies support negative health outcomes associated with family caregiving. A recent study showed that caregivers who provided 14 hours or more of care to their spouse per week had a lower risk of mortality than spouses who did not provide care (Brown et al., 2009).

Perceived health by caregivers may influence their reports of burden. Those caregivers who report more health symptoms have also reported higher levels of burden, isolation, disappointment, emotional involvement with the care recipient, and strain (Andren & Elmstahl, 2008). Adherence to a regular program of physical activity to promote health is also considered problematic for many caregivers (King & Brassington, 1997). Offering strategies for promoting health, self-efficacy, and self-care is an important role for the geropsychiatric nurse when caring for family caregivers.

Grief and the Family Caregiver

The concepts of loss, sorrow, and grief in caregivers of family members with dementia have been explored. Losses that are both psychological and social occur among caregivers before the physical loss of a loved one with dementia (Kuhn, 2001). Losses for spousal caregivers may include leisure time, companionship, financial well-being, and sexual intimacy, whereas losses for other family caregivers may be related to career and time for other family members (Kuhn). The losses

associated with family caregiving may result in feelings of sorrow and grief for the caregiver. Anticipatory grief is multifaceted and associated with the future loss of the family member and losses from the past and present (Holley & Mast, 2009). Chronic sorrow has been defined as the feelings of grief that occur as the result of the loss of the normal lifestyle of individuals with chronic health problems and their caregivers (Burke & Eakes, 1999). Grief is considered to be the behavioral, social, physical, and psychological response to loss (Kuhn).

Living with loss has been identified as an important theme among caregivers of family members with dementia (Moyle, Edwards, & Clinton, 2002). Anticipatory grief has been strongly associated with burden in caregivers (Holley & Mast, 2009). Geropsychiatric nurses have an important role in supporting family members with the anticipatory grieving of losses. Assisting caregivers with a redefinition of their relationship with the family member is important as losses from dementia progress. The loss of the previous relationship with the family member with dementia, changes in caregiver family, spousal, and work role, and loss of fulfillment of life expectations and transitions can all contribute to grief and depression for family caregivers. Changes in how the caregiver perceives the family member can affect how the caregiver perceives himself or herself because of the disruption in the previous predictable relationship (Hasselkus & Murray, 2007). The sense of helplessness that occurs and results in decreased control over one's life can be difficult for caregivers (Kuhn, 2001). Nursing sensitivity to these issues is essential to establish supportive and therapeutic relationships with family caregivers.

In a study that addressed the characteristics of grief among spouse and adult–child caregivers at each stage of dementia, Meuser and Marwit (2001) found that there were differences in the grief responses between these two groups of family caregivers. Early in the disease, spouse caregivers were more open and realistic about their partner's condition and burdens that may occur in the future, whereas adult–child caregivers minimized their feelings and did not accept early signs of dementia. Spouse caregivers expressed concern about the loss of companionship with their spouse, whereas adult–child caregivers were concerned about the loss of their own freedom and support from their siblings. Later in the disease, adult–child caregivers expressed a mix of anger, frustration, and resentment concerning mounting personal losses and a sense of having placed their lives on hold. Guilt over escapist thoughts (e.g., wishing the parent would die) and adequacy of care was also evident in some adult–child caregivers. These emotions were not found in spousal caregivers. Spouse caregivers were found to accept caregiving responsibilities with dignity and affection but experienced the highest level of grief on nursing home placement. Frustration and anger often accompanied nursing home placement for spouses, because they no longer identified themselves as a couple. However, adult–child caregivers experienced a decrease in anger during this phase of caregiving and reported more reflection and concern for their parent.

Because of the differences found in grief responses between adult–child and spouse caregivers at different stages of the disease, Meuser and Marwit (2001) proposed that interventions for caregivers be individualized and consideration be given to the stage of the disease and the relationship of the caregiver to the older adult with dementia. Anger management strategies, education, counseling, and opportunities for reflection may be beneficial interventions for family caregivers during various phases of the grief process, but because adult–child and spouse caregivers may experience the grief process differently depending on the progression of the disease, careful assessment of the grief response in the individual caregiver and appropriate targeting of the intervention are important.

The Marwit–Meuser Caregiver Grief Inventory (MM-CGI) is an instrument that may be helpful to the geropsychiatric nurse in assessing the grief response of the caregiver providing care to a family member with progressive dementia (Figure 15-2) (Marwit & Meuser, 2002). Testing has established that the instrument has a high internal consistency (Cronbach α = 0.96), and adequate test–retest reliability and concurrent validity. The instrument consists of 50 items, and the construct validity has been supported by a factor analysis that identified three factors explaining the items in the instrument.

The items that relate to the first factor are referred to as "Personal Sacrifice Burden" items. They focus on personal losses in the caregiver's life that occurred as a result of caregiving, such as loss of sleep and personal freedom. The second factor items are referred to as "Heartfelt Sadness and Longing" and relate to intrapersonal emotional reactions to caregiving that seem to be associated with grief. These items measure emotional reactions to the losses associated with a family member with dementia. The responses are personally based responses. The third factor items, the "Worry and Felt Isolation" items, are related to social support and losing the sense of connection with others (Marwit & Meuser, 2002). The factors are important because those items in Factor 1 and Factor 3 address areas of perceived loss and social isolation. Caregivers identifying problems in these areas may respond to cognitive–behavioral interventions. Caregivers with problems identified in Factor 2 may respond to interventions that are supportive, such as empathetic listening, because the items measure personal affective concerns (Marwit & Meuser, 2002).

A short form of the MM-CGI, the MM-CGI-SF, was developed by Marwit and Meuser (2005) and includes an 18-item scale derived from the 50-item MM-CGI (Figure 15-3). This may be a useful form for preliminary screening and for use in those who may have a decreased attention span and difficulty completing the 50-item form (Marwit & Meuser, 2005). Internal consistency was found to be high on the Heartfelt Sadness and Longing subscale (α reliability = 0.84), Personal Sacrifice Burden subscale (α reliability = 0.83), and the Worry and Felt Isolation subscale (α reliability = 0.78) when tested with 201 community-based spousal and adult child

FIGURE 15-2

MM Caregiver Grief Inventory

Instructions: This inventory is designed to measure the grief experience of *current* family caregivers of persons living with progressive dementia (e.g., Alzheimer's disease). Read each statement carefully, then decide how much you agree or disagree with what is said. Circle a number 1–5 to the right using the answer key below (For example 5 = Strongly Agree). It is important that you respond to all items so that the scores are accurate. Scoring rules are listed at the end.

1 = Strongly Disagree   2 = Disagree   3 = Somewhat Agree
4 = Agree   5 = Strongly Agree

1.	I've had to give up a great deal to be a caregiver.	1	2	3	4	5	A
2.	I miss so many of the activities we used to share.	1	2	3	4	5	B
3.	I feel I am losing my freedom.	1	2	3	4	5	A
4.	My physical health has declined from the stress of being a caregiver.	1	2	3	4	5	A
5.	I have nobody to communicate with.	1	2	3	4	5	C
6.	I don't know what is happening. I feel confused and unsure.	1	2	3	4	5	C
7.	I carry a lot of stress as a caregiver.	1	2	3	4	5	A
8.	I receive enough emotional support from others.	1	2	3	4	5	Cr
9.	I have this empty, sick feeling knowing that my loved one is "gone".	1	2	3	4	5	B
10.	I feel anxious and scared.	1	2	3	4	5	C
11.	My personal life has changed a great deal.	1	2	3	4	5	A
12.	I spend a lot of time worrying about the bad things to come.	1	2	3	4	5	C
13.	Dementia is like a double loss . . . I've lost the closeness with my loved one and connectedness with my family.	1	2	3	4	5	C
14.	I feel terrific sadness.	1	2	3	4	5	B
15.	This situation is totally unacceptable in my heart.	1	2	3	4	5	B

FIGURE 15-2

MM Caregiver Grief Inventory (continued)

16.	My friends simply don't understand what I'm going through.	1	2	3	4	5	C
17.	I feel this constant sense of responsibility and it just never leaves.	1	2	3	4	5	A
18.	I long for what was, what we had and shared in the past.	1	2	3	4	5	B
19.	I could deal with other serious disabilities better than with this.	1	2	3	4	5	B
20.	I can't feel free in this situation.	1	2	3	4	5	A
21.	I'm having trouble sleeping.	1	2	3	4	5	A
22.	I'm at peace with myself and my situation in life.	1	2	3	4	5	Cr
23.	It's a life phase and I know we'll get through it.	1	2	3	4	5	Cr
24.	My extended family has no idea what I go through in caring for him/her.	1	2	3	4	5	C
25.	I feel so frustrated that I often tune him/her out.	1	2	3	4	5	A
26.	I am always worrying.	1	2	3	4	5	C
27.	I'm angry at the disease for robbing me of so much.	1	2	3	4	5	B
28.	This is requiring more emotional energy and determination than I ever expected.	1	2	3	4	5	A
29.	I will be tied up with this for who knows how long.	1	2	3	4	5	A
30.	It hurts to put her/him to bed at night and realize that she/he is "gone."	1	2	3	4	5	B
31.	I feel very sad about what this disease has done.	1	2	3	4	5	B
32.	I feel severe depression.	1	2	3	4	5	C
33.	I lay awake most nights worrying about what's happening and how I'll manage tomorrow.	1	2	3	4	5	C

(continues)

FIGURE 15-2

MM Caregiver Grief Inventory *(continued)*

34.	The people closest to me do not understand what I'm going through.	1	2	3	4	5	C
35.	His/her death will bring me renewed personal freedom to live my life.	1	2	3	4	5	A
36.	I feel powerless.	1	2	3	4	5	B
37.	It's frightening because you know doctors can't cure this disease, so things only get worse.	1	2	3	4	5	B
38.	I've lost other people close to me, but the losses I'm experiencing now are much more troubling.	1	2	3	4	5	B
39.	Independence is what I've lost...I don't have the freedom to go and do what I want.	1	2	3	4	5	A
40.	I've had to make some drastic changes in my life as a result of becoming a caregiver.	1	2	3	4	5	A
41.	I wish I had an hour or two to myself each day to pursue personal interests.	1	2	3	4	5	A
42.	I'm stuck in this caregiving world and there's nothing I can do about it.	1	2	3	4	5	A
43.	I can't contain my sadness about all that's happening.	1	2	3	4	5	B
44.	What upsets me most is what I've had to give up.	1	2	3	4	5	A
45.	I'm managing pretty well overall.	1	2	3	4	5	Cr
46.	I think I'm denying the full implications of this for my life.	1	2	3	4	5	C
47.	I get excellent support from members of my family.	1	2	3	4	5	Cr
48.	I've had a hard time accepting what is happening.	1	2	3	4	5	B
49.	The demands on me are growing faster than I ever expected.	1	2	3	4	5	A
50.	I wish this was all a dream and I could wake up back in my old life.	1	2	3	4	5	B

FIGURE 15-2

MM Caregiver Grief Inventory *(continued)*

FAIR USE OF THE MM-CGI: The inventory was developed and pilot tested on two samples of dementia caregivers: 87 caregivers (45 adult child, 42 spouse) in the development phase and 166 (83 of each type) for pilot testing. Funding support came from the Alzheimer's Association (Grant 1999-PRG-1730). A 3-factor solution materialized (KMO = .889) and these factors are listed below. The authors consider this instrument to be part of the public domain. The authors would appreciate hearing feedback on how the scale is used. Researchers who wish to administer the inventory and/or modify it as part of a formal study are asked to notify the authors of their plans (Tom Meuser, Ph.D., meusert@abraxas.wustl.edu; 314-286-2992).

Meuser, T.M., & Marwit, S.J. (2001). A comprehensive, stage-sensitive model of grief in dementia caregiving. *The Gerontologist,* 41(5), 658–770. Marwit, S.J., & Meuser, T.M. (2002). Development and initial validation of an inventory to assess grief in caregivers of person with Alzheimer's disease. *The Gerontologist,* 42(6), 751–765.

Self-Scoring Procedure: Add the numbers you circled to derive the following sub-scale and total grief scores. Use the letters to the right of each score to guide you. **C Items with "r" afterwards must first be reversed scored (1 → 5, 2 → 4, 3 → 3, 4 → 2, 5 → 1) before adding to calculate your scores.**

Personal Sacrifice Burden *(A Items)* = _____
(18 items, M = 54.3, SD = 14, 1, Alpha = .93, Split-Half = 91)

Heartfelt Sadness and Longing *(B Items)* = _____
(15 Items, M = 48.2, SD = 11.1, Alpha = .90, Split-Half = .86)

Worry and Felt Isolation *(C Items)* = _____
(17 Items, M= 40.6, SD = 11.9, Alpha = .91, Split-Half = .91)

Total Grief Level *(Sum A + B + C)* = _____
(50 Items, M = 144, SD = 31.6, Alpha = .96, Split-Half = .87)

Plot your scores using the grid to the right. Make an "**X**" in the shaded section nearest to your numeric score for each sub-scale. This is your grief profile. Discuss the profile with your support group leader or counselor.

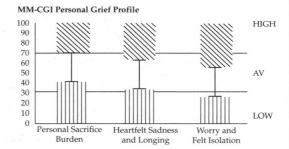

MM-CGI Personal Grief Profile

What do these scores mean?
Scores in the top area are higher than average based validation sample statistics (1 SD above the Mean). High scores may indicate a need for formal intervention or support assistance to enhance coping. Low scores in the bottom lined section (1 SD below the Mean) may indicate denial or a downplaying of distress. Low scores may also indicate positive adaptation if the individual is not showing other signs of suppressed grief. Average scores in the center indicate common reactions. These are general guides for discussion and support only—more research is needed on more specific interpretation issues.

Sources: Meuser, T. M., & Marwit, S. J. (2001). A comprehensive, stage-sensitive model of grief in dementia caregiving, *The Gerontologist,* 41(5), 658–670; and Marwit, S. J., & Meuser, T. M. (2002). Development and initial validation of an inventory to assess grief in caregivers of persons with Alzheimer's disease. *The Gerontologist,* 42(6), 751–765; Reprinted with permission of the authors and publisher.

FIGURE 15-3

Marwit-Meuser Caregiver Grief Inventory—Short Form (MM-CGI-SF)

MM Caregiver Grief Inventory – Short Form

Samuel J. Marwit, Ph.D., University of Missouri-St. Louis
Thomas M. Meuser, Ph.D., Washington University, St. Louis

Instructions: This inventory is designed to measure the grief experience of <u>current</u> family caregivers of persons living with progressive dementia (e.g., Alzheimer's disease). Read each statement carefully, then decide how much you agree or disagree with what is said. Circle a number 1-5 to the right using the answer key below (For example 5 = Strongly Agree). It is important that you respond to all items so that the scores are accurate. Scoring rules are listed below.

ANSWER KEY

1 = Strongly Disagree // 2 = Disagree // 3 = Somewhat Agree // 4 = Agree // **5 = Strongly Agree**

1	I've had to give up a great deal to be a caregiver.	1	2	3	4	5	A
2	I feel I am losing my freedom.	1	2	3	4	5	A
3	I have nobody to communicate with.	1	2	3	4	5	C
4	I have this empty, sick feeling knowing that my loved one is "gone".	1	2	3	4	5	B
5	I spend a lot of time worrying about the bad things to come.	1	2	3	4	5	C
6	Dementia is like a double loss…I've lost the closeness with my loved one and connectedness with my family.	1	2	3	4	5	C
7	My friends simply don't understand what I'm going through.	1	2	3	4	5	C
8	I long for what was, what we had and shared in the past.	1	2	3	4	5	B
9	I could deal with other serious disabilities better than with this.	1	2	3	4	5	B
10	I will be tied up with this for who knows how long.	1	2	3	4	5	A
11	It hurts to put her/him to bed at night and realize that she/he is "gone".	1	2	3	4	5	B
12	I feel very sad about what this disease has done.	1	2	3	4	5	B
13	I lay awake most nights worrying about what's happening and how I'll manage tomorrow.	1	2	3	4	5	C
14	The people closest to me do not understand what I'm going through.	1	2	3	4	5	C
15	I've lost other people close to me, but the losses I'm experiencing now are much more troubling.	1	2	3	4	5	B
16	Independence is what I've lost…I don't have the freedom to go and do what I want.	1	2	3	4	5	A
17	I wish I had an hour or two to myself each day to pursue personal interests.	1	2	3	4	5	A
18	I'm stuck in this caregiving world and there's nothing I can do about it.	1	2	3	4	5	A

Self-Scoring Procedure: Add the numbers you circled to derive the following sub-scale and total grief scores. Use the letters to the right of each score to guide you.

Personal Sacrifice Burden *(A Items)* = _____
(6 Items, M = 20.2, SD = 5.3, Alpha = .83, n = 292)

Heartfelt Sadness & Longing *(B Items)* = _____
(6 Items, M = 20.2, SD = 5.0, Alpha = .80, n = 292)

Worry & Felt Isolation *(C Items)* = _____
(6 Items, M = 16.6, SD = 5.2, Alpha = .82, n = 292)

Total Grief Level *(Sum A + B + C)* = _____
(18 Items, M = 57, SD = 12.9, Alpha = .90, n = 292)

Plot your scores using the grid to the right. Make an **"X"** nearest to your numeric score for each sub-scale heading. Connect the X's. This is your grief profile. Discuss this with your support group leader or counselor.

Author Note: This scale may be copied and freely used for clinical or supportive purposes. Those wishing to use the scale for research are asked to e-mail for permission: meusert@abraxas.wustl.edu (5/04)

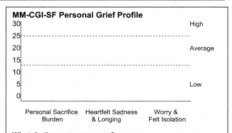

MM-CGI-SF Personal Grief Profile

What do these scores mean?
Scores in the top area are one standard deviation (SD) higher than average based on responses of other family caregivers (n = 292). High scores may indicate a need for formal intervention or support assistance to enhance coping. Low scores (one SD below the mean) may indicate denial or a downplaying of distress. Low scores may also indicate positive adaptation if the individual is not showing other signs of suppressed grief or psychological disturbance. Average scores in the center indicate common reactions. These are general guides for discussion and support only— more research is needed on specific interpretation issues.

caregivers of individuals with dementia (Sanders, Ott, Kelber, & Noonan, 2008). Twenty-two percent of the sample scored a high level of grief on the MM-CGI-SF. Those with high grief were primarily white (89%) and female (86%). Fifty-two percent were spouses and 52% were adult children, mostly daughters. This multimethod study showed that even though caregivers use coping strategies, such as social networks, spirituality, and pets, intense grief responses were still experienced by caregivers (Sanders et al.). The researchers recommended that professional support may be helpful to reduce feelings of guilt, lack of freedom, isolation, and loss (Sanders et al.). Geropsychiatric nurses and other nurses caring for caregiving families may be instrumental in providing the support needed for grieving family caregivers.

CAREGIVER ASSESSMENT AND THE GEROPSYCHIATRIC NURSE

It is important for the geropsychiatric nurse to assess the caregiver when the older adult with dementia is assessed. It is also essential that as part of the health history, all adults who undergo a health examination be screened for their involvement in caregiving. By identifying those adults who may be burdened by the caregiving role and who may be at risk for stress-related health problems, both physical and emotional, the nurse is better able to assess resource need and function in a supportive and educational role. All too frequently family caregivers receive health care but the potential burden of caregiving is not identified, resulting in the caregiver not receiving the care and support needed. The development of a caregiver and care recipient management plan may be effective in managing problems that affect both parties and may help to alleviate caregiver stress (Schulz et al., 1995).

The Modified Caregiver Strain Index (Thornton & Travis, 2003), which is a modification of the Caregiver Strain Index (Robinson, 1983), may be helpful in evaluating caregiver stress. The instrument serves as an assessment tool for geropsychiatric nurses to identify areas of strain that may indicate a need for intervention (Figure 15-4). Several domains of caregiver stress are explored including physical, social, employment, time, and financial. Caregivers with high scores have higher levels of caregiver strain (Sullivan, 2008). The internal reliability coefficient of the Modified Caregiver Strain Index was 0.90 and the test–retest reliability was strong at 0.88 (Thornton & Travis). The Caregiver Well-Being Scale and the MM-CGI, described previously in this chapter, are also helpful assessment tools, because they can assist nurses in targeting interactions so that issues for the caregiver can be explored and interventions that can address problem areas can be discussed. Each of the assessment instruments may be useful in the tailoring of counseling interventions by geropsychiatric nurses.

The assessment of caregiver need by the geropsychiatric nurse should also include how caregivers are coping with changes in their role as a caregiver. An instrument developed by Melillo and Futrell (1995) may be helpful in assessing the needs of family caregivers of older adults with dementia. This instrument provides a guideline for a comprehensive assessment of the caregiver including information about the caregiver's health status, employment, resources available, and relationship with the care recipient, and information about the type and amount of care provided. The instrument includes indicators about the type of education and referrals needed by the caregiver and provides space for the development of an assessment and care plan. The instrument may be helpful to nurses in assessing the need for professional caregivers in the home who may provide assistance to the family caregiver.

Caregivers have reported more sleep disturbances than noncaregivers (Vitaliano et al., 2009). Depression has been found to be predictive of poor sleep quality in caregivers (Rowe, McCrae, Campbell, Benito, & Cheng, 2008). Providing supervision at night may also interfere with sleep of caregivers. Assessing family caregivers for problems with sleep is an important role for the

FIGURE 15-4

Modified Caregiver Strain Index.

DIRECTIONS: Here is a list of things that other caregivers have found to be difficult. Please put a check mark in the columns that apply to you. We have included some examples that are common caregiver experiences to help you think about each item. Your situation may be slightly different, but the item could still apply.

	Yes, On a Regular Basis = 2	Yes, Some-times = 1	No = 0
My **sleep is disturbed** (*For example: the person I care for* is in and out of bed or wanders around at night)	___	___	___
Caregiving **is inconvenient** (*For example:* helping takes so much time or it's a long drive over to help)	___	___	___
Caregiving **is a physical strain** (*For example:* lifting in and out of a chair; effort or concentration is required)	___	___	___
Caregiving **is confining** (*For example:* helping restricts free time or *I* cannot go visiting)	___	___	___
There have been family adjustments (*For example:* helping has disrupted *my* routine; there has been no privacy)	___	___	___
There have been changes in personal plans (*For example: I* had to turn down a job; *I* could not go on vacation)	___	___	___
There have been other demands on my time (*For example:* other family members *need me*)	___	___	___
There have been emotional adjustments (*For example:* severe arguments *about caregiving*)	___	___	___
Some behavior is upsetting (*For example:* incontinence; *the person cared for* has trouble remembering things; or *the person I care for* accuses people of taking things)	___	___	___

FIGURE 15-4

Modified Caregiver Strain Index. *(continued)*

	Yes, On a Regular Basis = 2	Yes, Some-times = 1	No = 0
It is upsetting to find *the person I care for* has changed so much from his/her former self *(For example:* he/she is a different person than he/she used to be)	_____	_____	_____
There have been work adjustments *(For example: I have* to take time off *for caregiving duties*)	_____	_____	_____
***Caregiving* is a financial strain**	_____	_____	_____
***I feel* completely overwhelmed** *(For example: I* worry about *the person I care for*; *I have* concerns about how *I* will manage)	_____	_____	_____

(Sum responses for 'yes, on a regular basis' (2 pts each) and 'yes, sometimes' (1 pt each)

Total Score = _____

Source: Thornton, M., & Travis, S. S. (2003). Analysis of the reliability of the Modified Caregiver Strain Index. *Journal of Gerontology: Social Sciences, 58B*(2), S127–S132.

Words appearing in italics represent modifications from the original Caregiver Strain Index from Robinson, B. (1983). Validation of a caregiver strain index. *Journal of Gerontology, 38*, 344-348. Copyright by The Gerontological Society of America. Reprinted with permission.

nurse because sleep problems have been associated with decreased quality of life, health problems, and accidents (Resnick, Shaughnessy, & Simpson, 2005) and may place caregivers at a higher risk for adverse effects of caregiving.

One of the roles of the nurse may also include helping to coordinate formal services if needed. By evaluating caregivers on an ongoing basis, the nurse can assist the caregiver in better meeting his or her needs. The nurse may facilitate the use of respite care and provide encouragement to use available social support, including caregiver group support

(Ebersole, 2004). Nursing assessment of the caregiver can assist the nurse in recommending health promotion and preventive self-care activities that are individualized for each caregiver. Encouraging the caregiver to address his or her own health concerns and participating in health promotion and preventive health behaviors is important for the maintenance of the caregiver's support of the functionally impaired older adult in the home setting.

Targeting interventions to promote self-care activities in caregivers is an important nursing role. Interventions focused on increasing physical activity and exercise may be especially important in the prevention of chronic health problems in the older adult population and may assist the caregiver in maintaining optimal health (Matthews, Dunbar-Jacob, Sereika, Schulz, & McDowell, 2004).

Research has been reported that explores issues related to self-care and the family caregiver. Burton and colleagues (1997) found that caregivers who provide a high intensity of care were more likely to get inadequate rest and exercise, and forget to take prescription medication compared with noncaregivers. Acton (2002) also found that caregivers had more barriers to health promotion behaviors and practiced fewer self-care behaviors than noncaregivers. Caregivers who provide more ADL care, provide more hours of care, report more symptoms of depression, have less social support, and report less self-efficacy have been found to be at a higher risk for a decrease in self-care activities (Gallant & Connell, 1997). Evidence is conflicting, however, about the effect of caregiving on the caregivers' participation in self-care activities. Some researchers have found no evidence that caregivers had poorer self-care practices than noncaregivers. In fact, it has been proposed that caregivers may take better care of themselves because of the need to be able to provide care to the dependent family member. Findings have also supported that health-promoting behaviors may have a positive effect on caregiver stress (Acton). In a study comparing urban and rural spousal caregivers, no differences were found in health-promoting behaviors (Lee, 2009). The most common health-promoting behaviors were associated with stress management, spiritual growth, and interpersonal relationships. The least common health behaviors of spousal caregivers were related to physical activity and good nutrition (Lee).

INTERVENTIONS TO SUPPORT CAREGIVERS

Because of the high levels of burden, depression, and anxiety found in female caregivers, interventions to support women who provide care are very important. Male caregivers are also in need of support when providing care to family members, but it is not clear whether the interventions that are effective for female caregivers are effective in meeting the needs of male caregivers (Houde, 2002). Support groups may be helpful in assisting women to learn methods that are effective in providing care, and sharing concerns related to caregiving. Educational programs that address and promote preventive health behaviors may also be beneficial in preventing psychiatric symptoms by encouraging women to participate in self-care activities (Yee & Schulz, 2000). Skills training, individual and family psychotherapy, counseling, and respite care are also interventions that have been used as supportive interventions for family caregivers (Farran, 2001). Programs to enhance a caregiver's self-efficacy in caring for family members with dementia, including strategies to address problem behavior, may be helpful in preventing depression in family caregivers.

Technology is increasingly being used as a support for caregivers of older adults with dementia. Many organizations have developed resources for caregivers that are available for caregivers through the Internet. The U.S. Administration on Aging (AOA) provides information for caregivers through its Web site, www.aoa.gov. The Caregivers' Resource Room provides information about the AOA National Family Caregiver Support Program. This site provides important information links for both caregivers and professionals about issues of importance to caregivers. Other Web sites are available to assist caregivers with informational needs related to caregiving (Box 15-1).

There are also Web sites available that allow caregivers the opportunity to communicate with each other and offer support and suggestions. Chat rooms are available online where caregivers can communicate with others who are also providing care in the home. Using computer technology in the home can assist caregivers who have difficulty networking with other informal caregivers and who have inadequate support in the community to feel a sense of support without needing to leave the home environment. Computer use may help to prevent

BOX 15-1 WEB SITES TO ASSIST CAREGIVERS

National Family Caregivers Association (www.nfcacares.org)

- Current information about family caregiving for caregivers
- Tips for caregivers, including self advocacy
- News releases related to caregiving
- Publications to assist caregivers

Alzheimer's Association (www.alz.org)

- Detailed information about Alzheimer's disease, including warning signs, diagnosis, treatment, and stages
- Research information
- Many brochures available online in different languages
- Information about educational programs and local chapters
- Specific information for both family caregivers and professionals

National Alliance for Caregiving (www.caregiving.org)

- Information for both family caregivers and professionals
- Many resources available with links to multiple Web sites
- Tips for caregivers
- Information about international caregiving legislation

Family Caregiver Alliance (www.caregiver.org)

- Monographs related to caregiving
- Information about public policy and caregiving with policy briefs
- Newsletters for caregivers
- Fact sheets of interest to caregivers
- Online discussion groups for caregivers
- Caregiving information and advice

National Family Caregivers Association and National Alliance for Caregiving *Family Caregiving 101* **(www.familycaregiving101.org):** A basic online course for family caregivers that provides important information and strategies for family caregivers

AARP Caregiving Web site (www.aarp.org/relationships/caregiving): Timely articles, updates, and information for family caregivers

the sense of social isolation that occurs with many older caregivers who are unable to leave the home environment because of caregiving responsibilities.

A number of research studies have been developed to evaluate the use of interventions to support caregivers in the home. Resources for Enhancing Alzheimer's Caregiver Health (REACH) is a large multisite program, sponsored by the National Institute on Aging and the National Institute on Nursing Research. The purpose of this program is to evaluate the effectiveness of interventions to support family caregivers of those with Alzheimer's disease. A number of different interventions have been evaluated including psychoeducational and skill-based training, technology support systems, group support and family therapy, individual information and support, and environmental interventions (Schulz et al., 2003).

Interventions evaluated in the REACH study were a structural ecosystem (SET) and computer–telephone integrated system (CTIS), which when used together were shown to decrease the level of depression in both white non-Hispanic and Cuban American caregivers (Eisdorfer et al., 2003). The purpose of SET was to identify problems of caregivers and the resources available for the caregivers. Restructuring interactions linked to caregiver burden was an important goal. The CTIS supplemented SET by linking caregivers with family members and other resources. Results showed that SET and CTIS together had a positive impact on caregivers, but that the individual interventions alone did not have a significant impact on depression (Eisdorfer et al.).

The Environmental Skill-Building Program is another program evaluated under the REACH project (Gitlin et al., 2003). This program educated caregivers about the effect of the environment on behaviors and how to modify the environment to decrease problem behaviors. Strategies to maintain control and manage problems on a daily basis were also addressed. Results of this demonstration program showed a decrease in perceived burden and an improvement in the sense of well-being among caregivers (Gitlin et al.).

In a comparison of a Behavior Care intervention and Enhanced Care intervention, it was found that those caregivers who participated in the Behavior Care intervention had greater levels of distress and an increased risk of depression compared to those who participated in the Enhanced Care intervention (Burns, Nichols, Martindale-Adams, Graney, & Lummus, 2003). The Behavior Care intervention focused on the management of behavior problems in the care recipient only, whereas the Enhanced Care intervention also focused on the well-being of the caregiver. In the Behavior Care intervention, the caregiver's level of knowledge related to problem behaviors was assessed, and solutions to behavior problems and behavior management strategies were discussed. In the Enhanced Care intervention, not only were behavioral problems addressed, but cognitive–behavioral skills training, such as relaxation training and coping strategies, were included as important components in the program (Burns et al.).

In a telephone-based cognitive–behavioral intervention with rural caregivers that included both group and individual sessions, significant decreases were seen in caregiving-related problems, psychological caregiver distress, and subjective burden compared to caregivers who received routine education and support. Improvements were seen in perceived self-efficacy of caregivers (Glueckauf et al., 2007).

Many of the intervention programs that have been evaluated in the literature have been interventions that do not address the individualized needs of caregivers. It has been suggested that an individualized approach to targeting interventions to meet caregiver needs be adopted because the needs of caregivers are varied (Schulz et al., 2003). Although some caregivers may respond positively to group interventions, other caregivers may respond more favorably to individual counseling. An intervention using a multicomponent approach that is tailored using an individual risk profile is being evaluated in the follow-up study to REACH, called REACH II. This intervention focuses on several areas related to caregiver health outcomes, including self-care, emotional well-being, problem behaviors, social support, and safety (Schulz et al., 2003).

In a REACH II program, the REACH OUT program, positive outcomes were found in an intervention used by personnel in Area Agencies on Aging (Burgio et al., 2009). The intervention included a risk appraisal; education about caregiving, stress, and dementia; safety; caregiving health; behavior management; and stress management. Four hour-long home visits were made by trained case managers with three therapeutic phone calls. Those who participated in the program reported less subjective burden, less frustration, increased social support, improved self-rated health, fewer sleep problems, and a high level of satisfaction with the program (Burgio et al.).

Multicomponent approach studies have been found to have significant outcomes with a number of outcome measures including caregiver well-being, depression, self-efficacy, and burden (Parker, Mills, & Abbey, 2008). However, because of the wide variation in strategies used in multicomponent studies, analysis and comparison of results across studies is difficult. Factors that did not seem to be helpful to caregivers included only referring a caregiver to a support group, only providing self-help materials, or only offering peer support. Parker and colleagues identified factors that contributed to effectiveness of interventions as a result of a systematic review of the literature. Included in their recommendations were "provide opportunities within the intervention for the person with dementia as well as the caregiver to be involved, encourage active participation in educational interventions for caregivers, offer individualized programs rather than group sessions, provide information on an ongoing basis, with specific information about services and coaching regarding their new role, target the recipient particularly by reduction in behaviors" (p. 138). Etters, Goodall, and Harrison (2008) concluded from their literature review that nurses should develop and implement multicomponent interventions for caregivers because of their positive effects related to caregiver burden, depression, coping, and the delay of institutionalization of care recipients.

Interventions more readily available in the community that may be effective in addressing caregiver needs include support groups and respite or day-care programs. Support groups provide caregivers with emotional support by meeting with a group of other caregivers who may be experiencing similar stresses related to caregiving. Facilitating entry into a support group may be an important role of the geropsychiatric nurse. Caregivers may be hesitant to seek a support group and feel overwhelmed by arranging care for the person he or she is caring for so that attending the support group is possible. There are support groups that offer onsite care, and knowledge of these services is important for the nurse to share with caregivers. Support groups allow caregivers to exchange suggestions of strategies that have been helpful in the caring of their family member with dementia. Many support groups are coordinated by community agencies, local hospitals, or the Alzheimer's Association. Some support groups are helpful in that they teach caregivers skills that are important in caring for functionally impaired older adults in the home. Feeling that they have the skills necessary to provide care may help caregivers to minimize the stress associated with the need to provide care.

Men, who tend to discontinue caregiving sooner than women, may benefit from educational programs that teach skills, including direct personal care, such as bathing, dressing, feeding, and housekeeping skills. Studies have supported that male caregivers appreciate programs that provide advice and information about caregiving, and female caregivers have been shown to benefit from support groups that offer emotional support (Kaye, 1997). In a comparison of two interventions for male caregivers including videos, a workbook, and weekly telephone coaching sessions, and an educational booklet with biweekly check-in calls, improvements in levels of upset and annoyance with behavior problems, affect, and self-efficacy were noted with both interventions. No difference in outcomes was found, however, between the two interventions (Gant, Steffen, & Lauderdale, 2007). The researchers propose that there may need to be an increase in sensitivity in instruments that measure a male's reaction to caregiving, because many measures currently being used were developed for female caregivers (Gant et al.). With the increase in the number of male caregivers, there is still much to be learned about understanding male reactions to caregiving and developing interventions that support men who provide care to family members in the community.

An intervention that combined structured individual and family counseling, weekly support groups, and the availability of counselors by telephone was shown to decrease symptoms of depression in caregivers, and a delay in nursing home placement of care recipients with dementia (Mittelman, Roth, Haley, & Zarit, 2004). The counseling intervention was tailored to individual caregiver needs and included strategies for managing problem behaviors, communication and conflict resolution skills, improving support, and education and resource information about Alzheimer's disease.

Day care centers may provide respite for caregivers of older adults with dementia, and are especially helpful for caregivers who are employed and care for someone who cannot be left home alone during the day. Respite programs are programs that provide relief from care for the caregiver by providing care to the functionally impaired older adult. There are day care centers that specialize in the care of older adults with dementia. These centers can provide socialization for the older adult and decreased levels of stress in the family member providing the informal care in the home (Zarit, Stephens, Townsend, & Greene, 1998). Lower levels of stress and higher levels of psychological well-being have been found in those caregivers who use a day care program regularly compared to those who do not (Zarit et al.). Day care centers have been promoted for increasing the length of time that a caregiver provides care in the community;

however, McCann et al. (2005) found that care recipients who attend day care more days per week were at higher risk of nursing home placement.

Concern regarding day care services for the working caregiver may be the hours of operation and the cost. Many day care programs are open limited hours during the workday, such as 9 a.m. to 3 p.m. weekdays, which requires many working caregivers to rearrange work hours, arrange transportation to and from the day care center, or obtain additional coverage for care during the workday for the care recipient. Day care may not provide respite for working caregivers because of the limited hours of operation of some centers. This can add stress for the working caregiver, while at the same time bringing peace of mind knowing that the care recipient is not alone and is socially stimulated. Day care centers may be able to assist the family caregiver in seeking sources for financial assistance to cover transportation and day care costs. Additional resources to relieve caregiver stress and provide respite may need to be explored with working caregivers.

There are respite services available in some communities that provide care to older adults with dementia for more extended periods of time than day care centers. This service would provide care for weekends or weeks, allowing caregivers longer periods of time without providing care, so that they may vacation or have time to pursue individual interests. Respite services may help a caregiver to decrease the social isolation that sometimes occurs when caring for a family member with dementia. Knowing that their family member is being cared for in a safe environment enables the caregiver time to pursue his or her own interests and to socialize, which might not be possible without respite services. Despite potential benefits to the caregiver, these support services have been underused by family caregivers (McCabe, Sand, Yeaworth, & Nieveen, 1995). Reasons for poor utilization include a lack of knowledge and education related to needs (McCabe et al.), guilt (Rosenheimer & Francis, 1992), and concern regarding care provided by respite and community service programs (Collins,

Stommel, King, & Given, 1991). An important role for the geropsychiatric nurse is to be able to inform the caregiver of services available in the community that may provide respite and support, and educate the caregiver related to individual needs and the quality of services available. Exploring the services offered though places of worship, hospitals, nursing homes, and community service organizations, so that this information can be shared with caregivers, may help to empower caregivers to seek out services that will help them to fulfill the caregiving role and meet their own self-care needs. Helping caregivers to work through ambivalence about nursing home placement is also an important role. Hospice care for family members with end-stage dementia should also be explored with the caregiver (Kuhn, 2001). Hospice care can provide support to caregivers and palliative care to individuals with dementia in the final stages of life.

By providing assistance in the identification of available resources, the geropsychiatric nurse may be able to help prevent stress and burnout in family caregivers, which in turn may help to prevent institutionalization of the older adult with dementia. In addition to the resources listed previously, there is a wealth of information available online to assist family caregivers and to educate geropsychiatric nurses about issues related to family caregiving. Several additional resources available to the clinician may be found in the following list. Further reading about family caregiver concerns and issues will better prepare nurses to assume a more active role in advocating for the unmet needs of the family caregiver at the individual, community, state, and national level.

- Administration on Aging, *Elders and Families* (2009), www.aoa.gov/AoARoot/Elders_Families/index.aspx
- Centers for Disease Control and Prevention (CDC), *Caregiving: A Public Health Priority* (2009), www.cdc.gov/aging/caregiving/index.htm
- CDC and Kimberly-Clark Corporation, *Assuring Healthy Caregivers: A Public Health Approach to Translating Research into Practice: The RE-AIM Framework* (2008), www.cdc.gov/aging/pdf/caregiving_monograph.pdf
- Rosalynn Carter Institute for Caregiving, www.rosalynncarter.org

There is a need to provide emotional support to families providing care. Because assuming a new role of caregiver may be difficult for both parties involved, it is important for the nurse to be available for reinforcement and encouragement. Encouraging the family member with dementia to maintain independence for as long as possible is also an important role of the nurse (Ebersole, 2004). Establishing helping relationships and facilitating the grieving process for losses resulting from dementia require empathy, knowledge, skill, and the establishment of trust (Kuhn, 2001). The sharing of feelings related to the provision of care should be encouraged. Caregivers may need permission to discuss the losses associated with caregiving and should be provided with education about dementia and the grief process. They also may need help recognizing that grief is a normal response to losses experienced in the caregiving role.

Assisting caregivers to discuss needs with other family members and friends may help to mobilize support for the person assuming the primary responsibility for care. Places of worship often serve as sources of support for caregivers when they are aware of the need for support. Helping caregivers overcome the hesitancy to ask for help is an important role for nurses. Neighbors may also be a source of emotional support and provide a means for a caregiver to get respite. The use of all available resources and assistance should be encouraged.

The geropsychiatric nurse should allow caregivers the opportunity to verbalize anger toward the care recipient. Caregivers may feel anger, guilt, or helplessness because of personal losses resulting from caring for a family member with dementia. These feelings may be inappropriately directed toward the impaired family member. Feelings of anger may be conscious or unconscious but need to be addressed (Kuhn, 2001). The expression of negative feelings may assist the caregiver in diffusing anger and providing care in a more positive manner. It may also assist the nurse in identifying the need for resources that help to maintain the caregiving relationship. Because of the stress associated with caregiving and the multiple demands often experienced by caregivers, expressions of anger toward the care recipient may be an early indicator of the potential for abuse. Identifying unresolved anger and ineffective coping may be a first step in the prevention of an abusive caregiving relationship.

CASE STUDY

Louise was a 55-year-old married woman with two teenage daughters who had an active career and frequently worked from her home for long hours beyond the normal working day. Her mother with dementia had been cared for by her husband in the home they had owned for 40 years. When Louise's father died suddenly and unexpectedly, Louise stayed with her mother, who could not be left alone, in her parent's home for several days and then decided to move her mother into her own home. Soon after the move, Louise found that having her mother in her house was difficult because of her heavy work schedule and the inability to leave her mother alone, and because of behaviors associated with her dementia. The schedules of her husband and daughters were such that they were not home during the day. It was soon evident that the family dynamic in the house changed. Conversations between family members were difficult and Louise found herself hesitant to leave the house after work because of concern that she had left her mother too frequently during the week to tend to work responsibilities, and because she did not want to burden her husband and daughters with caregiving responsibilities. She discontinued attending church services because her mother was unwilling to attend, and withdrew from weekly quilting evenings she had with friends for many years. The dinners in restaurants she had enjoyed weekly with her husband also were discontinued. Conversations at the dinner table became difficult. Working at home was also difficult because of interruptions and concern that her mother had too little stimulation when she worked. Louise struggled with feelings of guilt and feeling sad and inadequate on a daily basis. When she spoke to her primary care provider about her daily episodes of crying and her heightened stress level, her provider told her to "Let me know if you start feeling worse." Louise later did enroll her mother in a day care program, but because the limited hours of operation (9 a.m. to 3 p.m.) did not cover the full workday, the day care did not alleviate Louise's stress or relieve stress associated with caregiving during the evening or weekend hours.

What intervention by a nurse during the transition phase immediately after Louise's father's death may have better prepared her and her family for the sudden responsibility of caring for her mother? What interventions or services may better help Louise to cope with the life change associated with caring for her mother? In contrast to the response by her primary care provider, how might a geropsychiatric nurse respond to the concerns expressed by Louise about her increased stress level?

SUMMARY

Nurses with knowledge and skills in geropsychiatric nursing can play a major role in the assessment and support of family caregivers of functionally impaired older adults in the home. The negative psychological effects of caregiving, which may include stress, burden, and grief reactions, can be adequately assessed by the geropsychiatric nurse, and appropriate interventions may be implemented effectively. Nursing intervention strategies, including counseling, emotional support, and mobilizing resources within the community, may help to promote well-being and a positive caregiving relationship for both the caregiver and functionally impaired family member. Nurses knowledgeable about the concerns and issues facing family caregivers today are needed to assume an advocacy role for family caregivers at the individual, community, state, and national level.

REFERENCES

AARP. (2009). *Caregiving in the U.S.* Retrieved January 25, 2010, from www.aarp.org/research/surveys/care/ltc/hc/articles/caregiving_09.htm

AARP Public Policy Institute. (2007). Valuing the invaluable: A new look at the economic value of family caregiving. Retrieved October 19, 2009, from http://assets.aarp.org/rgcenter/il/ib82_caregiving.pdf

Acton, G. (2002). Health-promoting self-care in family caregivers. *Western Journal of Nursing Research, 24*(1), 73–86.

Adams, K. (2006). The transition to caregiving: The experience of family members embarking on the dementia caregiving career. *Journal of Gerontological Social Work, 47*(3/4), 3–29.

Adams, K., McClendon, M., & Smyth, K. (2008). Personal losses and relationship quality in dementia caregiving. *Dementia, 7,* 301–319.

Alzheimer's Association. (2007). *Alzheimer's Association report: 2007 Alzheimer's disease facts and figures.* Retrieved January 3, 2010, from http://www.alz.org/national/documents/PR_FFfactsheet.pdf

Alzheimer's Association. (2009). Alzheimer's disease: Facts and figures: Executive summary. Retrieved January 3, 2010, from http://www.alz.org/national/documents/summary_alzfactsfigures2009.pdf

Amirkhanyan, A. A., & Wolf, D. A. (2003). Caregiver stress and noncaregiver stress: Exploring the pathways of psychiatric morbidity. *The Gerontologist, 43*(6), 817–827.

Andren, S., & Elmstahl, S. (2008). The relationship between caregiver burden, caregivers' perceived health and their sense of coherence in caring for elders with dementia. *Journal of Clinical Nursing, 17,* 790–799.

Bergman-Evans, B. (1994). Alzheimer's and related disorders: Loneliness, depression, and social support of spousal caregivers. *Journal of Gerontological Nursing, 20*(3), 6–16.

Berg-Weger, M., Rubio, D., & Tebb, S. (2001). The Caregiver Well-Being Scale revisited. *Health and Social Work, 25*(4), 255–263.

Berg-Weger, M., & Tebb, S. (1998). Caregiver well-being: A strengths-based case management approach. *Journal of Case Management, 7*(2), 67–73.

Bookwala, J. (2009). The impact of parent care on marital quality and well-being in adult daughters and sons. *Journal of Gerontology: Psychological Sciences, 64B*(3), 339–347.

Brown, S., Smith, D., Schulz, R., Kabeto, M., Ubel, P., Poulin, M., et al. (2009). Caregiving behavior is associated with decreased mortality risk. *Psychological Science, 20*(4), 488–494.

Bumagin, V. E., & Hirn, K. F. (2001). *Caregiving: A guide to those who give care and those who receive it.* New York: Springer.

Burgio, L., Collins, I., Schmid, B., Wharton, T., McCullum, D., & De Coster, J. (2009). Translating the REACH caregiver intervention for use by Area Agency on Aging personnel: The REACH OUT program. *The Gerontologist, 14*(1), 103–116.

Burke, M., & Eakes, G. (1999). Milestones of chronic sorrow: Perspectives of chronically ill and bereaved. *Journal of Family Nursing, 5*(4), 374–388.

Burns, R., Nichols, L. O., Martindale-Adams, J., Graney, M. J., & Lummus, A. (2003). Primary care interventions for dementia caregivers: 2–year outcomes from the REACH study. *The Gerontologist, 43*(4), 547–555.

Burton, L., Newsom, J., Schulz, R., Hirsch, C., & German, P. (1997). Preventive health behaviors among spousal caregivers. *Preventive Medicine, 26,* 162–169.

Cancian, F., & Oliker, S. (2000). *Caring and gender.* Thousand Oaks, CA: Pine Forge Press.

Carruth, A., Tate, U., Moffett, B., & Hill, K. (1997). Reciprocity, emotional well-being, and family functioning as determinants of family satisfaction in caregivers of elderly parents. *Nursing Research, 46*(2), 93–100.

Cho, S., Zarit, S., & Chiriboga, D. (2009). Wives and daughters: The differential role of day care use in the nursing home placement of cognitively impaired family members. *The Gerontologist, 49*(1), 57–67.

Clay, O., Roth, D., Wadley, V., & Haley, W. (2008). Changes in social support and their impact on psychosocial outcome over a 5-year period for African American and white dementia caregivers. *International Journal of Geriatric Psychiatry, 23,* 857–862.

Clyburn, L. D., Stones, M. J., Hadjistavropoulos, T., & Tuokko, H. (2000). Predicting caregiver burden and depression in Alzheimer's disease. *Journal of Gerontology: Social Sciences, 55B*(1), S2–S13.

Cohen, C., Colantonio, A., & Vernich, L. (2002). Positive aspects of caregiving: Rounding out the caregiving experience. *International Journal of Geriatric Psychiatry, 17*(2), 184–188.

Collins, C., Stommel, M., King, S., & Given, C. W. (1991). Assessment of the attitudes of family caregivers toward community services. *The Gerontologist, 31*(6), 756–761.

Cooper, C., Katona, C., Orrell, M., & Livingston, G. (2008). Coping strategies, anxiety and depression in caregivers of people with Alzheimer's disease. *International Journal of Geriatric Psychiatry, 23,* 929–936.

Ebersole, P. (2004). Relationships roles and transitions. In P. Ebersole, P. Hess, & A. S. Luggen (Eds.), *Toward healthy aging: Human needs and nursing response* (pp. 490–517). St. Louis, MO: Mosby.

Eisdorfer, C., Czaja, S. J., Loewenstein, D. A., Rubert, M. P., Argüelles, S., Mitrani, V. B., et al. (2003). The effect of family therapy and technology-based intervention on caregiver depression. *The Gerontologist, 43*(4), 521–531.

Etters, L., Goodall, D., & Harrison, B. (2008). Caregiver burden among dementia patient caregivers: A review of the literature. *Journal of the American Academy of Nurse Practitioners, 20,* 423–428.

Farran, C. J. (2001). Family caregiver intervention research: Where have we been? Where are we going? *Journal of Gerontological Nursing, 27*(7), 38–45.

Fingerman, K., Pitzer, L., Lefkowitz, E., Birditt, K., & Mroczek, D. (2008). Ambivalent relationship qualities between adults and their parents: Implications for well-being of both parties. *Journal of Gerontology: Social Science, 63B*(6), P362–P371.

Gallant, M. P., & Connell, C. M. (1997). Predictors of decreased self-care among spouse caregivers of older adults with dementing illnesses. *Journal of Aging and Health, 9*(3), 373–395.

Gant, J., Steffen, A., & Lauderdale, S. (2007). Comparative outcomes of two distance-based interventions for male caregivers of family members with dementia. *Journal of Alzheimer's Disease and other Dementias, 22*(2), 120–128.

Gaugler, J. E., Leitsch, S. A., Zarit, S. H., & Pearlin, L. I. (2000). Caregiver involvement following institutionalization: Effects of preplacement stress. *Research on Aging, 22*(4), 337–359.

Gilliam, C., & Steffen, A. (2006). The relationship between caregiving self-efficacy and depressive symptoms in dementia family caregivers. *Aging & Mental Health, 10*(2), 79–86.

Gitlin, L. N., Winter, L., Corcoran, M., Dennis, M. P., Schinfeld, S., & Hauck, W. W. (2003). Effects of the home environmental skill-building program on the caregiver-care-recipient dyad: 6–month outcomes from the Philadelphia REACH initiative. *The Gerontologist, 43*(4), 532–546.

Glueckauf, R., Sharma, D., Davis, W., Byrd, V., Stine, C., Jeffers, S., et al. (2007). Telephone-based cognitive-behavioral interventions for distressed rural dementia caregivers: Initial findings. *Clinical Gerontologist, 31*(1), 21–41.

Hasselkus, B., & Murray, B. (2007). Everyday occupation, well-being, and identity: The experience of caregivers in families with dementia. *The American Journal of Occupational Therapy, 61,* 9–20.

Hinton, L., Haan, M., Geller, S., & Mungas, D. (2003). Neuropsychiatric symptoms in Latino elders with dementia or cognitive impairment without dementia and factors that modify their association with caregiver depression. *The Gerontologist, 43*(5), 669–677.

Holley, C., & Mast, B. (2009). The impact of anticipatory grief on caregiver burden in dementia caregivers. *The Gerontologist, 49*(3), 388–396.

Hooyman, N., & Kiyak, H. A. (2002). *Social gerontology: A multidisciplinary approach.* Boston: Allyn & Bacon.

Houde, S. (2002). Methodological issues in male caregiver research: An integrative review of the literature. *Journal of Advanced Nursing, 40*(6), 626–640.

Johnson, R., & Lo Sasso, A. (2006). The impact of elder care on women's labor supply. *Inquiry, 43,* 195–210.

Kaye, L. (1997). Informal caregiving by older men. In J. Kosberg & L. Kaye (Eds.), *Elderly men: Special problems and professional challenges* (pp. 231–249). New York: Springer.

Kim, Y., & Schulz, R. (2008). Family caregivers' strains: Comparative analysis of cancer caregiving with dementia, diabetes, and frail elderly caregiving. *Journal of Aging and Health, 20,* 483–503.

King, A., & Brassington, G. (1997). Enhancing physical and psychological functioning in older family caregivers: The role of regular physical activity. *Annals of Behavioral Medicine, 16*(2), 91–100.

Knight, B., Longmire, C., Kim, J., & David, S. (2007). Mental health and physical health of family caregivers for persons with dementia: A comparison of African American and white caregivers. *Aging & Mental Health, 11*(5), 538–546.

Knussen, C., Tolson, D., Brogan, C., Swan, I., Stott, D., & Sullivan, F. (2008). Family caregivers of older relatives: Ways of coping and change in distress. *Psychology, Health, and Medicine, 13*(3), 274–290.

Kosberg, J., Kaufman, A., Burgio, L., Leeper, J., & Sun, F. (2007). Family caregiving to those with dementia in rural Alabama: Racial similarities and differences. *Journal of Aging and Health, 19*(3), 3–21.

Kuhn, D. (2001). Living with loss in Alzheimer's Disease. *Alzheimer's Care Quarterly, 2*(1), 12–22.

Lee, C. (2009). A comparison of health promotion behaviors in rural and urban community-dwelling spousal caregivers. *Journal of Gerontological Nursing, 35*(5), 34–40.

Lüscher, K., & Pillemer, K. (1998). Intergenerational ambivalence: A new approach to the study of parent-child relations in later life. *Journal of Marriage and the Family, 60,* 413–425.

Maio, G., Fincham, F., Regalia, C., & Paleari, F. (2004). Ambivalence and attachment in family relationships. In K. Pillemer & K. Lüscher (Eds.), *Intergenerational ambivalences: New perspectives on parent-child relations in later life* (pp. 285–312). Amsterdam, NY: Elsevier/JAI Press.

Martire, L. M., Parris Stephens, M. A., & Atienza, A. A. (1997). The interplay of work and caregiving: Relationships between role satisfaction, role involvement, and caregivers' well-being. *Journal of Gerontology: Social Sciences, 52B,* S279–S289.

Marwit, S. J., & Meuser, T. M. (2002). Development and initial validation of an inventory to assess grief in caregivers of persons with Alzheimer's disease. *The Gerontologist, 42*(6), 751–765.

Marwit, S. J., & Meuser, T. M. (2005). Development of a short form inventory to assess grief in caregivers of dementia patients. *Death Studies, 29,* 191–205.

Matthews, J., Dunbar-Jacob, J., Sereika, S., Schulz, R., & McDowell, B. (2004). Preventive health practices: Comparison of family caregivers 50 and older. *Journal of Gerontological Nursing, 30*(2), 46–54.

McCabe, B. W., Sand, B. J., Yeaworth, R. C., & Nieveen, J. L. (1995). Availability and utilization of services by Alzheimer's disease caregivers. *Journal of Gerontological Nursing, 21*(1), 14–22.

McCann, J., Hebert, L., Li, Y., Wolinsky, F., Gilley, D., & Aggarwal, N. (2005). The effect of adult day care services on time to nursing home placement in older adults with Alzheimer's disease. *The Gerontologist, 45*(6), 754–763.

Melillo, K. D., & Futrell, M. (1995). A guide for assessing caregiver needs: Determining a health history database for family caregivers. *Nurse Practitioner, 20*(5), 40–46.

MetLife Mature Market Institute & Life Plans Inc. (2006). *The MetLife study of Alzheimer's disease: The caregiving experience.* Westport, CT: MetLife Mature Market Institute.

Meuser, T. M., & Marwit, S. J. (2001). A comprehensive, stage-sensitive model of grief in dementia caregiving. *The Gerontologist, 41*(5), 658–670.

Mier, N. (2007). The caregiving experience among Hispanic caregivers of dementia patients. *Journal of Cultural Diversity, 14*(1), 12–18.

Mittelman, M. S., Roth, D. L., Haley, W. E., & Zarit, S. H. (2004). Effects of a caregiver intervention on negative caregiver appraisals of behavior problems in patients with Alzheimer's disease: Results of a randomized trial. *Journals of Gerontology: Psychological Sciences, 59B*(1), P27–P34.

Moyle, W., Edwards, H., & Clinton, M. (2002). Living with loss: Dementia and the family caregiver. *Australian Journal of Advanced Nursing, 19*(3), 25–31.

Mui, A. (1995). Caring for frail elderly parents: A comparison of adult sons and daughters. *The Gerontologist, 35*(1), 86–93.

National Academy on an Aging Society. (2000). *Helping the elderly with activity limitations: Caregiving, #7.* Washington, DC: Author.

National Alliance for Caregiving & AARP. (2004). *Caregiving in the U.S.* Retrieved January 3, 2010, from http://www.caregiving.org/data/04finalreport.pdf

Navaie-Waliser, M., Feldman, P., Gould, D., Levine, C., Kuerbis, A., & Donelan, K. (2002). When the caregiver needs care: The plight of vulnerable caregivers. *American Journal of Public Health, 92*(3), 409–413.

Neufeld, A., & Harrison, M. (2003). Unfulfilled expectations and negative interactions: Nonsupport in the relationships of women caregivers. *Journal of Advanced Nursing, 41*(4), 323–331.

Ory, M., Hoffman, R. R., Yee, J. L., Tennstedt, S., & Schulz, R. (1999). Prevalence and impact of caregiving: A detailed comparison between dementia and nondementia caregivers. *The Gerontologist, 39*(2), 177–185.

Ory, M., Yee, J., Tennstedt, S., & Schulz, R. (2000). The extent and impact of dementia care: Unique challenges experienced by family caregivers. In R. Schulz (Ed.), *Handbook on dementia caregiving* (pp. 1–32). New York: Springer.

Parker, D., Mills, S., & Abbey, J. (2008). Effectiveness of interventions that assist caregivers to support people with dementia living in the community: A systematic review. *International Journal of Evidence-Based Healthcare, 6*, 137–172.

Pillemer, K., & Suitor, J. (2008). Collective ambivalence: Considering new approaches to the complexity of intergenerational relations. *Journal of Gerontology: Social Sciences, 63B*(6), S394–S396.

Rabinowitz, Y., Mausbach, B., Thompson, L., & Gallagher-Thompson, D. (2007). The relationship between self-efficacy and cumulative health risk associated with health behavior patterns in female caregivers of elderly relatives with Alzheimer's dementia. *Journal of Aging and Health, 19*(6), 946–964.

Resnick, B., Shaughnessy, M., & Simpson, M. (2005). Sleep disorders of late life. In K. D. Melillo & S. Houde (Eds.), *Geropsychiatric and mental health nursing.* Sudbury, MA: Jones and Bartlett.

Robinson, B. (1983). Validation of a caregiver strain index. *Journal of Gerontology, 38,* 344–348.

Rosenheimer, L., & Francis, E. (1992). Feasible without subsidy? Overnight respite for Alzheimer's. *Journal of Gerontological Nursing, 18*(4), 21–29.

Rose-Rego, S., Strauss, M., & Smyth, K. (1998). Differences in the perceived well-being of wives and husbands caring for persons with Alzheimer's Disease. *Gerontologist, 38*(2), 224–230.

Rowe, M., McCrae, C., Campbell, J., Benito, A., & Cheng, I. (2008). Sleep pattern differences between older adult dementia caregivers and older adult noncaregivers using subjective and objective measures. *Journal of Clinical Sleep Medicine, 4*(4), 362–369.

Rubio, D. M., Berg-Weger, M., & Tebb, S. S. (1999). Assessing the validity and reliability of well-being and stress in family caregivers. *Social Work Research, 23*(1), 54–64.

Sanders, S., Ott, C., Kelber, S., & Noonan, P. (2008). The experience of high levels of grief in caregivers of persons with Alzheimer's disease and related dementia. *Death Studies, 32,* 495–523.

Scharlach, A., Kellam, R., Ong, N., Baskin, A., Goldstein, C., & Fox, P. (2006). Cultural attitudes and caregiver service use: Lessons from focus groups with racially and ethnically diverse family caregivers. *Journal of Gerontological Social Work, 47*(1/2), 133–156.

Schulz, R., Burgio, L., Burns, R., Eisdorfer, C., Gallagher-Thompson, D., Gitlin, L. N., et al. (2003). Resources for Enhancing Alzheimer's Caregiver Health (REACH): Overview, site-specific outcomes, and future directions. *The Gerontologist, 43*(4), 514–520.

Schulz, R., O'Brien, A. T., Bookwala, J., & Fleissner, K. (1995). Psychiatric and physical morbidity effects of dementia caregiving: Prevalence, correlates, and causes. *The Gerontologist, 35*(6), 771–791.

Seltzer, M., & Li, L. (2000). The dynamics of caregiving: Transitions during a three-year prospective study. *The Gerontologist, 40,* 165–178.

Son, J., Erno, A., Shea, D., Femia, E., Zarit, S., & Stephens, M. (2007). The caregiver stress process and health outcomes. *Journal of Aging and Health, 18,* 871–887.

Sugiura, K., Ito, M., Kutsumi, M., & Mikami, H. (2009). Gender differences in spousal caregiving in Japan. *Journal of Gerontology: Social Sciences, 64B*(1), 147–156.

Sullivan, M. (2008). Try this: The Modified Caregiver Strain Index (CSI). *AJN, 108*(9), 65–66.

Tebb, S. (1995). An aid to empowerment: A caregiver well-being scale. *Health and Social Work, 20*(2), 87–92.

Thornton, M., & Travis, S. S. (2003). Analysis of the reliability of the Modified Caregiver Strain Index. *Journal of Gerontology: Social Sciences, 58B*(2), S127–S132.

Vickrey, B., Strickland, T., Fitten, L., Adams, G., Ortiz, F., & Hays, R. (2007). Ethnic variations in dementia caregiving experiences: Insights from focus groups. *Journal of Human Behavior and Social Environment, 15*(2/3), 233–249.

Vitaliano, P., Zhang, J., Young, H., Caswell, L., Scanlan, J., & Echeverria, D. (2009). Depressed mood mediates decline in cognitive processing speed in caregivers. *The Gerontologist, 49*(1), 12–22.

Wallsten, S. S. (2000). Effects of caregiving, gender, and race on the health, mutuality, and social supports of older couples. *Journal of Aging and Health, 12*, 90–111.

White, T. M., Townsend, A. L., & Stephens, M. A. P. (2000). Comparison of African American and white women in the parent care role. *Gerontologist, 40*(6), 718–728.

Yates, M., Tennstedt, S., & Chang, B. (1999). Contributors to and mediators of psychological well-being for informal caregivers. *Journals of Gerontology: Psychological Sciences and Social Sciences, 54B*(1), P12–P22.

Yee, J., & Schulz, R. (2000). Gender differences in psychiatric morbidity among family caregivers: A review and analysis. *Gerontologist, 40*(2), 147–164.

Zarit, S. H., Stephens, M. A. P., Townsend, A., & Greene, R. (1998). Stress reduction for family caregivers: Effect of adult day care use. *Journals of Gerontology: Psychological Sciences and Social Sciences, 53B*, S267–S277.

Zarit, S. H., & Zarit, J. M. (1998). *Mental disorders in older adults: Fundamentals of assessment and treatment.* New York: Guilford Press.

16

Normal and Disordered Sleep in Late Life

Geoffry Phillips McEnany

Approximately one out of three adults experiences difficulty with sleep and nearly half of older adults report at least transient sleep difficulties. According to the National Sleep Foundation's *Sleep in America* poll (NSF, 2003), 44% of older persons experience one or more of the nighttime symptoms of insomnia at least a few nights per week. In a longitudinal study conducted by Byles and colleagues (2005) on the experience of insomnia in older women, most of the women with sleep problems (72%) spoke with a healthcare provider about the difficulty. Of the 72% of poor sleepers in that sample, 54% used sleeping medications to deal with the problem. Insomnia may be chronic (lasting over 1 month) or acute (lasting a few days or weeks) and is often related to an underlying cause, such as a medical or psychiatric condition. This research demonstrates how insomnia may be worse among older women compared to their male counterparts.

An increase in sleep-related drug sales also points to increasing struggles with insomnia in the United States. According to data from IMS Health, a healthcare information company, 56,287,000 prescriptions were dispensed in 2008 for sleep medications (Marcus, 2009). A study from Balkrishnan and colleagues using data from the National Ambulatory

Medical Care Survey from 1996 to 2001 (2005) provided some revealing and informative data. The study found that approximately 4.8 billion visits were made to physician offices in the United States and 94.6 million of these visits involved sleep-related complaints. Medications for sleep were prescribed for patients in 48% of the visits, totaling 45 million clinical contacts resulting in the prescription of sleep medications. Patients included in the data set sought help for sleep-related difficulties in outpatient physician offices. Elderly people, 65 and older, with private health insurance were more likely to receive benzodiazepines for insomnia, probably pointing to the vulnerability for insomnia in this cohort.

Lack of sleep can have a significant impact on quality of life. Insufficient and inefficient sleep can exacerbate underlying illness; alter both mood and behavior, particularly in those with cognitive impairment; and result in accidents (i.e., driving, falls, or household accidents). Unfortunately, sleep patterns in older adults are often ignored, especially when there are other acute or chronic illnesses being addressed during a typical office visit. To help older adults obtain and maintain optimal health, sleep and sleep patterns should be evaluated and aggressively managed.

PHYSIOLOGY OF SLEEP

Sleep and wakefulness are the products of a complex interplay of factors between the environment and the body's timing system. The underlying science of the body's timing system is referred to as "chronobiology" and is enacted in the observable behaviors associated with sleep and wakefulness. The commonly accepted theory of sleep–wake regulation is found in the Two Process Model of sleep and wakefulness, in which the two identified elements referred to are "homeostatic" and "circadian" processes. This model was developed and introduced by Borbely (1982) to facilitate an understanding of the processes involved in regulation of sleep and wakefulness.

The homeostatic process is driven by sleep debt and represents an underlying physiological need state. The further a person gets from his or her last sleep period, the sleepier he or she becomes, not dissimilar from hunger or thirst. According to the Two Process Model, after an adequate period of sleep, sleep debt is low because the need for sleep has been satisfied during the period of sleep. As the person remains awake, sleep debt builds and increases over the period of wakefulness. Sleep debt is identified in the experience of sleepiness. Fatigue is conceptually different than sleepiness, and this is an important distinction to make in clinical practice. Sleepiness is commonly defined as heaviness in the eyelid with difficulty keeping the eyes open to remain awake. Fatigue is a body symptom and is commonly seen in the experience of lethargy, low energy, and anergia. Sleepiness can happen in the absence of fatigue and vice versa.

The second dimension of the Two Process Model is circadian and refers to the role of circadian rhythms in the experience of sleep and wakefulness. All functions in the human body function rhythmically, whether they are cardiac, endocrine, respiratory, or other rhythms. All rhythms function synchronously, meaning that the peaks and nadirs of various biological rhythms occur in sequences that allow for the various functions of the body to occur in an adaptive fashion. The seat of the body's timing system is believed to be

located in the hypothalamus, and what is believed to be the main clock is referred to as the "suprachiasmatic nucleus" (SCN). The SCN is heavily influenced by the environment, particularly the presence of light, the most powerful influence on the functioning of the main body clock. Light is referred to as a "potent entrainer" of the circadian timing system, meaning that light triggers the enactment of rhythms related to wakefulness. Similarly, darkness activates the release of melatonin from the pineal gland, a small pine cone-shaped organ located near the center of the brain. Once melatonin is released by dim light, the melatonin quells the activating functions in the SCN and facilitates the onset of sleep. The response of the SCN is mediated by genetics and the expression of these clock-related genes (Piggins, 2002).

What happens to people who are blind, those who do not have the capacity to receive light? The seminal work done by Sack and colleagues (2000) provided evidence that melatonin rhythms in those who are totally blind are significantly altered in the absence of the daily benchmark provided to the circadian system with light. Consequently, the sleep of those with total blindness is often disturbed, characterized by difficulty with falling asleep at the desired time during the 24-hour day. In this placebo-controlled trial, Sack and colleagues (2000) demonstrated that a physiological "night" can be created in persons with total blindness by giving evening melatonin over a period of 3 weeks. This intervention seemed to have entrained the circadian system with melatonin rather than light and the consequence was a stable sleep period during the desired (night) sleep time.

The SCN regulates a complex series of rhythms, including sleep and wakefulness. Hormones and neurotransmitters control circadian oscillation and regulate timing of sleep, in conjunction with external cues (the light–dark cycle). The light–dark cycle is the primary synchronizer of endogenous circadian rhythms, and as such light acts as a benchmark of the circadian timing system. Light helps to maintain the alignment between the environmental day–night cycles with body rhythms. Anyone who has had jet lag or has had difficulty with getting restorative sleep during a period of nightshift work understands the experience of a desynchronization between the environmental day–night cycles and the internal workings of the body clocks. Body temperature fluctuations, and the release of cortisol and growth hormone, are also associated with the sleep–wake cycle. Melatonin, the hormone of darkness, is produced by the pineal gland and inhibits the major neurotransmitters associated with arousal: histamine, norepinephrine, dopamine, and serotonin in the presence of darkness. Most adults in nontropical areas are comfortable with 6.5 to 8 hours of sleep daily, taken in a single period (Vgontzas & Kales, 1999).

Combined, the homeostatic and circadian processes are responsible for the enactment of sleep and wakefulness. Sleep initiation relies heavily on sleepiness, reflected in a high homeostatic drive (sleep debt), whereas sleep maintenance relies on a low circadian drive. The model is depicted in Figure 16-1. Understanding the Two Process Model helps the advanced practice nurse to appreciate the influences involved in the regulation of sleep in elders. Clearly, the role of napping serves to reduce the homeostatic drive, creating potential difficulties with sleep. Other circadian influences can impact the quality of sleep maintenance (or staying asleep) or perhaps even more common among elders, the regulation of when the elder sleeps within the 24-hour circadian day. Examples of such shifts in when the person sleeps in a 24-hour period are seen in alterations in sleep patterning referred to as "phased-advanced" or "phase-delayed" sleep.

Phase-advanced sleep pattern refers to the enactment of the sleep period time occurring too early in the environmental day. In this circumstance, the shift in circadian rhythms for sleep occurs too early in the circadian day–night schedule. The observed behavior in the phase-advanced sleep pattern involves the person becoming sleepy earlier than the desired time, going to sleep earlier in the circadian day, and then awakening too

FIGURE 16-1

Differences in Rhythm Shape Between Morning and Evening Chronotypes.

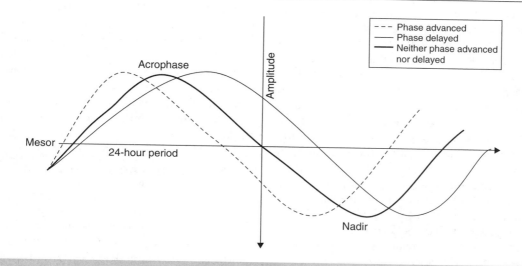

Source: Part 1: Rhythm and Blues Revisited: Biological Rhythm Disturbances in Depression. Geoffry McEnany. *Journal of the American Psychiatric Nurses Association,* 1996; 2; 15 DOI: 10.1177/107839039600200105. Published by Sage Publications on behalf of American Psychiatric Nurses Association.

early, possibly even during the very early morning hours (e.g., at 3 or 4 a.m.).

In the phase-delayed sleep pattern, the opposite is seen whereby the individual has difficulty getting to sleep and then has difficulty getting up in the morning at the desired time. Although this pattern is normal in adolescence, it may be seen in certain forms of psychiatric illness, such as bipolar disorder (Goodwin & Redfield, 2007). Figure 16-1 provides an example of circadian rhythm configuration across a 24-hour cycle, providing an example of phase-advanced and phase-delayed rhythm configurations.

Normal sleep consists of four to six behaviorally and electroencephalographically defined cycles (Vgontzas & Kales, 1999) (Box 16-1). Generally, adults pass through five phases of sleep: non–rapid eye movement (NREM) stages 1, 2, 3, and 4, and rapid eye movement (REM) sleep. NREM sleep begins with stage 1, the transitional period of drifting to sleep when one can be easily aroused. Stage 2 is light sleep, and stages 3 and 4 are progressively deeper and more restorative stages, when the pulse, respirations, and metabolism slow. NREM sleep could be characterized as an idling brain in an active body. For example, the person in NREM sleep may change positions in sleep. Dreaming is minimal in these NREM sleep stages.

REM sleep provides a sharp contrast to NREM sleep. REM sleep is characterized by active *electroencephalogram* (EEG) patterns and vital signs similar to that exhibited in a wakeful state, but with profound muscular relaxation (Hoffman, 2003). REM is the stage of sleep where most dream activity occurs, and large muscle paralysis and subsequent inactivity prevent the sleeping person from acting out dreams during this stage of sleep. In the absence of muscle paralysis, sleeping persons physically act out their dreams, usually harming their bed partners and often themselves. Such a pattern reflects a formal sleep disorder termed "REM sleep behavior disorder" (American Academy of Sleep Medicine, 1997).

The enactment of sleep stages across the night is referred to as "sleep architecture," which provides a map of the sequencing of sleep stages across the sleep period time. A number of influences can normatively or pathologically alter sleep architecture. One of the most influential normative sources of change in sleep architecture is aging. From a pathological perspective, there are many potential culprits including comorbid illnesses, medications, sleep deprivation, insomnia, and other formal sleep disorders as well as imposed conditions, such as shift work.

With aging, characteristic changes in sleep patterns occur. Overall, sleep tends to be less efficient with advanced age, although sleep requirements remain unchanged (generally 5–9 hours in most individuals). The first indices of sleep deterioration caused by aging actually occur between young adulthood (ages 16–25) and midlife (35–50) and are associated with a decline in growth hormone (Van Cauter, 2000). The second indication of sleep deterioration occurs after age 50, during the transition from midlife to late life. It includes decreased total sleep time, declining by about 27 minutes per decade; more frequent nocturnal awakening; a progressive decline in deeper stages of sleep (stages 3 and 4); more frequent and longer nighttime awakenings; and a significant reduction in REM sleep (Floyd, 2002). The loss of REM sleep seems to be associated with elevated evening levels of the stress-related hormone cortisol (Van Cauter). Further, older adults experience attenuation in a number of circadian rhythms including core body temperature and melatonin production. Consequently, these individuals tend to wake early in the morning when their body temperature is at the lowest point.

COMMON SLEEP DISTURBANCES IN OLDER ADULTS

Older adults may complain of sleep problems caused by underlying physiological or psychological issues, such as pain, anxiety, depression, shortness of breath, gastritis, or unrealistic sleep expectations (i.e., belief in the need to sleep for an undisrupted 8 hours). In addition, there are a

BOX 16-1 SLEEP CYCLES

Stage 1	Light sleep in which the individual drifts in and out of sleep and can be awakened easily
	Eyes move very slowly and muscle activity slows
	May experience sudden muscle contractions called hypnotic myoclonia, often preceded by a sensation of starting to fall
Stage 2	Eye movements stop and brain waves become slower, with occasional bursts of rapid waves called sleep spindles
Stage 3	Extremely slow brain waves called delta waves begin to appear, interspersed with smaller, faster waves
	Deep sleep, difficult to wake the individual
Stage 4	The brain produces delta waves almost exclusively
	Deep sleep, difficult to wake the individual
	No eye movement or muscle activity
	If awakened, the individual may feel groggy and disoriented for several minutes
Stage 5	Rapid eye movement (REM) sleep
	Breathing becomes more rapid, irregular, and shallow, eyes jerk rapidly in various directions, and the limb muscles become temporarily paralyzed
	Heart rate increases, blood pressure rises, and males develop penile erections
	If the individual awakens during REM sleep, he or she may recall dreams
	The first REM sleep period usually occurs about 70 to 90 minutes after falling asleep

number of specific sleep disorders that are known to present more frequently in older individuals.

Obstructive Sleep Apnea

The most common sleep-related problem is disturbed breathing, brought on by obstructive sleep apnea syndrome (OSAS). The development of OSAS seems to be age-dependent and male-dominant. The incidence is also higher in those individuals who are obese and have enlarged neck circumferences, although this is not always the case. Recent evidence suggests that diabetics may also be more likely to have this disorder (Marshall et al., 2008). Patients with sleep apnea snore very loudly and stop breathing for 10–30 seconds repeatedly through the night because of relaxation and collapse of the upper airway during REM sleep paralysis. The arterial desaturation stimulates surges in sympathetic activity, including increased heart rate and blood pressure, and muscle contraction of the chest, abdomen, and diaphragm. As those muscles are repeatedly and more forcefully stimulated, patients awaken and begin breathing again. Initially thought to be of significant consequence primarily to sleep-deprived partners, recent evidence suggests that patients with OSAS have significantly higher risk of medical comorbidity because of the sleep fragmentation and hypoxemia within the sleep period caused by the frequency and presence of the episodes of apnea.

Obesity, cardiovascular diseases, hypertension, metabolic dysfunction, and type 2 diabetes have been well documented with OSAS (Endeshaw, Bloom, & Bliwise, 2008; Lopez-Jimenez & Somers, 2006). More recently, data on the relationship between circadian regulation of sleep, melatonin, and breast cancer have raised significant concerns about the role of sleep dysregulation in the epigenesis of colon cancer as well (Blask, 2008). Of particular concern to nurses who work the nightshift, increased rates of breast cancer have been found compared to their dayshift-working counterparts (Straif, 2007). Initially, these findings were considered appreciable, although not definitive (Humm, 2005), but the perspective on the relationship between sleep and cancer is changing. In 2006, the International Agency for Research on Cancer, a dimension of the World Health Organization, made the determination that sleep-disrupting shift work is probably carcinogenic to humans, and as such added shift work to the list of level 2A carcinogens, akin to diesel exhaust and ultraviolet light (Humm, 2009; Straif). The implications of such findings for elders are not clear but point to some early work that speaks to the critical nature of sleep in disease regulation.

Treatment for Obstructive Sleep Apnea

Evaluation and treatment of OSAS should follow the evidence-based *Practice Parameters for the Medical Therapy of Obstructive Sleep Apnea* from the American Academy of Sleep Medicine (AASM) (Morganthaler, Kapen, et al., 2006). All patients with suspected OSAS should be evaluated at a sleep center to identify the cause and scope of problem. The treatment of choice for OSAS is a continuous positive airway pressure device. A small air compressor delivers pressurized air to the upper airway, forcing the airway to stay open by a face-fitting mask. Alternatives are dental devices (splint or mandibular advancement devices that move the jaw forward and are more effective in mild to moderate forms of obstructive sleep apnea) or surgical removal of soft tissues around the uvula and soft palate to enlarge the airway. This is rarely done, because most patients learn to tolerate a continuous positive airway pressure device (Dattilo & Drooger, 2004).

Restless Legs Syndrome

Approximately 9.8% of all older adults experience restless legs syndrome (RLS) (Rothdach, Trenkwalder, Haberstock, Keil, & Gerger, 2000), although this increases to 20% of those 80 years of age or older (Barthlen, 2002). Patients with RLS have uncomfortable sensations in the lower extremities, which they attempt to relieve by moving their legs during sleep, or rising and walking. These RLS-related sensations have been described as pulling or crawling and are only relieved with movement of the affected extremity, mainly between the knee and the foot. There are many possible causes of RLS in the adult population, although there is no definitive explanation. Strong associations with RLS include kidney failure, several nerve disorders, vitamin deficiencies, pregnancy, iron deficiency, and a number of medications. Antidepressants of the selective serotonin reuptake inhibitor class have been documented as a source of RLS (Ohayan & Roth, 2002). About 50% of those who have RLS have relatives with the same condition, leading to the perception that there may be a genetic predisposition to the disorder. It is more common in middle-aged or older adults. Patients with RLS experience delayed sleep or awakenings during the night. Almost 85–90% of patients with RLS also experience periodic limb movement disorder (PLMD) (National Center on Sleep Disorder Research, 2009).

Periodic Limb Movement Disorder

PLMD is characterized by episodes of repetitive limb movements caused by muscle contractions during sleep. Patients with PLMD kick or jerk their legs every 20–40 seconds, usually during NREM sleep stage 1 or 2. Those who have this problem may not awaken, or complain of any other symptoms besides daytime fatigue. The reason underlying the daytime fatigue is that with each episode of kicking, the person arouses out of sleep stage very briefly, often for only 1 or 2 seconds. These repeated arousals or small awakenings result in a reduction of sleep efficiency and the change in sleep efficiency is what is believed to be associated with daytime sleepiness and fatigue. Unfortunately, many cases go undetected if a sleep partner does not notice the leg movements.

Treatment of RLS and PLMD

Treatment for both RLS and PLMD should follow the evidence-based *Dopaminergic Treatment of Restless Legs Syndrome and Periodic Limb Movement Disorder* from the AASM (Henning, Allen, Earley, Piccietti, & Silber, 2004; Littner et al., 2004). The AASM practice parameters are based on evidence-based data stratified into levels I to V, with level I having the strongest evidence base for effectiveness and level V supporting the weakest evidence. These levels are determined in part by the quality of the studies supporting the evidence. For example, double-blind, placebo-controlled studies with larger samples produce the best evidence, with case studies demonstrating the weakest evidence, given the limitations of this type of research. The following recommendations from the AASM practice parameters (Henning et al.) suggest the use of the following medications in the treatment of RLS and PLMD: levodopa with decarboxylase inhibitor (Sinemet and others); dopamine agonists pramiprexole and pergolide (Mirapex and Permax, respectively); and dopamine agonist roprinole (Requip and others). Other dopamine agonists are used in the treatment of RLS and PLMD, such as talipexole and cabergoline, but the evidence does not support their routine use.

In the past, a number of medications were used to treat these conditions and drug classes included on the menu of options for treatment were opioids, such as codeine; benzodiazepines; and anticonvulsants (Minnick, 2003). Although these are still used in practice, the evidence base does not support their clinical applications in RLS or PLMD. Appropriate pharmacological treatment options for RLS or PLMD include the use of primary agents, such as dopamine precursors, dopamine-receptor agonists, opioids, benzodiazepines, and anticonvulsants (Minnick).

Insomnia

Insomnia is the single most common sleep complaint, occurs more frequently with increasing age, and has a preponderance for women (Paine, Gander, Harris, & Reid, 2004). Short-term insomnia may result from stressful life events, or with the recent onset of a medical disorder. Patients with mental health problems, such as depression or anxiety, may initially present with complaints of sleep disturbances best characterized by insomnia, such as difficulty with getting to sleep, with staying asleep, or with early morning awakening. Medical disorders are a very significant source of insomnia and as such need to be assessed routinely in the course of any patient evaluation. Sleep deprivation, possibly caused by insomnia or one of the other sleep disorders, is directly related to the increased vulnerability for weight gain, type 2 diabetes, hypertension, and the other medical comorbidities previously discussed. Those with underlying shortness of breath, paroxysmal nocturnal dyspnea, and gastroesophageal reflux disease are likely to suffer from insomnia because these medical problems are exacerbated with a recumbent posture and may interfere with falling asleep or staying asleep.

Treatment of Insomnia

Over the last decade, significant progress has been made in the area of evidence-based assessment and treatment of insomnia. The AASM has developed several evidence-based guidelines related to the assessment and treatment of insomnia since 1999 (Chessen, Anderson, et al., 1999). The current guideline, *Practice Parameters for the Psychological and Behavioral Treatment of Insomnia: An Update* (Morganthaler, Kramer, et al., 2006), provides the community standard related to the treatment of insomnia in its many manifestations.

ASSESSMENT OF SLEEP DISORDERS IN LATE LIFE

The initial approach that sleep specialists and researchers use to diagnose sleep disorders accurately includes a medical history, physical examination, and multiple questionnaires or sleep diaries, as listed next:

- Routine sleep patterns: normal bedtime and arising time
- Habits before bed (i.e., nighttime rituals and any food, drink, medications; use of alcohol or caffeine, amount and timing)
- Bedtime activities (i.e., activities once in the bed)
- Nocturnal awakenings
- Quality of sleep (subject can use 0–10 scale)
- Daytime sleepiness
- Daytime napping
- Environment at hour of sleep: light, noise, temperature
- Associated symptoms at hour of sleep: pain, anxiety, fear, shortness of breath

Lee and Ward (2005) provide an exceptionally well-organized and pragmatically focused approach to nursing assessment of sleep. In their publication, they have used the principles from the practice guidelines with a clear focus on concerns related to nursing assessment and sleep. This is a valuable resource for any advanced practice nurse working with elders because it provides clear guidelines as to the assessment of sleep and sleep dysregulation.

For older adults with cognitive impairment, or those in institutional settings, information should be obtained from families or other caregivers. When assessing a patient, it may be helpful to ask the patient if he or she specifically has any of the following problems: (1) not being able to fall asleep (sleep latency); (2) not being able to stay asleep (sleep efficiency); (3) early morning awakening; and (4) not feeling refreshed, or "waking up tired." A complete description of the history of the problem should follow. Insomnia can be a sleep disorder or a symptom of another health problem, and providers should pay careful attention to sleep complaints in the context of physical and emotional disorders. Patients with mental health problems, such as undiagnosed depression or anxiety, present with complaints of sleep disturbances, most commonly insomnia. Think of sleep dysregulation in many of the psychiatric disorders as being akin to chest pain in cardiac disease: it is a core dimension of the chronobiological dimension of the disease. However, given the nature of comorbid disease, obesity, and psychotropic medication–induced effects, assessment of sleep in those who have these illnesses is even more critical. Undiagnosed and untreated sleep dysregulation or sleep disorder only serve to perpetuate the course of the illness itself and worsen clinical outcome. Guidelines for taking a sleep history are as follows:

- Define the specific sleep problem
- Assess the onset and clinical course of the condition
- Evaluate 24-hour sleep–wakefulness patterns
- Question the bed partner
- Determine the presence of other sleep disorders
- Obtain a family history of sleep disorders

Diagnostic evaluations may include tests, such as the EEG, *electro-oculogram* (EOG), and *electro-myogram* (EMG), which are also used to measure sleep patterns. This type of testing requires significant involvement of the patient and would likely not be appropriate for the individual with cognitive impairment. An EEG records brain wave activity. Sensors placed on both sides of the temple are wired to a polygraph machine that displays brain activity. An EOG is a device that traces eye movements, which are particularly active during REM sleep. Muscle tension is measured using an EMG. Typical areas where EMG electrodes are placed are under the chin and on the legs.

A *polysomnogram* (PSG) is a comprehensive and noninvasive test that records vital signs and physiology during a night of sleep. The study includes results from the EEG, EMG, and EOG. It also measures respiratory airflow, blood oxygen saturation, pulse rate, heart rate, body position, and respiratory effort. The information is recorded and gathered throughout the night, and is used mainly to establish the underlying cause of the sleep disturbance.

The PSG is not appropriate for the evaluation of insomnia because often the self-report of the person parallels the findings on the PSG, namely longer sleep latency, middle of the night awakening, or early morning awakening. However, when other sleep disorders are suspected, such as RLS, PLMD, or OSAS, a PSG is clearly indicated and should be done. Although some insurers may require prior authorization for the PSG, generally there is no difficulty in securing the approval in light of a potential formal sleep disorder.

THERAPEUTIC NURSING INTERVENTIONS TO ADDRESS SLEEP DISORDERS

Before intervening in sleep dysregulation, it is important to know the practice guidelines that form the community standards related to sleep intervention. It is of great importance to follow the practice guidelines that have been developed by the AASM, which have been referenced here. These guidelines and the scope of the practice parameters can be reviewed at the AASM Web site (www.aasmnet.org).

A helpful model to understand sleep pattern disturbance among elders is referred to as the "Three P Model of Insomnia," developed by Spielman, Caruso, and Glovinsky (1987). This model helps the nurse to identify factors that are considered predisposing, precipitating, and perpetuating influences in insomnia. Predisposing factors refer to influences that may create a vulnerability to insomnia and include a history of being a light sleeper and a possible predisposition to anxiety or other conditions that lend themselves to insomnia. Precipitating factors include anything that could cause the onset of insomnia. These factors generally include acute stressors from any source, such as the death of a loved one, a new onset illness, a financial crisis, or other circumstances. Usually, the stressor leads to insomnia. In response, the affected individual attempts to compensate for the insomnia with behaviors that actually maintain the pattern of insomnia. Such behaviors include the use of alcohol as a sleep-inducer; use of long naps during the day to compensate for nighttime sleep disturbances; and remaining in bed for long periods of time at night when sleep is not happening, only to serve the function of becoming increasingly anxious about the inability to sleep. These factors together provide a sound foundation for understanding insomnia. It is not uncommon for nurses to assess elders who have had insomnia for long periods of time and have triggered the ongoing sleep disturbances with perpetuating behaviors.

Like any other intervention, treatment of sleep disturbance begins with a thorough evaluation. Having the patient complete a sleep diary for 1 to 2 weeks provides a very clear depiction of sleep–wake patterns and the quality of sleep hygiene practices. With these data, the nurse is able to formulate a plan to address the issues rationally and within an evidence-based framework. The National Sleep Foundation (www.sleepfoundation.org) and the public education arm of the AASM, Sleep Education (www.sleepeducation.org), provide excellent examples of sleep–wake diaries, sleep hygiene checklists, and resources for patients related to general sleep education.

Behavioral Interventions

The gold standard behavioral approach to insomnia is referred to as "cognitive–behavioral therapy for insomnia" (CBT-I). This multicomponent approach to insomnia addresses both behavioral patterning that perpetuates the insomnia, and patterns of perceiving and thinking about insomnia that may serve as perpetuating factors in the insomnia itself. The components of CBT-I are sleep hygiene, stimulus control, sleep restriction, CBT, and relaxation. The following information details the elements of CBT-I, beginning with behavioral interventions, followed by specific information related to cognitive strategies.

Sleep Hygiene

The bedroom environment is one of the most important factors that can influence or interfere with sleep. The environment should be quiet and dark with a comfortable temperature. Older adults should be instructed to use the bed only for sleep or sexual activity and avoid other activities, such as watching television, listening to the radio, or reading in bed. Bedtime snacks and eating before bed are a common nighttime ritual. Eating large meals in the evening before bedtime, however, can interfere with sleep onset. Food stimulates gastric acid production and lying down after a large meal can result in symptoms associated with gastric reflux. Instruct patients to eat evening meals at least 3 hours before bedtime and eat only a light snack before bed if they are hungry. Other dimensions of sleep hygiene include the avoidance of alcohol in the evening, avoiding exercise within several hours of bedtime, and abstaining from napping during the day.

Stimulus Control

The purpose of stimulus control is to maintain association of the bedroom with bed and sleep. With insomnia, it is not uncommon for persons dealing with this condition to find themselves tossing and turning across many nights and the association between bed and sound sleep and restoration is lost. Similarly, behaviors that are common to poor sleep hygiene contribute to this disconnect between bed and sleep. Stimulus

control addresses these patterns with recommendations to use the bedroom for sleep and sexual activity and to go to bed when sleepy.

Sleep Restriction

Commonly, those experiencing sleep-related disturbances, such as insomnia, remain in bed through the sleepless period. The consequence of this pattern is the erosion of the association between sleep and the bed and the enhancement of anxiety related to periods of sleeplessness with resulting reduction in the efficiency of sleep in general. Sleep restriction is used to restore sleep quality and to reinforce the relationship of sleep with the bedroom. The formulation of a sleep restriction plan is based on a sleep–wake diary, and if the clinician is unfamiliar with the intervention, it is best to seek consultation or clear instruction (Perlis, Smith, & Jungquist, 2005; Edinger & Carney, 2008).

The goal of sleep restriction is to ensure sleep for the period of time that the individual is in bed. If the person is in bed for 9 hours and only sleeping for 6 of those hours, then sleep restriction reduces the time in bed to the number of hours the person is actually sleeping. For many, this may seem counterintuitive as a treatment for insomnia, but referring to the Two Process Model of sleep regulation, this intervention aims to enhance the homeostatic drive, thus restoring sleep consolidation.

Sleep restriction requires the full participation of the person seeking treatment for the sleep disturbance. It requires commitment and dedication of the patient because it requires a manipulation of bedtime and wake time. Going back to the example of the person in bed for 9 hours and sleeping only 6, a regular bedtime and wake time are established that allow only for the person to be in bed for 6 hours. If the person's regular wake time is 7 a.m., then the bedtime for this person would be determined as 1 a.m., allowing for the 6 hours during which the person actually sleeps. Napping during the day is not allowed. These features combine enhanced sleep pressure, and although it may initially yield daytime sleepiness, sleep is forced into the allotted time for sleep. Once the person is sleeping soundly during the allotted time, the sleep period time is increased in 15-minute increments, providing that the person's sleep quality remains stable. Sleep should never be restricted to less than 5 hours, and this intervention should be used for insomnia alone. It is critical that other possible sources of sleep pattern disturbances be ruled out before applying this intervention. For example, if the source of the sleep disturbance is RLS, pain, gastric reflux, or other conditions, these must be treated first to ensure success of the behavioral sleep measures.

Cognitive–Behavioral Therapy for Insomnia

CBT is used to clarify the misconceptions about sleep and sleep disorders and change behaviors that interfere with the onset, duration, and quality of sleep. In addition to counseling and providing information about sleep and sleep disorders, educating patients about establishing a routine sleep and wake schedule and avoiding sleep-incompatible behaviors in the bed or bedroom, such as watching television in bed, can enhance sleep quality (Edinger, Wohlgemuth, Radtke, Mahr, & Quillian, 2001). These behavioral approaches are also referred to as good sleep hygiene techniques and are described in Box 16-2.

Perlis and colleagues (2005) and Edinger and Carney (2008) have led efforts internationally to educate health professionals on the appropriate assessment and intervention with cognitive behavioral approaches to insomnia. These books provide exceptional resources for clinicians to guide specific assessment and intervention with insomnia from a cognitive–behavioral perspective.

BOX 16-2 LIFESTYLE MODIFICATIONS AND SLEEP HYGIENE TO FACILITATE SLEEP

- Go to bed and get up at the same time every day.
- Avoid naps longer than about 20 minutes.
- Avoid caffeinated drinks after lunch.
- Remove the television and radio from the bedroom.
- Avoid alcohol in the evening.
- Avoid heavy meals within 3 hours of going to bed; have a light snack if hungry at this time.
- Do not lie in bed for a long time trying to go to sleep; after 30 minutes of trying to sleep, get up and do something quiet for a while, like reading or listening to quiet music, and then try again to fall asleep in bed (no radio, television, or reading).
- Keep room temperature sufficiently warm.
- Relieve pain using medication or positioning.
- Exercise every day for at least 20–30 minutes but avoid aerobic activity within 4 hours of going to bed.
- Use relaxation techniques, such as massage, aromatherapy, or deep breathing.
- Use light therapy, which involves sitting in front of a light box that emits a bright fluorescent light (usually 10,000 lux) for up to 2 hours a day (this intervention should be done in conjunction with a knowledgeable clinician).
- Try progressive muscle relaxation: patient tenses and relaxes various muscle groups.

Elders with sleep pattern disturbances require thorough assessment and intervention as outlined in the practice guidelines. The sleep of this cohort is complicated by several variables known to create disturbances in sleep: medical and psychiatric comorbidity, social isolation, financial and other stressors, and medications. Probably one of the greatest sources of sleep disturbance in elders is anxiety, often focused on sleep itself. If an elder expects to sleep in the same way that he or she did 10 years ago, given what is known about sleep pattern changes across the lifespan, then expectation will not meet experience in sleep. The best predictor of a bad night's sleep is anticipation of a bad night's sleep, and this very fact is often what drives insomnia in elders. Consequently, intervention strategies need to address the various causes of sleep disturbance, including anxiety. Perlis and colleagues (2005) and Edinger and Carney (2008) outline the dimensions of this intervention in a step-by-step process. If a referral is needed for this dimension of CBT-I, the nurse can check the AASM Web site (www.aasmnet.org) for available clinicians who are certified in behavioral sleep medicine.

Relaxation Techniques

Sleep induction depends on both the presence of sleepiness and a relaxed state. A prebedtime ritual of relaxation is helpful with sleep induction and should include activities that are nonstimulating. Minor daily stressors can have an impact on presleep arousal and subsequently reduce sleep onset, duration, and quality (Morin, Rodrigue, & Ivers, 2003). Relaxation techniques, such as progressive muscle relaxation and guided imagery, improve sleep quality by reducing presleep arousal (Richardson, 2003). With progressive muscle relaxation, patients are instructed to tense and then relax major muscle groups starting with the head and neck and working their way down to their feet (Cochran, 2003). Other methods include relaxing in a warm bath or shower or meditating before bedtime. Although the dimensions of CBT-I have been discussed, the other variables that impact sleep are outlined next.

Other Behavioral Influences on Sleep and Wakefulness: Complementary Therapies

Exercise

Inadequate levels of physical activity put older adults at significant risk for acute and chronic insomnia (Morgan, 2003). Regular exercise that includes aerobic activity, strength training, and stretching can improve sleep-onset latency, total sleep duration, and global sleep quality (Montgomery & Dennis, 2003). Regular exercise can also improve physiological factors that interfere with sleep onset, duration, and quality, such as chronic back pain (Van Tulder, Malmivaara, Esmall, & Koes, 2003) or depression (Penninx et al., 2002). To improve sleep, older adults should engage in 30–40 minutes of moderate-intensity endurance, resistance, and stretching activities at least 4 days a week, preferably in the morning and certainly 3–4 hours away from bedtime, although for many elders lack of exercise presents a greater risk factor for insomnia in this cohort (Ohayon & Vecchierini, 2005). Exercise programs, such as those provided by the National Institute on Aging (2001), provide older adults with a comprehensive program that is easy to follow. For more information, visit the Web site (http://www.nia.nih.gov/HealthInformation/Publications/ExerciseGuide/).

Light Therapy

In the assessment of the sleep of elders, it is not uncommon to observe patterns of sleeping characterized by going to bed too early and awakening too early. This pattern is referred to as a "phase-advanced sleep pattern," meaning that the circadian rhythms directing sleep and wake are occurring at an earlier than desired time. Alternatively, some elders may have a pattern of going to bed at a later time and awakening far later than the desired time. This is referred to as a "phase-delayed sleep pattern," implicating the occurrence of circadian rhythms at a later time than desired in the environmental day or night. In both of these cases, light therapy may be indicated to realign the body's clocks with the environmental time.

Light therapy to improve sleep onset and quality involves having the patient sit in front of a light device (light box, light therapy visor, or other forms of light therapy delivery systems). All of these devices emit bright fluorescent light (usually 10,000 lux or its equivalent), and the exposure is approximately 30–45 minutes (Bjorvatn & Pallesen, 2009). Application of light in the morning creates a phase advance of the circadian system and is used to treat such conditions as phase-delayed sleep–wake patterns. Light application in the morning reverses sleep patterns characterized by having difficulty getting to sleep at the desired bedtime with subsequent difficulty getting up in the morning at the desired time. The opposite is true for phase-advanced sleep patterns. Those who go to sleep too early in the evening, and who get up too early in the morning (sometimes in the middle of the night), benefit from bright light in the evening. Application of bright light in the evening phase delays the body's timing system and is used to treat phase-advanced sleep patterns. Phase-advanced sleep patterns are common among elders because of normative shifts in the body's timing system. Use of light therapy needs to be clearly understood before the clinician prescribes it as an intervention strategy. Light is the strongest zeitgeber (timekeeper) of the body's timing system and its application either naturally or artificially with light therapy equipment represents a powerful biologically active intervention. Light therapy has been successfully used for a number of conditions including jet lag, shift work sleep disorder, seasonal affective disorder, and other forms of depression. Among elders, it has been used to regulate sleep–wake cycles by exposure to artificial bright light in such settings as nursing homes and other care facilities (Thorpe, Middleton, Russell, & Stewart, 2000).

Light is measured in lux, and the standard for light therapy is 10,000 lux. The essential point here is that the lux intensity is proportional to the distance the light source is placed from the eyes. The effectiveness of light is dependent on the number of photons actually received at the retina. For example, if a light box with a capacity to deliver 10,000 lux at 24 inches from the eyes is moved back to 48 inches from the eyes, the lux intensity is divided by half. The effectiveness of light therapy is believed to be dependent on the intensity of the light and the duration of exposure. Commonly, 10,000 lux for 30–60 minutes is recommended in the morning for seasonal depression. In keeping with this use of a light therapy device, if the desired lux exposure is generally 10,000 lux for 30–60 minutes, but the person is unable to tolerate the intensity of the light, then it is acceptable to move the light source to 48 inches away from the person's eyes but double the exposure time. For elders, the *Practice Parameters for the Use of Light Therapy in the Treatment of Sleep Disorders* (Chesson, Littner, et al., 1999) offers evidence-based support for the use of light therapy in phase-advanced and phase-delayed sleep phase syndromes, jet lag, shift work, seasonal affective disorder, and non–24-hour sleep–wake syndrome. Light therapy continues to be useful in other conditions. For elders, the practice parameters support its use in insomnia, but other studies since the time of the publication of the parameters have also supported the use of light therapy in dementia (Deschenes & McCurry, 2009).

There are individuals for whom light therapy is not appropriate. If individuals have bipolar disorder, if their skin is sensitive to light, if they take medications that yield sensitivity to light, or if they have a condition in which light may possibly worsen the underlying condition, then they should avoid the use of light therapy. Additionally, light therapy is not without side effects. Common side effects include eyestrain or headache and rarely irritability may be seen.

As an alternative to the use of a light box, exposure to bright natural light helps maintain rhythm synchrony with environmental time cues. If a light box is used in lieu of natural light exposure, the exposure times are the same. For the elder who is experiencing a phase advance in sleep pattern, getting exposure to light in the evening for a half an hour or more helps to correct this pattern. For a phase-delayed pattern of sleep, a half an hour or more of light is helpful in restoring sleep–wake patterns closer to the desired schedule. A small body of literature points to the fact that elders who are in nursing facilities often get less than 30 minutes of exposure to natural light per day. Light produced by ordinary incandescent or fluorescent bulbs does not produce the quality or intensity of light needed to regulate circadian rhythm. Recent research has shown that exposure to all-day bright light in otherwise dimly lit nursing facilities yielded significant improvements in cognitive functioning, reduced depression, and enhanced self-care capacity (Riemersma-van der Lek et al., 2008).

Clinicians interested in the use of light therapy should be aware of the *Practice Parameters for the Use of Light Therapy in the Treatment of Sleep Disorders* (Chesson, Littner, et al., 1999). In consideration of using light therapy, the clinician needs to be familiar with the intervention and the principles underlying the use of light therapy. Reviewing the evidence base for light therapy by the available practice parameters is prudent and seeking consultation, if needed, is important.

There are many vendors who sell light therapy equipment and most offer a similar range of products with varying prices. In the United States, two established vendors include Bio-Brite and Apollo Lighting; additional vendors may be found at the North American Seasonal Light Device vendor site (http://www.geocities.com/hotsprings/7061/supplies.html). Light therapy equipment is classified as durable medical equipment and is often paid for through insurers. Clinicians may find it helpful to reference the light therapy practice parameters from AASM with insurers during the prior authorization process.

Massage Therapy

Massage therapy may be considered an adjunct intervention for disturbed sleep and uses manual soft tissue manipulation; it also includes holding, causing movement, or applying pressure to the body. The purpose of massage is to improve health and well-being (American Massage Therapy Association, 1999). Massage therapy is believed to

work by increasing the synthesis of endogenous opioids that inhibit pain by activating the descending pain inhibitory system and thereby reducing pain (Lund et al., 2002). Massage therapy is believed to reduce muscle tension and the overall stress that can interfere with the onset of sleep. In addition, massage therapy has been shown to improve sleep by reducing chronic lower back pain (Williamson, Fletcher, & Dawson, 2003; Wolsko, Eisenberg, Davis, Kessler, & Phillips, 2003). Family members and caregivers should be instructed in massage techniques to use at bedtime to enhance the quality of sleep.

Dietary Supplements

Herbal or natural products, which are categorized as dietary supplements by the Food and Drug Administration (FDA), are commonly used by older adults to facilitate sleep (Williamson et al., 2003). Although some research has supported the efficacy of herbal preparations, clinical trials on these products are limited and frequently show publication bias. However, an extensive and evidence-based resource is readily available on herbals in the *Physicians' Desk Reference for Herbal Medications* (Thomson Healthcare, 2007). In this book, established effectiveness of herbal preparations is determined by Commission E, a European-based institution that culls the evidence base on herbals and determines effectiveness of substances for intended uses. Additionally, it clearly speaks to potential drug interactions with established pharmaceuticals and spells out contraindications. In the United States, the present lack of quality control and standardization of herbal products may limit confidence in the use of herbals, but this in part is a consequence of the learning needs of the clinician as much as it is an issue of quality control of products. Of importance to the prescriber, it is critical to recognize that herbal products can affect cytochrome P-450 isoenzymes and either enhance or inhibit the metabolism of many medications (Scott & Elmer, 2002). Therefore, these products should be used with caution in older adults. Table 16-1 lists the herbal products that are commonly used to treat

TABLE 16-1

Herbal Products to Treat Sleep Disorders

Agent	Indications	Adverse Effects	Usual Dose	Drug Interactions	Efficacy
Melatonin	To induce sleep	Excessive drowsiness	5.4 mg	Fluvoxamine reduces the metabolism of melatonin by inhibiting CYP1A2 or CYP2C9 Reduces the antihypertensive effect of slow-release nifedipine	May be effective in treating jet lag and other sleep disorders
Kava kava	Anxiolytic Used in South Pacific as a recreational drink	Liver damage Long-term use at high doses is associated with dry skin, yellow discoloration of skin, ataxia, hair loss, partial hearing loss, decreased appetite, and weight loss	10–200 mg	Effects are enhanced when taken with alcohol or other medications that act on the central nervous system	Short-term use is effective in reducing anxiety Causes muscle relaxation and anticonvulsant action and may improve sleep onset
Chamomile	Induces sleep	Rare and usually allergic in nature	Two to four dried flowers qd-tid	May inhibit CYP 3A4 and decrease the metabolism of calcium-channel blockers, cisapride, lovastatin, and simvastatin	May have a mild hypnotic effect
Passion flower	Used as a sedative-hypnotic to induce sleep		0.25–1 g of dried herb as a tea; 0.5–1 ml liquid extract tid		
Ginseng	Used as a sedative, hypnotic, and anti-depressant activity	Insomnia, diarrhea, vaginal bleeding, severe headache, schizophrenia, and Stevens–Johnson syndrome		Decreases effects of warfarin	No evidence from clinical trials to support the use of ginseng for neuro-psychological symptoms
Lemon balm (Melissa officinalis L)	Anxiolytic, hypnotic, and analgesic effects	No serious side effects have been reported from ingestion	1–4 g daily	May potentiate the effects of other central nervous system depressants May interact with thyroid medication	May be an effective anxiolytic
Skull cap	Used as a sedative and anticonvulsant	Giddiness, confusion, sedation, seizures, and possibly hepatotoxicity	1–2 g of dried herb; 2–4 ml of liquid extract qd to tid		Effectiveness may depend of the species or part of the plant that is used

Sources: Ernst, E. (2002). The risk-benefit profile of commonly used herbal therapies: Gingko, St. John's wort, ginseng, Echinacea, saw palmetto, and kava. *Annals of Internal Medicine, 136*(1), 42–53; Scott, G., & Elmer, G. (2002). Update on natural product–drug interactions. *American Journal of Health Systems Pharmacy, 59*(5), 339–347; and Wong, A., Smith, M., & Boon, H. (1998). Herbal remedies in psychiatric practice. *Archives of General Psychiatry, 55*(1), 1033–1044.

sleep disorders. Common herbals used for their sedative–hypnotic properties include valerian, melatonin, kava kava, chamomile, and *Passiflora*.

INDICATIONS FOR PHARMACOLOGICAL THERAPIES

When behavioral interventions alone are not effective and impaired sleep is impacting quality of life, pharmacological therapies are indicated. Table 16-2 provides an overview of treatment options. Medication management of insomnia should supplement, not replace, behavioral interventions and complementary therapies. Identification and treatment of an underlying cause of insomnia, such as formal sleep disorders, medical or psychiatric comorbidity, pain, or medication-induced sleep problems, should be determined before intervention strategies are initiated. The clinical reasoning behind this plan recognizes that it is essential to understand the potential sources of sleep dysregulation and to address these issues in light of a plan to facilitate better sleep. For example, an iatrogenic insomnia caused by a medication is likely to be treated differently than sleep disturbance caused by poor sleep hygiene. As with any other intervention plan, if the diagnosis is incorrect, so is the appropriateness of the interventions. A plan that addresses the sources of the underlying sleep disturbance ensures greater success in conjunction with behavioral and complementary strategies. In any event, the use of standardized approaches to quality sleep should always be encouraged with proper sleep hygiene.

Pharmacological treatment of insomnia includes a wide range of indicated and off-label uses of drugs that have hypnotic properties. Those medications indicated by the FDA for the treatment of insomnia include five benzodiazepine receptor agonists (estazolam [ProSom], flurazepam [Dalmane], quazepam [Doral], temazepam [Restoril], and triazolam [Halcion]); three nonbenzodiazepine receptor agonists (eszopiclone [Lunesta], zolpidem [Ambien], and zaleplon [Sonata]); and one melatonin receptor agonist

(ramelteon [Rozerem]). Benzodiazepine receptor agonists are positive modulators and enhancers of γ-aminobutyric acid (GABA), the major inhibitory neurochemical in the central nervous system (CNS). One of the GABA receptors is the benzodiazepine receptor, and enhancement of the function of this receptor through neuroinhibitory influences enhanced sleep. All of the benzodiazepine receptor agonists have sedative–hypnotic properties, and these drugs rarely have the problems associated with off-label uses of medications, such as antihistamines, antidepressants, or antipsychotic medications, all of which usually have significant anticholinergic properties.

There are two major GABA receptors: $GABA_A$ and $GABA_B$. The sedative–hypnotics interact with the type A receptors to produce their effects on sleep. Medications from other drug classes interact with the benzodiazepine receptor and include barbiturates and alcohol. Some sedative–hypnotics, such as chloral hydrate, are categorized as nonbenzodiazepine, nonbarbiturate compounds, but the use of medications like chloral hydrate has become uncommon, given the safer alternatives in the newer sedative–hypnotic medications.

Benzodiazepine receptor agonists act at the limbic, thalamic, and hypothalamic levels of the CNS causing CNS depression and producing anxiolytic, sedative, hypnotic, skeletal muscle relaxant, and anticonvulsant effects. These drugs are metabolized in the liver, and their elimination half-life may be longer in older adults and in individuals with liver impairment. Consequently, these agents can potentially accumulate in the body with continued use. Flurazepam and quazepam have active metabolites that can also have long half-lives. The issue of metabolites is very important in elders inasmuch as these metabolites may be metabolized by P-450 enzymes that are not used to metabolize the parent compound. Therefore, the metabolites run the separate risk of causing drug–drug interactions that are not risks with the parent compound alone. A critical issue to bear in mind with the prescription of benzodiazepine receptor agonists is that of respiratory

TABLE 16-2

Pharmacological Management of Insomnia for Older Adults: Appropriate Dosage Recommendations

Drug Group	Dosing Recommendations (mg/d)	Half-Life	Side Effects by Drug Categories
Nonbenzodiazepine/Nonbarbiturates			
Chloral hydrate	250	4–8 hr	Dizziness
Ethchlorvynol (Placidyl)	200	10–20 hr	Weakness
Zolpidem (Ambien)	5	1.5–4.5 hr	Gastrointestinal irritation
Zaleplon (Sonata)	5	0.9–1.1 hr	Blurred vision
Eszopiclone (Lunesta)	1–3 mg before bedtime	Approximately 6 hr	Tolerance develops
			Headache
			Sleepiness
Benzodiazepines			
Estazolam (ProSom)*	0.5–1	8–24 hr	Daytime sedation
Flurazepam (Dalmane)	15	Long	Psychomotor impairment
Quazepam (Doral)	7.5–15	25–41 hr	Delirium
Temazepam (Restoril)	7.5–15	10–20 hr	
Triazolam (Halcion)*	0.0625–0.125	1.6–5.4 hr	
Antidepressants			
Amitriptyline (Elavil)	10–25	10–50 hr	Anticholinergic effects
Doxepin (Sinequan)	10–25, ≤ 75	6–8 hr	Orthostatic hypotension/dizziness
Trazodone (Desyrel)	25–50, ≤ 150	5–9 hr	Daytime sleepiness
Remeron (Mirtazapine)	7.5–15, ≤ 45	20–40 hr	
Antihistamines			
Diphenhydramine	25 mg	30–60 min	Tolerance develops in 1–2 weeks
			Daytime somnolence
			Anticholinergic effects
Melatonin Agonist			
Remalteon (Rozerem)	8 mg	30 min	Potential morning grogginess
Dizziness			

* Examples of triazolobenzodiazepines.

Source: Adapted from Semla, T. P., Higbee, M. D., & Beizer, J. L. (2009). *Lexi-Comp's Geriatric Dosage Handbook: Monitoring, Clinical Recommendations, and OBRA Guidelines* (14th ed.). Hudson, OH: Lexicom.

depression. These drugs should be prescribed with great caution in those with respiratory diseases, particularly such conditions as chronic obstructive pulmonary disease.

Off-label use of medications includes a broad range of drugs, such as alcohol, herbal preparations, melatonin, dietary supplements, over-the-counter sleeping aids, antihistamines, and antidepressants, and a number of other psychotropic drugs, such as sedating antipsychotic medications. In 2005, the National Institutes of Health convened a state-of-the-science conference to address manifestations and management of chronic insomnia in adults (NIH, 2005). The recommendations from this meeting were based on a clear review of evidence related to insomnia and its treatment. Specifically, the recommendations stated "Chronic insomnia is a major public health problem affecting millions of individuals, along with their families and communities. Little is known about the mechanisms, causes, clinical course, comorbidities, and consequences of chronic insomnia. Evidence supports the efficacy of cognitive-behavioral therapy and benzodiazepine receptor agonists in the treatment of this disorder, at least in the short term. Very little evidence supports the efficacy of other treatments, despite their widespread use. Moreover, even for those treatments that have been systematically evaluated, the panel is concerned about the mismatch between the potential lifelong nature of this illness and the longest clinical trials, which have lasted 1 year or less" (NIH, p. 15).

Considerations in the Prescription of Sedative Hypnotics in the Elderly

Given the sensitivities to medications that are common to many elders because of normal physiological changes in aging, it is wise for the nurse to follow the prudent recommendation of starting with low doses and moving slowly in dose titration. It is common for elders to take a number of medications, increasing the risk for drug–drug interactions. Drugs with anticholinergic properties (select antidepressants, antihistamines, and some antipsychotic medications) increase the risk

for confusion, dry mouth, constipation, or urinary retention. Other potential and significant issues with all sedative–hypnotics focus on safety concerns with an increased risk for sedation, habituation, potential for falls, and subsequent possible fracture and incapacity. Despite these issues, it is not uncommon to see pharmacological strategies implemented, often in the absence of behavioral interventions to effectively address the insomnia. Even in light of a black box warning on antipsychotic medication by the FDA, this class of medications is still prescribed for insomnia and sleep disturbances among elders (Kuehn, 2005).

What the NIH State of the Science conference recommendations on insomnia in adults point to is that the evidence base regarding effectiveness with sleeping medications supports the use of benzodiazepine receptor agonists, which includes medications whose chemical structure is either a true benzodiazepine (e.g., estazolam, flurazepam, quazepam, temazepam, and triazolam), or a nonbenzodiazepine receptor agonist (e.g., eszopiclone, zaleplon, and zolpidem). Other benzodiazepine receptor agonists are available, but these drugs are not indicated by the FDA as sedative–hypnotics (e.g., clonazepam, lorazepam, alprazolam, and diazepam).

All of the sedative–hypnotic medications approved by the FDA for insomnia are schedule IV and as such have abuse liability. All of these drugs hasten sleep onset, reduce awake time after sleep onset, and increase total sleep time. All of these drugs enhance GABA, the most abundant neuroinhibitory chemical in the CNS. All of these drugs have properties that are sedative, hypnotic, and anxiolytic, with muscle-relaxing and anticonvulsant properties.

Selection of a benzodiazepine receptor agonist (or medications indicated for insomnia that are in a different class) for sleep must be determined by the type of insomnia being treated. For example, difficulty falling asleep is best treated with a medication that has a short half-life. Hypnotics with moderate half-lives correct middle-of-the-night awakening, and the longer-acting medications are reserved for sleep pattern disturbances characterized by sleep disturbances in the lattermost part of the sleep period time. The longer-acting medications are more likely to be associated with residual daytime sedative effects; impaired psychomotor and mental performance; and subsequent ataxia, falls, and fractures (Gurvich & Cunningham, 2000). The elimination half-lives of the sedative–hypnotics are as follows: zaleplon, 1 hour; zolpidem, 2.5 hours; triazolam, 1.5–5.5 hours; eszopiclone, 6 hours; temazepam, 3.5–18.4 hours; estazolam, 18–24 hours; quazepam, 39 hours; and flurazepam, 47–100 hours. The prescriber of any sedative–hypnotic needs to be familiar with the half-life of the medication from the menu of choices. This knowledge allows for rational selection of a sedative–hypnotic to address the specific sleep pattern disturbance experienced by the person seeking treatment.

Although long-term treatment with sedative–hypnotics is not recommended, there may be circumstances where the use of sedative–hypnotics may be indicated. These circumstances include conditions where the insomnia cannot be altered, and in these cases longer-term use may be sanctioned and needed. As previously mentioned, it is critical to ensure that behavioral interventions aimed at the reduction of insomnia are implemented concurrently with the use of any medication used to enhance sleep quality and duration.

It is sound practice to question the contributing influences behind any insomnia, particularly if the use of sedative–hypnotics has been protracted over months or years. Revisiting the assessment of sleep throughout the course of routine care of elders is important. Polysomnographic evaluation of sleep is clearly indicated in light of a suspicion of a formal sleep disorder other than insomnia. An experienced clinician never worries alone. It is sound clinical practice to seek consultation around sleep evaluation if needed. In doing so, the duty to consult is met when the clinical presentation of a patient is unclear.

Additional Pharmacological Options for Sleep

In the section that follows, there is discussion of several agents that are rarely used in practice today, given the alternatives. However, because elders may have the same provider for decades with the possibility that the provider continues to prescribe through older practices, it is important to be aware of these medications. It is important to recognize, however, that these drugs are no longer first-line options for most persons, given the alternatives available and the evidence base that supports the current approaches to insomnia.

Chloral Hydrate

Chloral hydrate is a nonbenzodiazepine–nonbarbiturate sedative. The mechanism of action of chloral hydrate is unknown. This drug does decrease sleep latency and nighttime awakening with minimal effects on REM sleep. Chloral hydrate is absorbed readily and metabolized in the liver and kidney to active and inactive metabolites. The drug and the metabolites are excreted primarily in the urine, so that it should be avoided in patients with a creatinine clearance of less than 50 ml/min. This drug can result in significant sedation in older individuals, may be habit forming, and should be used cautiously in individuals prone to such addictions. Older individuals may become disoriented, sedated, ataxic, and dizzy, have nightmares, and complain of residual sleepiness with normal doses of chloral hydrate, making it a less desirable selection for elders.

Barbiturates

Barbiturates are classified into three groups: (1) short-acting (pentobarbital and secobarbital); (2) intermediate-acting (amobarbital, apropbarbital, and butabarbital); and (3) long-acting (phenobarbital and mephobarbital). The onset of action can range from 10–60 minutes, and the half-life of barbiturates ranges from 11–140 hours. All barbiturates have been shown to be relatively equivalent in efficacy. Barbiturates are indicated for the short-term treatment of insomnia because their efficacy does seem to diminish after 2 weeks and they have significant adverse drug side effects. Adverse effects associated with barbiturates include somnolence, confusion, and CNS depression. Residual sedation is not uncommon, particularly when used with older adults, and there may be acute changes in mood, impaired judgment, and impaired motor skills that can persist for hours. Because of this side effect profile, these drugs are not recommended as first-line treatment for insomnia in older adults, nor are they used with any frequency in practice, given the evidence-based recommendations and the option for safer alternatives for elders.

Antidepressants

Sedating antidepressants have been used to facilitate sleep among older adults, particularly those who also have concomitant depression. The drugs most commonly used to induce sleep include trazodone (Desyrel); low-dose amitriptyline (Elavil); or mirtazapine (Remeron). Mirtazapine, for example, when used in a small group of patients with known Alzheimer's disease, improved sleep patterns, decreased anxiety, and improved appetite (Raji & Brady, 2001). However, the benefits of using mirtazapine as a hypnotic are counterbalanced with risks of hyperlipidemia and significant weight gain.

Trazodone has been a commonly used off-label sedative–hypnotic medication. Its mechanism of action is complex and involves a number of neurochemical actions. Its sedating properties are most likely related to antagonism of $5HT_{2A}$ and antagonism of histamine receptor type 1. In a study by Saletu-Zyhlarz et al. (2002), trazodone was found to increase sleep efficiency and decrease wakefulness during the night and to reduce the chances for early morning awakening. Trazodone also improved subjective sleep quality, affectivity, numerical memory, and somatic complaints (Saletu-Zyhlarz et al.). However, results from such a study need to be evaluated in light of contradicting findings in other studies. For example, James and Mendelson (2004) report the findings of a 2-week, double-blind, placebo-controlled trial comparing the effectiveness of trazodone, 50 mg, zolpidem, 10 mg, and placebo. Results showed that in the first week there was a shorter time to falling asleep with both trazodone and zolpidem. However, results from the second week showed that there was shorter sleep latency with zolpidem, but trazodone was indistinguishable from placebo in its effect. As with any circumstance where research data are used to support or refute a clinical rationale for use of a medication, it is essential to critically analyze the studies from which the findings are derived. In any circumstance, sedating antidepressants should be used cautiously because they have significant anticholinergic side effects, including confusion, hypotension, dry mouth, constipation, and urinary retention, and they can exacerbate RLS and PLMD in some individuals.

Antihistamines

The histamine-1 receptor antagonist diphenhydramine (e.g., Benadryl) has been approved by the FDA for the treatment of insomnia. Many over-the-counter sleep aids contain diphenhydramine, alone or in combination with acetaminophen. Diphenhydramine antagonizes histamine at the H_1 receptor site and has a sedative effect, is well absorbed following oral administration, and has an onset of action of approximately 15–30 minutes. It is metabolized extensively in the liver and has a half-life of approximately 12–14 hours.

Although diphenhydramine is often assumed to be safe by many older individuals because it is sold over the counter, older adults should be informed about the potential side effects of sleep aids containing these drugs. Diphenhydramine is not only highly sedating but also has significant anticholinergic properties and causes dry mouth, constipation, dizziness, syncope, hypotension, constipation, and urinary retention. These side effects must be anticipated in individuals and treatment options provided. For example, older adults who have a history of urinary retention may note exacerbation of this problem when using diphenhydramine for sleep.

In 2005, the FDA approved a new sedative–hypnotic medication for insomnia, specifically indicated for difficulty falling asleep. The compound is ramelteon (Rozerem), and the mechanism of action of this compound is distinct among the sedative–hypnotic class of drugs. Unlike the other indicated sedative–hypnotics, ramelteon is the first nonscheduled medication for insomnia. Melatonin has three main receptor types, but types 1 and 2 are believed to be most influential in the circadian timing system. Type 1 receptors are involved in sleep promotion, whereas type 2 receptors are believed to have regulating influences on the circadian timing system but are not necessarily involved in sleep. Ramelteon is a selective melatonin MT_1/MT_2 receptor agonist. These receptors have high concentrations in the suprachiasmatic nucleus, considered to be the seat of the major clock in the circadian timing system. At the dose prescribed for sleep (8 mg), ramelteon is not believed to significantly affect the type 2 receptors. It is a strong P-450 1A2 inhibitor and as such it should never be combined with fluvoxamine. There is no evidence of abuse liability with this medication. It needs to be used with caution in people with mild hepatic impairment and should not be used for those diagnosed with severe hepatic impairment. It has no respiratory depressant effect, but to date it has not been studied in people with chronic obstructive pulmonary disease (Takeda Pharmaceuticals America, 2005).

Consideration for Use of Sedative Hypnotics Among Institutionalized Older Adults

The Centers for Medicare and Medicaid Services has published guidelines for the use of sedative–hypnotics in institutionalized older adults (i.e., in nursing facilities). These guidelines recommend that the drugs be used for 10 days and then attempts should be made to decrease or eliminate use. Specific doses of agents for use with older adults have been recommended, and use should not exceed these dosages (Table 16-2). It is strongly recommended that alternatives to sleeping agents be incorporated into care, particularly behavioral sleep measures, as previously discussed.

Discontinuation of Sedative–Hypnotics

In discontinuing sedative–hypnotic medications, there are two important things to consider. The first is the chance for physiological withdrawal, particularly if the medication has been in regular use by the person over a longer period of time. It is well established that rapid withdrawal of CNS depressants leads to the opposite effect, namely excitability and irritability. As such, planning a rational taper of medications is essential, and this taper should be paired with behavioral interventions to facilitate sleep. As a general principle, it is helpful to acknowledge that nothing can be taken away without replacing it with something else, and in the case of careful sedative–hypnotic withdrawal, implementing behavioral sleep measures is a sound replacement for the medication when possible. Additionally, it is important to realize that the role of expectation is significantly influential in the outcome of any sleep-related intervention. Being attentive to the person's expectations of medication withdrawal and implementation of behavioral measures is critical to the success of the treatment plan.

Benzodiazepines that have shorter half-lives (estazolam, temazepam, and triazolam) are more likely to be associated with rebound anxiety and insomnia after discontinuation (Wang, Bohn, Glynn, Mogun, & Avorn, 2001). Discontinuation of triazolam and estazolam is more likely to be associated with delirium in older adults than other benzodiazepines (Wang et al.). This is particularly true when the drug is used in greater-than-recommended doses and over a longer period of time. For patients on chloral hydrate, attempts to discontinue use should be done by tapering the dose initially and weaning the individual off this agent. Withdrawal symptoms (convulsions, tremor, vomiting, and sweating) can occur following abrupt discontinuation of any benzodiazepine. The more severe withdrawal symptoms usually have been seen in patients who received excessive doses over an extended period of time.

Individual plans for scheduled medication tapers should be determined based on the type of medication that the patient has been taking, the doses of the medication, and the duration of the exposure to the medication. Seeking consultation on planned tapers of medications that pose clinical risk (e.g., protracted use of a benzodiazepine) may be helpful and provide greater margins of safety in the treatment plan. When planning a medication taper, it needs to be done with the full engagement of the patient. It is the responsibility of the advanced practice nurse to assess other medications that could possibly interfere with a planned withdrawal of sedative–hypnotic medications. Box 16-3 lists those medications that can aggravate sleep disorders in older adults.

Although individuals are often willing to work with providers to eliminate or alter prescribed medications, alcohol, caffeine, and nicotine are generally less likely to be discontinued altogether by these individuals. Changing beliefs and attitudes about sleep and poor sleep habits can be a slow and often difficult process. Using a step approach and establishing patient-centered short- and long-term goals can facilitate behavior change. For example, a history and physical may reveal that an individual is currently a smoker, drinks two to four alcoholic beverages in the evening to relax, and does not engage in regular exercise. Although changing all three of these behaviors may be an appropriate long-term goal, breaking this long-term goal into smaller short-term goals is less challenging and results in greater outcomes over time.

ENVIRONMENTAL APPROACHES IN INSTITUTIONAL SETTINGS

Institutionalized older adults are required to adopt the schedule and nighttime routine set by the facility and the nursing staff. Decisions that individuals usually make independently, such as when to go to bed, when to rise, and when to eat, are too often made by the staff. This change in routine can have a serious impact on the sleep–wake cycle of older adults and may result in impaired overall quality of sleep. Creating an environment in institutions where residents have the freedom to decide their

BOX 16-3 DRUGS THAT DECREASE SLEEP

Prescribed	Over-the-Counter
Antidepressants	Histamine-2 receptor blockers
Antihypertensives	Smoking cessation aids
Antineoplastics	Nicotine
Bronchodilators	Some herbs and supplements
CNS stimulants	Nonsteroidal anti-inflammatory drugs
Corticosteroids	Alcohol
Diuretics	Caffeine
	Anticholinergics
	Decongestants

own wake time, bedtime, and nap time can have a positive effect on sleep and also provides a level of control to the individual, which in fact may reduce dissatisfaction and struggles over bedtime scheduling. Adjusting nighttime routines in institutions to reduce the number of times residents are awakened for care-related activities may increase the total sleep time and the amount of uninterrupted sleep (Eser, Khorshid, & Cinar, 2007).

PATIENT EDUCATION AND COUNSELING

Patients with sleep disorders need encouragement and education on how to incorporate the use of a variety of techniques to facilitate sleep: behavioral sleep measures, such as sleep hygiene, stimulus control, complementary treatments, environmental interventions, and short-term use of medications if necessary. Specific information regarding medication management is particularly important. Patients should be informed that some medications that are prescribed to treat comorbid conditions may create the possibility for drug interactions with other medications that the person may be taking. It is the responsibility of the advanced practice nurse to be aware of these potential interactions and to take measures to reduce risk associated with the use of multiple medications. A table of such drug interactions could be reviewed with the patient as appropriate (medicine.iupui.edu/flockhart). The bioavailability of zolpidem and zaleplon is significantly reduced when given with food and should not be taken within 2 hours of an evening snack. Dosage adjustments may be needed in these situations. Patients should be informed that barbiturates, available in liquid, tablet, and intravenous preparations, are well known to interact with other CNS depressants. Moreover, these drugs can interact with anticoagulants, antihistamines, narcotics, alcohol, and tranquilizers. Dosage adjustments should be considered when used with these other agents, and for any patient who has liver or renal impairment.

REFERRAL AND CONSULTATION

Identification of problems, such as depression, alcohol abuse, or chronic pain, that impact sleep may be best managed through referrals to appropriate pain clinics that often collaborate with psychiatric clinical nurse specialists or psychiatric nurse practitioners (or other appropriate mental health professional) for individual or group therapy. The pain clinics offer the expertise focused on the treatment of pain-related conditions, and the psychiatric nursing resources provide expertise in coping, adjustment, and consultation around areas of medication management that overlap with the purview of the pain specialist. In addition, support groups for specific problems, such as RLS and insomnia, may be useful in helping these individuals or their caregivers best manage and cope with both the underlying disorder and the associated problem with sleep.

EVALUATION OF TREATMENT EFFECTIVENESS WITH FOLLOW-UP

Follow-up is particularly important for older adults with sleep disorders because of the negative clinical consequences of not doing so, namely perpetuation of the sleep disorder itself, and potentially poor clinical outcomes for comorbid conditions. Treatment plans to decrease medication use as soon as there is evidence that the underlying cause of the insomnia is resolving is in keeping with evidence-based recommendations and enhances more positive clinical outcomes. At the same time, patients need to be encouraged to continue with appropriate sleep hygiene techniques and the use of behavioral sleep measures to promote positive health outcomes. Healthy practices, such as exercise and limited use of alcohol, along with complementary treatments, are likely to improve clinical outcomes. In so doing, older adults will enjoy optimal sleep, which should improve their overall health and quality of life.

CASE STUDY: THE BEST PREDICTOR OF A BAD NIGHT'S SLEEP IS ANTICIPATION OF A BAD NIGHT'S SLEEP: THE ILLUSTRATIVE CASE OF MS. W.

Ms. W. is an 82-year-old widow who presents repeatedly in her primary care physician's office for treatment of a number of somatic complaints including shortness of breath, chest pain, abdominal pains, and "difficulty with sleeping." The nurse practitioner working with Ms. W. conducted thorough assessments of the presenting complaints, only to find negative workups across the board for the respiratory, cardiac, and abdominal complaints. The primary care physician corroborated the findings of the workups. Her sleep-related complaints were characterized mainly by difficulty falling asleep; short sleep period time (5–6 hours); some middle of the night awakening to use the bathroom; followed by returning back to sleep and then awakening around 4 a.m. with an inability to get back to sleep. Given the nature of her complaints (and high recidivism related to the same), the nurse practitioner involved in her care referred her for psychiatric treatment.

She lives with her son and his family in a large home. During the day, she is left by herself because all of the other family members in the house work full time. She stays at home to care for the family's two dogs. She loves the dogs and by her report, they love her. Her relationship with her family is functional, although she is quick to point out that "they try to control my life and always are telling me what I ought to be doing." There is no evidence of abuse and she corroborates the same.

Her sleep–wake diaries over 7 days (search www.sleepfoundation.org or www.sleepeducation.com for examples of diaries) show that she indeed does get up at 4 a.m. but tosses and turns and becomes frustrated with her inability to sleep. At 6 a.m., she gets out of bed and feeds her two dogs, prepares breakfast, and reads the morning paper. At 9 a.m. every day, she watches a church service on the television. She often falls asleep during the sermon part of the televised service, waking up after about 45 minutes. She then usually goes for a 20-minute walk with the dogs, then returns and makes lunch. The afternoon is usually filled with a standard routine of saying prayers for 30 minutes, followed by some telephone calls to friends and then some knitting. She "just rests" her eyes on the sofa for about 30 minutes each day. At 5:30 p.m. her family comes home, she helps with dinner, and watches television in the evening with them during which time she sometimes falls asleep "just for a couple minutes" and then finally gets up from the sofa at 9:45 p.m., gets ready for bed, and then goes to bed. She is quick to say that she is "constantly worried" about not getting enough sleep and fears that her nights will be tortured by uncontrollable periods of wakefulness, followed by days filled with low energy.

Medically, she is generally healthy and takes a proton pump inhibitor for gastroesophageal reflux disease. She has no allergies. She does not drink alcohol, use tobacco, or use any over-the-counter drugs by her report. Her self-care is very good.

From a psychiatric perspective, she has a long history of dysthymic disorder, generalized anxiety disorder, and panic without agoraphobia. She meets diagnostic criteria for somatization disorder. She sees a psychiatric clinical nurse specialist for both psychotherapy and medication management. The focus of the therapy is both cognitive and supportive. Her medication regimen includes

CASE STUDY: THE BEST PREDICTOR OF A BAD NIGHT'S SLEEP IS ANTICIPATION OF A BAD NIGHT'S SLEEP: THE ILLUSTRATIVE CASE OF MS. W. *(continued)*

mirtazapine, 15 mg at bedtime. Additionally, she has a prescription for clonazepam, 0.5 mg tablets to be used in 0.25-mg doses once or twice daily, if needed. With that prescription, she rarely uses it during the day but feels anxious about her sleep if she does not take it at night. She has no side effects with the medication and has not had any symptoms of dizziness or ataxia. Her falls risk is very low. Although she has some residual symptoms related to mood and anxiety, she is not willing to accept medication adjustments at this time. Currently, her mood is not depressed, although there is evidence of mild to moderate underlying anxiety. She has had no panic episodes for over a year. Her somatic symptoms wax and wane, usually worsening with stressors. Her current diagnosis is as follows:

Axis I: Dysthymic disorder
            Generalized anxiety disorder
            Panic disorder without
            agoraphobia
            Somatization disorder
            Insomnia related to psychiatric
            illnesses

Axis II: Dependent features; does not
            meet criteria for any formal
            axis II disorder

Axis III: Gastroesophageal reflux disease

Axis IV: Family stressors, chronic psychiatric illness

Axis V: 60

How would you approach this woman's sleep-related concerns if she were to present herself in your practice? A good place to start is with the evaluation, which should include the elements noted next. It is important to use the evidence-based guidelines to facilitate accurate assessment and intervention. In this case, using *Practice Parameters for the Psychological and Behavioral Treatment of Insomnia: An Update* (Morganthaler, Kramer, et al., 2006) is a great place to start (check www.aasmnet.org for parameters).

Evaluation of Sleep/Wake Patterns with the Use of Diaries for at Least 7 Days

Rule out formal sleep disorders, such as OSAS, RLS, and PLMD. Using the Pittsburgh Sleep Quality Index (Buysse, Reynolds, Monk, Berman, & Kupfer, 1989) is a sound approach to the assessment of sleep in clinical populations. It is a self-rated questionnaire that assesses sleep quality and disturbances over a 1-month time interval. Nineteen individual items generate seven component scores: subjective sleep quality, sleep latency, sleep duration, habitual sleep efficiency, sleep disturbances, use of sleeping medication, and daytime dysfunction. The sum of scores for these seven components yields one global score (Buysse et al.). Assess the level of sleepiness that she is experiencing with the Epworth Sleepiness Scale (available at http://www.sleepeducation.com/SleepScale.aspx).

Formulate a plan that uses a multicomponent approach (CBT-I) including sleep hygiene, stimulus control, assessment of the need for sleep restriction, relaxation, and CBT-I. Combined, these interventions modify or correct the perpetuating factors of the insomnia. Given the chronicity of the sleep pattern, the process will take time, and this issue needs to be addressed in the course of the work. It is likely that reinforcement of the principles of CBT-I will be important to sustain results with the interventions.

REFERENCES

Ambien, G. D. Searle, Product Information. (Last updated July 29, 2004). Retrieved July 31, 2004, from http://www.rxlist.com/generic/zolpid.htm

American Academy of Sleep Medicine. (1997). *International classification of sleep disorders: Diagnostic and coding manual, revised*. Chicago: American Academy of Sleep Medicine.

American Massage Therapy Association. (1999). *Massage therapy: Enhancing your health with therapeutic massage*. [Online]. Retrieved February 2004, from http://www.amtamassage.org/publications/enhancing-health.htm

Balkrishnan, R., Rasu, R. S., & Rajagopalan, R. (2005). Physician and patient determinants of pharmacologic treatment of sleep difficulties in outpatient settings in the United States. *Sleep, 28*(6), 715–719.

Barthlen, G. (2002). Sleep disorders: Obstructive sleep apnea syndrome, restless legs syndrome, and insomnia in geriatric patients. *Geriatrics, 57*(11), 34.

Bjorvatn, B., & Pallesen, S. (2009). A practical approach to circadian rhythm sleep disorder. *Sleep Medicine Reviews, 13*, 47–60.

Blask, D. E. (2008). Melatonin, sleep disturbance and cancer risk. *Sleep Medicine Reviews, 13*(4), 257–264.

Borbely, A. A. (1982). A two process model of sleep regulation. *Human Neurobiology, 1*(3), 395–404.

Buysse, D. J., Reynolds, C. F., Monk, T. H., Berman, S. R., & Kupfer, D. J. (1989). Pittsburgh Sleep Quality Index: A new instrument for psychiatric practice and research. *Psychiatry Research, 28*, 193–213.

Byles, J. E., Mishra, G. D., & Harris, M. A. (2005). The experience of insomnia among older women. *Sleep, 28*(8), 972–979.

Chesson, A. L., Anderson, W. M., Littner, M., Davila, D., Hartse, K., Johnson, S., et al. (1999). Practice parameters for the nonpharmacologic treatment of chronic insomnia. *Sleep, 22*(8), 1128–1133.

Chesson, A. L., Littner, M., Davila, D., Anderson, W. M., Grigg-Danberger, M., Hartse, K., et al. (1999). Practice parameters for the use of light therapy in the treatment of sleep disorders. *Sleep, 22*(5), 641–660.

Cochran, H. (2003). Diagnose and treat primary insomnia. *The Nurse Practitioner, 28*(9), 15–27.

Dattilo, D. J., & Drooger, S. A. (2004). Outcome assessment of patients undergoing maxillofacial procedures for the treatment of sleep apnea: Comparison of subjective and objective results. *Journal of Oral & Maxillofacial Surgery, 62*(2), 164–168.

Deschenes, C. L., & McCurry, S. M. (2009). Current treatments for sleep disturbances in individuals with dementia. *Current Psychiatry Reports, 11*(1), 20–26.

Edinger, J. D., & Carney, C. (2008). *Overcoming insomnia: A cognitive-behavioral therapy approach therapist guide*. New York: Oxford University Press.

Edinger, J., Wohlgemuth, W., Radtke, R., Mahr, G., & Quillian, R. (2001). Cognitive behavioral therapy for treatment of chronic primary insomnia: A randomized controlled trial. *JAMA, 285*(14), 1856–1864.

Endeshaw, Y. W., Bloom, H. L., & Bliwise, D. L. (2008). Sleep-disordered breathing and cardiovascular disease in the Bay Area Sleep Cohort. *Sleep, 31*(4), 563–568.

Eser, I., Khorshid, L., & Cinar, S. (2007). Sleep quality of older adults in nursing homes in Turkey: Enhancing the quality of sleep improves quality of life. *Journal of Gerontological Nursing, 33*(10), 42–49.

Floyd, J. A. (2002). Sleep and aging. *Nursing Clinics of North America, 37*(4), 719–731.

Goodwin, F. K., & Redfield, K. R. (2007). *Manic-depressive illness: Bipolar disorders and recurrent illness* (2nd ed.). New York: Oxford University Press.

Gurvich, T., & Cunningham, J. A. (2000). Appropriate use of psychotropic drugs in nursing homes. *American Family Physician, 61*(5), 1437–1446.

Henning, W. A., Allen, R. P., Earley, C. J., Piccietti, D. L., & Silber, M. H. (2004). An update on the dopaminergic treatment of restless legs syndrome and periodic limb movement disorder. *Sleep, 27*(3), 560–583.

Hoffman, S. (2003). Sleep in the older adult: Implications for nurses. *Geriatric Nursing, 24*, 210–214.

Humm, C. (2005). In the dark. *Nursing Standard, 19*(24), 20–21.

Humm, C. (2009). Occupational hazard: working nights can seriously damage your health—in fact it has now been classified as a carcinogen. *Nursing Standard, 23*(20), 20.

James, S. P., & Mendelson, W. B. (2004). The use of trazodone as a hypnotic: A critical review. *Journal of Clinical Psychiatry, 65*(6), 752–755.

King, A., Oman, R., Brassington, G., Bliwise, D., & Haskell, W. (1997). Moderate-intensity exercise and self-rated quality of sleep in older adults: A randomized controlled trial. *JAMA, 277*(1), 32–37.

Kuehn, B. M. (2005). FDA warns that antipsychotic drugs are risky for elders. *JAMA, 293,* 2462.

Lee, K. A., & Ward, T. M. (2005). Critical components of a sleep assessment for clinical practice settings. *Issues in Mental Health Nursing, 26*(7), 739–750.

Littner, M. R., Kushida, C., Anderson, W. M., Bailey, D., Berry, R. B., Hirshkowitz, M., et al. (2004). Practice parameters for the dopaminergic treatment of restless legs syndrome and periodic limb movement disorder. *Sleep, 27*(3), 557–559.

Lopez-Jimenez, F., & Somers, V. K. (2006). Stress measures linking sleep apnea, hypertension and diabetes: AHI vs arousals vs hypoxemia. *Sleep, 29*(6), 743–744.

Lund, I., Yu, L. C., Uvnas-Moberg, K., Wang, J., Yu, C., Kurosawa, M., et al. (2002). Repeated massage-like stimulation induces long-term effects on nociception: Contribution of oxytocinergic mechanisms. *European Journal of Neuroscience, 16,* 330–338.

Marcus, M. B. (2009). Economy doing a number on people's sleep. Retrieved March 3, 2009, from http://www.usatoday.com/news/health/2009-03-01-sleep-economy_N.htm

Marshall, N. S., Wong, K. H., Liu, P. Y., Cullen S., Knuiman, M. W., & Grunstein, R. R. (2008). Sleep apnea as an independent risk factor for all-cause mortality: The Busselton Health Study. *Sleep, 31*(8), 1079–1085.

Minnick, M. E. (2003). Restless legs syndrome: Recognition and management in primary care. *Advance for Nurse Practitioners, 11*(3), 71–75.

Montgomery, P., & Dennis, J. (2003). Physical exercise for sleep problems in adults aged 60+ (Cochrane Review). *The Cochrane Library, 3.* Retrieved February 8, 2004, from http://www.update-software.com/abstract/ab003404.htm

Morgan, K. (2003). Daytime activity and risk factors for late-life insomnia. *Journal of Sleep Research, 12,* 231–238.

Morganthaler, T. I., Kapen, S., Chiong, T. L., Allessi, C., Boehlecke, B., Brown, T., et al. (2006). Practice parameters for the medical therapy of obstructive sleep apnea. *Sleep, 29*(8), 1031–1035.

Morganthaler, T., Kramer, M., Alessi, C., Friedman, L., Boehlecke, B., Brown, T., et al. (2006). Practice parameters for the psychological and behavioral treatment of insomnia: An update. An American Academy of Sleep Medicine Report. *Sleep, 29*(11), 1415–1419.

Morin, C., Rodrigue, S., & Ivers, H. (2003). Role of stress, arousal, and coping skills in primary insomnia. *Psychosomatic Medicine, 65,* 259–267.

National Center on Sleep Disorder Research. (2009). *Restless leg syndrome/periodic limb movement disorder.* Retrieved May 10, 2009, from http://www.nhlbi.nih.gov/health/prof/sleep/res_plan/section5/section5d.html

National Institute on Aging. (2001). *Exercise: A guide from the National Institute on Aging.* Retrieved February 2004, from http://www.nia.nih.gov/exercisebook//

National Sleep Foundation. (2003). *Sleep poll in America 2003: Sleep and aging.* Retrieved July 2009, from http://www.sleepfoundation.org/article/sleep-america-polls/2003-sleep-and-aging

National Sleep Foundation. (2009). Sleep and aging. Retrieved January, 2009, from http://www.sleepfoundation.org/site/apps/nlnet/content2.aspx?c=huIXKjM0IxF&b=4821453&ct=6426833

NIH State-of-the-Science Conference Statement on manifestations and management of chronic insomnia in adults. *NIH Consensus of the State of the Science Statements 2005 June 13–15. 22*(2), 1–30.

Ohayan, M. M., & Roth, T. (2002). Prevalence of restless leg syndrome and periodic limb movement disorder in the general population. *Journal of Psychosomatic Research, 53,* 547–545.

Ohayon, M. M., & Vecchierini, M. F. (2005). Normative sleep data, cognitive function and daily living activities in older adults in the community. *Sleep, 28*(8), 981–989.

Paine, S. J., Gander, P. H., Harris, R., & Reid, P. (2004). Who reports insomnia? Relationships with age, sex, ethnicity, and socioeconomic deprivation. *Sleep, 27*(6), 1163–1169.

Penninx, B. W., Rejeski, W. J., Pandya, J., Miller, M. E., Di Bari, M., Applegate, W. B., et al. (2002). Exercise and depressive symptoms: A comparison of aerobic and resistance exercise effects on emotional and physical function in older persons with high and low depressive symptomatology. *Journals of Gerontology, 57B,* 124–132.

Perlis, M. L., Smith, M. T., & Jungquist, C. (2005). *Cognitive behavioral treatment of insomnia.* New York: Springer-Verlag.

Piggins, H. D. (2002). Human clock genes. *Annals of Medicine, 34,* 394–400.

Raji, M. A., & Brady, S. R. (2001). Mirtazapine for treatment of depression and comorbidities in Alzheimer's disease. *Annals of Pharmacotherapy, 35*(9), 1024–1027.

Richardson, S. (2003). Effects of relaxation and imagery on the sleep of critically ill adults. *Dimensions of Critical Care Nursing, 22*(4), 182–190.

Riemersma-van der Lek, B. A., Swaab, D. F., Twisk, J., Hol, E. M., Hoogendijk, W. J., & Van Someren, E. J. (2008). Effect of bright light and melatonin on cognitive and noncognitive function in elderly residents of group care facilities: A randomized controlled trial. *JAMA, 299*(22), 2642–2655.

Rothdach, A. J., Trenkwalder, C., Haberstock, J., Keil, U., & Gerger, K. (2000). Prevalence and risk factors of RLS in an elderly population: The MEMO study. *Neurology, 54*(5), 1064–1068.

Sack, R. L., Brandes, R. W., Kendall, A. R., & Lewy, A. J. (2000). Entrainment of free-running circadian rhythms by melatonin in blind people. *New England Journal of Medicine, 343*, 1070–1077.

Saletu-Zyhlarz, G. M., Abu-Bakr, M. H., Anderer, P., Gruber, G., Mandl, M., Strobl, R., et al. (2002). Insomnia in depression: Differences in objective and subjective sleep and awakening quality to normal controls and acute effects of trazodone. *Progress in Neuropsychopharmacology Biology Psychiatry, 26*(2), 249–260.

Scott, G. N., & Elmer, G. W. (2002). Update on natural product: drug interactions. *American Journal of Health Systems Pharmacology, 59*(4), 339–347.

Semla, T. P., Higbee, M. D., & Beizer, J. L. (2009). *Lexi-Comp's geriatric dosage handbook: Monitoring, clinical recommendations, and OBRA guidelines* (14th ed.). Hudson, OH: Lexicom.

Spielman, A. J., Caruso, L. S., & Glovinsky, P. B. (1987). A behavioral perspective on insomnia treatment. *Psychiatric Clinics of North America, 10*, 541–553.

Straif, K. (2007). Carcinogenicity of shift work, painting and fire-fighting. *Lancet Oncology, 8*(12), 1065–1066.

Takeda Pharmaceuticals America. (2005). Rozerem prescribing information. Lincolnshire, IL: Author.

Thomson Healthcare. (2007). *PDR for herbal medicines* (4th ed.). Montvale, NJ: Thomson Healthcare.

Thorpe, L., Middleton, J., Russell, G., & Stewart, N. (2000). Bright light therapy for demented nursing home patients with behavioral disturbance. *American Journal of Alzheimer's Disease and Other Dementias, 15*(1), 18–26.

Van Cauter, E. (2000). Slow wave sleep and release of growth hormone. *JAMA, 284*(21), 2717–2718.

Van Tulder, M., Malmivaara, A., Esmall, R., & Koes, B. (2003). Exercise therapy for low back pain (Cochrane Review). *The Cochrane Library, 3.* Retrieved February 2004, from http://www.update-software.com/abstract/ab000335.htm

Vgontzas, A. N., & Kales, A. (1999). Sleep and its disorders. *Annual Review of Medicine, 50*, 387–400.

Wang, P., Bohn, R., Glynn, R., Mogun, H., & Avorn, J. (2001). Hazardous benzodiazepine regimens in the elderly: Effects of half life dosage and duration on risk of hip fracture. *American Journal of Psychiatry, 158*, 892–898.

Williamson, A., Fletcher, P., & Dawson, E. (2003). Complementary and alternative medicine. Use in an older population. *Journal of Gerontological Nursing, 29*(2), 20–28.

Wolsko, P., Eisenberg, D., Davis, R., Kessler, R., & Phillips, R. (2003). Patterns and perceptions of care for treatment of back and neck pain: Results of a national survey. *Spine, 28*, 292–297.

17

Pathological Gambling Among Older Adults

Cindy Sullivan Kerber

The expansion of legalized gambling, beginning in the mid-1970s, increased gambling opportunities across the nation, with the most dramatic change in frequency of gambling observed in the growing older adult population. Research indicates that visits to casinos by older adults have doubled since 1975 (American Gaming Association, 2001). Increased access to gambling venues has had a greater impact on the frequency of gambling. The National Opinion Research Center (NORC) indicates that more people gamble today than in the past (NORC, 1999). As adults reach retirement age, they generally have more time for leisure and social activities, and the potential for gambling-related problems consequently becomes greater (Gosker, 1999). Problems related to gambling may be alleviated by primary care psychiatric assessment that differentiates between recreational and problem gambling behaviors, and by educating older adults and care providers, such as activity directors at senior centers.

Gambling can be an innocent recreational activity for many individuals. However, as the availability of gambling opportunities has increased, so too have the problems associated with excessive or compulsive gambling. When gambling becomes more than an occasional entertainment option (Lucke & Wallace, 2006; NORC, 1999; Shaw, Forbush, Schlinder, Rosenman, & Black, 2007) problems arise, resulting in increased stress, financial strains, disagreements with family, trouble at work, and legal difficulties. Unlike problem gambling, recreational gambling may not be associated with problems in older adults. In fact, older adult recreational gamblers report better health than nongamblers even though they have similar levels of chronic illness (Desai, Desai, & Potenza, 2007). For some, however, gambling becomes a compulsive, pathological behavior. The transition between recreational gambling and problem gambling can be difficult to detect.

PREVALENCE OF PATHOLOGICAL GAMBLING

Prevalence studies for pathological gambling began in the 1970s as an increasing number of states legalized gambling. In 1998, a project requested by the National Gambling Impact Study Commission used the NORC screen (NORC/DSM-IV, NODS) to study the prevalence of pathological gambling in the United States. Eighty-six percent of U.S. citizens had gambled at some time in their lives, with 63% reporting that they had gambled in the past year. Using the NODS in a telephone interview, researchers recorded that 0.8% of interviewees scored in the pathological gambler range (NORC, 1999). Welte, Barnes, Wieczorek, Tidwell, and Parker (2001) conducted a telephone survey using both the NODS and the South Oaks Gambling Screen (SOGS). Scores consistent with pathological gambling were identified in 1.9% of respondents.

In his critique of epidemiological studies, Lesieur (1994) argues that research studies had underestimated the incidence of problem and pathological gambling. Concerned that these studies were not comprehensive, he stated that supplemental surveys were needed to obtain data from inpatient and intensive outpatient treatment programs and from prison and jail populations. Lesieur also pointed out that military personnel and the homeless had been excluded from epidemiological studies. The exclusion of these high-risk populations, he argued, had led to an underestimation of the proportion of the population that may be problem or pathological gamblers. This argument is supported by Lepage, Ladouceur, and Jacque (2000), who found that 17.2% of individuals who relied on a community agency for food, material assistance, or lodging scored in the pathological gambling range on the SOGS.

PATHOLOGICAL GAMBLING AMONG OLDER ADULTS

No age group is immune to problem gambling, but older adults seem to be among the most vulnerable. A national study of older adults (Welte et al., 2001) found that 1.2% of older adults over age 60 have current problem or pathological gambling. Regional studies found even higher rates. Researchers from the University of Nebraska (McNeilly & Burke, 2001) studied 315 older adults from gambling venues and within the community. Older adults at casinos were more likely to have gambling problems (17%) than those surveyed in the community (4%). Older adults cited relaxation,

boredom, passing time, and getting away for the day as motivations for gambling. Bazargan, Bazargan, and Akanda (2000) studied 80 older adults living independently at two senior citizen centers that provide inexpensive or free trips to gambling sites. They found 17% of the older adult population to be heavy to pathological gamblers, 19% to be light to moderate gamblers, and 64% to be nongamblers or occasional gamblers.

As the prevalence of older adult gambling increases, the problems associated with excessive gambling also increase. According to NORC (1999), gamblers' bets increase with age. Older adults with retirement money, some with lump-sum amounts, are vulnerable to gambling. Casinos market to senior centers near the third of the month, when seniors receive their Social Security checks (Gosker, 1999). They entice older adults by offering affordable trips, free drinks, meal tokens, and medication discounts. Trips to casinos have become popular day trips for senior centers. Stewart and Oslin (2001) found that 65% of losses in Atlantic City casinos were incurred by older adults.

Several factors increase risks of problem gambling for older adults. A study by Burge, Pietrzak, Molina, and Petry (2004) found that individuals who began gambling earlier in life, compared with late-onset gambling, gambled more frequently and were at greater risk for psychiatric and medical problems later in life. Preston, Shapiro, and Keene (2007) found that older adults who gambled as a primary form of recreation were four times more likely to have gambling problems, and those who played video poker were twice as likely to be at risk. Zaranek and Chapleski (2005), in their study of 1410 community-dwelling adults age 60 and older, found that those who visited a casino more than once a month were more likely to report poorer mental health, lower incomes, and social support.

Wiebe and Cox (2005) telephone-interviewed 1000 adults age 60 and older to determine prevalence of gambling problems and sociodemographic gambling patterns. Of those interviewed, 75% had gambled in the past year. Only 2.8% scored in the problem and pathological gambling range. These researchers cite underendorsement as a concern because "lying about gambling" is a diagnostic criterion. Sociodemographic characteristics indicate those with SOGS scores of 5 or more were most often smokers. Also, there is a threefold increase in gambling problems for older adults who spend more than 1 hour a week gambling.

ASSESSMENT AND DIAGNOSIS OF PATHOLOGICAL GAMBLING IN THE GENERAL POPULATION

There is an urgent need to increase clinicians' awareness of the prevalence, diagnosis, healthcare concerns, and treatment for patients with pathological gambling (Petry & Armentano, 1999). For comprehensive assessment of problem gambling behaviors, SOGS is most often used (Figure 17-1). SOGS, developed in the 1980s and revised in 1993 (Lesieur & Blume, 1993), has been the primary tool for screening problem and pathological gambling. It is a valid and reliable 20-item screen that has been used in various studies, including epidemiological studies in the United States and Canada. Wiebe and Cox (2005) examined the frequency of items endorsed by older adults on the SOGS. Of the criteria, "missed work to gamble" was rarely endorsed, which is typical of a mostly retired population. Refinement of this tool to more closely address the older adult would be beneficial because there are no tools specifically designed to screen older adults. The three most commonly endorsed behaviors are gambling more than intended, trying to win back lost money, and guilt related to gambling.

NODS is also a comprehensive assessment (Gerstein et al., 1999; Toce-Gerstein, Gerstein, & Volberg, 2003) (Figure 17-2). It is a shorter instrument and was developed to reflect closely the *Diagnostic and Statistical Manual of Mental Disorders-IV* (DSM-IV) criteria. According to the DSM-IV-TR (American Psychiatric Association [APA], 2000), the diagnosis of pathological gambling is an illness within the category of impulse-control disorders and is based on the following 10

criteria. A pathological gambler has persistent and recurrent maladaptive gambling behavior as indicated by five or more of these criteria (APA, 2000, p. 674):

- Is preoccupied with gambling (e.g., preoccupied with reliving past gambling experiences, handicapping or planning the next venture, or thinking of ways to get money with which to gamble)
- Needs to gamble with increasing amounts of money in order to achieve the desired excitement
- Has repeated unsuccessful efforts to control, cut down, or stop gambling
- Is restless or irritable when attempting to cut down or stop gambling
- Gambles as a way of escaping from problems or of relieving a dysphoric mood (e.g., feelings of helplessness, guilt, anxiety, depression)
- After losing money gambling, often returns another day to get even ("chasing" one's losses)
- Lies to family members, therapists, or others to conceal the extent of involvement with gambling
- Has committed illegal acts such as forgery, fraud, theft, or embezzlement to finance gambling
- Has jeopardized or lost a significant relationship, job, or educational or career opportunity because of gambling
- Relies on others to provide money to relieve a desperate financial situation caused by gambling.

ASSESSMENT AND DIAGNOSIS OF PATHOLOGICAL GAMBLING AMONG OLDER ADULTS

Older adults tend not to seek help for addictions in behavioral health settings (Stewart & Oslin, 2001). Therefore, Unwin, Davis, and De Leeuw (2000) recommend screening patients for pathological gambling especially when financial problems, alcoholism, or depression are present. A method of assessment recommended by Potenza et al. (2002) suggests that practitioners ease into the assessment by identifying gambling as a common

---

FIGURE 17-1

Assessment of Pathological Gambling: South Oaks Gambling Screen

---

This is a questionnaire about types of gambling, the incidence of gambling and related behaviors. Please answer each item as it relates to you. Thank you.

1. Please indicate which of the following types of gambling you have done in your lifetime. For each type, mark one answer: "not at all," "less than once a week," or "once a week or more."

	Not at all	Less than once a week	Once a week or more	
a.	❏	❏	❏	play cards for money
b.	❏	❏	❏	bet on horses, dogs, or other animals (at OTB, at the track, or with a bookie)
c.	❏	❏	❏	bet on sports (parlay cards, with a bookie, or at jai alai)
d.	❏	❏	❏	played dice games (including craps, over and under, or other dice games) for money
e.	❏	❏	❏	gambled in a casino (legal or otherwise)
f.	❏	❏	❏	played the numbers or bet on lotteries
g.	❏	❏	❏	played bingo for money
h.	❏	❏	❏	played the stock, options and/or commodities market
i.	❏	❏	❏	played slot machines, poker machines, or other gambling machines
j.	❏	❏	❏	bowled, shot pool, played golf, or played some other game of skill for money
k.	❏	❏	❏	pull tabs or "paper" games other than lotteries
l.	❏	❏	❏	gambled on internet
m.	❏	❏	❏	some form of gambling not listed above (please specify) _____

2. What is the largest amount of money you have ever gambled with on any one day?
   ❏ never have gambled
   ❏ $1 or less
   ❏ more than $1 up to $10
   ❏ more than $10 up to $100
   ❏ more than $100 up to $1000
   ❏ more than $1000 up to $10,000
   ❏ more than $10,000

FIGURE 17-1

Assessment of Pathological Gambling: South Oaks Gambling Screen *(continued)*

3. Check which of the following people in your life has (or had) a gambling problem.
   ❏ father ❏ mother ❏ brother or sister ❏ grandparent
   ❏ my spouse/partner ❏ my children ❏ another relative
   ❏ a friend or someone else important in my life ❏ does not apply

4. When you gamble, how often do you go back another day to win back money you lost?
   ❏ never
   ❏ some of the time (less than half the time) I lost
   ❏ most of the time I lost
   ❏ every time I lost

5. Have you ever claimed to be winning money gambling but weren't really? In fact, you lost?
   ❏ never (or never gamble)
   ❏ yes, less than half the time I lost
   ❏ yes, most of the time

6. Do you feel you have ever had a problem with betting money or gambling?
   ❏ no
   ❏ yes, in the past, but not now
   ❏ yes

CIRCLE YES OR NO FOR EACH OF THE FOLLOWING:

7. Did you ever gamble more than you intended to?
   yes   no

8. Have people criticized your betting or told you that you had a gambling problem, regardless of whether or not you thought it was true?
   yes   no

9. Have you ever felt guilty about the way you gamble or what happens when you gamble?
   yes   no

10. Have you ever felt like you would like to stop betting money or gambling but didn't think you could?
    yes   no

(continues)

FIGURE 17-1

Assessment of Pathological Gambling: South Oaks Gambling Screen *(continued)*

---

11. Have you ever hidden betting slips, lottery tickets, gambling money, I.O.U.s or other signs of betting or gambling from your spouse, children, or other important people in your life?

    yes   no

12. Have you ever argued with people you live with over how you handle money?

    yes   no

13. (If you answered yes to question 12): Have money arguments ever centered on your gambling?

    yes   no

14. Have you ever borrowed from someone and not paid them back as a result of your gambling?

    yes   no

15. Have you ever lost time from work (or school) due to betting money or gambling?

    yes   no

16. If you borrowed money to gamble or to pay gambling debts, who or where did you borrow from? (check "yes" or "no" for each)

	No	Yes
a. from household money	❑	❑
b. from your spouse	❑	❑
c. from other relatives or in-laws	❑	❑
d. from banks, loan companies, or credit unions	❑	❑
e. from credit cards	❑	❑
f. from loan sharks	❑	❑
g. you cashed in stocks, bonds, or other securities	❑	❑
h. you sold personal or family property	❑	❑
i. you borrowed on your checking account (passed bad checks)	❑	❑
j. you have (had) a credit line with a bookie	❑	❑
k. you have (had) a credit line with a casino	❑	❑

17. About how much money do you owe which is possibly a result of gambling? _____

18. At what age did you first gamble? _____

FIGURE 17–1

Assessment of Pathological Gambling: South Oaks Gambling Screen *(continued)*

South Oaks Gambling Screen Score Sheet
Scores on the SOGS itself are determined by adding up the number of questions which show an "at risk" response:

Questions 1, 2, & 3 not counted:
- ❏ Question 4 —most of the time I lose or every time I lose
- ❏ Question 5 — yes, less than half the time I lose or yes, most of the time
- ❏ Question 6 — yes, in the past but not now or yes
- ❏ Question 7 — yes
- ❏ Question 8 —yes
- ❏ Question 9 — yes
- ❏ Question 10 — yes
- ❏ Question 11 — yes

Question 12 not counted
- ❏ Question 13 — yes
- ❏ Question 14 — yes
- ❏ Question 15 — yes
- ❏ Question 16a — yes
- ❏ Question b — yes
- ❏ Question c — yes
- ❏ Question d — yes
- ❏ Question e — yes
- ❏ Question f — yes
- ❏ Question g — yes
- ❏ Question h — yes
- ❏ Question i — yes

Question 16j & k not counted

_____ Total (there are 20 questions which are counted)

0 = no problem

3–4 = some problem

5 or more = probable pathological gambler

Source: Lesieur, H. R., & Blume, S. B. (1993). Revising the South Oaks Gambling Screen in a different setting. *Journal of Gambling Studies, 9*, 213–223. Reprinted with permission.

> **FIGURE 17-2**

The NORC Diagnostic Screen for Gambling Problems

INSTRUCTIONS: For each question asked, circle YES or NO. When interview is complete, for questions for which R said YES, mark the corresponding box in the right-hand margin, ignoring items that do not have a corresponding box. Add up the number of marked boxes to determine R's score. A score of 0 indicates that results are not consistent with problematic levels of gambling. A score of 1 or 2 means that results are consistent with mild but subclinical risk for gambling problems. A score of 3 or 4 indicates results are consistent with moderate but subclinical gambling problems. A score of 5 or higher means that results are consistent with a likely diagnosis of pathological gambling, consistent with the diagnostic criteria of the DSM-IV. The highest score possible is 10.

1. Have there ever been periods lasting 2 weeks or longer when you spent a lot of time thinking about your gambling experiences, or planning out future gambling ventures or bets?
   ❑ yes   SKIP TO 3   1 ❑
   ❑ no   GO TO 2

2. Have there ever been periods lasting 2 weeks or longer when you spent a lot of time thinking about ways of getting money to gamble with?
   ❑ yes   2 ❑
   ❑ no

3. Have there ever been periods when you needed to gamble with increasing amounts of money or with larger bets than before in order to get the same feeling of excitement?
   ❑ yes   3 ❑
   ❑ no

4. Have you ever tried to stop, cut down, or control your gambling?
   ❑ yes   GO TO 5
   ❑ no   SKIP TO 8

5. On one or more of the times when you tried to stop, cut down, or control your gambling, were you restless or irritable?
   ❑ yes   5 ❑
   ❑ no

6. Have you ever tried *but not succeeded* in stopping, cutting down, or controlling your gambling?
   ❑ yes   GO TO 7
   ❑ no   SKIP TO 8

7. Has this happened three or more times?
   ❑ yes   7 ❑
   ❑ no

8. Have you ever gambled to relieve uncomfortable feelings such as guilt, anxiety, helplessness, or depression?
   ❑ yes   SKIP TO 10   8 ❑
   ❑ no   GO TO 9

FIGURE 17-2

The NORC Diagnostic Screen for Gambling Problems (continued)

9. Have you ever gambled as a way to escape from personal problems?
   ❑ yes
   ❑ no   9 ❑

10. Has there ever been a period when, if you lost money gambling one day, you would often return another day to get even?
    ❑ yes
    ❑ no   10 ❑

11. Have you ever lied to family members, friends, or others about how much you gamble or how much money you lost on gambling?
    ❑ yes   GO TO 12
    ❑ no   SKIP TO 13

12. Has this happened three or more times?
    ❑ yes
    ❑ no   12 ❑

13. Have you ever written a bad check or taken money that didn't belong to you from family members or anyone else in order to pay for your gambling?
    ❑ yes
    ❑ no   13 ❑

14. Has your gambling ever caused serious or repeated problems in your relationships with any of your family members or friends?
    ❑ yes   SKIP TO 17
    ❑ no   GO TO 15   14 ❑

15. Has your gambling ever caused you any problems in school, such as missing classes or days of school or your grades dropping?
    ❑ yes   SKIP TO 17
    ❑ no   GO TO 16   15 ❑

16. Has your gambling ever caused you to lose a job, have trouble with your job, or miss out on an important job or career opportunity?
    ❑ yes
    ❑ no   16 ❑

17. Have you ever needed to ask family members or anyone else to loan you money or otherwise bail you out of a desperate money situation that was largely caused by your gambling?
    ❑ yes
    ❑ no   17 ❑

Source: Gerstein, D., Volberg, R., Toce, M., Harwood, H., Johnson, R., Buie, T., et al. (1999). *Gambling Impact and Behavior Study: Report to the National Gambling Impact Study Commission*. Chicago: National Opinion Research Center. The NORC NODS instrument is in the public domain.

recreational activity. Then, they should follow up with a conversation that identifies a potential correlation between gambling and health problems, identifies a concern for the individual's health, and avoids labeling. Older adults may not recognize gambling activities as problematic, and if they do they may feel shame. Stewart and Oslin (2001) suggest a direct approach of asking clients, such as, "What type of gambling do you do?" If the patient offers information about gambling behaviors, they suggest following this with the Lie/Bet questionnaire (Johnson, Hamer, Nora, & Tan, 1997), which consists of two questions: (1) Have you ever had to lie to people important to you about how much you gamble?; and (2) Have you ever felt the need to bet more and more money?

This two-question screen has shown both sensitivity and specificity in identifying pathological gamblers. If a client answers yes to either of the Lie/Bet questions, Stewart and Oslin (2001) recommend that practitioners follow with a review of the DSM-IV criteria for verification of the diagnosis. The pathological gambling diagnostic screens (SOGS, NODS, and Lie/Bet), although not designed specifically for older adults, are considered tools of choice for the adult population in general (Johnson et al., 1997).

A study by Volberg (2003) of gambling and problem gambling among seniors in Florida sought to improve methods to identify older adults with problem gambling behaviors. Two topics to assess, which were endorsed by 95% of older adults who identified any gambling problem, were borrowing from or using credit cards to gamble and experiencing feelings of shame related to gambling. Older adults who gamble are at higher risk for depression and suicide compared to other age groups (McKeown, Cuffe, & Schulz, 2006). Because problem gambling behavior will likely increase suicide risk, assessment of older adult gamblers for suicide risk is vital.

Mental health concerns, such as anxiety, distractibility, increased isolation, and depressed mood, are common psychological signs of pathological gambling. Problem and pathological gambling is often comorbid with other mental illnesses. Kerber, Black, and Buckwalter (2008), in a sample of 40 recovering pathological gamblers, found 82.5% experience an Axis I disorder with depression, alcohol dependence, panic, and generalized anxiety disorder being among the most common. In addition, 60% experienced personality disorders with obsessive-compulsive, avoidant, and depressive being most common. Black and Moyer (1998), in their study of 30 individuals with pathological gambling, found a lower prevalence of lifetime mood disorders (60%) and a higher percentage of personality disorders (87%). They found obsessive–compulsive and avoidant to be among the most common. Their study also found higher prevalence of schizotypal and paranoid personality disorders. In addition, other impulse-control disorders, such as compulsive shopping and sexual behavior, were common.

Older adults should also be assessed for gambling problems when taking medication for restless leg syndrome and Parkinson's disease. Pathological gambling and other impulse control disorders, such as sexual addiction and compulsive shopping, have been reported to be associated with use of dopaminergic drugs (Burn & Troster, 2004). These effects are potentially reversible with discontinuation of the medication. Dodd et al. (2005) cited that the selective dopamine D_3 agonist pramipexole (Mirapex) was most often implicated.

THERAPEUTIC NURSING INTERVENTIONS FOR PROBLEM AND PATHOLOGICAL GAMBLING

Limited research has been done to identify specific treatments for problem and pathological gambling. However, as the number of pathological gamblers has increased, so has interest in how best to treat this illness. Outpatient treatment, through counseling and Gamblers Anonymous (GA), is the most common treatment (NORC, 1999) although other approaches, including individual and group therapy, support groups, and pharmacotherapy, have been used to treat problem and pathological gambling. Only a few studies have evaluated the effectiveness of treatments, and none has focused specifically on older adults.

Support Groups

The support group for people with gambling pathology is GA (1998). Advanced practice nurses should provide information about GA support groups and availability of meetings for their patients. Contact information is available on the GA Web site (http://www.gamblersanonymous. org). The information provided includes a meeting directory icon listing meetings by state. GA, like Alcoholics Anonymous, uses a 12-step program and supports abstinence as a means to recovery. Nurses can refer patients to GA and their family members to Gam-Anon and Gam-A-Teen. GA is free, and evidence-based outcomes were better for GA members than for those participating in cognitive behavioral therapy (Leung & Cottler, 2009).

Indications for Pharmacological Therapies

There are only a few pharmacological studies of pathological gambling, with no studies focused specifically on older adults. Leung and Cottler (2009) found mood stabilizers and opiate antagonists have been used to treat pathological gambling in their review of recent gambling studies. For example, in a double-blind study of 77 pathological gamblers, naltrexone (Narcan) was found to significantly reduce gambling urges and euphoria associated with gambling over placebo (Grant, Kim, & Hartman, 2008). Black, Shaw, and Allen (2008) in an open clinical trial of carbamazepine (Tegretol) found a decrease in gambling urges and behaviors, such as time spent gambling, money lost, and urges to gamble. Topiramate (Topamax), lithium carbonate (Eskalith), and valproate (Depakote) were found to alleviate gambling problems at a rate similar to fluvoxamine (Luvox) and significantly more than placebo group (Leung & Cottler).

Zimmerman, Breen, and Posternak (2002) found that gamblers both with and without major depressive disorder responded to citalopram (Celexa). Black (2004) gave bupropion (Wellbutrin) to 10 persons with pathological gambling. Seven were judged to have had much or very much improvement, indicating that their gambling behavior was significantly better controlled. In contrast, olanzapine (Zyprexa), a second-generation, atypical antipsychotic approved to treat mood disorders, was found to be no more effective than placebo, and haloperidol (Haldol), an older antipsychotic, may actually increase desire to gamble (Leung & Cottler, 2009).

Counseling

Individual or group counseling can be of help to those with gambling problems. Most counselors recommend combining counseling with enrollment in GA. Interventions for pathological gambling, such as relapse prevention, problem solving, and social skill training, are common to both pathological gambling and other addictions (Tavares, Zilberman, & el-Guebaly, 2003). Most common methods of maintaining abstinence cited by greater than one half of problem gamblers was to participate in a different activity and recall problems associated with gambling. Other, less frequently, endorsed techniques are sense of pride over not gambling, social support, and cognitive strategies (Petry, 2005).

Psychotherapy techniques specific to pathological gambling should address cognitive distortions. Gamblers believe that their actions, betting choices, or personal attributes are likely to influence outcomes. Individual counseling aims to help the client identify irrational, fantasy-based ways of thinking about gambling, and then replace those beliefs with a realistic understanding of the randomness, unpredictability, and independence of events that could change the lifestyle of the gambler (Ladouceur, Sylvain, Boutin, & Doucet, 2002). Cue exposure, whether in vivo or imagined, may help clients deal with gambling triggers (Tavares et al., 2003). In the elderly population it is important to differentiate the altered cognitions seen in pathological gambling from other mental conditions, such as depression and dementia.

Ideally, a pathological gambler should be treated by an advanced practice nurse or counselor who is certified to treat gambling problems. The National Council on Problem Gambling (NCPG) offers certification for training and 2000 hours of supervised clinical practice (NORC, 1999). The NCPG Web site (http://www.ncpgambling.org) offers information about how to identify and treat gambling problems. They also offer a certification program for counselors wishing to specialize in the treatment of pathological gambling. Certified counselors can be found at the NCPG Web site by city and state.

Alternative Therapies

Natural recovery from addictive disorders is becoming increasingly recognized as a common occurrence (McCartney, 1996). Hodgins and el-Guebaly (2000) compared natural and treatment-assisted recovery from gambling problems among resolved and active gamblers. They speculated that because natural recovery can occur from alcohol problems and most smokers quit on their own, a natural recovery phenomenon also may occur with gambling. They cited two major reasons for quitting: negative emotions (e.g., anxiety, depression, and guilt) and financial constraints. The two actions taken by the natural recovery group were stimulus control (avoiding gambling activities and advertisements) and new activities to replace gambling.

Education

Education about the risks of gambling is highly recommended for older adults given the reported risk of addiction (American Gaming Association, 2001; Higgins, 2001). An educational program for seniors should identify recreational gambling as an activity that may lead to gambling problems. An older adult member of a local GA group can offer valuable information to residents and a personal contact to meetings. Common problems for older adults are spending more than intended, feelings

of guilt, credit card debt, and lying to others about gambling. Copies of the SOGS with a self-scoring sheet are available online at: http://www.stopgamblingnow.com/sogs_print.htm. Local GA meetings can be found online or by calling a local addiction treatment center. Higgins recommends a gambling education program for seniors, especially those living in residential communities. She also recommends peers to serve as mentors on gambling trips sponsored by senior centers.

EVALUATION OF TREATMENT EFFECTIVENESS WITH FOLLOW-UP

Treatment effectiveness can be measured by the following outcomes (Blaszczynski & Silove, 1995). If treatment is effective, the client

■ Avoids exposure to gambling cues, situations, and other gamblers
■ Participates in stress management or relaxation training if coping with stress by gambling
■ Seeks treatment if dysphoric or depressed through counseling and/or antidepressants
■ Challenges false beliefs, attitudes, and expectations regarding gambling
■ Participates in marriage or family counseling to reestablish trust between partners
■ Accepts financial responsibility to meet financial obligations without gambling
■ Develops nongambling leisure activities
■ Addresses addiction to alcohol or other drugs if present
■ Attends GA meetings and spouse or significant other attends GamAnon meetings.

RELATED ISSUES PERTAINING TO PROBLEM AND PATHOLOGICAL GAMBLING IN OLDER ADULTS

The increased use of computers and Internet services by older adults has introduced a newer type of gambling. Internet gambling is available to those who want to place a bet without leaving home. Online gambling offers unprecedented access, and individuals are lured to "just play for fun" initially. Pop-up advertisements then encourage "playing for real," which requires only a credit card number. The companies running gambling Web sites are based outside the United States, therefore avoiding the illegalities of their operation (Tresniowski et al., 2003).

Trips to casinos seem to be affordable and especially enticing to those on a fixed income, but this form of recreation is not without risk. These outings are popular offsite activities for those attending senior centers (McNeilly & Burke, 2001). They provide a day out, socialization, reasonably priced meals, and a chance to win money. Older adults cited motivations for gambling as relaxation, escaping boredom, passing time, and getting away for the day (McNeilly & Burke). Activity directors at senior centers may encourage residents to attend for the social benefit and to obtain a reasonably priced meal. In addition, some casinos provide bus service if there are enough individuals to fill the bus, so an added benefit is that there may be no financial obligation from the senior center. However, the risks may easily outweigh the benefits at several levels. Individuals at senior centers most likely do not know where to go for help, how to identify problems, or what treatments are available to treat gambling problems. Senior centers may be at risk for sending residents into an environment to participate in a potentially addictive activity. If a resident loses large sums of money on center-sponsored trips, family members may consider the center responsible for the residents' losses. These centers are not likely to have an outing to the local tavern and would not take a known alcoholic to a bar; however, they might not be aware that they are taking a problem or pathological gambler to the casino.

CASE STUDY

Meredith is almost 60 years old, a divorced patient with hypertension, obesity, and chronic pain, and a smoker. She tells you that she has withdrawn money from her retirement account to gamble, that there is no penalty to withdraw funds after age 59.5, and she has spent $84,000 in the past 4 months. She has $3000 remaining. She gambles nearly daily, sometimes over lunch. She is worried about losing her job. She tells you her mother died 3 weeks ago.

On examination, Meredith seems tired but neatly groomed. Her affect is blunted. Thoughts are logical but sometimes tangential. She wonders why she is not more upset over her mother's death. She denies current suicidal thoughts but follows that should she lose her job, she would not have a reason to live. What other assessment questions would you ask? What issue in the above scenario is of highest priority, and why?

SUMMARY

Given the increase in problem and pathological gambling, it is crucial for nurses to assess older adults for possible gambling problems and provide treatment for pathological gambling and comorbid illnesses. Treatment for pathological gambling is available from certified counselors and by attending GA meetings. For every older adult with gambling pathology, careful assessment for depression and for possible suicidal thoughts or plans is vital. Nurses in senior centers or faith-based and residential communities have an opportunity to communicate the risks and dangerous effects of gambling to older adults and recreational directors. Increased public awareness of the impact of pathological gambling on the individual and family must be communicated. In the future, community planning could focus on the development of more social alternatives for seniors.

REFERENCES

American Gaming Association. (2001). *State of the states: The AGA Survey of Casino Entertainment.* Washington, DC: Author.

American Psychiatric Association. (2000). *Diagnostic and statistical manual of mental disorders* (4th ed., Rev. ed.). Washington, DC: Author.

Bazargan, M., Bazargan, S., & Akanda, M. (2000). Gambling habits among aged African Americans. *Clinical Gerontologist, 22*(3/4), 51–62.

Black, D. W. (2004). An open-label trial of bupropion in the treatment of pathological gambling. *Journal of Clinical Psychopharmacology, 24,* 108–109.

Black, D. W., & Moyer, B. A. (1998). Clinical features and psychiatric comorbidity of subjects with pathological gambling behavior. *Psychiatric Services, 49*(11), 1434–1439.

Black, D. W., Shaw, M. C., & Allen, J. (2008). Extended release carbamazepine in the treatment of pathological gambling: An open-label study. *Progress in Neuro-Psychopharmacology & Biological Psychiatry, 32,* 1191–1194.

Blaszczynski, A., & Silove, D. (1995), Cognitive and behavioral therapies for pathological gambling. *Journal of Gambling Studies, 11,* 195–220.

Burge, B. N., Pietrzak, R. H., Molina, C. A., & Petry, N. M. (2004). Age of gambling initiation and severity of gambling and health problems among older adult problem gamblers. *Psychiatric Services, 55*(12), 1437–1439.

Burn, J. D., & Troster, A. I. (2004). Neuropsychiatric complications of medical and surgical therapies for Parkinson's disease. *Journal of Geriatric Psychiatry and Neurology, 17,* 172–180.

Desai, R. A., Desai, M. M., & Potenza, M. N. (2007). Gambling, health and age: Data from the national epidemiologic survey on alcohol and related conditions. *Psychology of Addictive Behaviors, 2*(4), 431–440.

Dodd, M. L., Klos, K. J., Bower, J. H., Geda, Y. E., Josephs, D. A., & Ahlskog, E. (2005). Pathological gambling caused by drugs used to treat Parkinson disease. *Archives of Neurology, 62,* 1377–1381.

Gamblers Anonymous. (1998). *Gamblers Anonymous: A new beginning.* Los Angeles: Gamblers Anonymous.

Gerstein, D., Volberg, R., Toce, M., Harwood, H., Johnson, R., Buie, T., et al. (1999). *Gambling impact and behavior study: Report to the National Gambling Impact Study Commission.* Chicago: National Opinion Research Center and partners. Retrieved July 12, 2004, from http://www.purl.oclc.org/norc/dlib/ngis.htm

Gosker, E. (1999). The marketing of gambling to the elderly. *The Elder Law Journal, 7,* 185–216.

Grant, J. E., Kim, S. W., & Hartman, B. K. (2008). A double-blind placebo-controlled study of the opiate antagonist naltrexone in the treatment of pathological gambling urges. *Journal of Clinical Psychiatry, 69,* 783–789.

Higgins, J. (2001). A comprehensive policy analysis of and recommendations for senior center gambling trips. *Journal of Aging & Social Policy, 12*(2), 73–91.

Hodgins, D. C., & el-Guebaly, N. (2000). Natural and treatment-assisted recovery from gambling problems: A comparison of resolved and active gamblers. *Addiction, 95*(5), 777–789.

Johnson, E. E., Hamer, R., Nora, R. M., & Tan, B. (1997). The lie/bet questionnaire for screening pathological gamblers. *Psychological Reports, 80,* 83–88.

Kerber, C. S., Black, D. W., & Buckwalter, K. (2008). Comorbid psychiatric disorders among older adult pathological gamblers. *Issues in Mental Health Nursing, 29,* 1018–1028.

Ladouceur, R., Sylvain, C., Boutin, C., & Doucet, C. (2002). *Understanding and treating the pathological gambler.* Quebec, Canada: Wiley.

Lepage, C., Ladouceur, R., & Jacque, C. (2000). Brief report prevalence of problem gambling among community service users. *Community Mental Health Journal, 36*(6), 597–601.

Lesieur, H. R. (1994). Epidemiological surveys on pathological gambling: Critique and suggestions for modification. *Journal of Gambling Studies, 10,* 385–398.

Lesieur, H. R., & Blume, S. B. (1993). Revising the South Oaks Gambling Screen in a different setting. *Journal of Gambling Studies, 9,* 213–223.

Leung, K. S., & Cottler, L. B. (2009). Treatment of pathological gambling. *Current Opinion in Psychiatry, 22*(1), 69–74.

Lucke, S., & Wallace, M. (2006). Assessment and management of pathological and problem gambling among older adults. *Geriatric Nursing, 27*(1), 51–57.

McCartney, J. (1996). A community study of natural change across the addictions. *Addiction Research, 4*, 65–83.

McKeown, R. E., Cuffe, S. P., & Schulz, R. M. (2006). US suicide rates by age group, 1970-2002: An examination of recent trends. *American Journal of Public Health, 96*(10), 1744–1751.

McNeilly, D. P., & Burke, W. J. (2001). Gambling as a social activity of older adults. *International Journal of Aging and Human Development, 52*(1), 19–28.

National Opinion Research Center (NORC). (1999). *Gambling Impact and Behavior Study.* Chicago: National Opinion Research Center.

Petry, N. (2005). *Pathological gambling: Etiology, comorbidity, and treatment.* Washington, DC: American Psychological Association.

Petry, N., & Armentano, C. (1999). Prevalence, assessment and treatment of pathological gambling: A review. *Psychiatric Services, 50*, 1021–1027.

Potenza, M., Fiellin, D. A., Heninger, G. R., Rounsaville, B. J., & Mazure, C. M. (2002). Gambling: An addictive behavior with health and primary care implications. *Journal of General Internal Medicine, 17*(9), 721–732.

Preston, F. W., Shapiro, P. D., & Keene, J. R. (2007). Successful aging and gambling predictors of gambling risk among older adults in Las Vegas. *American Behavioral Scientist, 51*(1), 102–121.

Shaw, M., Forbush, K., Schlinder, J., Rosenman E., & Black, D. W. (2007). The effect of pathological gambling on families, marriages, and children. *CNS Spectrums, 12*(8), 615–622.

Stewart, D., & Oslin, D. (2001). Recognition and treatment of late-life addictions in medical settings. *Journal of Clinical Geropsychology, 7*(2), 145–158.

Tavares, H., Zilberman, M. L., & el-Guébaly, N. (2003). Are there cognitive and behavioural approaches specific to the treatment of pathological gambling? *Canadian Journal of Psychiatry, 48*(1), 22–28.

Toce-Gerstein, M., Gerstein, D., & Volberg, R. (2003). A hierarchy of gambling disorders in the community. *Addiction, 98*(12), 1661–1672.

Tresniowski, A., Arias, R., Morrison, M., Billups, A., Bass, S., Howard, C., et al. (2003, October 13). Gambling online: How to go deep into debt without ever leaving your living room. *People*, 119–122.

Unwin, B. K., Davis, M. K., & De Leeuw, J. B. (2000). Pathologic gambling. *American Family Physician, 61*(3), 741–749.

Volberg, R. A. (2003). *Gambling and problem gambling among seniors in Florida.* Maitland, FL: Florida Council on Compulsive Gambling.

Welte, J., Barnes, G., Wieczorek, W., Tidwell, M. C., & Parker, J. (2001). Alcohol and gambling pathology among US adults: Prevalence, demographic patterns and comorbidity. *Journal of Studies on Alcohol and Drugs, 62*, 706–712.

Wiebe, J. M., & Cox, B. J. (2005). Problem and probable pathological gambling among older adults assessed by the SOGS-R. *Journal of Gambling Studies, 21*(2), 205–221.

Zaranek, R. R., & Chapleski, E. E. (2005). Casino gambling among urban elders: Just another social activity? *Journal of Gerontology Social Sciences, 60B*(2), S74-S81.

Zimmerman, M., Breen, R. B., & Posternak, M. A. (2002). An open-label study of citalopram in the treatment of pathological gambling. *Journal of Clinical Psychiatry, 63*(1), 44–48.

18

Elder Mistreatment

Terry Fulmer
Jamie Blankenship
Angela Chandracomar
Nina Ng

Elder mistreatment (EM) is a major healthcare problem that can lead to severe physical disability, psychological problems, and even death in the older adult. Surgeon General Louis Sullivan played a major role in "medicalizing" the issue, which has helped sensitize American healthcare professionals to the important role they have in assessing and managing cases of EM (Sullivan, 1992). Although legal definitions of EM vary from state to state, EM is generally considered to include intentional actions that cause harm or create serious risk of harm (whether or not harm is intended) to a vulnerable elder by a caregiver or other person who is in a trust relationship to the elder, or failure by a caregiver to satisfy the elder's basic needs or to protect him or her from harm (National Research Council, 2003).

EM is the outcome of abuse, neglect, exploitation, or abandonment of older adults by a known caregiver. The definition is distinct from "stranger violence," which does not entail a caregiving relationship. Spouse abuse in older adults may be a longstanding issue but is generally not considered particular to older adults in the EM literature. There is also a lack of consensus about whether self-neglect, the failure of a mentally competent elder to protect himself or herself from harm, is a subcategory of EM. The National Center on Elder Abuse and various states include it in the definition of EM because outcomes may be similar to mistreatment by caregivers (National Center on Elder Abuse, 2005). However, the Panel to Review Risk and Prevalence of Elder Abuse and Neglect (National Research Council, 2003) considers self-neglect as a separate domain from EM, albeit one that also often warrants intervention. Unfortunately, the construct of EM is often lumped in with the overall category of family violence, which does little to further education and knowledge generation in this distinctly important area (American Medical Association National Advisory Council on Violence and Abuse, 2008). Finally, summary papers on family violence that do reference EM reflect the paucity of data-based papers written over the past 10 years (Draucker, 2002).

TYPES OF EM

EM occurs in both domestic and institutional settings, although much of the research on the causes and outcomes has focused on the domestic setting. Table 18-1 lists several different subtypes of EM that clinicians should recognize.

TABLE 18-1

Subtypes of EM

Type of Mistreatment	Definition	Examples
Physical abuse	Acts of violence that may result in pain, injury, impairment, or disease	Pushing, slapping, striking, improper use of restraints, force-feeding
Sexual abuse	Sexual contact or exposure without the older person's consent or when the person is incapable of giving consent	Unwanted touching, sexual assault battery, rape, coerced nudity
Physical neglect	Failure to provide for the needs of an older person that may result in harm	Failure to provide clothing, food, shelter, hygiene; withholding of health maintenance care, social interaction
Psychological abuse	Infliction of mental anguish, pain, or distress on an older person	Harassment, intimidation, threats, isolating the person, treating the person like a child
Psychological neglect	Failure to provide the older person with sufficient social stimulation	Leaving the person alone, ignoring the person, giving the "silent treatment," failure to provide news or companionship
Financial/material abuse or exploitation	Misuse of the older person's funds, income, or assets	Stealing money, cashing the person's checks for personal gain, forging the person's signature on documents, improper use of guardianship or power of attorney

Source: Adapted from American Medical Association (1992). *Diagnostic and treatment guidelines on elder abuse and neglect* (p. 9). Chicago: Author. Adapted with permission.

INCIDENCE AND PREVALENCE

Precise estimates on the number of cases of EM are difficult to obtain for a variety of reasons, including the social stigma and fear of retribution from the abuser. In a classic study on prevalence, EM was estimated at 32 per 1000 in a community-based random sample survey (Pillemer & Finkelhor, 1988). Laumann and colleagues documented a prevalence of 9% for verbal mistreatment, 3.5% for financial mistreatment, and 0.2% for physical mistreatment by family members, using the National Social Life, Health and Aging Project (Laumann, Leitsch, & Waite, 2008). Barriers to the conduct of national prevalence studies include the cost of the undertaking, and the lack of consensus of what constitutes an exact case. Further, a major barrier in determining the true number of cases of EM is the fact that many cases are never reported. Some states do not record separate data on elders, nor are the reports uniform across states for accurate data collection (Jogerst et al., 2003). In the only study of its kind, it was noted that only 21% of EM cases were reported and substantiated by Adult Protective Services (APS) agencies (National Center on Elder Abuse at The American Public Human Services Association in Collaboration with Westat, 1998). By using hypothetical case vignettes, another study discovered significant differences in EM reporting thresholds between APS and hospice palliative care professionals, with the hospice palliative care group underreporting (Liao, Jayawardena, Bufalini, & Wiglesworth, 2009). There are scant data to help understand how nurses across settings report or underreport EM.

POPULATION AT RISK

Risk factors for EM include low socioeconomic status; low educational level; impaired functional or cognitive status; and a history of domestic violence, stressful events, and depression in the older adult or caregiver (Dyer, Pavlik, Murphy, & Hyman, 2000; Lachs & Pillemer, 2004). EM victims are more likely to be female (Dunlop, Rothman, Condon, Hebert, & Martinez, 2000), over 80 years old (National Center on Elder Abuse at The American Public Human Services Association in Collaboration with Westat, 1998; Teaster, Roberto, Duke, & Myeonghwan, 2000), and live with the caregiver who is mistreating them (Lachs & Pillemer; Pillemer & Finkelhor, 1988). Furthermore, chronic disabling illnesses that impair function have been shown to be a risk factor for mistreatment. However, greater social support has recently been shown to be somewhat protective against EM (Dong & Simon, 2008). Lower risk has been associated with a number of social support constructs, including having a person to listen or talk to, receive good advice from, and show love and affection toward.

There are several characteristics that have been shown to be more common among perpetrators of EM. These individuals are more likely to have impairment, such as mental illness, depression, or substance abuse (Brownell, 1999; Cohen, Llorente, & Eisdorfer, 1998; Lachs & Pillemer, 2004; Pillemer & Finkelhor, 1989; Reis & Nahmiash, 1998). They are also more likely to be financially dependent on the older adult (Brownell; Pillemer & Finkelhor, 1989; Seaver, 1996; Wolf & Pillemer, 1997). Many studies have reported that most perpetrators are male, particularly in cases of sexual abuse (Brownell; Ramsey-Klawsnik, Teaster, Mendiondo, Marcum, & Abner, 2008).

THEORIES OF EM

The etiology of EM has been examined through a number of different theories and models. "Transgenerational" violence, a phenomenon whereby children who were abused grow up and mistreat their abusive parents, has been postulated as a possible theory (O'Malley, O'Malley, Everitt, & Sarson, 1984). Others theorize that psychopathology of the abuser may be a contributing factor. Perpetrators have been shown to be more likely to have substance abuse issues and psychopathology (Lachs & Fulmer, 1993). Caregiver stress may also account for cases of EM. Caregivers may become overburdened or overwhelmed by their caregiving responsibilities, which may cause them to become violent. The phenomenon of "generational inversion," where children must suddenly reverse their roles and become the caregiver instead of being cared for by the parent, may also be a contributing factor to caregiver stress, thereby increasing the potential of EM (Steinmetz, 1990). Another theory of etiology for EM includes dependency as a central issue. Older adults who are dependent on their caregivers for activities of daily living and instrumental activities of daily living are more vulnerable to being mistreated (Lachs & Pillemer, 2004). Caregivers who are emotionally or financially dependent on the older adult they care for are more likely to become perpetrators of EM. This is sometimes described as a "web of dependency," in which the victim and perpetrator are equally dependent on one another, thereby creating a situation that can give rise to EM (O'Malley, Everitt, O'Malley, & Campion, 1983). Lastly, it has been noted that isolation plays a key role in EM. With no outsider to monitor their quality of life, isolated older adults are at greater risk for EM and are less likely to be identified by the healthcare system or reporting agencies (National Center on Elder Abuse at The American Public Human Services Association in Collaboration with Westat, 1998).

INSTITUTIONAL MISTREATMENT

EM in nursing homes often involves an overworked caregiver in an underfunded care environment (Lindbloom, Brandt, Hough, & Meadows, 2007). In a classic survey of nursing home staff, 10% of the staff members reported committing an act of physical abuse against a resident in the previous year, and 40% admitted to having committed an act of psychological abuse. Moreover, 81% had witnessed at least one incident of psychological abuse by another staff member and 36% had witnessed at least one incident of physical abuse (Pillemer & Moore, 1989). In this study, older adult aggressiveness was a predictor of physical and psychological abuse by staff members, and abusers were more likely to be younger than non-abusers. With a sample of 183 caregivers recruited from seven long-term care facilities, a more recent study found that caregivers who work fewer hours with less education and fewer social resources had more work stress and showed higher levels of psychological abuse behavior when caring for older adults (Joshi & Flaherty, 2005; Wang, Lin, Tseng, & Chang, 2009).

Reporting of EM in nursing homes is a problem, and long delays in the reporting of incidents are common (U.S. General Accounting Office Report to Congressional Requesters, 2002). For instance, great delays were reported in the length of time it takes for nursing homes to report incidents of EM to law enforcement and state agencies, in addition to the time it takes state survey agencies to follow up and make determinations about reports of mistreatment (U.S. General Accounting Office Report to Congressional Requesters). These delays in reporting hamper efforts of state survey agencies to collect evidence and may put other nursing home residents at risk for mistreatment. No federal law requiring criminal background checks of nursing home employees exists, although several states require background checks and have proposed a federal Patient Safety and Abuse Prevention Act that would mandate background checks of employees (Library of Congress, 2008).

The Minimum Data Set requirements for long-term care facilities, which include a section on resident abuse, have done much to improve EM assessment (Centers for Medicare and Medicaid Services, 2006). Every institution is required to have new employees complete in-service training on resident abuse initially and annually thereafter. All staff members are instructed on the institutional guidelines for reporting suspected EM.

Reasons have been suggested as to why there are delays in reporting EM in nursing homes. Staff members may fear losing their jobs or facing reprisal by other staff members and management if they report EM. Residents may be afraid of retribution, and family members may fear having to find a new nursing home for the resident. Finally, managers of nursing homes may want to avoid adverse publicity (Burgess, Dowdell, & Prentky, 2000). These are unacceptable reasons for the lack of EM reporting and could ultimately result in state agencies penalizing the institution for noncompliance or even obstruction of justice. Reporting EM should be presented as a positive feature in all nursing homes that strive to create a safe and supportive environment.

CLINICAL PRESENTATIONS

History

Successful assessment for EM begins with a thorough history. Unless older adults are asked directly about it, they are unlikely to discuss a history of mistreatment. When obtaining a history, a nurse has a number of appropriate opportunities to ask the older adult about EM, and the nurse should use his or her own judgment with regard to the timing based on the rapport he or she has established with the older adult. In a busy emergency department setting, EM should be explored during the history taking. After review of the chief complaint, it is appropriate to ask about physical violence in the same context as one would ask about guns in the home, drugs and alcohol history, and other high-risk or dangerous aspects of a person's life. The nurse should be direct and help the older adult by using such phrases as "Is there any family violence you would like to talk about?" and "Have you ever been abused by any of your family members or friends? Any physical abuse? Emotional abuse?"

As with any thorough history, when there is a positive response to a screening question, the nurse should continue to determine the onset of the problem, the circumstances, the length of time it has been occurring, characteristics of the problem, associated or aggravating issues that precipitate the abuse, factors that relieve the situation, and appropriate types of interventions based on the individual's life circumstances.

The Institute of Medicine discusses screening assessments in Appendix A of its 2002 report (Institute of Medicine, 2002), and a review article with a succinct analysis of available instruments was published in *The Journal of the American Geriatrics Society* (Fulmer, Guadagno, Bitondo Dyer, & Connolly, 2004). The American Medical Association has published diagnostic and treatment guidelines on elder abuse and neglect (American Medical Association, 1992) that are extremely useful in developing an approach to screening for EM.

The clinician is urged to incorporate routine questions related to EM into his or her daily practice and to pay special attention to older adults who have cognitive impairment, which is a risk factor for EM. In the case where older adults do not hear well or have conditions that might impair their ability to communicate, such as Parkinson's disease or a cerebral vascular accident, it is even more important to obtain accurate information from the patient's health history. In the event that

information is not obtained during the first interview, the nurse should establish a follow-up plan to obtain the additional data as soon as possible. This may require an interdisciplinary approach. For example, if the emergency department nurse does not get the answer to an EM screening question, he or she should contact the social worker who would be in touch with the older adult on the unit, or who will communicate with the older adult after discharge, so that eventually all of the facts can be obtained and a follow-up plan can be developed as needed (Box 18-1).

In an older adult with severe dementia, the nurse needs to seek out a proxy who can comment on the possibility of EM. It is very important for the nurse to be sensitive to the fact that proxies could potentially be the abusers and that caution should be exercised to avoid creating a dangerous situation for the elderly patient. It is extremely important that the nurse determine how serious and dangerous the current situation is for the older adult. For example, in the clinic or emergency department, when the older adult is being treated and released, an alternative plan needs to be developed if the patient is at risk for injury and harm from EM. Such a plan needs to be created rapidly

BOX 18-1 SCREENING QUESTIONS

- Has anyone at home ever hurt you?
- Has anyone ever touched you without your consent?
- Has anyone ever made you do things you didn't want to do?
- Has anyone taken anything that was yours without asking?
- Has anyone ever scolded or threatened you?
- Have you ever signed any documents that you didn't understand?
- Are you afraid of anyone at home?
- Are you alone a lot?
- Has anyone ever failed to help you take care of yourself when you needed help?

Source: Adapted from American Medical Association. (1992). *Diagnostic and treatment guidelines on elder abuse and neglect* (p. 9). Chicago: Author. Adapted with permission.

to avoid having the older adult return to an unsafe situation (Weinberg Center for Elder Abuse at The Hebrew Home for the Aged at Riverdale, 2009). In some circumstances, shelters may be needed, or it may be necessary to arrange for a protective service admission into the hospital (Cohen et al., 2002). All of this needs to be done in the context of state reporting laws and in the context of the older adult's rights and wishes. There are mandatory EM reporting laws in 46 states (Capezuti, Brush, & Lawson, 1997; Jogerst et al., 2003; Roby & Sullivan, 2000). Protocols need to be followed not only for the state requirements, but also within the context of any institutional guidelines at the hospital, clinic, or practice setting.

The nurse needs to safeguard the older adult from care plans that are not in his or her best interest or that are contrary to the older adult's wishes. For example, older adults who have cognitive impairment and live in a home with an abusive relative may be reviewed for nursing home placement (Centers for Medicare and Medicaid Services, 2006). Although there are times when this may be appropriate, it should not be considered the only possible plan of care. Older adults should not be forced out of their homes because of another person's detrimental behavior. Depending on the situation, it may be possible to alleviate the situation through adult day health services or home care services, while still allowing the elder to maintain independence and live at home. In some cases, adult children misuse the resources and the living spaces of their parents in a negative way that disrupts the older adults' lives. Steps can be taken to obtain restraining orders against adult children or other individuals who are harming the older adult. Older adults often feel guilty about doing this to a relative, even when they are clearly being mistreated. Therefore, they may benefit from counseling to help them more fully understand the situation and the risks involved.

EM cases are complicated and require a team approach that involves multidisciplinary assessment and regular team follow-up to ensure the older adult's well-being. The Hartford Institute for Geriatric Nursing (2009) suggests that nurses and other healthcare professionals should be educated to detect cases of EM. Clergy, health service administrators, physicians, psychologists, rehabilitation therapists, social workers, community practitioners, care providers, dentists, and geriatric care managers may be involved in the team approach (Hartford Institute for Geriatric Nursing). With increased awareness from this array of professionals, more cases of abuse will be detected and more victims will be provided with help. Legal services or police protection may be needed and will require expertise from the team to be alert for any signs of depression, suicidal tendencies, or self-neglect in these potentially devastating circumstances.

Physical Examination

Once the history has been completed, a physical examination should be conducted in a comprehensive manner to determine if there are any signs of EM. Box 18-2 provides an overview of high-risk signs for physical abuse, neglect, financial and material abuse, and neglect and violation of rights.

Given comorbidities and use of multiple medications, the older adult may experience physical signs that can be misconstrued as EM. For example, a bruise may be misinterpreted as a sign of abuse while in fact, the older adult may be on an anticoagulant, or have a history of falls, which may be the cause of bruising. The nurse should therefore question the older adult about the causes of any suspicious bruises or skin lesions. Older adults who are incontinent may have urine burns or excoriations on their skin as a result of neglect. The causes of these findings should be explored thoroughly to determine if neglect exists. In the past, clinical assessment of older adults has been extraordinarily "forgiving" of symptoms, such as dehydration, skin tears, poor hygiene, and other presentations, that would never be overlooked in a younger person. A physical assessment of an older adult requires precise documentation of findings that may indicate that the elder is a victim of abuse or neglect.

BOX 18-2 EXAMPLES OF HIGH-RISK SIGNS AND SYMPTOMS

Abuse	Unexplained bruises, repeated falls, laboratory values inconsistent with history, fractures or bruises in various stages of healing (any report by patient of being physically abused should be followed up immediately)
Neglect	Listlessness, poor hygiene, evidence of malnourishment, inappropriate dress, decubiti, urine burns, reports of being left in an unsafe situation, reports of inability to get needed medications
Exploitation	Unexplained loss of Social Security or pension checks, any evidence that material goods are being taken in exchange for care, any evidence that personal belongings of elder (house, jewelry, or car) are being taken over without consent or approval of elder

Other High-Risk Situations

- Drug or alcohol addiction in the family
- Isolation of the elder
- History of untreated psychiatric problems
- Evidence of unusual family stress
- Excessive dependence of elder on caretaker

Source: Adapted from Fulmer, T., & O'Malley, T. (1987). *Inadequate care of the elderly: A health care perspective on abuse and neglect* (pp. 18–19). New York: Springer. Adapted with permission.

Psychological Assessment

A psychological assessment for EM is extremely important and needs to be done with precision and specificity. In many cases, it is useful to contact a psychiatric liaison nurse, a social worker, a psychiatrist, or another mental health professional to conduct the assessment of symptoms in the context of the older patient's mental health. In some cases, the symptoms or behavior may be long-standing and result from childhood trauma or child abuse. The Childhood Trauma Questionnaire (Bernstein & Fink, 1998) is a useful screening instrument for determining if an older adult suffered from traumatic life circumstances during childhood that have left him or her with issues that still remain unresolved. This instrument has been used and validated with older adult samples including health maintenance organization members, female pain patients, adult psychiatric outpatients, and adult substance abusers. The instrument can be used in adult populations to assess for traumatic histories and formulate a treatment plan (Bernstein & Fink).

Laboratory and Diagnostic Testing

Laboratory tests for older adults should be selected and conducted based on the history and presentation in the clinical setting. Routine blood work should be ordered as appropriate for annual physical examinations. When signs of EM are evident, as in severe dehydration or multiple bruises, radiographs or blood chemistries should be obtained to explore the presentation more thoroughly. If an older adult presents with an open wound that seems to be untreated, a culture of that wound may be required.

EVALUATION AND REFERRAL

Whenever an older adult screens positive for EM, the nurse needs to be knowledgeable about the state reporting laws, the institutional guidelines in the workplace, and the follow-up required to ensure the well-being of the adult. The APS network in the United States is extremely effective in following up on suspected cases of EM and, in some cases, can provide support services that can create a safer home environment for the adult. Community-based services, such as respite care, hospice care, adult day health care centers, and less formal organizations, such as church groups, can all serve as useful interventions in cases of EM. The Alzheimer's Association, with its extensive network of chapters throughout the United States, is an excellent resource for older adults and their families or caregivers who need support and guidance in understanding community services.

LEGAL CONSIDERATIONS

When a nurse obtains a positive history of EM, he or she needs to work with the administration of his or her organization to determine the best way to engage law enforcement and legal assistance. Assault and battery are against the law, and the procedures for working with the police should be known in advance. Rape is a felony and should never be labeled as a type of EM without following the appropriate rape procedures already in place for any other age group. Careful documentation of the history, the physical assessment, and the laboratory findings in such cases cannot be underscored enough. For an in-depth review of legal responses to abuse of older adults, Otto (2005) has compiled case studies from the courts that are extremely instructive.

PREVENTION

Every time an older adult presents in any nursing care setting, there is opportunity to screen for EM and to teach older adults that they have the right to live a life free from fear of mistreatment. It is helpful to have distributable teaching materials that can provide the older adult with contact information that can be used should they become victims of EM or have questions or concerns regarding EM. In some circumstances, the older adult may disclose a history of EM and yet demand that "no one be told," or refuse services. This presents an ethical dilemma for any nurse who is concerned about the older adult. The fear of discharging an older adult to an unsafe setting or leaving a person in his or her residence when there is known abuse is antithetical to good nursing practice. However, in the absence of dementia or other serious cognitive impairments, the older adult has the right to self-determination no matter how objectionable it is to the nurse. In such situations, teaching materials with contact telephone numbers that can be used on a 24-hour emergency basis are essential in the clinical interaction. It is tempting for any clinician to assume cognitive impairment when the older adult chooses an EM situation over a protected environment, but it is nevertheless a possibility. In these circumstances, counseling services should be obtained to address the nature of the EM situation and to suggest alternatives to the older adult.

In cases of EM where the older adult does have documented dementia or cognitive impairment, a geropsychiatric consultation is needed. Geropsychiatric nurses are in a unique position to complete a detailed assessment and diagnose impairments that preclude self-determination at a given moment. Regular reevaluation of cognitive status is mandatory given the fluctuating cycles that take place over time. The plan of care is highly dependent on the context including the site of care, the residence of the older adult, his or her living circumstances, and any guardianship or conservatorship proxies in place. When an elder is screened and diagnosed in the emergency department, concern regarding a treat-and-release situation is especially high. Plans for follow-up should be carefully coordinated with home care nursing and social services. Older adults need to be informed that nurses are mandatory reporters for suspected EM and that appropriate reports will be made. The older adult should also be informed that if APS makes contact, he or she may refuse services at that time. If there is suspected criminal activity, such as assault or theft, police will be contacted. This may be distressing for the older adult, just as it is to parents when child abuse reports are made. Nurses can alleviate some of the tension by explaining that their actions are being made in good faith.

▍CASE STUDY

D.M., a 73-year-old woman, was brought to the emergency department (ED) by an ambulance at 5:00 p.m. presenting with dehydration after her neighbor found her unconscious on her bathroom floor. The patient was oriented only to self. D.M. has a history of depression, hypertension, and hyperlipidemia. She also had an open reduction internal fixation of the right femur 5 months ago after falling and presently requires a cane to help her ambulate.

On assessment, the triage nurse discovered a 1-cm laceration on D.M.'s forehead and multiple bruises along both arms in different phases of healing. When questioned about her bruises, D.M. initially refused to discuss the issue, but later stated, "Oh, I'm just so clumsy. I hit my head on the bathroom sink and I occasionally bump into things without even noticing. It's nothing to worry about, really." The triage nurse documented her physical assessment, including her vital signs (blood pressure 88/50, heart rate 110, temperature 99°F oral, and RR 24), and quickly sent D.M. into the ED so she could triage the next patient.

As D.M. slowly regained orientation, the receiving registered nurse discovered that the patient was home alone when she slipped and hit her head on the bathroom sink. The patient also revealed that she lives in an apartment with her 42-year-old daughter, Nora, who is single, has a history of alcohol dependence, and works 6 days a week from 9 a.m. to 5 p.m. as a clerical assistant at a nearby hospital. In addition, Nora babysits her neighbor's children several times per month. Although D.M. has no problem performing activities of daily living, she is dependent on her daughter for financial assistance, grocery shopping, and transportation to medical appointments.

At the start of the night shift, the receiving registered nurse in the ED reviewed D.M.'s admitting assessment and became concerned when D.M. refused to have anyone call her daughter to pick her up, or when he inquired further about the nature of the bruises along her arms. He also noticed that the bruises resemble a grabbing pattern on several locations on the patient's arms. After some hesitation, the ED nurse reported his suspicion of abuse and neglect to APS and asked the social worker to talk with D.M.

1. What factors surrounding D.M.'s physical, social, and environmental disposition indicate suspicion for EM (i.e., neglect or abuse)?

2. What factors precipitate underreporting of EM by healthcare providers?

3. What are appropriate levels of intervention and services that should be provided to the older adult suspected of being a victim of EM?

4. What EM indicators might the triage nurse miss?

SUMMARY

EM presents major challenges for both the older adult and the nurse. Comprehensive assessment, sensitivity, care planning, and follow-up are pivotal elements in the health outcomes of the older adult.

ACKNOWLEDGMENTS

The authors acknowledge a previous version of this chapter, which was written by Terry Fulmer, PhD, RN, FAAN, Lisa Guadagno, MPA, and Marguarette M. Bolton, BA, and express their appreciation to Laura Pennace for her assistance in preparing the manuscript.

REFERENCES

American Medical Association. (1992). *Diagnostic and treatment guidelines on elder abuse and neglect.* Chicago: American Medical Association.

American Medical Association National Advisory Council on Violence and Abuse. Policy Compendium. (2008). Retrieved June 15, 2009, from http://www.ama-assn.org/ama1/pub/upload/mm/386/vio_policy_comp.pdf

Bernstein, D., & Fink, L. (1998). *Childhood Trauma Questionnaire: A retrospective of self-report.* San Antonio, TX: Psychological Corporation.

Brownell, P. (1999). Mental health and criminal justice issues among perpetrators of elder abuse. *Journal of Elder Abuse & Neglect, 11*(4), 81–94.

Burgess, A. W., Dowdell, E. B., & Prentky, R. A. (2000). Sexual abuse of nursing home residents. *Journal of Psychosocial Nursing, 38*(6), 10–18.

Capezuti, E., Brush, B. L., & Lawson, W. T. (1997). Reporting elder mistreatment. *Journal of Gerontological Nursing, 23*(7), 24–32.

Centers for Medicare and Medicaid Services. (2006). *Minimum Data Set (MDS) long term care user's facility manual.* Baltimore: DHHS.

Cohen, D., Llorente, M., & Eisdorfer, C. (1998). Homicide-suicide in older persons. *The American Journal of Psychiatry, 155*(3), 390–396.

Cohen, H. J., Feussner, J. R., Weinberger, M., Carnes, M., Hamdy, R. C., Hsieh, F., et al. (2002). A controlled trial of inpatient and outpatient geriatric evaluation and management. *New England Journal of Medicine, 346*(12), 905–912.

Dong, X., & Simon, M. A. (2008). Is greater social support a protective factor against elder mistreatment? *Gerontology, 54*(6), 381–388.

Draucker, C. B. (2002). Domestic violence: The challenge for nursing. *Online Journal of Issues in Nursing, 7*(1), Manuscript 1. Retrieved June 1, 2010, from www.nursingworld.org/MainMenuCategories/ANAMarketplace/ANAPeriodicals/OJIN/TableofContents/Volume72002/No1Jan2002/DomesticViolenceChallenge.aspx

Dunlop, B., Rothman, M. B., Condon, K. M., Hebert, K. S., & Martinez, I. L. (2000). Elder abuse: Risk factors and use of case data to improve policy and practice. *Journal of Elder Abuse & Neglect, 12*(3/4), 95–122.

Dyer, C. B., Pavlik, V. N., Murphy, K. P., & Hyman, D. J. (2000). The high prevalence of depression and dementia in elder abuse or neglect. *Journal of the American Geriatrics Society, 48*(2), 205–208.

Fulmer, T., Guadagno, L., Bitondo Dyer, C., & Connolly, M. T. (2004). Progress in elder abuse screening and assessment instruments. *Journal of the American Geriatrics Society, 52*(2), 297–304.

Fulmer, T., & O'Malley, T. (1987). *Inadequate care of the elderly: A health care perspective on abuse and neglect.* New York: Springer.

Hartford Institute for Geriatric Nursing. Elder mistreatment. Retrieved March 11, 2009, from http://www.hartfordign.org/continuing_ed/elder_mistreatment

Institute of Medicine. (2002). *Confronting chronic neglect: The education and training of health professionals on family violence.* Washington, DC: National Academy Press.

Jogerst, G. J., Daly, J. M., Brinig, M. F., Dawson, J. D., Schmuch, G. A., & Ingram, J. G. (2003). Domestic elder abuse and the law. *American Journal of Public Health, 93*(12), 2131–2136.

Joshi, S., & Flaherty, J. H. (2005). Elder abuse and neglect in long-term care. *Clinics in Geriatric Medicine, 21*(2), 333–354.

Lachs, M. S., & Fulmer, T. (1993). Recognizing elder abuse and neglect. *Clinical Geriatric Medicine, 9*(3), 665–681.

Lachs, M. S., & Pillemer, K. (2004). Elder abuse. *Lancet, 364*(9441), 1263–1272.

Laumann, E. O., Leitsch, S. A., & Waite, L. J. (2008). Elder mistreatment in the United States: Prevalence estimates from a nationally representative study. *Journals of Gerontology Series B: Psychological Sciences and Social Sciences, 63*(4), S248–S254.

Liao, S., Jayawardena, K. M., Bufalini, E., & Wiglesworth, A. (2009). Elder mistreatment reporting: Differences in the threshold of reporting between hospice and palliative care professionals and adult protective service. *Journal of Palliative Medicine, 12*(1), 64–70.

Library of Congress. (2008). Senate Report 110–474: Patient Safety and Abuse Prevention Act (2nd ed.) Max Baucus (Editor). Committee on Finance. U.S. Senate, Washington, DC. Retrieved March 11, 2009, from http://www.thomas.gov/cgi-bin/cpquery/T?&report=sr474&dbname=110&

Lindbloom, E. J., Brandt, J., Hough, L. D., & Meadows, S. E. (2007). Elder mistreatment in the nursing home: A systematic review. *Journal of the American Medical Directors Association, 8*(9), 610–616.

National Center on Elder Abuse. (2000–2005). Self-neglect: An update of the literature 2000–2005. Retrieved June 13, 2009, from http://www.ncea.aoa.gov/ncearoot/Main_Site/library/CANE/CANE_Series/CANE_selfneglectupdate.aspx

National Center on Elder Abuse at The American Public Human Services Association in Collaboration with Westat, Inc. (1998). *The National Elder Abuse Incidence Study: Final report.* Washington, DC: National Aging Information Center.

National Research Council. (2003). Elder mistreatment: Abuse, neglect, and exploitation in an aging America. Panel to review risk and prevalence of elder abuse and neglect. R. J. Bonnie & R. B. Wallace (Eds.). Committee on National Statistics and Committee on Law and Justice, Division of Behavioral and Social Sciences and Education. Washington, DC: National Academies Press.

O'Malley, T. A., Everitt, D. E., O'Malley, H. C., & Campion, E. W. (1983). Identifying and preventing family-mediated abuse and neglect of elderly persons. *Annals of Internal Medicine, 98*(6), 998–1005.

O'Malley, T. A., O'Malley, H. C., Everitt, D. E., & Sarson, D. (1984). Categories of family-mediated abuse and neglect of elderly persons. *Journal of the American Geriatrics Society, 32*(5), 362–369.

Otto, J. M. (2005). *Abuse and neglect of vulnerable adult populations.* Kingston, NJ: Civic Research Institute.

Pillemer, K. A., & Finkelhor, D. (1988). The prevalence of elder abuse: A random sample survey. *Gerontologist, 28*(1), 51–57.

Pillemer, K. A., & Finkelhor, D. (1989). Causes of elder abuse: Caregiver stress versus problem relatives. *American Journal of Orthopsychiatry, 59*(2), 179–187.

Pillemer, K. A., & Moore, D. W. (1989). Abuse of patients in nursing homes: Findings from a survey of staff. *Gerontologist, 29*(3), 314–320.

Ramsey-Klawsnik, H., Teaster, P. B., Mendiondo, M. S., Marcum, J. L., & Abner, E. L. (2008). Sexual predators who target elders: Findings from the first national study of sexual abuse in care facilities. *Journal of Elder Abuse & Neglect, 20*(4), 353–376.

Reis, M., & Nahmiash, D. (1998). Validation of the indicators of abuse (IOA) screen. *Gerontologist, 38*(4), 471–480.

Roby, J. L., & Sullivan, R. (2000). Adult protection service laws: a comparison of state statutes from definition to case closure. *Journal of Elder Abuse & Neglect, 12*(3/4), 17–51.

Seaver, C. (1996). Muted lives: Older battered women. *Journal of Elder Abuse & Neglect, 8*(2), 3–21.

Steinmetz, S. K. (1990). Elder abuse by adult offspring: The relationship of actual vs. perceived dependency. *Journal of Health and Human Resources Administration, 12*(4), 434–463.

Sullivan, L. (1992). *Nursing home resident protection.* Retrieved April 22, 1999, from http://www.hhs.gov/news.../pre1995pres/92025.txt

Teaster, P., Roberto, K., Duke, J., & Myeonghwan, K. (2000). Sexual abuse of older adults: Preliminary findings of cases in Virginia. *Journal of Elder Abuse & Neglect, 12*(3/4), 1–16.

U.S. General Accounting Office Report to Congressional Requesters. (2002). *Nursing homes: More can be done to protect residents from abuse.* Washington, DC: GAO-02-312.

Wang, J. J., Lin, M. F., Tseng, H. F., & Chang, W. Y. (2009). Caregiver factors contributing to psychological elder abuse behavior in long-term care facilities: A structural equation model approach. *International Psychogeriatrics, 21*(2), 314–320.

Weinberg Center for Elder Abuse at The Hebrew Home for the Aged at Riverdale. Elder abuse services. Retrieved June 29, 2009, from http://www.elderserve.org/details.asp?ID=10

Wolf, R. S., & Pillemer, K. A. (1997). The older battered woman: Wives and mothers compared. *Journal of Mental Health & Aging, 3*(3), 325–336.

19

End of Life

Michelle Doran
Karyn Geary

Over the past century, how and where people die has changed dramatically. Before World War II, people usually died in the comfort of their own home, cared for by family members. Deaths often occurred rapidly as a result of communicable illnesses or acute events. In 1900, the average life expectancy for both men and women was less than 50 years of age (Berry & Matzo, 2004; Bookbinder & Kiss, 2001). In the earlier half of the 1900s, infant and childhood death was not an uncommon experience for a family to endure, with 53% of all deaths occurring in children under the age of 15 (Krisman-Scott, 2003). In the absence of advanced medical technology, symptom management was a major focus of care. Families were skilled at providing the care and attention necessary for achieving comfortable, peaceful, and dignified death experiences for their loved ones. Death was accepted to be as much a part of life as birth. Families embraced the opportunity to provide meaningful end-of-life care (Sherman & Laporte, 2001).

By the mid-1900s, several developments had taken place that contributed to changing the death experience in the United States. Growth in science and industry resulted in improved living and working conditions. Disease prevention, treatment, and life-saving or prolonging treatments evolved with the development of vaccinations, antibiotics,

cardiopulmonary resuscitation (CPR), advances in surgery, and anesthesia. As a result, the focus of care shifted from symptom management to curative interventions. With these changes patients, families, and healthcare professionals not only began to have higher expectations for curable illnesses, but also for those that were incurable. Death became equated with medical failure. Medical treatments were sought that resulted in a shift for the dying from care at home to hospitalization. End-of-life care became the responsibility of healthcare providers who often were not educated in care of the dying and hospitals that were ill equipped to meet the complex physical, emotional, and spiritual needs of the terminally ill (Bookbinder & Kiss, 2001; Ferrell, Virani, & Grant, 1999; Krisman-Scott, 2003; Rabow, Hardie, Fair, & McPhee, 2000; Super, 2001).

With advances in medical technology and treatments, many other aspects of dying were impacted. Infant and childhood mortality rates decreased markedly and causes of death changed dramatically. In the first half of the 1900s, most deaths were the result of influenza and pneumonia. Death from communicable disease became far less common with developments in sanitation, antibiotics, and immunizations (Berry & Matzo, 2004; Bookbinder & Kiss, 2001; Krisman-Scott, 2003). As a result, people began to live longer with chronic,

423

degenerative, and progressive illnesses. By 2006, the 10 leading causes of death in the United States (in rank order) were identified as: heart disease, malignant neoplasms, cerebrovascular diseases, chronic lower respiratory diseases, accidents or unintentional injuries, diabetes mellitus, Alzheimer's disease, influenza/pneumonia, kidney disease, and sepsis. These diseases accounted for close to 80% of all deaths. This, coupled with increased life expectancies and a growing, aging population, resulted in larger numbers of older Americans experiencing a longer, slower dying process (Amella, 2003; Heron et al., 2009).

Changes, such as the decline in infant and childhood mortality, mobility of society, distancing of extended families, late experiences with death, and hospitalization of the dying, resulted in Americans becoming estranged from death. These factors and medical advances made it easier for patients, families, and healthcare providers to deny the inevitability of death. It became common practice to use aggressive technology and curative therapies in patients with incurable illness. It was not unusual for patients to be kept alive with technology with the expectation that developments for a cure could be in progress. In the 1960s, families and professionals began to question the medicalization of the dying and the technical, depersonalized deaths occurring in hospitals. In 1969, Dr. Elizabeth Kubler-Ross published her best-selling work on dying patients, *On Death and Dying*, which revealed the tragedy of the hospitalized dying experience and the inability of the American healthcare system to focus on appropriate care when cure was no longer possible.

It is overwhelmingly clear that care for the dying in this country remains inadequate and much work remains to be done. Nurses in general and advanced practice nurses, particularly those with expertise in palliative care, have been recognized as an essential resource for meeting the complex needs of dying patients and their families. One key component of nurses' willingness to actively take part in end-of-life care comes with the acceptance of death as a natural part of the life cycle. With this acceptance, a journey of

growth can begin with the recognition of death as an opportunity and achievement, rather than a medical failure. Nursing professionals are crucial in ensuring that patients and families are not deprived of such opportunities for growth at the end of life (Byock, 1997; Weigel, Parker, Fanning, Reyna, & Gasbarra, 2007).

GOLD STANDARD FOR END-OF-LIFE CARE: HOSPICE AND PALLIATIVE CARE

Hospice

Hospice began in the United States as a grassroots movement to improve the quality of care being provided to dying patients and surviving families. The contemporary hospice movement, founded by Dame Cicely Saunders in London in the 1950s and 1960s, continues to be the gold standard for end-of-life care. Dame Saunders was instrumental in the development of the first organized hospice program in the United States, which opened in Connecticut in 1975 (Egan & Labyak, 2001; Krisman-Scott, 2003). At the center of hospice care is the belief that dying is a normal part of the life cycle. When cure is no longer possible or realistic, focusing on curative care becomes inappropriate. Instead, patients elect to focus on quality of remaining life, relief of suffering, and symptom control. An interdisciplinary hospice team helps not only with physical care, but also psychosocial and spiritual support, and grief and bereavement for surviving family members. Hospice teams include physicians, nurses, chaplains, social workers, nursing assistants, bereavement counselors, and volunteers. The plan of care is based on knowledge of patient and family preferences and goals of end-of-life care.

The delivery of hospice care can occur in a variety of settings. Most hospice care continues to be provided in the home setting by family and friends. However, as the population ages, hospices are serving an older-adult population who can no longer live alone or with frail caregivers. In such cases, the definition of "home" may commonly be a rest home, assisted living facility, or nursing home. In addition, inpatient hospital hospice units and hospice residences are emerging as other options for patients who are no longer able to stay in their own homes at end of life. Hospice services are available to patients of any age, religion, race, illness, and financial situation. Many hospice programs provide free care to specific patients without insurance or financial resources.

The Medicare Hospice Benefit provides hospice care to patients who elect it and are certified to be terminally ill with a prognosis of 6 months or less if the disease runs its usual course. Under the Medicare Hospice Benefit, beneficiaries elect to receive noncurative treatment and services for a variety of life-limiting illnesses ranging from cancer to dementia. The Medicare Hospice Benefit includes home visits by the interdisciplinary team, medical equipment, medical supplies, medications that relate to the hospice diagnosis, volunteer and bereavement support, and therapy services, when appropriate. The benefit reimburses for inpatient care in a variety of settings when patients are very close to end of life or have acute symptoms that require intensive management for a limited time, usually a few weeks. Additionally, the routine hospice benefit covers services delivered in a variety of settings including home, nursing home, assisted living, and residences, but does not cover room and board. Patients and families are also eligible for respite care in a Medicare-approved facility for up to 5 days at a time. Patients continue to receive hospice care for their illnesses as long as these services remain appropriate, which can range from days to months to years. Patients may revoke their hospice benefit at any time. Various insurance companies are realizing the importance of hospice and include a hospice benefit similar to the Medicare benefit.

Palliative Care

Palliative care is specialized, interdisciplinary care for patients with serious, life-limiting, or chronic debilitating illnesses. It involves the comprehensive management of the patient's physical, psychological, social, and spiritual needs. The goal of palliative care is to maximize quality of life through expert control of pain and other distressing physical symptoms, management of psychosocial stressors, and attention to spiritual needs. The original model of palliative care is hospice care. However, unlike hospice care, palliative care can occur any time during a patient's illness, even if life expectancy extends to years and aggressive or curative treatment is being pursued. Typically, the intensity and range of palliative interventions change as the illness progresses and the complexity of care increases. Palliative care continues to mature from a grass-roots field of end-of-life care into a freestanding healthcare service (Symes & Bruce, 2009). Palliative care services developed primarily within large healthcare institutions, whereas hospice care developed in communities (Symes & Bruce).

Palliative medicine and nursing are well established specialties in Great Britain and Australia. In more recent years, palliative care has been emerging as a distinct medical and nursing specialty in the United States. The number of palliative care programs in this country continues to grow. Palliative care is being offered in specialized inpatient units, in the form of consultative services in acute, long-term care, and home settings, and in outpatient clinics. Physicians and nurses with specialized training and experience are eligible to sit for board certification in palliative care. Palliative care should be provided by a specially trained, interdisciplinary team that includes physicians, nurses, social workers, and chaplains.

There is overwhelming evidence that most healthcare providers in general receive little or no training in pain and symptom management and other complex issues related to end-of-life care. As a result, there is often unfamiliarity with concepts of advanced pain and symptom control and discomfort with complex topics, such as prognostication, communicating bad news, resuscitation wishes, artificial nutrition and hydration (ANH), placement of feeding tubes, implications of initiating and withdrawing treatments, medical futility, resolving communication conflicts, and discussions surrounding burdens versus benefits of treatments. In addition, because of the complexity and time intensity of these discussions, primary care providers are often left without the proper time to facilitate these lengthy, emotional discussions. With advanced training and certification, palliative care providers are the ideal specialists to be consulted to provide this level of care in conjunction with the primary healthcare team. Geropsychiatric nurses may be important members of the palliative care team providing mental health services to older adults with psychiatric or mental health problems and their families.

Barriers to Quality Care at End of Life

Despite the fact that hospice care is the gold standard for end of life and that it is widely available in the United States, many barriers prevent uniform access. Perhaps the most eye-opening recognition of these barriers came with the results of the Study to Understand Prognoses and Preferences for Outcomes and Risks of Treatments (SUPPORT, 1995). SUPPORT was a 5-year study of more than 9000 hospitalized adults with one or more of nine life-threatening cancer and noncancer diagnoses. All of the patients involved were terminally ill and had predictable courses of illness. The objective of the study was to improve end-of-life decision making and reduce the frequency of a mechanically supported, painful, and prolonged process of dying. The goal was to develop a model intervention that would improve the frequency and effectiveness of communication between physicians and patients about medical decisions. This landmark study provided overwhelming empirical evidence that detailed many problems with end-of-life care of seriously ill, hospitalized patients.

SUPPORT data suggested that most of the patients who participated in the study died in the hospital under unfavorable conditions. Almost half of all "do not resuscitate" orders were written within the last 2 days of life, and for patients preferring "do not resuscitate" status, less than 50% of their physicians were aware of this preference. Almost half of patients spent more than 8 days at the end of life in an intensive care unit receiving mechanical ventilation or in a comatose state. For 50% of patients who had been conscious at the end of life, families reported at least half of their final days were spent in moderate to severe pain. The study demonstrated that well-planned interventions did not improve outcomes, because patients in the intervention group did not have better experiences than the control group. The findings from this study have contributed to the development of many initiatives to improve the care of the dying.

The inadequacy of care of the dying in the United States was further documented in 1997 when the Institute of Medicine published a report that summarized the priorities necessary for improving end-of-life care. Four major barriers to quality end-of-life care were identified: (1) many people suffer at end of life because they do not receive appropriate palliative care or they receive inappropriate or ineffective care; (2) legal, organizational, and financial barriers prevent excellent end-of-life care; (3) physicians, nurses, and other healthcare professionals do not receive proper education and training to care for dying patients and their families; and (4) there is insufficient knowledge to guide consistent practice of evidence-based care at end of life (Field & Cassel, 1997).

Misperceptions by healthcare providers and the public in general about hospice and palliative care services remain a tremendous barrier to adequate end-of-life care. Many providers believe that hospice is for patients with a cancer diagnosis only or those very close to death. Hospice and palliative care experts are often called in very late, when patients are expected to live days to weeks rather than months. At this point, services become focused on crisis work because of limited time with dying patients and surviving family members. The challenge is to educate healthcare providers to refer patients early, so they can benefit from the full range of services for months rather than days. Most providers are unfamiliar with the National Hospice Organization's specific guidelines for noncancer diagnoses. This includes eligibility for patients with heart failure, dementia, terminal debility, and all advanced diseases. Improving the awareness among providers and the general public can improve use of the hospice benefit.

ADVANCE-CARE PLANNING

Advance-care planning enables patients to consider and communicate preferences regarding medical interventions that relate to illnesses and end-of-life care. Typically, patients make decisions with regard to specific life-sustaining therapies, such as CPR and mechanical ventilation, or about the general level of care they wish to receive, such as life-prolonging or palliative care (Lamont & Siegler, 2000). Additionally, discussions about advance-care planning involve appointing a person as decision maker in the event the patient becomes unable to communicate.

The Patient Self-Determination Act of 1990 guarantees the right of patients to determine the kinds of medical care they will and will not want if they lose the capacity to participate in decision making by virtue of disease progression or other causes (Grant, 1992). Healthcare providers are required to discuss and document such advance directives. Despite the Patient Self-Determination Act, and the widely held notion that completing advance directives is important to providing good medical care, few people have done so. According to the U.S. Living Will Registry (2000), only 20% of the general population had an advance directive. Another survey demonstrated that 16% of the public have engaged in these discussions with their healthcare providers and 11% have completed an advance directive (Schlegel & Shannon, 2000).

The two types of advance directives are the durable power of attorney for health care and the living will. The durable power of attorney for health care, also known as the "healthcare proxy," is a simple legal document naming an agent to make decisions relating to medical care in the event that the patient becomes unable to communicate preferences. Any competent adult 18 years of age or older can fill out a healthcare proxy. The document becomes legal when completed by the person and does not require an attorney. It is essential that the patient discuss his or her wishes for specific medical care with the designated agent. The agent's role is to make decisions with

regard to particular medical treatments, based on the patient's previous stated preferences and wishes. If the patient did not specify specific treatment preferences, the proxy should use substituted judgment to make decisions.

The living will is a legal statement that lists specific treatments and preferences by the individual patient. Patients are given the opportunity to think about specific medical interventions in the event of terminal illness, imminent death, vegetative state, and other specific states of health. The legalities of living wills may vary from state to state. Although this specific advance directive may not be legally binding in many states, it can be helpful in guiding care. Providers should familiarize themselves with their individual state laws in relation to such advance directives.

There are numerous barriers to providers and patients participating in advance care planning. These discussions can be time consuming and are often not reimbursed (Butterworth, 2003). Patients' preferences for end-of-life care are often misunderstood or misinterpreted, as demonstrated by the SUPPORT study. Discussing end-of-life issues forces providers to face their own mortality, which can be a deterrent to engaging in such discussions (Buttersworth). The general public often shares unrealistic expectations of medical interventions in relation to terminal illness. Lack of education for providers is a common barrier to advance-care planning. According to one study, only 26% of providers have received any end-of-life training in their educational programs (Schlegel & Shannon, 2000). Additionally, the cultures of healthcare systems, and patients' individual cultural beliefs, are a common obstacle to engaging in planning.

A prevalent impediment to advance-care planning is the public's misconception of the success rate for CPR, mechanical ventilation, and other aggressive interventions. In contrast to popular belief, resuscitation is not an easy procedure with a high success rate. It is known that CPR under the best circumstances has a survival rate of about 15% (Cranston, 2001). Furthermore, CPR is fraught with a variety of complications including rib fractures, major heart or lung injuries, or ending up in a persistent vegetative state (Cranston). Patients at end of life, with advanced illnesses, have little to no chance of survival by having CPR performed, and in such cases CPR may violate a patient's right to die with dignity. The literature supports the notion that for CPR to have any remote possibility of success, the event must be witnessed and unexpected, meaning that terminally ill patients without vital signs do not have any possible life-saving benefit from CPR (Gordon, 2003). If it is clear that death is approaching and the goals of care have been identified as comfort focused, then CPR is not an appropriate medical intervention and healthcare providers should recommend against such an intervention. Artificial ventilation is also not considered appropriate treatment for terminally ill patients who are nearing the end of life. If artificial ventilation fails to benefit the patient, and the process of death is proceeding, such interventions should be discontinued or withheld and the focus of care should be on aggressive comfort interventions. Discussions should take place in advance with patients and families based on preferences, values, and goals of care.

Artificial nutrition and hydration (ANH) at end of life is a twentieth-century technology. ANH has been considered a necessary component to good medical care, with the primary intention of benefiting patients. Withholding or withdrawing hydration is a difficult issue for many providers, perhaps because offering food and fluids is linked to sustaining life and providing patient care (Bennett, 2000). It is almost reflexive for healthcare providers and families to request such interventions for patients who lose the ability to swallow, although the evidence base for using such techniques is weak at best. When a person is approaching death, ANH can be potentially harmful and may provide little to no benefit to patients and at times may make dying more uncomfortable (AAHPM, 2006).

There are numerous benefits of terminal dehydration found in the literature. Many of the potential benefits of dehydration include decreased pain

or no pain because of the anesthetic effect that electrolyte imbalances may provide. At the end of life, the brain converts the derivative of metabolic fat to γ-hydroxybutyrate, a substance with anesthetic properties (Fox, 1996). Electrolyte imbalances may serve as a natural anesthetic, facilitating a reduction in pain medication (Sutcliffe, 1994). Decreased urine output is a beneficial side effect of becoming fluid deficient at the end of life. Reduced urine output lessens incontinence, decreases the need for catheterization, and preserves skin integrity. Dehydration at the end of life decreases pharyngeal, pulmonary, and gastrointestinal secretions, leading to reduction in nausea, emesis, and pulmonary congestion (Meares, 1994; Zerwekh, 1983). Parenteral fluid and nutrition can cause discomfort with repeated venipunctures and iatrogenic infections (HPNA, 2003). Having an intravenous line is invasive, and terminally ill patients may need to be restrained because of the risk of injury from pulling at the line. It is also argued that the dying patient experiences multisystem failure, so electrolyte balance may be impossible to maintain even in the presence of artificial hydration (Sutcliffe).

There is limited support in the literature for using ANH at the end of life. Two common reasons for using it are concerns for discomfort related to thirst and dry mouth. Some authors propose thirst is attributable to a feeling of dry mouth, rather than to actual dehydration (Sutcliffe, 1994). Most experts agree that such oral discomfort can be eased with saliva substitutes, moisturizers, mouth care, ice chips, and petroleum jelly. Some medical consequences of dehydration at end of life include confusion, restlessness, and neuromuscular irritability (Huffman & Dunn, 2002). Occasionally, patients may benefit from a trial of intravenous fluids at end of life, to improve renal clearance when opioid metabolite accumulation is the suspected cause of confusion, or when patients have rapid fluid loss resulting in syncope and confusion (Huffman & Dunn).

In providing care to terminally ill patients close to the end of life, only essential medications should be administered (Cherny, Coyle, & Foley, 1996). These include medications for treatment of pain and other common symptoms. Medications that are offering no benefit to the patient should be discontinued. Antibiotic use at the end of life is often an issue met with controversy. In some cases, oral antibiotics may be a useful adjunct when the goal is palliation of the symptoms of infection, versus eradication of the infection. Oral antibiotics may be useful to reduce tachypnea, cough, sputum, fever, and shaking chills associated with infections. However, if antibiotics cause increased burden and physical distress because of nausea, diarrhea, or pruritis, for example, they should be discontinued. Parenteral antibiotic use is often not indicated unless there is an identified organism, there are clear goals to be met, the likelihood of success is high, and the patient is expected to live long enough to achieve the benefits of treatment.

DETERMINING PROGNOSIS

One hundred percent of patients will die. Ten percent will die suddenly, but 90% will at some point need terminal medical care (Plonk & Arnold, 2005). Medical science is poor at predicting how and when patients will die (Plonk & Arnold). Prognostication, or estimating life expectancy, is crucial in clinical practice, particularly in regards to end-of-life care. Accurate prediction of life expectancy is important for both providers and patients to make good clinical decisions when dealing with terminal illness (Christakis, 1999; SUPPORT, 1995). Prognostication involves exploring the natural history or clinical course of a particular disease, determining its average prognosis in most patients, and then applying it to a specific patient and his or her treatment decisions. However, true prognosis can never be absolutely established. Diagnosis, treatment, and prognosis are interrelated, although diagnosis and treatment receive much more attention in patient care, medical education, and research.

Prognosis is often linked to ethical decisions in clinical practice. It may affect decisions to initiate, withhold, or withdraw life-sustaining treatments in the terminally ill. Patients want information regarding prognosis to evaluate treatment decisions and determine when they should be referred for hospice care. With the lack of or an inaccurate prognosis, patients may receive unnecessary or burdensome rather than beneficial treatments. Unfortunately, no established method exists to definitively determine prognosis. Aside from disease-specific criteria, functional status and nutritional status can be good predictors of prognosis. Patients and families should understand that prognostication is not an exact science and can vary widely from one patient to another, particularly with chronic, progressive illness. Patients and families may need prognostic information to make and complete important plans, such as saying goodbye, completing relationships, writing wills, arranging finances, and making funeral plans (AAHPM, 2003). See Box 19-1 for the American Nurses Association's position on the role of the nurse in end-of-life decision making.

Despite the complexity inherent in the issue of prognostication, a more simplistic approach can serve as a beginning step toward improving end-of-life care and opportunities. With each patient encounter, consider the question "Would I be surprised if this patient died in the next few months?" Those who may be sick enough to die should be informed and counseled about possibilities to eliminate misconceptions and anxiety. Efforts should focus on prioritizing the patient's concerns, which may include symptom control, family support, and advance-care planning or spiritual issues. To understand the patient clearly, the nurse should ask "What do you hope for as you live with this condition? What do you fear?" Patients should understand that it is often difficult to know when death is close and should be asked to contemplate "If you were to die soon, what would be left undone?" Prognostication can help providers and patients to focus on life yet to be lived and what can be done to make it better (Lynn, Schuster, & Kabcenell, 2000).

BOX 19-1 ANA POSITION STATEMENTS ON NURSES' ROLE IN END-OF-LIFE DECISIONS

The American Nurses Association (ANA) (1996) has developed position statements on the nurses' role in end-of-life decisions, including:

Nursing and the Patient Self-Determination Acts—11/18/91
The American Nurses Association (ANA) believes that nurses should play a primary role in implementation of the Patient Self-Determination Act, passed as part of the Omnibus Budget Reconciliation Act of 1990. It is the responsibility of nurses to facilitate informed decision-making for patients making choices about end-of-life care. The nurse's role in education, research, patient care, and advocacy is critical to implementation of the Patient Self-Determination Act within all health care settings.

Pain Management and Control of Distressing Symptoms in Dying Patients—12/5/03
In the context of the caring relationship, nurses perform a primary role in the assessment and management of pain and other distressing symptoms in dying patients. Therefore, nurses must use effective doses of medications prescribed for symptom control and nurses have a moral obligation to advocate on behalf of the patient when prescribed medication is insufficiently managing pain and other distressing symptoms. The increasing titration of medication to achieve adequate symptom control is ethically justified.

Forgoing Nutrition and Hydration—4/2/92
The American Nurses Association (ANA) believes that the decision to withhold artificial nutrition and hydration should be made by the patient or surrogate with the health care team. The nurse continues to provide expert care to patients who are no longer receiving artificial nutrition and hydration.

Nursing Care and Do-Not-Resuscitate Decisions—12/2003
The appropriate use of DNR orders, together with adequate palliative end of life care, can prevent suffering for many dying patients who experience cardiac/pulmonary arrest. As the primary continuous HCP in health care facilities, the nurse must be involved in the planning as well as the implementation of resuscitation decisions. Clear DNR policies at the institutional level that include the basic features that ANA recommends will enable nurses to effectively participate in this crucial aspect of patient care.

Assisted Suicide—12/8/94
The American Nurses Association (ANA) believes that the nurse should not participate in assisted suicide. Such an act is in violation of the Code for Nurses with Interpretive Statements (Code for Nurses) and the ethical traditions of the profession. Nurses, individually and collectively, have an obligation to provide comprehensive and compassionate end-of-life care which includes the promotion of comfort and the relief of pain, and at times, forgoing life-sustaining treatments.

Active Euthanasia—12/8/94
The American Nurses Association (ANA) believes that the nurse should not participate in active euthanasia because such an act is in direct violation of the Code for Nurses with Interpretive Statements (Code for Nurses), the ethical traditions and goals of the profession, and its covenant with society. Nurses have an obligation to provide timely, humane, comprehensive and compassionate end-of-life care.

Source: American Nurses Association. (1996). Position statements on nurse's role in end-of-life decisions. Washington, DC: Author. Retrieved June 7, 2009, from http://www.nursingworld.org. Reproduced with permission.

PATIENT–FAMILY ASSESSMENT

The number one priority in patient assessment in end-of-life care is to identify areas of suffering so that appropriate plans for symptom relief can be formulated and necessary interdisciplinary team members can be consulted, such as palliative care specialists, psychiatric specialists, chaplains, or social workers (Lee & Washington, 2008). To ensure a holistic assessment, the American Medical Association's Education for Physicians on End-of-Life Care Curriculum (EPEC, 1999) has developed an assessment tool made up of nine dimensions. The assessment dimensions include illness and treatment summary, physical, psychological, decision making, communication, social, spiritual, practical, and anticipatory planning for death. A few of these dimensions are addressed next in detail.

Physical assessment in end-of-life care is primarily concerned with physical symptoms and how they impact on an individual's daily life and ability to function. There is less focus on physical assessment from an anatomic or organ system approach, because the major relevance in palliative care is the control of symptoms. Symptoms, such as pain, that are poorly managed prevent patients from achieving quality of remaining life and participating in meaningful activities as end of life approaches. Some commonly encountered symptoms in advanced terminal illness are pain, fatigue, dyspnea, insomnia, anorexia, nausea, constipation, anxiety, depression, and delirium. Inquiry about each symptom is crucial. The patient's self-report and self-measurement of the intensity or severity of the symptom should be accepted because these are subjective phenomena.

Performing a psychological assessment is essential to providing good care at end of life. Nurses may begin to make some notes at the beginning of the interview. Observations should be made about cognitive status, mood, and presence of any confusion or delirium and these should be addressed if noted. History should be gathered about past or present mood disorders. Screening questions about suicidal ideation may be appropriate. Assessing for anxiety, depression, and delirium is essential, with more in-depth assessments using validated tools. It is essential for the nurse to address common fears, such as loss of control, loss of dignity, loss of independence, loss of relationships, becoming a burden, and physical suffering. Individuals also commonly face unresolved issues in personal matters and relationships as end of life approaches. Sometimes these issues may prevent patients from achieving a peaceful frame of mind. Identification of these issues allows for development of an individualized care plan. Referral should be considered in any situation in need of higher levels of psychiatric expertise, preferably to providers also skilled in end-of-life care.

Spiritual assessment is essential to understanding the role of religion in a patient's life and the resources that affiliation may bring. Past spiritual involvement, and current desires, should be explored. Questioning should explore whether the patient would like a chaplain to visit, and whether there are any important religious rituals to honor. It should be recognized that some patients might experience significant spiritual growth at end of life, whereas others may struggle with spiritual distress. Spiritual crises may arise as people face death and begin to question the meaning and purpose in life. Patients may also question their faith or express guilt and a desire for forgiveness. Others may feel abandoned by God. Spiritual needs may be assessed through such questions as "Are you a spiritual person?" "What role does religion play in your life?" "Have you thought about what will happen after you die?" or "Have you tried to make sense of what's happening to you?" The identification of spiritual suffering is crucial and enables obtaining appropriate religious support and resources for comprehensive spiritual care.

Assessment of decision-making capacity follows naturally from the psychological assessment. Even patients with some degree of mental compromise may show clear insight into information and may be able to give meaningful consent. To assess a patient's decision-making capacity, it must be determined whether the patient can understand that he or she is authorizing the decision, can demonstrate rational use of the information including risks, can demonstrate insight into the possible consequences of the decision, and that the decision is made without the influence of coercion. In the absence of capacity, an authorized proxy must decide on the patient's behalf using the patient's prior stated preferences or substituted judgment. Goals of care should be discussed with the patient and family so they may be tailored to matters of personal meaning. Patients may be asked, "What are the most important things to be accomplished?" Common responses may include aggressive symptom management or the desire to prolong life until an important event, such as a family wedding or anniversary. Advance-care planning for future medical care should also be addressed. Preferences should be discussed, preferably in the presence of the future proxy decision maker, in the event that there may be a time when the patient may not be able to make decisions. Having already identified goals of care makes it easier for the patient to make decisions about future medical care that may or may not help to achieve individual goals.

PAIN

Pain can be defined in many ways, although most succinctly it is "whatever the person says it is, experienced whenever they say they are experiencing it" (McCaffery & Pasero, 1999). Dame Cicely Saunders correctly noted that pain at the end of life can be physical, emotional, social, or spiritual (Plonk & Arnold, 2005). It is a completely subjective experience and patient self-reports remain the only valid measure of pain. Some patients may not be able to report their pain, and in such cases it is acceptable to ask family and caregivers if they believe the person is in pain. Adequate relief of pain begins with comprehensive assessment. Assessment parameters should include pain history, onset, location, intensity, quality, pattern, aggravating or alleviating factors, medication history, and meaning of the pain to the patient. Whenever possible, it is best to ask patients to quantify pain severity with a validated tool, such as a 0–10 intensity rating scale. A thorough medication history should be taken to determine what medications have already been tried, at what

doses and timing intervals. Any report of allergic reaction to analgesics should be explored because true allergies are rare and the experience may have been a manageable side effect, such as nausea. Physical examination should focus on nonverbal pain cues, inspection of site or sites of pain, palpation, auscultation, percussion, and focused neurological examination as needed, if there is suspicion for neuropathic pain or neurological compromise. Nonpharmacological approaches to terminal discomfort include excellent nursing care, skin care, repositioning, massage, music, Reiki, and many other supportive interventions. Pharmacological principles and therapies are numerous and beyond the scope of this chapter.

THE DYING PROCESS

The art of nursing care includes the opportunity to be present when a patient is actively dying. This can be both a time of grief and sorrow, and a time of love and personal growth for all involved. As a patient's illness progresses and death nears, the focus of care changes. The philosophy of care shifts from living well and quality of life to the process of dying well. Physical, social, and spiritual needs change as the end of life grows closer. Pain and symptom management issues become more complex and involving hospice and palliative care experts becomes essential to good end-of-life care.

It is often difficult for healthcare providers to recognize and acknowledge imminently approaching death. This may be a self-protective mechanism used by providers, patients, and families. However, in an era of technically disguised dying, the dying process may be surprisingly difficult to recognize (Dunn & Milch, 2002). One of the most reliable signs that a patient is dying is their own report. It is important for healthcare providers to pay close attention, because patients often allude to when they anticipate dying. Sometimes patients who are very near death relate having visions of people who are deceased waiting in the room. They may have conversations with people who are not visible. These experiences may be comforting to both patients and families at the end of life.

Although prognosticating when death will occur is often inaccurate, there are some predictable signs that death is nearing. Commonly, physical changes can assist patients and families in the preparation for death. Months before death may occur, patients may become more withdrawn. Patients may begin to decrease their food and fluid intake and require more sleep. When death draws closer, within days to weeks, patients commonly are profoundly weak, often becoming bedbound. At this point, patients become dependent with all care, including feeding and continence. Additionally, there may be a reduction in awareness, disinterest in food and fluids, and dysphagia. Skin often becomes clammy and appearance changes from pale to mottled (Moneymaker, 2005; Pitorak, 2003). Mottling, a sign that death is imminent, is secondary to decreases in the peripheral circulation. It is commonly seen first on the heels of the patient and over bony prominence. Agitation and restlessness in the final hours of life are common symptoms. This may be caused by medications, electrolyte imbalances, organ failure, infections, or various other reasons (Pitorak). Approaching death exhibits the following changes (Dunn & Milch, 2002):

Changes consistent with death approaching within weeks to days

Progressive, profound weakness

Bedbound

Increased sleeping

Disinterest in food and fluids

Dysphagia

Weakening voice

Inability to close eyes

Incontinence

Oliguria

Diminished attention span

Vivid dreams

Reports of seeing previously deceased people

Speech content containing references to home or travel to a final destination

Changes consistent with death approaching within hours

Cheyne-Stokes respirations

Apnea

Mottling

Cool skin

Restlessness, agitation

Death rattle

Hypotension

Tachycardia

No radial pulse

Death vigils are an important opportunity for friends and families to begin the grieving process. Sitting at the bedside and being present can be the greatest gift to those in the process of dying. Often time is spent sharing memories, telling stories, and touching the dying individual. Nurses should encourage and take part in death vigils when appropriate. It is believed that hearing is the last remaining sense, so continual communication with the dying patient should be encouraged, even when comatose. It is essential that discussions are held with patients and families before the dying process regarding where they wish to die, whom they would like present, and whether they would like to listen to music and if so what type. Immediately after the patient dies, it is important that the healthcare team allow time for family members and friends to spend with the patient's body.

GRIEF AND BEREAVEMENT

Two very important aspects of end-of-life care are often overlooked. First, nursing care and responsibilities to the patient and family do not come to an end on the death of the patient. Second, a bereavement needs assessment of the family and friends of the dying patient should ideally begin at the time of diagnosis and continue throughout the course of the illness. Bereavement is the range of emotions and behavior a person experiences when he or she suffers a loss, particularly the death of another person. It consists of the grief a person feels and the outward expression of mourning exhibited. It occurs over the period of time that it takes to experience grief of the loss, and to adjust to life without the deceased. Grief is the emotional response or reaction that occurs as a result of the loss (Corliss, 2001; Egan & Arnold, 2003; Potter, 2001). All dying patients may feel loss because of many factors, such as loss of physical control or function, loss of independence, loss of employment and finances, and eventually loss of life. Grief is often felt by patients and families in response to these losses and in response to approaching death. Grief and bereavement are normal, individualized experiences and processes. Resolution of grief is often dependent on support and resources available to aid in dealing with grief. Bereavement care should be offered to friends and family before death to increase support and information to try to prevent complicated grief and bereavement (Egan & Arnold; Hebert, Schulz, Copeland, & Arnold, 2009).

There are various types of grief and nurses should be able to assess for and determine the type to implement appropriate interventions. Anticipatory grief usually occurs before a loss, such as at the time of diagnosis. It may occur in response to anticipated or actual loss of health, function, or independence. Anticipatory grief may provide some benefits, such as providing time for acknowledgment of death, preparation for death, adaptation to change that will occur over the course of an illness, and resolution of conflicts.

Normal or uncomplicated grief is characterized by expected emotional and behavioral responses to a loss. Responses to loss may be physical, psychological, cognitive, or spiritual. The responses vary widely among individuals in terms of coping strategies, expressions, and behaviors. They are influenced by past experience with loss and death, and cultural and social factors (Clements et al., 2003; Corliss, 2001).

Complicated grief may occur if reactions persist over long periods of time, are overwhelming, or interfere with physical or emotional well-being. Some manifestations of complicated grief include severe or prolonged depression, suicidal ideation, extreme isolation, or avoidance of any reminder of the deceased. Some risk factors for complicated grief include sudden or traumatic death, multiple losses, unresolved grief from earlier losses, suffering at end of life by the loved one, lack of supports, and lack of faith beliefs (Zhang, El-Jawahri, & Prigerson, 2006). Complicated grief may be further subdivided into chronic, delayed, exaggerated, masked, and disenfranchised grief. Chronic grief may begin as normal grief but persists over an excessively long period of time. Delayed grief occurs when normal grief reactions are suppressed or postponed, either consciously or subconsciously, to avoid the pain of the loss. Exaggerated grief is characterized by the use of potentially harmful coping strategies or self-destructive behavior in an attempt to alleviate pain. It may manifest as substance abuse, suicidal ideation or attempts, or unsafe sex practices. Masked grief results when a person is unaware that his or her ability to function normally is being affected by their response to loss. Manifestations may include maintaining physical distance, avoiding relationships, and rejecting help (Arnold & Egan, 2004; Ferris, Von Gunten, & Emanuel, 2003). Disenfranchised grief occurs when a loss has been experienced and cannot be openly acknowledged or shared because the relationship has not been accepted by or revealed to family or friends. People who may be at risk for this type of grief include gay and lesbian partners. It is often manifested as anger, sadness, and isolation (Egan & Arnold, 2003).

Nursing assessment of grief should include the patient, family, significant others, friends, and professional caregivers, such as nursing home or home care staff. Ideally, it should start at the time of diagnosis of serious illness and should continue throughout the course of the illness. Following the death of the patient, it should extend into the bereavement period for the survivors. Following assessment, bereavement interventions should be implemented to facilitate the grieving process. This should start with helping survivors to recognize that grief is a normal response and that there is no standard or "right" way to grieve. It is helpful for survivors to understand that the symptoms of grief that they may be experiencing are expected, such as trouble sleeping or concentrating or sudden waves of sadness or emotion. Education should include information, such as the fact that grieving may go on for months to years and may become more intense or resurface on significant dates, such as holidays, birthdays, or the anniversary of the death (Egan & Arnold, 2003). Nursing interventions should include facilitation of identification and expression of feelings, which may help survivors manage stress and deal with the emotional pain that is a necessary component of grief. Facilitation of and participation in funerals, memorial services, or other rituals are important bereavement interventions to help survivors acknowledge the death and memorialize their loved one (Arnold & Egan, 2004).

There are generally four tasks that bereaved persons must complete to deal with their loss in an effective manner. The first task involves realizing and accepting that the loss or death has actually occurred. Second, it is important that they are able to experience the pain that the loss has caused. Third, they need to acknowledge how the loss is significant to them and how it is going to impact their lives. Finally, as grief evolves, they need to be able to concentrate their energy into new relationships and activities. Although these tasks may seem simple to approach, they can be extremely difficult for emotionally overwhelmed, grieving individuals without appropriate support from caregivers, friends, and family (Ferris et al., 2003).

▌ CASE STUDY 1

An 82-year-old woman with widely metastatic breast cancer to bone, pleura, and brain has been admitted to the hospital. She has had multiple rounds of chemotherapy and whole-brain radiation since her initial diagnosis in 2002. She is married with three grown children and has been admitted to the hospital for further management of her severe pain, anxiety, and dyspnea related to her disease. Over the past 6 months she has become much weaker, spending more time in bed or in a chair. She has had several falls at home and lost approximately 25 pounds in the past 2 months. There have been several discussions with the patient and her family related to end-of-life issues and a possible hospice referral. The patient and her family have adamantly refused to consider the possibility of death approaching.

What resources may be helpful for the patient and family during this difficult time? How would you address the care of this patient if you were the geropsychiatric nurse caring for this patient?

▌ CASE STUDY 2

A 72-year-old woman with severe cardiomyopathy, congestive heart failure, and an ejection fraction of 20% is being seen in an outpatient psychiatric care facility because of her severe depression, anxiety, and insomnia. She has been widowed for the past 3 years and is accompanied by her two supportive nieces. She lives in a senior housing facility but has had several admissions to the hospital and local rehabilitation facilities because of her progressive weakness. She was recently admitted to the geropsychiatric unit because of her statements about wishing to die.

What would be your approach to caring for this woman? Describe resources that would assist in addressing the needs of this patient and family. Discuss appropriate follow-up for this patient in relation to her mental health needs.

FUTURE END-OF-LIFE CARE

The future of end-of-life care remains ever-changing. End-of-life care will become more significant as the population ages. The trend will continue to change from dying in hospital settings to dying in homes, nursing homes, and various other settings. Interventions will be developed and terminal illnesses may transition to chronic illnesses. Although the medical community searches for a quick fix to the inevitable mortality through the discovery of miracle cures for terminal illness, little discussion takes place about the alternatives for care of persons who will not survive their disease, known as "palliative care" (Walsh & Gordon, 2001). Palliative care must become a healthcare priority, and public policy and healthcare funding must be redirected to respond (Walsh & Gordon). This includes more research to guide pain and symptom management, and quality end-of-life care. The research committee of the Hospice and Palliative Nurses Association has set forth a research agenda for 2009 to 2012 to provide a focus for nurse researchers for well designed studies to obtain evidence-based information necessary for optimal care of the terminally ill and their families (Campbell et al., 2009).

Healthcare providers are all faced with many challenges within the healthcare system. A major challenge ahead is the rapidly growing population of aging, chronically, and terminally ill people in the United States. Americans are living longer in general and living longer with complex, debilitating illness. As a result, there is an increased need for specialized pain and symptom control and complex care discussions and planning. A challenge in meeting this need is the scarcity of healthcare providers with the expertise required providing this level of care (Kapo, Morrison, & Liao, 2007). The "Promoting Excellence in End-of-Life Care" national program of the Robert Wood Johnson Foundation (2002), "dedicated to long-term changes in health care to improve care of the dying and their families" (para. 11), has examined this issue and recognizes that nurses, and especially advanced practice nurses with expertise in palliative care, represent a crucial resource for meeting the needs of chronically and terminally ill Americans and their families. Since 2001, the Robert Wood Johnson Foundation has provided funding for a national education program on end-of-life care for nurses known as the End-of-Life Nursing Education Consortium. In 2007, a specialty curriculum for this program was developed regarding geriatric end-of-life care and palliative care, which is working to prepare nurses to meet the needs of this ever-growing, unique population (Malloy, Virani, Kelly, Harrington-Jacobs, & Ferrell 2008).

REFERENCES

Amella, E. (2003). Geriatrics and palliative care: Collaboration for quality of life until death. *Journal of Hospice and Palliative Nursing, 5*(1), 40–48.

American Academy of Hospice and Palliative Medicine (AAHPM). (2003). *Pocket guide to hospice/palliative medicine.* Glenview, IL: Author.

American Academy of Hospice and Palliative Medicine. (2006). Position statement: Statement on the use of nutrition and hydration. Retrieved November 5, 2009, from http://www.aahpm.org/positions/nutrition.html

American Nurses Association. (1996). *Position statements on the nurse's role in end-of-life decisions.* Washington, DC: Author.

American Nurses Association. (2005). Code of ethics for nurses with interpretive statements. Kansas City, MO: Author. Retrieved November 5, 2009, from http://nursingworld.org/ethics/code/protected_nwcoe813.htm

Arnold, R., & Egan, K. (2004). Suffering, loss, grief, and bereavement. In M. Matzo & D. Sherman (Eds.), *Gerontologic pallative care nursing* (pp. 148–164). St. Louis, MO: Mosby.

Bennett, J. A. (2000). Dehydration: Hazards and benefits. *Geriatric Nursing, 21*(2), 84–88.

Berry, P., & Matzo, M. (2004). Death and an aging society. In M. Matzo & D. Sherman (Eds.), *Gerontologic palliative care nursing* (pp. 31–51). St. Louis, MO: Mosby.

Bookbinder, M., & Kiss, M. (2001). Death and society. In M. Matzo & D. Sherman (Eds.), *Palliative care nursing: Quality care to the end of life* (pp. 89–117). New York: Springer.

Butterworth, A. M. (2003). Reality check: Ten barriers to advance planning. *The Nurse Practitioner, 28*(5), 42–43.

Byock, I. (1997). *Dying well: Peace and possibilities at the end of life.* New York: Berkley.

Campbell, M., Happ, M., Hultman, T., Kirchhoff, K., Mahon, M., Murray Mayo, M., et al. (2009). The HPNA research agenda for 2009-2012. *Journal of Hospice and Palliative Nursing, 11*(1), 10–18.

Cherny, N. I., Coyle, N., & Foley, K. M. (1996). Guidelines in the care of the dying cancer patient. *Hematology/Oncology Clinics of North America, 10*(1), 261–287.

Christakis, N. (1999). *Death foretold: Prophecy and prognosis in medical care.* Chicago: University of Chicago Press.

Clements, P., Vigil, G., Manno, M., Henry, G., Wilks, J., Das, S., et al. (2003). Cultural perspectives of death, grief, and bereavement. *Journal of Psychosocial Nursing and Mental Health Services, 41*(7), 18–26.

Corliss, I. (2001). Bereavement. In B. Ferrell & N. Coyle (Eds.), *Textbook of palliative nursing* (pp. 352–362). New York: Oxford University Press.

Cranston, R. E. (2001). Advance directives and "do not resuscitate" orders. Retrieved December 22, 2003, from http://www.cbhd.org/resources/endoflife/cranston_2001-12-14.htm

Dunn, G., & Milch, R. (2002). Is this a bad day, or one of the last days? How to recognize and respond to approaching demise. *Journal of American College of Surgeons, 195*(6), 879–887.

Education for Physicians on End-of-Life Care Curriculum (EPEC). (1999). *Whole patient assessment. Trainer's guide.* Chicago: American Medical Association.

Egan, K., & Arnold, R. (2003). Grief and bereavement care: With sufficient support, grief and bereavement can be transformative. *American Journal of Nursing, 103*(9), 42–52.

Egan, K., & Labyak, M. (2001). Hospice care: A model for quality end-of-life care. In B. Ferrell & N. Coyle (Eds.), *Textbook of palliative nursing* (pp. 7–26). New York: Oxford University Press.

Ferrell, B., Virani, R., & Grant, M. (1999). Analysis of end-of-life content in nursing textbooks. *Oncology Nursing Forum, 26,* 869–876.

Ferris, F., Von Gunten, C., & Emanuel, L. (2003). Competency in end-of-life care. *Journal of Palliative Medicine, 6*(4), 605–613.

Field, M., & Cassel, C. (Eds.). (1997). *Approaching death: Improving care at the end of life.* Committee on Care at the End of Life, Division of Health Care Services, Institute of Medicine. Washington, DC: National Academy Press.

Fox, E. T. (1996). IV hydration in the terminally ill: Ritual or therapy. *British Journal of Nursing, 5*(1), 41–45.

Gordon, M. (2003). CPR in long-term care: Mythical benefits or necessary ritual? *Annals of Long-Term Care, 11*(4), 41–49.

Grant, K. D. (1992). The Patient Self-Determination Act: Implications for physicians. *Hospital Practice, 27*(44), 44–48.

Hebert, R., Schulz, R., Copeland, V., & Arnold, R. (2009). Preparing family caregivers for death and bereavement: Insights from caregivers of terminally ill patients. *Journal of Pain and Symptom Management, 37*(1), 3–12.

Heron, M., Hoyert, D., Murphy, S., Xu, J., Kochanek, K., & Tejada-Vera, B. (2009). Deaths: Final data for 2006. *U.S. Department of Health and Human Services; National Vital Statistics Report, 57*(14), 1–135.

Hospice and Palliative Nurses Association. (2003). *Position statement on artificial nutrition and hydration.* Retrieved June 23, 2003, from http://www.hpna.org/position_artificialnutrition

Huffman, J. L., & Dunn, G. P. (2002). The paradox of hydration in advanced terminal illness. *Journal of American College of Surgeons, 194*(6), 835–839.

Kapo, J., Morrison, L., & Liao, S. (2007). Palliative care of the older adult. *Journal of Palliative Medicine, 10*(1), 185–209.

Krisman-Scott, M. (2003). Origins of hospice in the United States. *Journal of Hospice and Palliative Nursing, 5*(4), 205–210.

Kubler-Ross, E. (1969). *On death and dying.* New York: Macmillan.

Lamont, E., & Siegler, M. (2000). Paradoxes in cancer patients' advance care planning. *Journal of Palliative Medicine, 3*(1), 27–35.

Lee, N., & Washington, G. (2008). Management of common symptoms at end of life in acute care settings. *The Journal for Nurse Practitioners, 4*(8), 610–615.

Lynn, J., Schuster, J., & Kabcenell, A. (2000). *Improving care for the end of life: A sourcebook for health care managers and clinicians.* New York: Oxford University Press.

Malloy, P., Virani, R., Kelly, K., Harrington-Jacobs, H., & Ferrell, B. (2008). Seven years and 50 courses later: End-of-Life Nursing Education Consortium continues commitment to provide excellent palliative care education. *Journal of Hospice and Palliative Nursing, 10*(4), 233–239.

McCaffery, M., & Pasero, C. (1999). *Pain clinical manual* (2nd ed.). St. Louis, MO: Mosby.

Meares, C. J. (1994). Terminal dehydration: A review. *American Journal of Hospice and Palliative Care, 11*(3), 10–14.

Moneymaker, K. A. (2005). Understanding the dying process: Transition from final days to hours. *Journal of Palliative Medicine, 8*(5), 1079

Omnibus Budget Reconciliation Act of 1990. (Publication No. 101-508, Sect. 4206, 4751)

Pitorak, E. F. (2003). Care at the time of death. *American Journal of Nursing, 103*(7), 42–52.

Plonk, W. M., & Arnold, R. M. (2005). Terminal care: The last weeks of life. *Journal of Palliative Medicine, 8*(5), 1042–1054.

Potter, M. (2001). Loss, suffering, bereavement, and grief. In M. Matzo & D. Sherman (Eds.), *Palliative care nursing: Quality care to the end of life* (pp. 275–321). New York: Springer.

Promoting Excellence in End of Life Care. (2002). *A position statement from American nursing leaders: Recommendations.* Retrieved August 3, 2004, from http://www.PromotingExcellence.org

Rabow, M., Hardie, G., Fair, J., & McPhee, S. (2000). End-of-life care content in 50 textbooks from multiple specialties. *JAMA, 283*, 771–778.

Schlegel, K. L., & Shannon, S. E. (2000). Legal guidelines related to end-of-life decisions: Are nurse practitioners knowledgeable? *Journal of Gerontological Nursing, 26*(9), 14–24.

Sherman, D., & Laporte, M. (2001). Palliative care nursing: Changing the experience of dying in America. In M. Matzo & D. Sherman (Eds.), *Palliative care nursing: Quality care to the end of life* (pp. xvii–xxiv). New York: Springer.

Super, A. (2001). The context of palliative care in progressive illness. In B. Ferrell & N. Coyle (Eds.), *Textbook of palliative nursing* (pp. 27–36). New York: Oxford University Press.

SUPPORT Principal Investigators. (1995). A controlled trial to improve care for seriously ill hospitalized patients: The Study to Understand Prognoses and Preferences for Outcomes and Risks of Treatments (SUPPORT). *JAMA, 274*(20), 1591–1598.

Sutcliffe, J. (1994). Terminal dehydration. *Nursing Times, 90*(6), 60–63.

Symes, A., & Bruce, A. (2009). Hospice and palliative care: What unites us, what divides us. *Journal of Hospice and Palliative Nursing, 11*(1), 19–26.

U.S. Living Will Registry (2000). U.S. Living Will Registry helps hospitals educate public about advance directives. Retrieved December 24, 2004, from www.livingwillregistry.com/pr_hospital.shtm

Walsh, D., & Gordon, S. (2001). The terminally ill: Dying for palliative medicine? *American Journal of Hospice and Palliative Care, 18*(3), 203–205.

Weigel, C., Parker, G., Fanning, L., Reyna, K., & Gasbarra, D. B. (2007). Apprehension among hospital nurses providing end of life care. *Journal of Hospice and Palliative Nursing, 9*(2), 86–91.

Zerwekh, J. V. (1983). The dehydration question. *Nursing, 13*(1), 46–51.

Zhang, B., El-Jawahri, A., & Prigerson, H. (2006). Update on bereavement research: Evidence based guidelines for the diagnosis and treatment of complicated bereavement. *Journal of Palliative Medicine, 9*(5), 1188–1203.

20

Social, Health, and Long-Term Care Programs and Policies Affecting Mental Health in Older Adults

Kathy J. Fabiszewski

Mental health is the successful performance of mental function, resulting in productive activities, fulfilling relationships with other people, and the ability to adapt to change and to cope with adversity; from early childhood until late life, mental health is the springboard of thinking and communication skills, learning, emotional growth, resilience, and self-esteem (Satcher, 2000).

One of the most important items on the current U.S. domestic policy agenda is how to organize, finance, and deliver high-quality, cost-effective, health care including community-based social programs and long-term care. Mental health care is an essential component of overall health care. The landscape of health care is changing, driven, in part, by population demographics. The aging of the U.S. population is one of the major public health challenges of the 21st century. The age 65 years and older population is increasing at a faster rate than the total population. From 1950 to 2006, the total U.S. population increased from 151 to 199 million persons. During the same period, the 65–74 years age group grew from 8 to 19 million persons, and the population age 75 years and older increased the fastest, rising from 4 to 18 million persons (National Center for Health Statistics, 2008).

By 2029, all of the baby boomers (those born in the post–World War II period 1946 to 1965) will be 65 years of age and older. As a result, the population age 65–74 years will increase from 6 to 10% of the total population between 2006 and 2030. As the baby boomers age, the population 75 years and older will rise from 6% in 2006 to 9% of the population by 2030 and will continue to grow to 12% in 2050. By 2040, the population age 75 years and older will exceed the population 65–74 years of age (National Center for Health Statistics, 2008).

Two factors will combine to double the population of Americans age 65 years and older during the next 25 years: greater longevity and the aging of the baby boomer cohort. By 2030, an estimated 71 million Americans age 65 years and older will account for nearly 20% of the United States population (Centers for Disease Control and Prevention & the Merck Company Foundation, 2007).

Healthcare costs, which are already high, will be affected by the increasing number of Americans age 65 years and older. The United States spent $2.2 trillion on health care in 2007 with adults 65 years and older averaging $8776 per person in 2006 (The Henry J. Kaiser Family Foundation, 2009). Currently, more than two thirds of healthcare costs are for treating chronic illnesses. Among older Americans almost 95% of healthcare expenditures are for chronic disease care (Centers for Disease Control and Prevention & the Merck Company Foundation, 2007). One quarter of older adults today experience some chronic mental disorder, including dementia. By 2040, it is projected that more than 15 million older adults, nearly double the current number, will suffer a mental illness (Jeste et al, 1999; President's New Freedom Commission on Mental Health, Subcommittee on Older Adults and Mental Health, 2003). Thus, although the disease burden of mental illness is enormous and is expected to increase in the future, mental health disorders must be viewed like other chronic medical conditions as highly treatable, and attention to mental health must be incorporated across the life span.

Older adults suffer from many of the same mental disorders as their younger counterparts. The risk of depression in older adults increases with physical illness, functional impairment, inadequately treated pain, and multiple medical comorbidities. For example, depression can strike an older adult after he or she has suffered a hip fracture or myocardial infarction or has been diagnosed with cancer. Frasure-Smith, Lesperance, Juneau, Talajic, and Bourassa (1999) found that the onset of depression post–myocardial infarction was associated with a fourfold increase in death. The highest suicide rates in the United States are found in white men older than 85 years (Kochanek, Murphy, Anderson, & Scott, 2004). Aging-associated psychosocial factors, such as retirement, financial difficulties, bereavement, and physical disability, may contribute to the development of very-late-onset schizophrenia-like psychosis (Howard, Rabins, Seaman, Jeste, & The International Late Onset Schizophrenia Group, 2000). However, the prevalence, nature, and course of each disorder might be very different in older adults and assessment and management strategies are complicated by medical comorbidities, inadequate social support systems, and in some cases lack of appropriately aggressive treatment (Sullivan, 2008). Millions of older Americans (the frail elderly,

disabled and chronically ill persons, and mentally ill individuals) have difficulty living fully independent lives. Yet, despite the impact of mental illness on functional status, fewer than half of all older adults with mental illnesses receive any mental health services (Klap, Unroe, & Unutzer, 2003).

Mental illness in the older adult is often underdiagnosed. The most common mental illnesses in the older adult population include anxiety disorders, depressive disorders, dementia, and schizophrenia (U.S. Department of Health and Human Services [DHHS], SAMHSA, Center for Mental Health Services, 2007). Eleven percent of men and 17% of women in the United States age 65 and older have clinically relevant depressive symptoms. This percentage increases to 19% for both genders older than age 85 years (Federal Interagency Forum on Aging-Related Statistics, 2008). Although an estimated 2 million adults age 65 years and older in the United States have depressive illnesses, another 5 million may have "subsyndromal" depression (U.S. DHHS, SAMHSA, Center for Mental Health Services). Data collected by the Centers for Disease Control and Prevention's Behavioral Risk Factor Surveillance System suggested that among Americans age 65 years or older, the prevalence of frequent mental distress, defined as having 14 or more mentally unhealthy days caused by stress, depression, and problems with emotions in the previous month, ranged from 5.9% for non-Hispanic whites to 11.2% for Hispanics (Centers for Disease Control and Prevention & the Merck Company Foundation, 2007).

An estimated 5.3 million people in the United States are living with Alzheimer's disease (Alzheimer's Association, 2009). In addition, as many as 58% of Americans between the ages of 75 and 89 may be affected by Alzheimer's disease (Hebert, Scherr, Bienias, Bennett, & Evans, 2003); 20% of older adults suffer from some sort of anxiety; and approximately 1% are diagnosed with schizophrenia (National Institute on Aging, 1993).

This chapter discusses social, health, and long-term care programs and policies affecting mental health in older adults.

ROLE OF THE PROFESSIONAL NURSE

Nurses have become increasingly involved not only in the clinical assessment and management of mental health issues of older adults but also in affecting health policy change. Never has mental healthcare policy been more political and in need of bipartisanship. As the demographics of aging populations evolve, technological advances soar, and life expectancy rises, professional nursing remains politically dynamic and responsive to the needs and demands for health care in the fastest growing segment of our population, the oldest–old. Nurses have never been more cognizant of barriers to mental health care including geographic access, limited funding and resources, and workforce issues. Not only is there a dramatic shortfall in healthcare professionals with expertise in geriatrics and mental health, but there are inadequate support services to informal caregivers (President's New Freedom Commission on Mental Health, Subcommittee on Older Adults and Mental Health, 2003).

In upholding the *Scope and Standards of Gerontological Nursing Practice* (American Nurses Association [ANA], 2001) and the *Scope and Standards of Advanced Practice Registered Nursing* (ANA, 1996), professional nurses engaged in gerontological practice are expected to ". . . identify the settings in which services may be safely and appropriately delivered" to the older adult and ". . . propose alternatives for continuity of care for long term needs" (ANA, 2001, p. 15). To uphold these standards, it behooves nurses to understand mental health policy and how it translates into programs and services that impact the delivery of effective, high-quality health care for older adults.

Among the over 40,000 clinical nurse specialists (CNS) currently in practice across the United States, close to 7000 are nationally credentialed by the American Nurses Credentialing Center as psychiatric mental health CNSs (American Nurses Credentialing Center, 2008). The clinical practice of psychiatric-mental health nursing occurs at two levels: basic and advanced. Advanced practice nurses (APNs) can subspecialize in such areas as

geropsychiatric nursing. However, no specialty national certification exists for either APNs in gerontological nursing who subspecialize in geropsychiatric mental health nursing or for their APN counterparts in psychiatric nursing who subspecialize in gerontological nursing. Many APNs specialize in the consultation–liaison role in which the APN provides a service and consultation to elderly clients who are physically ill and experiencing psychiatric problems or their caregiver (American Psychiatric Nurses Association, 1995).

Nurses engaged in clinical geropsychiatric practice use evidence-based critical thinking that embodies the well documented relationship between mental disorders on both quality of health care and outcomes. Nurses know, for example, that late life depression is both underdiagnosed and inadequately treated (Unutzer, 2007) (older adults with significant depression have total healthcare costs that are approximately 50% higher than those without depression [Unutzer et al., 1997]) and recognize that older individuals with chronic health conditions, such as heart disease, cancer, and arthritis, have better outcomes and treatment compliance if co-occurring mental health disorders are identified and treated effectively (Lantz, 2002; Lin et al., 2003). Rathmore, Wang, Druss, Masoudi, and Krumhole (2008) found that 17% of patients with heart failure had a mental illness diagnosis. Yet, this subgroup of patients received poorer care during hospitalization and had a greater risk of death and hospital readmission. Because older adults with mental illnesses generally experience high medical comorbidity (Goldman, 1999) and are at increased risk of poor recovery (Pennix et al., 2001), the demand for professional nurses with geropsychiatric expertise and a strong advocacy posture is high and is likely to increase in the decades ahead.

Among the health policy priorities for geropsychiatric nurses is the achievement of mental health parity. Mental health parity is critical to a sound and effective healthcare delivery system (American Association for Geriatric Psychiatry, 2007). Older individuals with mental illness must be afforded the same quality of health care as their counterparts with medical illness. The Mental Health Parity Act (MHPA), signed into federal law in 1996, and renewed annually by Congress since 2001, required that annual or lifetime dollar limits on mental health benefits be no lower than any such dollar limits for medical and surgical benefits offered by a group health plan or health insurer (U.S. Department of Labor, 2009). The intent of this legislation was to establish parity or equivalence in coverage for both physical and mental illness, but in reality the law until recently had done little to ensure that coverage for treatment of mental illness is adequate (O'Sullivan & Krauss, 2007). Loopholes in the MHPA allowed Medicare and other group health plans to institute such practices as higher patient copayments, higher deductibles, and restricted numbers of outpatient visits and inpatient hospital days for treatment of mental illness in contrast to physical illness. Furthermore, plans could specify which illnesses will or will not be covered and many exclude such diagnoses as alcohol and chemical dependency and recurrent depression (O'Sullivan & Krauss). In addition, employers with fewer than 50 employees have been exempt from the requirements of the MHPA, further limiting access to mental health services.

Enacted into law on October 3, 2008, The Wellstone-Domenici Parity Act amended the MHPA and ended health insurance benefits inequity between mental health and substance abuse disorders and medical and surgical benefits for group health plans with more than 50 employees effective January 1, 2010 (American Psychological Association Practice Organization, 2008). Opponents to mental health parity suggest that coverage of mental health services will exponentially and unfairly increase premiums for all health plan enrollees. Scientific and economic projections indicate, however, that instituting equal coverage for the care of mental illness will result in lower overall healthcare costs (American Association for Geriatric Psychiatry, 2007).

Professional nursing has also advanced its research agenda in mental health and aging. In their study of the effect of nurse staffing and education on the outcomes of surgical patients with comorbid serious mental illness, Kutney-Lee and Aiken (2008), for example, found that in addition to presenting a higher risk of adverse events, the care of seriously mentally ill patients involved greater use of hospital resources and higher costs because stays are longer. In their study, a higher level of nurse staffing had a stronger effect on prevention of death among patients with serious mental illness than among those without serious mental illness. Length of stay for patients with serious mental illness was shorter in hospitals with higher proportions of baccalaureate-prepared nurses (Kutney-Lee & Aiken).

Given the significant impact that mental illness has on the health and function of older adults, the need for effective and humane policy that guides the design and delivery of mental health care for all age groups and generations at the local, state, and national levels has long been recognized in the profession of nursing. Unfortunately, most policies that have the greatest effects on the health and welfare of the mentally ill are made outside the mental health arena and often outside of health care. As a result, the quantity and quality of mental health care that older adults can access and receive across the healthcare continuum has historically been suboptimal. There is a desire and a need for many changes, but the existing financing, delivery, regulation, and evaluation of implemented social and mental health programs and services create another dimension of health care for nursing scrutiny. From this scrutiny many mental health policy questions arise including:

Does the current reimbursement system adequately provide for older adults with mental illness? . . . in the community? . . . in institutions?

To what extent do mental health care programs and private third party payers cover the services of nursing professionals?

To what extent is the quality and cost of primary and mental health care delivered by professional nurses comparable to that of other providers?

How can mental wellness best be integrated into primary healthcare practice for the older adult?

What lessons can be learned about the impact of state variations in Medicaid reimbursement rates and mental health outcomes in older adults?

In what ways can professional nurses promote parity in mental health care and eliminate disparities in mental health care?

How can professional nurses play a role in expediting and maximizing recovery from mental illness in the older adult population?

Policy making for persons with mental illness is a very challenging process because sociocultural, environmental, and even geographic factors weigh so heavily on how the illness is experienced and how life experiences shape what is believed to be the best approach to care and treatment. Policies that address this parity are needed but are only one piece of a very complex and convoluted puzzle (Smoyak, 2000). Nurses interested in client advocacy should be aware of the emerging issues that challenge their best efforts and must continue finding ways to meet client's needs even when policies seem to make this impossible (Edmunds, 2003). By recognizing both the strengths and weaknesses in the mental health system and by creatively educating and advocating for clients attempting to access care and services, the professional nurse is able to optimize use of available resources. The politically dynamic nurse no longer uncritically accepts mediocrity, the status quo, simply because of knowledge about skyrocketing healthcare costs. Nurses know that healthcare, and in particular mental healthcare, reform is badly needed. Unfortunately, reforms are often driven and shaped by economic and political considerations and not by coherent, internally consistent healthcare policy.

FEDERAL PROGRAMS SUPPORTING AND FINANCING MENTAL HEALTH CARE

The federal government provides an extensive range of programs that support and finance mental health care to meet the complex needs of adults with serious mental illnesses. Unfortunately, the responsibility for these programs is scattered across many departments and agencies, resulting in the "layering on" of multiple, well-intentioned programs without overall direction, coordination, or consistency (President's New Freedom Commission on Mental Health, 2003). "The current mental health service delivery system is inadequate and unprepared to address the needs associated with the anticipated growth in the number of older persons requiring treatment for late-life mental disorders" (President's New Freedom Commission on Mental Health, Subcommittee on Older Adults and Mental Health, 2003, p. 1). An integrated system that effectively addresses the needs of people with mental illnesses, especially older adults who may coexperience physical frailty, functional impairment, and financial limitation, must include a comprehensive range of mental health services including ancillary supports, such as housing, education, substance abuse treatment, income support, and other basic services. Yet, the lack of federal program focus on adults, and in particular older adults, with serious mental illnesses has resulted in a mental health system that is severely fragmented and uncoordinated because of the underlying structural, financial, and organizational inconsistencies or conflicts that exist in the programs that support it (President's New Freedom Commission on Mental Health).

Furthermore, there is a paucity of programs targeted specifically to meeting the needs of older adults with mental health problems. This paucity has contributed to both the gap between the need for mental health services and the availability and quality of those services and a mismatch between covered services and preferred services (President's New Freedom Commission on Mental Health, Subcommittee on Older Adults and Mental Health, 2003). Additional barriers to service may stem from misconceptions about aging, stigma (because of mental illness and advanced age), discrimination, poverty and isolation among older adults, and out-of-date Medicare policies (President's New Freedom Commission on

Mental Health, Subcommittee on Older Adults and Mental Health; U.S. DHHS, SAMHSA, Center for Mental Health Services, 2007). In addition, a lack of adequate preventive interventions and programs that aid in the early identification of geriatric mental illness exists (President's New Freedom Commission on Mental Health, Subcommittee on Older Adults and Mental Health). "The tragic consequences of system fragmentation and service gaps have produced unnecessary human suffering, disability, homelessness, criminalization of mental illnesses, and other severe consequences" (President's New Freedom Commission on Mental Health, 2003, p. i). Some have portrayed federal programs as isolated funding streams that are difficult or impossible to coordinate, generating a large ad-ministrative burden for state and local agency and provider staff, and denying consumers and family members access to integrated and essential services (President's New Freedom Commission on Mental Health).

The financing of mental health care amounts to billions of dollars annually in the United States. Sources of funding include Medicaid, Medicare, the Department of Veterans Affairs (DVA), state agencies, local agencies, foundations, and private insurance. Unfortunately, each source of funding of mental health care has its own complex, sometimes contradictory, set of rules. Taken as a whole, the system is supposed to function in a coordinated manner; it is supposed to deliver optimal treatments, services, and supports, but it often falls short (President's New Freedom Commission on Mental Health, 2003).

Over 40 programs exist in the federal program armamentarium to support and finance mental health care in general. Those programs specifically targeting mental health and older adults are displayed in Figure 20-1. Each program varies in terms of who or what entity is eligible to receive funds, the allowable uses of funds, the application process, the payment methodology, and funding requirements or limitations. Some programs provide grants to states, localities, private providers, or public providers; others offer direct services, funds, or income directly to

individuals; and others are flexible so that funds can be distributed to either entities or individuals. "Despite the existence of many Federal programs, all too often Federal funds are unavailable to meet even the most basic needs of consumers and families" (President's New Freedom Commission on Mental Health, 2003, p. ii). There is a consensus among providers, advocates, and policymakers that the system could improve. The following are descriptions of the few social, health, and long-term care programs among the 40 that have direct applicability to older adults with mental illness (President's New Freedom Commission on Mental Health).

Administration on Aging: State and Community Programs

The Older Americans Act authorizes and funds a range of programs that offer services and opportunities for older Americans, especially those at risk of losing their independence. The Administration on Aging (AoA) budget totals $1,491,343,000 (AoA, 2009). As part of the Omnibus Appropriations Act of 2009 signed into law by President Barack Obama, the AoA budget for fiscal year 2009 is nearly $78 million above the fiscal year 2008 budget (AoA, 2009). Under Title III, State and Community Programs, the AoA works closely with its nationwide network on aging composed of Regional Offices, State Agencies on Aging, and Area Agencies on Aging, to plan, coordinate, and develop community-level systems of services designed to assist older persons at risk of losing their independence (AoA, 2009).

The AoA awards Title III funds to 57 state Agencies on Aging, based on the number of older persons residing in the state, to plan, develop, and coordinate systems of supportive in-home and community-based services for older persons. States receive funds on a formula grant basis. All individuals age 60 and over are eligible for services, although priority is given to those with the greatest economic and social need with particular attention to low-income minority older persons. There are no mandatory fees for services. Older persons are,

---

Sample of Major Federal Programs Supporting and Financing Mental Health Care for Older Adults

---

Center for Mental Health Services, SAMHSA, DHHS
PATH (Projects for Assistance in Transitioning from Homelessness)
CMHS Block Grant (Community Mental Health Services)
AIMI (Protection and Advocacy for Individuals with Mental Illness

HUD
Emergency Shelter Grants
Shelter Plus Care
Section 811 Supportive Housing for Persons with Disabilities
Supportive Housing Program for the Homeless
232 Mortgage Insurance

Other Agency Programs
Community Health Centers (HRSA, DHHS)
Veteran Health Benefits (DVA)
Administration on Aging State Grants and Community Programs (AoA)

Administration for Children and Families, DHHS
Social Services Block Grant, Title XX

CMS, DHHS
Medicaid, Title XIX
Medicare, Title XVIII

Social Security Administration
SSI
SSDI

Source: From "Major Federal Programs Supporting and Financing Mental Health Care," adapted from the President's New Freedom Commission on Mental Health, 2003. Retrieved February 3, 2010, from http://www.mentalhealthcommission.gov/reports/Fedprograms_031003.doc

---

however, encouraged to contribute to help defray the costs of services. Core service activities include the following (AoA, 2009):

1. Supportive services
   - Access services (transportation, outreach, information and assistance, and case management)
   - In-home services (homemaker and home health aides, chore maintenance, and supportive services for families of older individuals with Alzheimer's disease)
   - Community services (adult day care, legal assistance, and recreation)
2. Congregate and home-delivered meals
3. In-home services for frail elderly
4. Disease prevention and health promotion services (support to public health and educational organizations, community-based agencies, hospitals and medical institutions, and senior centers)

Area Agencies on Aging may be contacted for information and referral to services for older adults in the community. In addition, a nationwide toll free hotline may be found at www.aoa.gov, which provides information about assistance for older individuals anywhere in the nation (AoA, 2009).

Community Health Centers

Community health centers (CHCs) provide primary and preventive healthcare services to people living in rural and urban medically underserved communities where economic, geographic, or cultural barriers limit access to primary health care for a substantial portion of the population. Major CHC activities include provision of primary and preventive health care; outreach; pharmacy services; linkage to other services, such as welfare income assistance, Medicaid, mental health, substance abuse treatment, and nutrition programs; and specialty care services, including mental health services. CHCs deliver care regardless of clients' ability to pay. Charges for healthcare services are income-based, with services to the poorest clients provided at no cost.

In 2009, the U.S. Department of Health and Human Services released $338 million, made available by the American Recovery and Reinvestment Act, to expand CHCs and serve increased numbers of medically uninsured patients during the nation's economic downturn. This will be accomplished through Increased Demand for Services grants. Citing the increasing number of Americans joining the ranks of the medically uninsured and turning to CHCs for care, Increased Demand for Services grants were distributed to 1128 CHCs to create and retain over 6000 CHC positions. CHCs served more than 16 million patients in 2007, 40% of whom had no health insurance (Health Resources and Services Administration, 2009). No data are available to ascertain how many of the individuals served by CHCs were older adults or afflicted with mental illness.

The Health Resources and Services Administration assists in the preparation of program applications, providing consultation about grants administration and managing the grant process. The method of payment is direct grants from Health Resources and Services Administration to CHC grantees.

Community Mental Health Block Grants

The Community Mental Health Services Block Grant is authorized by Part B of Title XIX of the Public Health Service Act and is the single largest federal contribution dedicated toward improving mental health service systems in the United States (President's New Freedom Commission on Mental Health, 2003). Because what is effective in one state may not be effective in another, this formula grant to states supports delivery of a broad range of community mental health services determined by the individual states. The goal of the grant is to improve community-based services and reduce reliance on hospitalization. Community Mental Health Services Block Grants create federal-state partnerships not only to support existing public services but also to encourage the developments of creative and cost-effective systems of community-based care for persons with serious mental disorders (U.S. Department of Health and Human Services, 2004). Although there are no provisions requiring tailored outreach to the older adult, this program supports comprehensive, community-based systems of care for adults with serious mental illnesses and represents the major federal effort to work in partnership with the states to plan and deliver state-of-the-art systems of community-based mental health services for adults aimed at reducing reliance on hospitalization.

HUD Section 232: Mortgage Insurance for Board and Care, Assisted-Living, and Other Facilities

U.S. Department of Housing and Urban Development (HUD) Section 232 provides government-backed mortgage loan insurance to facilitate the construction and rehabilitation, acquisition, or refinancing of nursing homes, intermediate care facilities, board and care homes, and assisted-living and other facilities. "Eligible mortgage borrowers include investors, builders, developers, public entities and private non-profit corporations and associations" (President's New Freedom Commission on Mental Health, 2003, p. 8). Eligible residents under HUD Section 232 must require skilled nursing, custodial care, assistance with activities of daily living, or be eligible to live in facilities insured under this program.

Under the American Recovery and Reinvestment Act of 2009, $13.61 billion was designated for projects and programs administered by HUD. The funding is designed to assist those hardest hit by the U.S. economic crisis. This includes $1.5 billion invested in preventing homelessness and enabling the rapid rehousing of homeless families and individuals including homeless veterans and homeless mentally ill individuals (U.S. HUD, 2009).

Medicaid (Title XIX)

Medicaid (Title XIX of the Social Security Act) is 56 jointly administered state and federal welfare entitlement programs that pay for medical assistance for certain individuals and families with low income and resources. "Medicaid is the largest single payer for mental health services in the United States—providing services and supports for 58 million adults and children" (Centers for Medicare and Medicaid Services [CMS], 2009b, para. 1). Medicaid is the largest source of funding for medical and healthcare services for the poorest Americans (Hoffman, Klees, & Curtis, 2008) and is the third largest source of health insurance in the United States behind Medicare and employer-sponsored coverage (Center for Medicare and Medicaid Services, 2004). Although the CMS officially presides over Medicaid, each state administers its Medicaid program under broad federal guidelines. Because latitude is provided to the states in the design of their Medicaid programs, each state establishes its own eligibility standards; determines the type, amount, duration, and scope of services provided; and sets a different Medicaid formula for benefits and for the rates of federal reimbursement.

Medicaid does not provide medical assistance for all poor persons (Hoffman et al., 2008). Medicaid programs provide: (1) health insurance for low-income families and for disabled individuals (Supplemental Security Income [SSI] eligible); (2) long-term care (community-based or institutional) for older adults, the blind, and disabled individuals; and (3) supplemental copayment coverage for low-income Medicare beneficiaries (dual eligibility). Payment methodologies may vary and are state determined based on broad federal limits. States may impose nominal deductibles, coinsurance, or copayments on some Medicaid beneficiaries (Hoffman et al., 2008).

The Deficit Reduction Act of 2005 (Public Law 109-171) refined Medicaid eligibility requirements for Medicaid beneficiaries by tightening standards for citizenship and immigration documentation and by modifying the requirements for long-term care eligibility. Now, the look-back period for determining community spouse income and assets is lengthened to 60 months (from 36 months previously) and individuals whose homes exceed $500,000 in values are disqualified (Hoffman et al., 2008).

Medicaid provides a comprehensive package of basic health insurance benefits for most categorically needy populations. In general, each state must cover 10 categories of "mandatory services" identified in statute if federal matching funds are to be received. Among included services are inpatient and outpatient hospital services, physician and APN services, laboratory and radiology services, home health care for persons eligible for skilled-nursing services, and nursing facility services. In addition, states have the discretion to cover one or more of up to 33 "optional services" under Medicaid including case management services, personal care services, transportation services, prescription drugs, and a variety of professional services (including psychologist services) (President's New Freedom Commission on Mental Health, 2003).

The Balanced Budget Act of 1997 (Public Law 105-33) included a state option known as Programs of All-Inclusive Care for the Elderly. This program is a national, innovative, long-term care model that provides a community-based alternative to institutional care for older adults who require a facility level of care. Programs of All-Inclusive Care for the Elderly offers and manages all Medicare and Medicaid services including medications, environmental modification, and nontraditional services needed to provide preventive, rehabilitative, curative, and supportive care in adult day health centers, homes, hospitals, and nursing homes (Centers for Medicare and Medicaid Services, 2009c; Hoffman et al., 2008).

The Medicaid program is a key source of support for low-income older adults with mental illness. Although some mental health services are included among the "mandatory services" (e.g., limited outpatient mental health services and inpatient psychiatric care) required by federal law, most community-based mental health services are among the various "optional services" that states may choose to include in their Medicaid programs. Optional mental health services that states may provide include care by APNs, psychologists, clinic services, and inpatient hospital and nursing facility services for individuals 65 years of age and older in an institution for mental diseases, case management services, and community-supported living arrangements. In practice, because states have primary responsibility for the care and financing of persons with severe mental illness, most states have made extensive use of optional Medicaid benefits to provide services for the mentally ill population. In addition to the traditional fee-for-service model, some state Medicaid programs provide mental health services through contracts with managed care organizations (MCOs), such as HMOs, prepaid health plans, or comparable entities (Centers for Medicare and Medicaid Services, 2004). The purpose of managed care programs is to enhance access to quality care in a cost-effective manner. In 2007, 64% of Medicaid beneficiaries were enrolled in some form of managed care program (Hoffman et al., 2008).

Medicaid is the dominant payer for state mental health services. Medicaid now funds more than one half of all mental health services administered by states and could account for two thirds of such spending by 2017 (Buck, 2003). Ten percent of all Medicaid dollars were spent on mental health services in 2003 (Mark et al., 2007). According to the American Association for Geriatric Psychiatry (2007), in the current U.S. economic climate, proposals to cap or cut Medicaid funding or eligibility would likely result in fewer low-income elders receiving mental health services and more restrictions on the services that are available. Spending increases in the Medicaid program continue to grow at a rapid pace, and states have already instituted cutbacks in Medicaid coverage prompted by widespread budget deficits and Medicaid funding shortfall (American Association for Geriatric Psychiatry).

State Medicaid agencies are playing an increasing role in funding, managing, and monitoring public mental health services in states. In their 50-state survey of how state Medicaid agencies are exercising their responsibilities for mental health services, Verdier and Barrett (2008) found that Medicaid and mental health agencies were located within the same umbrella agency in 28 states, potentially facilitating collaboration. Because Medicaid plays a key role in funding state mental health services, interagency collaboration and optimal alignment of Medicaid and mental health responsibilities are now and will continue to be in the future critical in determining how Medicaid funds are spent (Verdier & Barrett).

Currently, over 56 million Americans receive Medicaid benefits including low-income adults, people with severe disabilities, and low-income Medicare beneficiaries known as "dual eligibles." In the absence of Medicaid, most of its beneficiaries would join the ranks of the nearly 46 million uninsured Americans (The Kaiser Commission on Medicaid and the Uninsured, 2009).

About 70% of Medicaid spending is attributed to older adults and people with disabilities. Although these beneficiaries comprise only about 25% of all Medicaid enrollees, their intense needs translate into high costs to the program.

Although aggregate Medicaid costs are high, the program administrative costs are low, and Medicaid acute care spending per capita has been rising more slowly than private insurance premiums (The Kaiser Commission on Medicaid and the Uninsured, 2009).

Medicare (Title XVIII)

As part of the Social Security Amendments of 1965, Medicare's enactment established a national health insurance program for the elderly and, ultimately, for other vulnerable Americans. Medicare is administered nationally by the CMS. Medicare is a broad but limited package of health insurance benefits for (1) persons age 65 and older; (2) severely disabled persons younger than age 65 (Social Security Disability Insurance definition); and (3) people of any age with end-stage renal disease. It provides acute care to older adults and the disabled regardless of income. Unlike Medicaid, Medicare has national eligibility, coverage, and reimbursement standards. The program offers two basic choices to enrollees: Standard Medicare, also known as the Original Medicare Plan (traditional or fee-for-service Medicare); and Medicare Advantage Plans (which are an alternative to traditional Medicare and include Managed Medicare Care Plans and Medicare Private Fee for Service Options).

Standard Medicare is offered nationwide and is comprised of two main parts. Part A (hospital insurance) provides hospital insurance that helps pay for most inpatient hospital care and care in skilled nursing facilities, hospice care, and some home health care. Part A benefits are provided automatically and free of premiums to eligible individuals (i.e., most people with any work history). In 2010, eligible individuals are required to pay a $1100 deductible for each benefit period (Centers for Medicare and Medicaid Services, 2009f). The amount of this deductible changes from year to year. Part B (supplementary medical insurance) is optional and provides medical insurance that helps pay for physician/APN services, outpatient hospital care, and some medical and

home health services not covered by Part A. "In 2010, beneficiaries pay the first $155 yearly for Part B covered services or items" (Centers for Medicare and Medicaid Services, 2010, p. 121). The monthly premium for 2010 remains unchanged from 2009 at $96.40 (Centers for Medicare and Medicaid Services, 2009f). This monthly premium usually changes from year to year. Almost all Medicare enrollees in Part A choose to enroll in Part B.

A third component of Medicare, sometimes known as Part C, is the Medicare Advantage Program. Established as the Medicare + Choice program by the Balanced Budget Act of 1997 and later renamed and modified by the Medicare Prescription Drug, Improvement, and Modernization Act (MMA) of 2003, the Medicare Advantage program expands Medicare beneficiaries' options for participation in private-sector health plans, such as health maintenance organizations (HMOs), preferred provider organizations, and other certified coordinated healthcare plans that meet standards set forth in the MMA (Hoffman et al., 2008). Medicare Advantage plans are offered by private companies and organizations and are required to provide, at a minimum, those services covered by Part A and B, except hospice care (Hoffman et al.). That is, the same benefits and coverage rules that apply to fee-for-service enrollees apply, but additional benefits, over and above what Standard Medicare covers, such as outpatient prescription drugs, eyeglasses, hearing aids, and others services, may also be provided. Capitated payments to the plans provide an incentive to avoid expensive services, particularly inpatient hospital admissions, by encouraging early identification of health problems among patients and proactive management. For example, the resources devoted to screening and self-care may reduce the use of a hospital, and transportation to obtain outpatient mental healthcare costs less in a taxi or van than in an ambulance, particularly when the destination is a healthcare provider's office rather than an emergency department (HMO Workgroup on Care Management, 1998).

Medicare Advantage plans are offered in many but not all areas of the country. Within Medicare

Advantage plans, each participating healthcare organization receives a capitated payment or predetermined lump sum from Medicare for the healthcare services for each enrolled beneficiary (usually paid per member per month), regardless of the number of healthcare encounters the client requires. Providers establish their own payment agreements with the health plans. Beneficiaries pay monthly premiums and nominal copayments for services. No Medigap policy is necessary. The capitation method of payment introduces flexibility in the financing and delivery of care that is not present under the fee-for-services method.

A fourth part of Medicare, Part D, also established by the MMA in 2006, is a voluntary prescription drug benefit for people on Medicare that helps pay for prescription medications not covered by Parts A or B. Part D provides subsidized access to prescription drug coverage, on payment of premium, on a voluntary basis, for all Medicare beneficiaries, with premium and cost-sharing subsidies for low-income enrollees (Hoffman et al., 2008). Although Part D covers most FDA-approved prescription medications, most Part D plans establish their own formularies for their prescription drug coverage.

Federally approved, private, fee-for-service plans in Medicare's Part D prescription drug program have a gap or "doughnut hole" in coverage. Medicare pays 75% of eligible drug costs after a deductible, up to a $2250 limit. Coverage then ends until the beneficiary's expenses reach $5100 (at which point Medicare pays 95% of eligible prescription drug costs). This leaves many beneficiaries in a predicament: in addition to paying premiums for the Part D insurance, many incur thousands of dollars in out-of-pocket costs for medications they simply cannot afford. Many older adults are forced to make decisions regarding their medication based exclusively on their finances rather than on therapeutic efficacy (American Association for Geriatric Psychiatry, 2007).

Chen et al. (2008) studied the impact of the Medicare Part D prescription drug benefit on psychoactive medication use and the consequent financial burden for community-based older adults.

Findings revealed that in the first year implementation of Part D, the proportion of out-of-pocket payment in total pharmacy reimbursement decreased 18% for antidepressants and 21% for antipsychotics. Older adults used more of these medications in 2006 than they had in 2005. In contrast, the out-of-pocket expenses for older adult benzodiazepine users increased 19% compared to the out-of-pocket cost incurred in the year before Medicare Part D implementation. Overall, the investigators concluded that although Part D improved access to psychotropic medications covered under plans by reducing out-of-pocket expenses, the financial burden related to excluded medications including benzodiazepines increased (Chen et al.).

The Medicare Prescription Drug Improvement and Modernization Act also provides for the development of a research agenda on outcomes and clinical effectiveness in relation to the Medicare prescription drug benefit. Unfortunately, this provision has not yet been funded.

Many beneficiaries with Standard Medicare electively purchase Medigap insurance. Medigap insurance covers expenses not reimbursed by Parts A or B. Persons eligible for Medicare with low incomes or assets may also qualify for Medicaid coverage. Such beneficiaries are categorized as being dual-eligible.

As an alternative to nursing home care, Medicare now offers Social Managed Care Plans in four locations in the United States (Centers for Medicare and Medicaid Services, 2009d) including Kaiser Permanente in Portland, OR; SCAN in Long Beach, CA; Elderplan in Brooklyn, NY; and the Health Plan of Nevada in Las Vegas, NV. These plans offer extensive health benefits not provided through Medicare alone. They provide the full range of Medicare benefits offered by standard managed care plans plus additional services, such as care coordination; prescription drug benefits; chronic care benefits covering short-term nursing home care; and a full range of home and community services including adult day care, respite care, homemaker, personal care services, and medical transportation (Centers for Medicare and Medicaid Services, 2009d). All Social Managed

Care Plans have different requirements for premiums and copayments for certain services.

Standard Medicare covers outpatient and inpatient psychiatric care and mental health care in a partial hospitalization psychiatric program if a healthcare provider certifies that inpatient treatment would be required without it. Medicare pays for mental health services provided by certain specialty providers, such as psychiatrists; psychiatric APNs (both CNSs and nurse practitioners [NP]); clinical psychologists; and clinical social workers (Centers for Medicare and Medicaid Services, 2009f). Unfortunately, up until 2010 ". . . most outpatient mental health services are subject to higher beneficiary co-payments than other outpatient care (50/50 co-payments for mental health versus 80/20 for other covered benefits). Inpatient mental health care is limited to a lifetime maximum of 190 days of care in a specialty psychiatric hospital" (President's New Freedom Commission on Mental Health, 2003, p. 52).

In 2008, Congress enacted legislation to equalize cost sharing for mental and physical health services in group health plans and in the Medicare Part B program. This law reduces coinsurance in the Medicare program for outpatient mental health services from 50% to 20%. This is equivalent to the Medicare Part B coinsurance rate for medical and surgical services. This law (The Wellstone-Domenici Parity Act of 2008) will be phased in over 5 years starting in 2010 (Trivedi, Swaminathan, & Mor, 2008). Also, in 2008, Congress approved the Emergency Economic Stabilization Act, which mandates insurance parity in cost sharing and visit restrictions for mental health and medical services among group health plans covering more than 50 employees beginning in 2010 (Trivedi et al.).

Medicare is a major payer in the U.S. healthcare system. In 2008, almost 45 million elderly and disabled people were enrolled in one or both of Parts A and B, and over 9 million individuals chose to participate in a Medicare Advantage plan. Medicare spending has increased about ninefold in the past two decades, from $37 billion in 1980 to $336 billion in 2005 (Medicare Payment Advisory Commission, 2006). In 2007, Medicare Part A benefits alone totaled $200.2 billion; Part B benefits totaled $176.4 billion that same year; Part D benefits totaled $48.6 billion; and total Medicare expenditures were $431.5 billion (Hoffman et al., 2008).

By 2030 the number of Americans covered by Medicare will nearly double to 90 million or 26% of the population. Unlike Medicaid, Medicare does not pay for long-term care, either in the community or in institutional-based setting when care is primarily used for assisting patients with activities of daily living that could be provided by informal or nonprofessional caregivers. Other noncovered healthcare needs include dental care, dentures, corrective lenses, and hearing aids, unless they are covered as part of a private health plan under the Medicare Advantage program.

In 2008, Medicare approved payment mechanisms for clinicians to address smoking cessation and alcohol and substance abuse (Centers for Medicare and Medicaid Services, 2009e). Current Procedural Terminology has added new codes for smoking cessation counseling and for alcohol or substance abuse screening and brief interventions (Buppert, 2009). In addition, Medicare will pay for eight face-to-face smoking and tobacco use cessation counseling sessions in a 12-month period if ordered by a Medicare-recognized practitioner. Two attempts are covered each year, with each attempt including a maximum of four intermediate or intensive sessions. The beneficiary may receive another eight sessions during a subsequent year after 11 full months have passed since the first Medicare-covered session. The diagnosis code should reflect the patient's condition as adversely affected by tobacco use or as being treated with a therapeutic agent whose metabolism or dosing is affected by tobacco use (Buppert, 2009).

Projects for Assistance in Transition from Homelessness

Of the 600,000 Americans that are homeless on any given night, an estimated 33% have serious mental illnesses and more than one half have alcohol or drug-related problems (President's New Freedom Commission on Mental Health,

2003). Projects for Assistance in Transition from Homelessness was established in 1990 to address the multiple needs of people who are homeless and mentally ill. It provides formula grants to states and territories, which are required to match funds with $1 for every $3 received in federal funds. Projects for Assistance in Transition from Homelessness develops innovative programs for persons with mental illness who are homeless. Such services as outreach, screening and diagnosis, rehabilitation, community mental health treatment, case management, and limited housing assistance are available to individuals with severe mental illness including those with co-occurring substance abuse disorders who are homeless or at risk of becoming homeless. Individual states and territories determine the payment methodology.

Protection and Advocacy for Individuals with Mental Illness

Protection and Advocacy for Individuals with Mental Illness state formula grants support Protection and Advocacy systems designated by the Governor of each state to protect and to advocate for the rights of persons diagnosed with a significant mental illness or emotional impairment. Grants support Protection and Advocacy systems to pursue administrative, legal, and legislative activities or other remedies to redress complaints of abuse, neglect, and civil rights violations.

Service beneficiaries include those who are diagnosed with a significant mental illness or emotional impairment by a mental health professional; inpatients or residents in public or private residential facilities that provide care or treatment to individuals with mental illness; residents in a community-based setting, including their home; and those who were abused, neglected, or had their rights violated or were in danger of abuse, neglect, or rights violations while receiving care or treatment in a public or private residential facility (President's New Freedom Commission on Mental Health, 2003).

Social Service Block Grant (Title XX)

"The Social Services Block Grant (SSBG) program provides formula grants to states for the provision of social services directed at achieving economic self-support or self-sufficiency, preventing or remedying neglect, abuse, or the exploitation of adults, preventing or reducing inappropriate institutionalization, and securing referral for institutional care, where appropriate" (President's New Freedom Commission on Mental Health, 2003, p. 60). Social Services Block Grant allocations are determined by a statutory formula based on each state's population. States are fully responsible for determining the use of their funds.

Supplemental Security Income (Title XVI)

SSI is a federal income supplement program that provides monthly financial assistance payments to individuals who are aged, blind, or disabled and have little or no income to meet basic needs (e.g., food, clothing, and shelter). In March of 2009, SSI provided an average monthly payment of $503.70 per individual plus Medicaid and Food Stamp Program eligibility to approximately 7.6 million recipients (Social Security Administration, 2009). Income limits are state determined. Payments are sent to eligible individuals monthly from the Social Security Administration.

Almost 30% of SSI beneficiaries in 2009 were age 65 years and older (Social Security Administration, 2009). More than one third (38%) of all adult beneficiaries were eligible because of mental disorders. Overall, approximately 1.2 million adult beneficiaries were disabled for reasons of mental disorders (President's New Freedom Commission on Mental Health, 2003).

Department of Veterans Affairs

The U.S. DVA was established in 1989 succeeding the Veterans Administration. It is the second largest of the 15 Cabinet departments and operates nationwide programs for health care, financial assistance, and burial benefits at 1200 inpatient and outpatient healthcare facilities in the United States.

All veterans of active duty in the U.S. Armed Services are potentially eligible for health benefits through the DVA. The DVA delivers health care through a network of 153 medical centers, 731 community-based outpatient clinics, 135 nursing homes, 209 readjustment counseling centers, and 47 domiciliaries (U.S. Department of Veterans Affairs, 2009). There are an estimated 25 million veterans alive, with more than 7.8 million enrolled to receive DVA healthcare benefits. The aging of the veteran population is a major issue confronting the DVA. About 9.2 million veterans are age 65 or older, representing 35% of the total veteran population. By 2020 the proportion of older veterans will increase dramatically to 51% of the total population. More than 100,000 homeless veterans receive DVA health care and benefits. About 45% of homeless veterans suffer from mental illness and over 68% suffer from alcohol or drug abuse problems. Thirty-three percent have both psychiatric and substance abuse disorders. The DVA offers a spectrum of geriatric and extended care services to veterans with nearly 65,000 veterans receiving long-term care annually through inpatient programs of the DVA or state veterans homes (U.S. Department of Veterans Affairs).

The Veterans Health Care Eligibility Reform Act of 1996 created a standard enhanced health benefits plan available to enrolled veterans that provides health services that promote, preserve, and restore health with no prescribed day or visit limits. Those eligible include veterans discharged from active military service under honorable conditions. If discharged after September 7, 1980, a minimum service of 2 years is required. Once enrolled, veterans can receive care anywhere in the DVA system. In general, mental health benefits provided within the Medical Benefits Package are quite comprehensive. A substantial percentage of DVA healthcare service and funds are used for psychiatric care.

In 2010, in addition to $1.4 billion provided for Veterans Administration projects in the American Recovery and Reinvestment Act of 2009, projected spending on the DVA will increase from $97.7 billion in 2009 to $112 billion in 2010 (VA Media Relations, 2009). The DVA enhanced overall mental health resources by over $500 million in fiscal year 2007 to meet the needs of veterans of all service eras with mental illness and emotional needs (U.S. Department of Veterans Affairs, 2009).

The new budget supports additional specialty care in both mental health and aging through new initiatives, including the development of four Veterans Administration Centers of Excellence and 10 Mental Illness Research, Education, and Clinical Centers (U.S. Department of Veterans Affairs, 2009). The mission of the Centers of Excellence and Mental Illness Research, Education, and Clinical Centers is to develop new knowledge about mental illness and to improve clinical care to veterans with mental illness including Alzheimer's disease, substance abuse disorders, and depression. Most services are provided through DVA-operated facilities. Recipient cost sharing varies based on the service received and eligibility status of the individual.

Senior Centers

Social issues and physical and mental health problems affect the overall health of older adults. Senior centers, through positive social interaction, play a vital role in promoting healthy and successful aging and, along with Meals-On-Wheels, adult day care, transportation, and companion services, help to improve the quality of life of older adults. In the current climate of economic downturn, many state and local municipalities are confronting increased caseloads and shrinking budgets. Services most commonly provided at senior centers include routine health screening; physical fitness programs; health promotion activities; nutritional screening and educational services; health risk assessments; and mental health screening, education, and referral (under the Administration on Aging State and Community Programs). Participation in senior centers may decrease the inappropriate use of healthcare providers, emergency departments, and hospitals. The centrality of social ties to the health and well-being of older adults cannot be overemphasized.

Substance Abuse and Mental Health Services Administration

SAMHSA is the U.S. Department of Health and Human Services government agency that specializes in producing publications, resources, and referrals for individuals including low income and uninsured clients seeking mental health care, and those seeking substance abuse (drug and alcohol) treatments. Information is available at www.find-treatment.samhsa.gov. This site allows the geropsychiatric nurse to enter his or her practice site zip code to generate a full list of treatment facilities, including those with free or sliding-scale alcohol abuse services (1-888-ASK-HRSA).

In recent years, one of SAMHSA's highest priorities has been addressing the needs of older adults with mental illness with particular emphasis on overcoming stigmatization and discrimination against older Americans with mental illnesses. Strategies implemented to eliminate stigma have included a community-based campaign to empower and educate older adults with mental illness, those who work with older adults, those who volunteer to help them, and those who provide physical and mental health care; and education of the public on mental health and aging, delivering positive messages about mental health and aging by way of the media (advertising in print, on radio, and on television).

Another SAMHSA initiative, as part of its "science to service" strategy is the development and implementation of Evidence-Based Practice Implementation Resource Kits, including the Illness Management and Recovery Kit, the Family Psychoeducation Kit, the Co-occurring Disorders: Integrated Dual Diagnosis Kit, and The Assertive Community Treatment Kit. These kits provide a resource to encourage the use of evidence-based practices in mental health and include information sheets for all stakeholder groups; videos (introductory and practice demonstration); and manuals for

practitioners (Substance Abuse and Mental Health Services Administration, 2009a).

The Center for Mental Health Services is a component of SAMHSA, established by Congress in 1992 to lead federal efforts to treat mental illness through the promotion of mental health and by preventing the development or worsening of mental illness whenever possible. This agency's goals are to play a leadership role in delivering mental health services, generate and apply new knowledge, and establish national mental health policy. This is accomplished by helping states improve and increase the quality and range of their treatment, rehabilitation, and support services for those with mental illness, their families, and communities through outreach and case management. Among its 16 division offices are the Division of Service and Systems Improvement, the Division of State and Community Systems development, and the Associate Director for Organization and Financing (Substance Abuse and Mental Health Services Administration, 2009b).

REIMBURSEMENT ISSUES FOR THE GEROPSYCHIATRIC NURSE

According to the Fellows of the American Academy of Nurse Practitioners (2002), NPs should be at the forefront of health care and ". . . will be the skilled providers of health care services to vulnerable populations who have little or no access to care, as well as those who are insured through employers, the government or other private pay health care systems" (Fellows of the American Academy of Nurse Practitioners, p. 2). It is incumbent on geropsychiatric nurses and APNs to understand reimbursement of mental healthcare services to older adults. This is important not only as clinicians, but for advocacy, case management, and health policy researcher and analyst role functions. Most older adults seeking psychiatric health care have a third-party payer. There are three primary categories of third party payers that reimburse healthcare providers for mental health services: (1) MCOs;

(2) federally funded programs (Medicare, Medicaid); and (3) indemnity insurance companies.

Federally Funded Programs (Medicare, Medicaid) and APNs

The Balanced Budget Act of 1997 made direct Medicare reimbursement for APNs possible. It is the responsibility of each provider submitting claims to become familiar with Medicare and Medicaid coverage and requirements (National Heritage Insurance Company, 2009). To receive reimbursement from Medicare for professional services provided, an APN must be a registered professional nurse authorized by the state in which services are provided to practice as a NP or as a CNS; must be certified by a recognized national certifying body, such as the American Nurses Credentialing Center or the American Academy of Nurse Practitioners, that has established standards for NPs or CNSs; and must possess a Master's degree in Nursing or a Doctor of Nursing Practice degree. In addition, the NP or CNS must work collaboratively with a physician. Collaboration is defined as being ". . . a process in which an NP (or CNS) works with one or more physicians to deliver health care services, with medical direction and appropriate supervision as required by the law of the State in which the services are furnished" (National Heritage Insurance Company, p. 10).

There are two possible arrangements by which an APN may be reimbursed for services provided to a Medicare enrollee. The first is when Medicare reimburses the APN directly on a fee-for-service basis through a local Medicare carrier agency. Self-employed APNs may bill directly for their services under their own Medicare provider number and receive 85% of the physician fee schedule for the billed procedure (Massachusetts Coalition of Nurse Practitioners, 2003). The Massachusetts Coalition of Nurse Practitioners will be publishing an updated version of the guidebook in 2010. Readers may refer to *Getting Started: A To Do List For Graduate Nurse Practitioners in Massachusetts*, which is available on the Massachusetts Coalition of Nurse Practitioners Web site at www.mcnp.org/for_students.php

Alternatively, when employed by a physician or a practice, an APN may bill Medicare under the physician provider number and receive 100% of the physician charge subject to "incident to" provisions. "Incident to" provisions imply that the services are provided as an integral, although incidental, part of the physician's personal professional services in the course of diagnosis or treatment of an injury or illness. This care is limited to situations in which there is direct physician supervision of the service (i.e., a physician is on the premises and is immediately available to provide assistance and direction [National Heritage Insurance Company, 2009]).

The second reimbursement arrangement is when the Medicare beneficiary is enrolled in a capitated Medicare Advantage program, such as an HMO or MCO. In this scenario, Medicare pays the organization a lump sum for the healthcare services of the beneficiary and the HMO or MCO, in turn, pays the provider a predetermined capitated fee per member per month, regardless of how many times the client is seen (Hoffman et al., 2008). To succeed in this type of arrangement, the APN must proactively manage acute and chronic health conditions to maximize cost-effective use of services.

APNs, like other providers, can decide annually whether they want to participate in Medicare in a given year. In 2003, almost 90% of Medicare providers enrolled to treat Medicare beneficiaries chose participating status and nearly 95% of Medicare claims were submitted by participating providers. Participating providers are paid using a higher fee schedule than used for nonparticipating providers, but agree to accept assignment and to bill beneficiaries only for the 20% copayment. As part of the Medicare Prescription Drug, Improvement and Modernization Act of 2003, CMS increased payments to more than 875,000 healthcare providers for services under the Medicare Physician Fee Schedule by an average of more than 1.5%. This change was implemented to provide healthcare professionals with higher payments to create incentives for APNs and other providers to continue to treat Medicare beneficiaries.

The same two reimbursement arrangements apply to Medicaid reimbursement. To receive reimbursement under Medicaid, an APN must apply and be accepted as a Medicaid provider by the state Medicaid agency. In the state of Massachusetts, for example, APNs may enroll as Medicaid (Mass-Health) providers if the APN is a member of a private practice group, not salaried by a hospital, and compensated by the group practice in the same manner as the physicians and other APNs in the practice; or if the APN is a member of a group practice that solely comprises APNs; or if the APN is in a solo APN private practice (Massachusetts Coalition of Nurse Practitioners, 2003). Medicaid then pays 80% of the fee-for-service rates set for physicians and these rates vary from state-to-state (Phillips, 2009). To provide care to a Medicaid client enrolled in an HMO, an APN must apply and be admitted to the provider panel of the HMO within which the client is enrolled (Buppert, 1998). Some states have Medicaid waivers from the federal government that allow the states to enroll all Medicaid patients in MCOs.

One of the biggest challenges to APNs is ensuring that Medicaid regulations are applied correctly. Although Medicare tends to be consistent and homogeneous, Medicaid may have heterogeneous influences based on variability in state government views and perspectives. In addition, public policy is subjected to various orientations, such as those concerned with cure and rehabilitation versus those concerned with chronic care or palliative care. The National Heritage Insurance Company's Education and Outreach Unit has developed a guide to provide APNs with Medicare Part B nonphysician reimbursement and billing information (National Heritage Insurance Company, 2009). This manual can be accessed at http://www.medicarenhic.com/providers/pubs/nonphyguide.pdf

Another helpful resource is the Medicare Learning Network, which now has an APN Web page that provides access to Medicare fee-for service program topics. From this Web page, APNs can keep abreast of policy and operational updates specific for their profession. One of the featured educational resources is an interactive Web-based training program. It outlines the qualifications of APNs, describes collaboration and supervision requirements for Medicare reimbursement, lists Medicare billing requirements for APNs, and identifies links to Medicare manuals and other resources. The Web page is at http://www.cms.hhs.gov/MLNProuducts/70_APNPA.asp

Managed Care Organizations

When an APN gains admission to an MCO provider panel, the designation Primary Care Provider is awarded, as is a contract for providing care, credentialing, directory listing, and reimbursement (Buppert, 1998). MCOs sell a priced package of health services to their clients who may be employers, individuals, or government agencies, such as the state Medicaid agency or Medicare. A client signs up for a particular plan and offers that plan to "members," who often share the cost of the plan (Buppert).

The American Psychiatric Nurses Association in its position paper on managed care points out that managed care is based on health rather than on illness. Managed care increases access to appropriate mental health care and supports meaningful participation of consumers and families (American Psychiatric Nurses Association, 2007).

Indemnity Insurance Companies

An indemnity insurance company pays for the health care of its beneficiaries but does not deliver the care directly (e.g., Blue Cross, Blue Shield). Indemnity insurance companies privately credential individual providers, including APNs, as they deem necessary to meet the needs of their clientele. These companies pay APN's claims on a per-visit or per-procedure basis. The APN submits a bill to the insurance company and is reimbursed by a fee schedule based on "usual and customary" charges. Some companies reimburse at higher rates than others. The APN has the option of billing a predetermined price and is able to charge or balance bill the patient for the difference.

CREATING A MENTAL HEALTH POLICY AGENDA FOR OLDER ADULTS

A significant effort is underway to overhaul the nation's healthcare system. President Barack Obama has set aside $634 billion as a down payment for reforming healthcare finance and delivery. Nevertheless, the trends are alarming. Forty-seven million Americans are without health insurance (compared to 37 million in 1993). This is despite the nation's $2.5 trillion health care spending (up from $912 billion in 1993). This translates to $8160 spent per person, compared to $3468 per person in 1993. The country spends nearly twice as much per capita as the rest of the industrialized world, yet has lower life expectancy and higher mortality rates among children. There is a shortage of primary healthcare providers and emergency departments are swamped (Toedtman, 2009). This also leaves 47 million uninsured Americans to seek their own services, often unaffordable.

Serious debate about how mental health fits into the U.S. national health reform agenda has not occurred in many years (Koyanagi, 2009). Mental illness in older adults is associated with both increased healthcare use and costs (President's New Freedom Commission on Mental Health, Subcommittee on Older Adults and Mental Health, 2003). Although it is clear that older adults experience many of the same mental health issues that confront other age groups in society and that mental illness contributes to increased morbidity and mortality as well as decreased quality of life in the aging population, many obstacles to full inclusion of mental health in healthcare reform continue to exist. These barriers include a system that is a confusing mix of uncoordinated public and private services, a system that is not responsive to consumers, cost-shifting, an overemphasis on institutional care, and poor quality of care with an imbalance between pharmacotherapy and psychotherapeutic counseling (Koyanagi). Effectively advocating for optimal mental health services requires a comprehensive understanding of these general and systemic barriers older adults face in accessing mental health care. Furthermore, assessment and management strategies are complicated by underdiagnosis of mental disorders by healthcare providers, multiple medical comorbidities, multiple losses, inadequate social support systems, lack of access to clinicians skilled in psychotherapeutic counseling of elders, and in some cases lack of appropriately aggressive treatment (Sullivan, 2008). Despite many positive and promising changes, and despite efforts to ease the stigma of mental illness, the nation's mental healthcare system remains in need of a fundamental transformation, one that prizes recovery instead of simply managing daily symptoms (Krisberg, 2003). The reality is that recovery is necessary to achieve cost-effectiveness.

The New Freedom Commission on Mental Health, created by President George W. Bush in April of 2002, was charged with examining the country's mental health delivery system. The final report of the Commission (2003) addressed six overarching goals: (1) to help Americans understand that mental health is essential to overall health; (2) to make mental health consumer-driven and family-driven; (3) to eliminate racial and ethnic disparity in mental health; (4) to achieve early mental health screening, assessment, and referral; (5) to ensure that excellent mental health care is delivered and that research is expedited; and (6) to promote the use of technology to access mental health care and information on mental health (President's New Freedom Commission on Mental Health, 2003).

The Commission's Subcommittee on Older Adults (2003) identified three main priorities to enhance mental health care for older adults: (1) improving access and continuity, (2) improving quality, and (3) developing workforce and caregiver capacity. Focusing on these themes, three primary policy options for improving mental health service delivery were identified: (1) revision of policy and reimbursement to improve access and continuity of services by supporting comprehensive outreach mental health services in home and community-based settings where older adults seek services and reside; (2) development and implementation of a national initiative to implement evidence-based practices in geriatric mental health care; and (3) development of a workforce with specialized training in gerontology and geriatric mental health care (President's New Freedom Commission on Mental Health, Subcommittee on Older Adults and Mental Health, 2003).

These initiatives encompass a broad spectrum of services and programs that encompass "outreach services, including community education and training, prevention and intervention efforts, and screening and early identification; comprehensive home- and community-based services, including integration with primary care, case management, peer- and consumer-run services, caregiver supports, crisis services, and long-term care; and policy and legislative changes that address the problems of workforce development, funding, research, coalition building, and integrated service systems" (U.S. DHHS, SAMHSA, Center for Mental Health Services, 2007, p. 15).

Additionally, more recent mental health policy reform imperatives championed by the National Conference of State Legislatures (2009) include federal mental health policy and programs that provide federal assistance to states for the development of a continuum of care, ranging from home and community-based programs to institutional care, for all mentally ill individuals in the least restrictive setting; providing states the flexibility to design and implement cost-effective, evidence-based alternatives to institutional care; providing mechanisms for coordination of services to the mentally ill; developing flexible financing mechanisms under Medicare and Medicaid for the provision of mental health care in alternative settings; and encouraging the inclusion of coverage of mental health services in private health insurance policies (National Conference of State Legislatures).

Although myths that mental health care is not valuable have largely been dispelled and evidenced-based treatment recommendations for mental illness are as readily available as they are for medical-surgical services, little has changed since the final report of the New Freedom Commission on Mental Health was issued in 2003. There is still consensus that achievement of these goals will improve the lives of millions of citizens now living with mental illnesses. However, questions about the quality of mental health care and the value of healthcare spending are also at issue in the current economic downturn.

Mental health integration is a concept related to full integration or mainstreaming of mental health and substance abuse care in single delivery system within primary healthcare settings. It is a comprehensive approach not only to promoting the health of individuals, families, and communities based on communication and coordination of evidence-based primary care and mental health services but to providing insurance coverage for all appropriate services. The integration of mental health into primary care simply means to treat mental health like any other health condition. An estimated 50–70% of primary healthcare visits are related to mental health issues including stress, anxiety, or depression (American Psychological Association, 2004). Mental health integration is one example of quality healthcare delivery redesign that is evidence-based and outcomes-oriented and follows a standardized quality process that facilitates communication and coordination, based on consumer and family preferences and sound economics (Reiss-Brennan, 2004).

Three models proposed by the AoA for integrating primary care and mental health include (1) the attached mental health professional model in which a primary care office or clinic has a formal affiliation with a mental health professional to provide screening, psychotherapeutic counseling sessions, and psychopharmacotherapy; (2) the consultation liaison model in which there is close collaboration between mental health clinicians and primary care providers; and (3) the community mental health teams model in which multidisciplinary teams serve within the community for assessments, education, and consultation with primary care and other agencies (Administration on Aging, 2001).

Barriers to integration efforts include the lack of a well-coordinated national effort to improve the quality of mental health and substance abuse services in primary health care or to improve the quality of primary healthcare services available in specialty mental healthcare services. Strategies identified to overcome these barriers include:

- Identify champion leaders
- Establish community coalitions
- Provide consumer access to health information
- Enact measurement standards
- Build flexible information systems (Reiss-Brennan, 2004)
- Promote basic education of all primary healthcare providers in mental healthcare provision
- Encourage enhanced continuing professional development of primary healthcare providers

The prevention of mental illness may be possible for some older adults and might be provided through health reform and through expansions of the public health system. In addition, addressing the mental health needs of individuals with chronic physical illnesses can improve outcomes and should be discussed as part of the wellness agenda (Koyanagi, 2009). Recovery from mental illness must be a goal of the U.S. healthcare system.

Mental health problems in the older adult are pervasive and adversely affect health and often lead to disability. The mental health issues of older adults have not been adequately addressed, which has had an adverse effect on quality of life. Geropsychiatric nurses should assume a leadership role in defining and mobilizing practices for quality mental health care. Focusing views on health policy for older adults may reshape current thinking and decision making related to this important issue. Policy agenda considerations in planning holistic mental health care for an aging society include the following:

Clinical

- Establishing Centers of Excellence for geriatric mental health care
- Identifying best practice models for depression, dementia, substance abuse, and schizophrenia in older adults
- Implementing and evaluating clinical practice guidelines
- Establishing methods to improve care coordination and case management
- Designing staffing models to optimize the provision of mental health care
- Defining unique interdisciplinary collaboration strategies in geriatric mental health care
- Exploring collaborative practice models and opportunities for the geriatric APN
- Improving and increasing benefits (pharmacy, psychotherapy, and social support services)
- Eliminating disparities in the clinical care of older adult patients with coexisting medical and psychiatric illness

Academic

- Designing clinical faculty practice models in mental health care to older adults
- Promoting blended APN role development
- Facilitating caregiver and consumer education and advocacy
- Establishing municipal, regional, and national mental healthcare consortia
- Establishment of funding incentives for mental health professional education across disciplines

Research

- Developing quality indicators for treatment of mental illness in acute- and long-term care settings
- Designing and conducting outcomes research in geriatric mental health care
- Planning, implementing, and evaluating mental health service delivery programs particularly as they pertain to service integration

- Preventing mental illness in the elderly
- Maintaining cognitive function in the elderly
- Exploring links between cognitive decline and dementia
- Testing creative financing and service delivery models for mental health care
- Improving quality of mental health care in nursing homes
- Assessing the public's perceptions about mental health in the older adult

Policy

- Assessing use patterns of acute- and long-term care services
- Exploring integrated service delivery models in long-term care (community versus institutional care)
- Designing local, regional, statewide, and national initiatives
- Enhancing access to mental health care
- Linking health care and social programs to help professionals and organizations cope with mental illness
- Eliminating disparities in the delivery of quality mental health care
- Developing national strategies for suicide prevention and alcohol dependence elimination
- Screening for mental illness and for medical comorbidities in all primary care and mental health settings
- Testing financing reform initiatives in the provision of mental health care
- Promoting interagency collaboration
- Publicizing the effectiveness of risk factor identification and intervention
- Networking with professional nursing organizations who champion mental health parity

Healthcare reform remains high on the U.S. domestic policy agenda. Professional nurses have key positions in influencing health policy, advocacy, and research. Influence begins with awareness, creating networks, developing partnerships, and getting involved. The challenge for geropsychiatric nurses is to tailor these goals into policy reform initiatives that benefit a historically underserved population: older Americans, and in particular, older Americans with mental illness. Research related to geropsychiatric and mental health nursing and policies affecting older adults remains a priority.

Reform begins with interventions to identify and optimally treat mental illness with individual clients in clinical practice. In turn, change evolves at the local and regional levels with awareness of the needs of those afflicted with mental illness at the community level. This must involve all constituencies with a stake in mental health care: clients, families, healthcare professionals, institutions, policymakers, and society. Targeting outreach and proactive interventions toward high-intensity, high-cost users of Medicare expenditures may enhance both quality of care and cost effectiveness.

Geropsychiatric and mental health nurses can support older adults in getting the best possible care by delineating the issues, exploring options, and promoting quality mental health care to policymakers. Quality of life in older adults with mental illness, and outcomes associated with the implementation of social, health, and long-term care programs for older adults need systematic evaluation. Partnerships between nurse researchers and healthcare policy analysts, and interdisciplinary efforts in practice and research related to mental illness and aging, are needed as the 21st century unfolds. Geropsychiatric and mental health nurses in advanced practice roles are in key positions to facilitate positive changes in mental health policy for older adults through advocacy in policy issues at the local, state, and national levels.

It is imperative for gerontological nurses to embrace the importance of social policy, and how programs and services, and their reimbursement, impact the quality of mental health care older adults can access and receive. Nursing's agenda encompasses access, quality, research, and education. Research is a priority that must be addressed even in the face of the nation's economic crisis and budget constraints.

REFERENCES

Administration on Aging. (2001). *Older adults and mental health: Issues and opportunities.* Rockville, MD: Administration on Aging.

Administration on Aging. (2009). *AoA programs.* Retrieved April 15, 2009, from http://www.aoa.gov

Alzheimer's Association. (2009). *2009 Alzheimer's disease: Facts and figures.* Retrieved January 18, 2010, from http://www.alz.org/alzheimer's_disease_facts figures.asp

American Association for Geriatric Psychiatry. (2007). *Legislative and regulatory agenda, 110th Congress, 2007-2008.* Retrieved December 3, 2008, from http://www.aagpgpa.org/advocacy

American Nurses Association. (1996). *Scope and standards of advanced practice registered nursing.* [Brochure]. Washington, DC: Author.

American Nurses Association. (2001). *Scope and standards of gerontological nursing practice.* [Brochure]. Washington, DC: Author.

American Nurses Credentialing Center. (2008). *Certification.* Retrieved February 5, 2009, from http://www.nursecredentialing.org/Certification/PoliciesServices/Statistics.aspx

American Psychiatric Nurses Association. (1995). *Prescriptive authority for advanced practice psychiatric nurses.* Retrieved January 18, 2009, from http://www.apna.org/i4a/pages/index.cfm?pageid=3339

American Psychiatric Nurses Association. (2007). *Role of psychiatric-mental health nurses in managed care.* Retrieved August 1, 2009, from http://www.apna.org/i4a/pages/index.cfm?pageid=3344

American Psychological Association. (2004). *The costs of failing to provide appropriate mental health care.* Washington, DC: Author.

American Psychological Association Practice Organization. (2008). *Summary of the Wellstone-Domenici Mental Health Parity and Addictions Equity Act of 2008.* Retrieved June 6, 2009, from http://www.apapractice.org/apo/in_the_news/parity_summary.GenericArticle.Single.article Link.GenericArticle.Single.file.tmp/Summary OfTheNewParityLaw.pdf

Buck, J. A. (2003). Medicaid, health care financing trends, and the future of state-based public mental health services. *Psychiatric Services, 54*(3), 969–975.

Buppert, C. (1998). Reimbursement for nurse practitioner services. *The Nurse Practitioner, 23*(1), 67–81.

Buppert, C. (2009). Billing for efforts to eradicate unhealthy habits. *Nurse Practitioner World News, 14*(1/2), 1–7.

Centers for Disease Control and Prevention & The Merck Company Foundation. (2007). *The state of aging and health in America 2007.* Whitehouse Station, NJ: The Merck Company Foundation. Retrieved January 15, 2009, from http://www.cdc/gov/aging

Centers for Medicare and Medicaid Services. (2004). *The Chronic Care Improvement Program.* Retrieved May 1, 2004, from http://www.cms.hhs.gov/medicare reform/ccip

Centers for Medicare and Medicaid Services. (2009a). *MLN products. Advanced practice nursing/physician assistant (APN/PA).* Retrieved February 3, 2010, from http://www.cms.hhs.gov/MLNProducts/70_APNPA.asp

Centers for Medicare and Medicaid Services. (2009b). *Medicaid. Mental health service. Overview.* Retrieved January 18, 2010, from http://www.cms.hhs.gov/MHS/

Centers for Medicare and Medicaid Services. (2009c). *Medicare. Program of All Inclusive Care for the Elderly (PACE).* Retrieved January 18, 2010, from http://www.cms.hhs.gov/PACE/

Centers for Medicare and Medicaid Services. (2009d). *Nursing homes. Alternatives to nursing home care.* Retrieved April 1, 2009, from http://www.medicare.gov/Nursing/Alternatives/SHMO.asp

Centers for Medicare and Medicaid Services. (2009e). *Preventive services. Smoking cessation.* Retrieved July 15, 2009, from http://www.medicare.gov/health/smoking.asp?Language=English

Centers for Medicare and Medicaid Services. (2009f). *Statistics.* Retrieved April 1, 2009, from www.cms.gov

Centers for Medicare and Medicaid Services. (2010). *Medicare and you 2010.* Retrieved August 5, 2010, from http://www.medicare.gov/publications/pubs/pdf/10050.pdf

Chen, H., Nwangwu, A., Aparasu, M., Essien, E., Sun, S., & Lee, K. (2008). The impact of Medicare Part D on psychotropic utilization and financial burden for community-based seniors. *Psychiatric Services, 59*(10), 1191–1197.

Edmunds, M. (2003). Medicaid patients bear brunt of budget cuts. *The Nurse Practitioner, 28*(12), 11.

Federal Interagency Forum on Aging-Related Statistics. (2008). *Older Americans 2008: Key indicators of well-being.* Federal Interagency on Aging-Related Statistics. Washington, DC: U.S. Government Printing Office. March 2008. Retrieved January 18, 2009, from http://www.agingstats.gov/agingstatsdotnet/main_site/data/2008_Documents/OA_2008.pdf

Fellows of the American Academy of Nurse Practitioners. (2002). *Nurse practitioner practice in 2012.* Retrieved July 15, 2009, from http://aanp.org/NR/rdonlyres/F63161AC-B9DC-4F35-AC28-846DA2ED2908/33/ThinkTankWhitePaper2012March03.pdf#search="reimbursement"

Frasure-Smith, N., Lesperance, F., Juneau, M., Talajic, M., & Bourassa, M. G. (1999). Gender, depression, and one-year prognosis after myocardial infarction. *Psychosomatic Medicine, 61,* 26–30.

Goldman, L. S. (1999). Medical illness in patients with schizophrenia. *Journal of Clinical Psychiatry, 60*(Suppl. 21), 10–15.

Health Resources and Services Administration. (2009). *HHS releases $338 million to expand community health centers, serve more patients.* Retrieved April 1, 2009, from http://www.hhs.gov/news/press/2009pres/20090327a.html

Hebert, L. E., Scherr, P. A., Bienias, J. L., Bennett, D. A., & Evans, D. A. (2003). Alzheimer's disease in the US population. *Archives of Neurology, 60*(8), 119–122.

HMO Workgroup on Care Management. (1998). Essential components of geriatric care provided through health maintenance organizations. *Journal of the American Geriatrics Society, 46*(3), 303–308.

Hoffman, E. D., Klees, B. S., & Curtis, C. A. (2008). *Brief summaries of Medicare & Medicaid, Title XVIII and Title XIX of The Social Security Act as of November 1, 2008.* Retrieved November 1, 2008, from http://www.cms.hhs.gov/MedicareProgramRatesStats/Downloads/MedicareMedicaidSummaries2008.pdf

Howard, R., Rabins, P. V., Seeman, M. V., Jeste, D. V., & the International Late-Onset, Schizophrenia Group. (2000). Late-onset schizophrenia and very-late onset schizophrenia-like psychosis: An international consensus. *The American Journal of Psychiatry, 157*(2), 172–178.

Jeste, D. V., Alexopoulos, G. S., Bartels, S. J., Cummings, J. L., Gallo, J. J., Gottlieb, G. L., et al. (1999). Consensus statement on the upcoming crisis in geriatric mental health: Research agenda for the next 2 decades. *Archives of General Psychiatry, 56,* 848–853.

Klap, R., Unroe, K. T., & Unutzer, J. (2003). Caring for mental illness in the United States: A focus on older adults. *American Journal of Geriatric Psychiatry, 11,* 517–524.

Kochanek, K. D., Murphy, S. L., Anderson, R. N., & Scott, C. (2004). Deaths: Final data for 2002. *National Vital Statistic Reports, 53*(5), 1–115.

Koyanagi, C. (2009). Economic grand rounds: Can we learn from history? Mental health in health care reform revisited. *Psychiatric Services, 60*(1), 17–20.

Krisberg, K. (2003). Presidential Commission calls for U.S. mental health care reform. *The Nation's Health, 33*(7), 1–6.

Kutney-Lee, A., & Aiken, L. A. (2008). Effect of nurse staffing and education on the outcomes of surgical patients with co-morbid serious mental illnesses. *Psychiatric Services, 59*(12), 1466–1469.

Lantz, M. S. (2002). Depression in the elderly: Recognition and treatment. *Clinical Geriatrics, 10*(10), 18–24.

Lin, E. H. B., Katon, W., Von Korff, M., Tang, L., Williams, J. W., Kroenke, K., et al. (2003). Effect of improving depression care on pain and functional outcomes among older adults with arthritis: A randomized controlled trial. *JAMA, 290*(8), 2428–2434.

Mark, T. L., Levit, K. R., Coffey, R. M., McKusick, D. R., Horwood, H. J., King, E. C., et al. (2007). *National expenditures for mental health services and substance abuse treatment, 1993-2003.* SAMHSA Publication No. SMA 07-4227, Rockville, MD: Substance Abuse and Mental Health Services Administration.

Massachusetts Coalition of Nurse Practitioners. (n.d.). *Getting started: A to do list for graduate nurse practitioners in Massachusetts.* Retrieved February 3, 2010, from www.mcnp.org/for_students.php

Massachusetts Coalition of Nurse Practitioners. (2003). *Guide to nurse practitioner practice in Massachusetts.* Littleton, MA: Author.

Medicare Payment Advisory Commission. (2006). *A data book: Healthcare spending and the Medicare program.* Retrieved December 1, 2008, from http://www.cdc.gov/brfss

National Center for Health Statistics. (2008). *Health, United States 2008 with chartbook.* Hyattsville, MD: U.S. Department of Health and Human Services.

National Conference of State Legislatures. (2009). *Mental health policy.* Retrieved May 10, 2009, from http://www.ncsl.org/statefed/Health.HTM#Long TermCare

National Heritage Insurance Company. (2009). *Physician assistant, nurse practitioner & clinical nurse specialist billing guide.* Retrieved August 1, 2009, from http://www.medicarenhic.com/providers/pubs/nonphy guide.pdf

National Institute on Aging. (1993). *Discoveries in health for aging Americans. Special report on aging 1993.* Washington, DC: U.S. Department of Health and Human Services.

O'Sullivan, C. K., & Krauss, J. B. (2007). True mental health parity: A long overdue public health policy. *American Journal of Nursing, 77*(3), 77–80.

Pennix, B. W., Beekman, A. T., Honig, A., Deeg, D. J., Schoevers, R. A., van Eijk, J. T., et al. (2001). Depression and cardiac mortality: Results from a community-based longitudinal study. *Archives of General Psychiatry, 58*, 221–227.

Phillips, S. (2009). Legislative update 2009: Despite legal issues, APNs are still standing strong. *Nurse Practitioner, 34*(1), 19–41.

President's New Freedom Commission on Mental Health. (2003). *Major federal programs supporting and financing mental health care.* Retrieved February 3, 2010, from http://www.mentalhealthcommission. gov/reports/Fedprograms/031003.doc

President's New Freedom Commission on Mental Health, Subcommittee on Older Adults and Mental Health. (2003). *Anil Godbole and Francis Murphy, Co-Chairs. An outline for the draft report of the Subcommittee on Older Adults.* Retrieved January 18, 2010, from http://www.mentalhealthcommission.gov/subcommittee/Sub_Chairs.htm

Rathmore, S. S., Wang, Y., Druss, B. G., Masoudi, F. A., & Krumhole, H. M. (2008). Mental disorders, quality of care, and outcomes among older patients hospitalized with heart failure: An analysis of the National Heart Failure Project. *Archives of General Psychiatry, 65*(120), 1402–1408.

Reiss-Brennan, B. (2004). Introduction to mental health care in primary care settings. National Mental Health Information Center. Retrieved January 10, 2009, from http://mentalhealth. samhsa.gov/publications/allpubs/SMA06-4195/chapter12.asp

Satcher, D. S. (2000). Executive summary: A report of the Surgeon General on mental health. *Public Health Reports, 115*(1), 89–101.

Smoyak, S. (2000). The history, economics, and financing of mental health care. Part 3: The present. *Journal of Psychosocial Nursing, 38*(11), 32–38.

Social Security Administration. (2009). *Social Security Disability Insurance Program.* Retrieved July 15, 2009, from http://www.ssa.gov/policy/docs/statcomps/ssi_monthly/2009-03/

Substance Abuse and Mental Health Services Administration. (2009a). *Assertive Community Treatment Knowledge Informing Transformation Kit (ACT KIT).* Retrieved July 15, 2009, from http://mental health.samhsa.gov/cmhs/CommunitySupport/toolkits/community

Substance Abuse and Mental Health Services Administration. (2009b). *Center for Mental Health Services.* Retrieved July 15, 2009, from http://mentalhealth.samhsa.gov/cmhs/

Sullivan, G. (2008). Complacent care and the quality gap. *Psychiatric Services, 59*(12), 1367.

The Henry J. Kaiser Family Foundation. (2009). *Health care costs: A primer.* [Report #7670-02]. Retrieved February 2, 2009, from www.kff.org

The Kaiser Commission on Medicaid and the Uninsured. (2009). *Medicaid: A primer 2009.* [Report #7334-03]. Retrieved February 2, 2009, from www.kff.org

Toedtman, J. (2009, April). Fixing health care—the sequel. *American Association of Retired Persons Bulletin, 3.*

Trivedi, A. N., Swaminathan, S., & Mor, V. (2008). Insurance parity and the use of outpatient mental health care following a psychiatric hospitalization. *JAMA, 300*(24), 2879–2885.

Unutzer, J. (2007). Clinical practice. Late-life depression. *New England Journal of Medicine, 357*(22), 2269–2276.

Unutzer, J., Patrick, D. L., Simon, G., Grembowski, D., Walker, E., Rutter, C., et al. (1997). Depressive symptoms and the cost of health services in HMO patients aged 65 years and older. *Journal of the American Medical Association, 277*, 1618–1623.

U.S. Department of Health and Human Services. (2004). *Community integration for older adults with mental illnesses: Overcoming barriers and seizing opportunities.* U.S. DHHS Pub. No. (SMA) 05-4018. Rockville, MD: Center for Mental Health Services, Substance Abuse and Mental Health Services Administration.

U.S. Department of Health and Human Services, SAMHSA, Center for Mental Health Services.

(2007). *Older adults and mental health: A time for reform. A guide for mental health planning and advisory councils.* Washington, DC: Author.

U.S. Department of Housing and Urban Development. (2009). *HUD implementation of the Recovery Act.* Retrieved April 1, 2009, from www.hud.gov/recovery/arract2009.cfm

U.S. Department of Labor. (2009). *Fact sheet: The Mental Health Parity Act.* Retrieved July 1, 2009, from http://www.dol.gov/ebsa/newsroom/fsmhparity.html

U.S. Department of Veterans Affairs. (2009). Retrieved April 1, 2009, from www.va.gov/healtheligibility

VA Media Relations. (2009). President's 2010 budget requests strongly supports VA programs: Funding plan improves access, modernizes technology. *VA Media Relations,* February 26, 2009.

Verdier, J., & Barrett, A. (2008). How Medicaid agencies administer mental health services: Results from a 50-state survey. *Psychiatric Services, 59*(10), 1203–1206.

21

Envisioning the Future of Geropsychiatric Nursing

Kathleen C. Buckwalter

Cornelia Beck

Lois K. Evans

Many changes have taken place since the term "geropsychiatric nursing" first appeared in the Cumulative Index to Nursing and Allied Health Literature in 1977 (Beck, 1988, p. 841). We remain very optimistic about the future of geropsychiatric nursing, but there is still much to be done. "Nurses must work to create the professional and political will to avoid a crisis in long-term care. We must work to create models of care that are appropriate for the elderly and their families; pursue adequate funding and reimbursement for programming and services; support the preparation and retention of adequate numbers of qualified nursing providers; increase our research to assess the effectiveness of care strategies; increase our emphasis on health promotion, community-based services, and continuity of care; and strengthen the gerontological and professional ethics content of our curricula" (Maas & Buckwalter, 1996, p. 247). At a seminal conference focused on the future of geropsychiatric nursing held in 2005 in Philadelphia (Puentes & Evans, 2006), a panel of nurse experts charged the audience to infiltrate geropsychiatric nursing everywhere; to role model and advocate; and to work for legal, policy, and financial mandates that

will help the field reach a level that can really make a difference in the lives of older Americans. The panelists also identified the many challenges that remain: to tackle mental health disparities in older adults; to demonstrate cost benefit of mental health nursing services for this population; to adapt an evidence base for application to new settings of care; to conduct research and evolve education for geropsychiatric nursing practice; and to develop a critical mass of nurses with knowledge and skill to provide mental health care to older adults, potentially certifying specialists in the field. We envision changes and innovations in geropsychiatric nursing education, research, and practice to meet the "broad-based psychosocial, psychiatric, neurobiological and medical knowledge necessary to meet the mental health needs of the elderly" (Wakefield, Buckwalter, & Gerdner, 1998, p. 914). Space limitations prohibit an exhaustive review of these changes, so this discussion is limited to the following areas: new service delivery models and setting for care; needed research; emphasis on translation of research into practice; need to prepare more nurses with geropsychiatric expertise; and health promotion and disease prevention.

NEW SERVICE DELIVERY MODELS AND SETTINGS FOR CARE

Older adults, and especially those with mental health needs, use a high percentage of healthcare services across the continuum of care, ranging from community-based to long-term care services. However, because the focus of the healthcare system is primarily on acute and physical care, the current system is unprepared to care adequately for elders with chronic care and mental health needs. To address this issue, geropsychiatric nurses must play an active role in the transformation of the current fragmented healthcare system. Maas (2004) called for new paradigms of care that are holistic, with an array of strategies that meet the needs of older adults and include higher staff to resident ratios, health promotion, prevention of illness and disability, management of chronic illness, assistance with functional independence, and prevention of avoidable medical errors. Nowhere is this more true than in the long-term care system, where shortcomings are visible, serious, and costly. Nonetheless, despite strong evidence of the positive influence of nurse practitioners with geriatric and psychiatric skills on resident outcomes and cost-effectiveness, they are still underutilized in long-term care systems.

Nursing Homes

Approximately 80% of persons who reside in nursing homes (NHs) have a diagnosable psychiatric disorder, with dementia being the most prevalent. Indeed, the prevalence of mental illnesses among NH residents is growing so dramatically that the Office of the Inspector General dubbed these nursing facilities "de facto psychiatric hospitals" (Vickery, 2003). And yet, despite this high prevalence, and associated behavioral problems, most residents who need mental health services do not receive them (Bartels, Moak, & Dums, 2002). Further, half of NHs report inadequate access to psychiatric consultation and 75% are unable to obtain the consultation and educational services

they need to provide effective behavioral interventions for residents (Reichman et al., 1998). Currently, three primary models of mental health service delivery in NHs have been identified (Bartels et al.): (1) psychiatrist-centered, (2) multidisciplinary team, and (3) nurse-centered models. The nurse-centered models emphasize consultation to NH personnel and the education of direct care staff to provide mental health interventions within the home. A train-the-trainer approach is used, in which geropsychiatric nurses outside of the NH provide ongoing training and consultation to staff who then become internal "experts" responsible for the training of others in the facility (Smith, Mitchell, Buckwalter, & Garand, 1994; Smith, Mitchell, & Buckwalter, 1995; Pajarillo, Sers, Ryan, Headley, & Nalven, 1997). To address current unmet needs for the delivery of mental health services to NHs, we foresee the emergence of more nurse-centered models of care, and an enhanced role for geropsychiatric nurses as members of interdisciplinary teams.

One promising new initiative was formed in 2007 as the Nursing Home Collaborative (NHC), which in 2009 became the Sigma Theta Tau International (STTI) Nursing Home Collaborative. The goals of this program are to improve the quality of nursing care for, and quality of life of, NH residents through organizational and human capital development strategies, and to strengthen the professional practice of nursing in these facilities. Within STTI, a suite of products and services is currently under development, in collaboration with the John A. Hartford Centers of Geriatric Nursing Excellence, to strengthen the professional practice of nursing in NHs. An important focus of STTI/NHC is the key leadership role of registered nurses in providing quality resident care, in concert with culture change values. Development of a business plan and business case for the products and services is underway, and over the next five years STTI/NHC will test products and services and their delivery to the NH industry. Both directly and indirectly, outcomes from STTI/NHC should improve the mental health care of older adults in long-term care facilities, by creating new care delivery models, decreasing staff turnover, and increasing competencies of the workforce in NHs.

Another related initiative to be completed in 2010 is the Golden Living project, a collaboration of the John A. Hartford Foundation Centers of Geriatric Nursing Excellence at the Universities of Iowa and Arkansas. This project is developing recommendations for dementia care best practices, including required staffing, staff competencies, and staff training materials for special care and traditional units serving persons with dementia. Recommendations will be based on a review and synthesis of research, expert clinical judgments, and the work the Alzheimer's Association and other groups have done in compiling best practices and training.

Assisted Living Facilities

A rapidly growing segment of the care continuum is assisted living (AL) residences, currently serving more than 1 million older adults, with that number on the rise (Arehart-Treichel, 2003; Assisted Living Federation of America, 2009). Reported rates of dementia among residents of AL settings are high, yet vary widely from 34–68% (Rosenblatt et al., 2004). More than 30% of all AL residences have dedicated dementia units, with growth in the number of dementia-specific facilities predicted in the future. Despite the increasing role played by AL residences in dementia care, much about them remains unknown.

Indeed, especially given the increasing acuity levels of residents and the prevalence of dementia and psychiatric disorders in this population, AL residents may have many unmet needs, particularly those associated with maintaining health and function (Boustani et al., 2005; Maas & Buckwalter, 2006; Rosenblatt et al., 2004; Zimmerman et al., 2005). Insufficient numbers of staff with inadequate preparation and training to deal with cognitive and emotional challenges in this population may lead to compromised quality of care and premature transfer to NHs and place residents of ALs at high risk for developing or worsening of cognitive and psychological disorders. Geropsychiatric nurses can play a pivotal role in changing patterns and quality of care in these fast-growing residential settings. Before effective health promotion and disease-related interventions can be developed for residents in AL, more needs to be understood about the levels of cognitive and mental health impairment in these settings.

Geropsychiatric Inpatient Units

To accommodate the unique problems and mental health needs of older adults, specialized geriatric psychiatric inpatient units and services have been developed. However, too little is known about how many or what types of services are available nationwide, information that is essential for establishing best practices for these inpatient units, providing a foundation of knowledge on which staff can build, and promoting networking among nurses who share common goals and needs (Smith, Specht, & Buckwalter, 2005). Geropsychiatric nurses need to determine the current state of the art for inpatient geropsychiatric units to develop specialized staff orientation and training that addresses both geriatric and psychiatric care needs, and to acknowledge the importance of interdisciplinary care in treating these complex patients, many of whom present with medical comorbidities.

Regrettably, posthospitalization success is often limited, suggesting that improved understanding and communication between nurses working in NHs, home care, and hospital inpatient units are needed to solve the "revolving door" syndrome associated with transfer trauma for geropsychiatric patients. More joint conferences and other means of information sharing, problem solving, and networking between geriatric and psychiatric nurses are warranted (Smith, Buckwalter, & Maxson, 2002; Stevenson & Naylor, 2005). In addition, a recent study comparing patient and family satisfaction using telemedicine in a rural geropsychiatric unit to onsite psychiatric care found high satisfaction levels, good use, and effectiveness using telemedicine applications from the inpatient site (Holden & Dew, 2008).

Co-located and Integrated Primary Care and Mental Health Services

The lack of adequately trained geriatric mental health professionals is compounded by the fact that older adults seldom acknowledge their mental health problems or self refer to psychiatric service settings because of barriers, such as stigma, geographic access, limited funding and resources, and workforce issues. Even when mental health services are available, they are not used by older adults. Less than 3% of elders report seeing a mental health professional for treatment, and only half of those who acknowledge mental health problems receive any kind of psychiatric treatment. Indeed, the primary care system has been called the "de facto mental health delivery system" (Peek & Heinrich, 2000) in that it manages, either directly or indirectly, about 30% of all patients with mental disorders. A recent study of Medicare utilization found that advanced practice nurses provide a sizeable proportion of elders' mental health care, especially in rural areas (Hanrahan & Sullivan-Marx, 2005). Undiagnosed and untreated mental disorders, such as depression and anxiety, can lead to increased disability, premature death, increased morbidity, increased risk of institutionalization, and a significant decrease in an elder's quality of life (Gold, Kilbourne, & Valenstein, 2008; Morris, 2001). Therefore, better integration of mental health and primary care for older people with mental illness is needed. Geropsychiatric nurses can play a pivotal role in promoting collaborative, cooperative approaches among health, mental health, primary care and community and institutional care service providers, consumers, and family members so that the system as a whole can deliver more effective and consistent services to mentally ill elders that supports their functional status and quality of life (Cotroneo, Kurlowicz, Outlaw, Burgess, & Evans, 2001). Findings from the IMPACT study (Unutzer et al., 2002), a randomized controlled trial that enrolled 1801 older

adults from 18 primary care clinics in five states, showed substantial and persistent reductions in symptoms of depression (Hunkeler et al., 2006) and improved physical functioning (Callahan et al., 2005). Nurses played an important role in this primary care–based intervention as depression care managers.

New Settings of Geropsychiatric Nursing Care

Kaas and Beattie (2006) argue for the critical role geropsychiatric nurses can play in more nontraditional care settings, such as prisons and homeless shelters, where inhabitants are characterized by high levels of mental health problems and limited resources are available for psychiatric treatment. The inmate population is growing in both numbers and age (Loeb & AbuDagga, 2006), and with this increase comes the challenge of more older prisoners with mental and neurological disorders and a greater need for end-of-life and palliative care. Loeb (2009) suggests infusing advanced practice geropsychiatric nurses, among others, into prison settings as a cost-effective solution to the disease burden of older prisoners. A significant number of older persons discharged from the criminal justice system wind up in homeless shelters with chronic, complex health issues, including substance abuse and mental illness. Geropsychiatric nurses can provide targeted outreach services to this underserved population, including detection, treatment, and referral services (Garibaldi, Conde-Martel, & O'Toole, 2005).

EXPANDED ROLES

Geropsychiatric nurses are likely to be called on to take more of a clinical leadership and case management role in the future, to act as "bridge builders" of understanding across specialties, and as advocates for integration of mental health into a primary care framework to enhance the overall health and functioning of vulnerable elders (Cotroneo et al., 2001) and during end-of-life care. In their review of future models of geropsychiatric nursing care, Kaas and Beattie (2006) discuss how geropsychiatric nurses will increasingly serve in a variety of independent practice roles, and collaborative and consultative roles. They will be active in geropsychiatric nurse consultation services to hospitals, particularly their geropsychiatric units and emergency departments; NHs, including their special care units; and AL facilities. As the number of older persons in hospitals increases, there will likely be more geropsychiatric units without walls as described by Nadler-Moodie and Gold (2005). As the number of older adults in home care increases, it is hoped that multiple examples of psychiatric home care will be seen. Nurses will increasingly become geropsychiatric product line managers for healthcare systems that are establishing geropsychiatric units or dementia care units. They will be active in determining cost-containment strategies while preserving quality care in the cost-driven healthcare reform process and will serve as advocates for the most vulnerable special care elder populations, such as minorities, the homeless, rural elders, developmentally disabled elders, those living alone, and the oldest–old.

They will also be increasingly called upon to use telehealth and other technology-based approaches and delivery methods to provide education and care for patients and their families in distant and underserved communities (Buckwalter, Davis, Wakefield, Kienzle, & Murray, 2002). There may even be a new specialization of a nurse geropsychtechnologist, who uses technology to develop new geropsychiatric services. In the role of cybertherapist, we may see nurses specializing in delivering geropsychiatric care through such avenues as using interactive voice response telephone sessions to provide self-assessments; conducting remote video home visits; videophone-assisted individual, group, or family therapy; or using smart home technology to monitor patients (Mahoney, 2005).

NEEDED RESEARCH

In their review of the state of geropsychiatric nursing science, Kolanowski and Piven (2006) evaluated the knowledge base in 17 discrete clinical areas and identified specific gaps. In each of these areas there remain an insufficient number of rigorous, well-powered randomized clinical trials to allow the meta-analysis needed to support evidence-based practice (EBP). We need to be better able to distinguish the emotional adjustment to late-life losses from the pathological sadness of depression and to distinguish the depression that often accompanies the progression of dementia from an underlying diagnosis of depression. An underresearched area is that of anxiety in older adults, specifically the role of medical comorbidities and aging in the occurrence of anxiety. Other areas greatly in need of nursing research are substance abuse, severe mental illness, and sleep. In each of these areas, data are needed on how ethnicity and race influence not only the expression of symptoms, but also help-seeking behaviors. More focus on prevention research is also needed, such as programs to promote cognitive functioning. In the area of caregiving research, more attention needs to be given to the role of grandparenting, particularly in populations where older adults are assuming heavy parenting responsibilities. Each of these areas of research needs to include the multiple settings in which older adults live, such as AL and retirement communities.

As knowledge continues to develop about the role of genetics in mental illness, geropsychiatric nursing research needs to incorporate this new knowledge into studies. Similarly, rapid advances in the area of neuroimaging hold great promise for better understanding of the mechanisms by which interventions work. The emerging fields of behavioral economics and neuroeconomics can also be applied to understand the decisions that older persons make about their mental health. Behavioral economics applies scientific research on human and social, cognitive, and emotional factors to better understand the economic decisions made by consumers, and neuroeconomics uses neuroimaging to examine the activation of brain regions as people make choices, as in the work of Bickel et al. (2007) on drug addiction.

It is incumbent on geropsychiatric nurses to then use their research findings to change regulatory and reimbursement policies and to support improved mental health services to elders (Bartels et al., 2002). To achieve this goal, geropsychiatric nurses need to develop more evidence-based protocols to guide their practice and undertake more translation research.

EMPHASIS ON TRANSLATION OF RESEARCH INTO PRACTICE

Three decades ago the need for greater use of research findings in practice was identified as 1 of the 15 priorities in clinical nursing research (Lindeman, 1975). Since that time, the emphasis on EBP has generated a greater demand for nurses to use research to guide practice (Janken & Dufault, 2002). Despite regulatory and professional standards that address EBP, use of research in practice remains sporadic at best (Kirchhoff, 2004). EBP is defined as the conscientious and judicious use of current best evidence, in conjunction with patient values and clinical expertise, to guide healthcare decisions (Sackett, Straus, Richardson, Rosenberg, & Haynes, 2000). It encompasses dissemination of scientific knowledge and other types of evidence, critique and synthesis of the evidence, determining applicability of the evidence in practice, developing an EBP standard, implementing the EBPs, and evaluating changes in practice. The National Institutes of Health has recognized the need for bringing new treatments more efficiently and quickly to patients by establishing Clinical and Translational Science Awards. Their goal is to link about 60 institutions together to energize clinical and translational science (National Center for Research Resources, 2009). Geropsychiatric nurses need to be involved in these Clinical and Translational Science Awards and foster a focus on geropsychiatric issues. Other important roles for geropsychiatric nurses are facilitating the testing of selected EBP protocols in clinical sites, taking an active role with providers to promote adoption of EBPs, and creating EBP centers of excellence in acute and long-term care settings that can serve as exemplars for the provision of evidence-based care for mentally ill older adults.

To assist with the translation effort, the *American Journal of Nursing* joined with the Hartford Institute for Geriatric Nursing at New York University's College of Nursing to publish the "Try This: Best Practices in Nursing Care of Older Adults" series of assessment tools, many of which are relevant for geropsychiatric nursing practice and research. A companion series of translation-focused articles and demonstration videos on the care of older adults, called "How to Try This," is also available. The goal of this effort is to provide nurses with information that is accessible, easily understood, and easily implemented. More information on these free, Web-based offerings is available at www.NursingCenter.com/AJNolderadults or www.hartfordign.org/Resources/Try_This_Series. The Hartford Institute for Geriatric Nursing provides a number of other resources for geropsychiatric nurses in the form of evidence-based geriatric protocols and topics for the management of common syndromes and conditions (http://consultgerirn.org/resources/geriatrics_topics/). These include protocols on delirium, dementia, depression, elder mistreatment and abuse, family caregiving, physical restraints, sexuality issues in aging, and substance abuse.

Similarly, the Research Dissemination Core of the University of Iowa's Gerontological Nursing Interventions Research Center has published 33 evidence-based nursing practice protocols designed to promote adoption of evidence-based interventions to improve care of older adults. Many of these protocols, which have been accepted by the National Guidelines Clearinghouse (www.guidelines.gov), are also relevant for geropsychiatric nursing practice, and cover many of the same topics as available in the Hartford Institute protocols, such as acute confusion and delirium, Alzheimer's disease and chronic dementing illnesses, bathing persons with dementia, detection of depression in both cognitively intact and cognitively impaired older adults, elderly suicide, secondary prevention, restraints, wandering, and family involvement in care for persons with dementia. Quick reference guides are available for many of the evidence-based protocols, which can be accessed at the following Web site: www.nursing.uiowa.edu/centers/gnirc/disseminatecore.htm

NEED TO PREPARE MORE GEROPSYCHIATRIC NURSES

Nurses are still struggling with the issue of what it means to be a geropsychiatric nurse, and what qualifications and educational background are needed to best care for older adults with complex psychiatric and comorbid medical problems. Indeed, the number of currently practicing geropsychiatric nurses is unknown, in part because there is neither a certification procedure nor registry. One thing, however, is certain: the demand for specialists in the care of mentally ill and cognitively impaired elders will only increase in the coming years as the baby boom generation cares for aging parents, begins to think about their own retirement and old age, and places financial demands on the health and mental health systems. The expectations and demands of "boomers" for rational and responsive systems of care will be enormous. Our current "systems" of elder care are unlikely to meet those demands, in large part because of the inadequate numbers of nurses prepared to care for the elderly, and especially for those suffering from mental and neurological disorders.

In that approximately 20% of older adults experience specific mental disorders that cannot be considered part of the normal aging process, nurses will require a greater understanding of the behavioral science of aging to function as effective practitioners (McBride, 2000), knowledge not only of the unique presentation of psychiatric disorders in later life, but also aspects of normal aging, disease and disabilities associated with aging, psychopharmacology, genetics and pharmacogenetics, a more integrated view of wellness and illness, and cultural differences among minority aged (Morris, 2001). Traditional geriatric nursing programs lack adequate content related to the assessment and management of psychosocial and psychiatric needs of older adults. Neither do they prepare nurses to intervene using successful individual, group,

family, and pharmacological strategies. Similarly, most psychiatric nursing programs fail to provide adequate information on the unique needs of the older adult. Thus, despite tremendous advances in the field, geropsychiatric mental health education for nurses remains sorely inadequate (Kurlowicz, Puentes, Evans, Spool, & Ratcliffe, 2007), and Morris and Mentes (2006) recommended development of core content for all levels of education. Integration of geropsychiatric content is required in basic educational programs, and in specialty programs at the advanced practice level. Further, more programs emphasizing geropsychiatric nursing are needed, and the number of such high-quality programs is expanding. For example, Case Western Reserve University Frances Payne Bolton School of Nursing has incorporated more geriatric mental health content into the GNP curriculum, and the University of Arkansas for Medical Sciences College of Nursing has implemented a five-credit geropsychiatric course focus as part of its geriatric nurse practitioner program to prepare practitioners to address better a comprehensive array of mental and physical health needs of older adults. Similarly, the University of Michigan School of Nursing has developed a specialized concentration in geropsychiatric nursing that augments existing programs and uses distance-learning strategies, and the University of Nebraska Medical Center College of Nursing has five courses in its advanced geropsychiatric nursing practice focus area (Algase, Souder, Roberts, & Beattie, 2006).

A number of other excellent courses, programs, and post-baccalaureate and post-master's certificate programs have recently been implemented or are under development. Implementing one of the major strategies that evolved from the Philadelphia national conference mentioned previously (Puentes, Buckwalter, & Evans, 2006), we have embarked on an ambitious journey to enhance the mental health of older Americans by improving the educational preparation of nurses at all levels. With funding from the John A. Hartford Foundation, leaders at the Universities of Arkansas for Medical Sciences, Iowa, and Pennsylvania are implementing a Geropsychiatric Nursing Collaborative, housed at the American Academy of Nursing. Beginning with development of enhancements to existing competency statements for entry level and advanced practice nurses, the goal is to collect and adapt curriculum materials and resources that faculty can use to help students learn the requisite knowledge and skills. These materials will be made easily accessible from a Web site and a train-the-trainer model will be used with faculty to facilitate broad implementation. Timing is everything, and this project benefits from the headway made by the recently completed Geriatric Nursing Education Consortium (American Association of Colleges of Nursing and the John A. Hartford Institute for Geriatric Nursing) in which hundreds of baccalaureate faculty from across the nation were trained to integrate and teach geriatric content, including geriatric mental health. It further benefits from recent consensus reached at the national level on the roles and population foci for advanced practice nursing; in this new regulatory model, gerontology (and by extension, geriatric mental health) will be required as didactic and clinical content in all programs whose graduates may care for older adults (Stanley, 2009).

HEALTH PROMOTION AND DISEASE PREVENTION

Geropsychiatric nurses are concerned with both the prevention of health problems in older adults and their families and the care of those who have emotional, behavioral, and mental disorders in a variety of community-based and institutional settings (Wakefield et al., 1998). Much of the specialty focus to date, however, has been on the care of frail and cognitively impaired elders. With increases in active life expectancy, and growing ethnic diversity among the elderly population, this focus may change to a greater emphasis on maintaining vitality and health and restorative models of care in well older adults, those who have the physical, mental, social, and spiritual function or resources to meet the needs of everyday living (Belza & Baker, 2000). Emphasis on physical exercise, cognitive exercise,

self-efficacy, and learned resourcefulness enhancement as components of routine "mental health hygiene" (Cohen, 2005) may become the norm. Greater attention to the developmental and psychoeducational needs of well elders is required. Further, development and evaluation of innovative mental health wellness centers and services, and provision of adequate support systems (e.g., transportation, recreation, and nutrition) and trained providers will help ensure that older adults can attain and maintain optimal mental health, remain actively engaged in their communities, feel a sense of personal control over their lives, and enjoy life-long good interpersonal relationships (Belza & Baker). Because functional status is strongly impacted by coping styles, social support, and affective status, it seems likely that geropsychiatric nurses will play a key role in optimizing the mental health of well elders. For example, they might provide preretirement counseling services, conduct mental health screening, lead problem-solving and assertiveness groups, and train peer counselors at community centers.

CONCLUSION

Geropsychiatric nursing will not only survive, but will thrive in years to come. The evidence mounts as we meet with new graduates who are choosing a career in geropsychiatric nursing, talk with nursing leaders at conferences, create geropsychiatric enhancements to extant competencies, read the enhanced quantity and quality of the literature addressing geropsychiatric nursing issues, review innovative proposals submitted by nurses for private and federal funding to support their research related to care of mentally ill elders, and see the improvements that are slowly taking place in healthcare environments for elders. It is truly an exciting time to be a geropsychiatric nurse. We feel fortunate to have "gotten in on the ground floor" of geropsychiatric nursing more than 25 years ago, and to bear witness to current and promised developments in new service delivery models and settings for care, expanded roles for geropsychiatric nurses in clinical practice, and enhancements to nursing education and the conduct and translation of research.

REFERENCES

Algase, D. L., Souder, E., Roberts, B., & Beattie, E. (2006). Enriching geropsychiatric nursing in advanced practice nursing programs. *Journal of Professional Nursing, 22*(2), 129–136.

Arehart-Treichel, J. (2003). Many assisted-living residents not getting depression help. *Psychiatric News, 38*(22), 27.

Assisted Living Federation of America. (2009). What is assisted living? Retrieved June 22, 2009, from http://www.alfa.org/alfa/What_is_Assisted_Living1.asp?SnID=1880353361

Bartels, S. J., Moak, G. S., & Dums, A. R. (2002). Mental health services in nursing homes: Models of mental health services in nursing homes: A review of the literature. *Psychiatric Services, 53*(22), 1390–1396.

Beck, C. K. (1988). The aged adult. In C. K. Beck, R. P. Rawlins, & S. R. Williams (Eds.), *Mental health-psychiatric nursing* (2nd ed., pp. 840–864). St. Louis, MO: Mosby.

Belza, B., & Baker, M. W. (2000). Maintaining health in well older adults: Initiatives for schools of nursing and the John A. Hartford foundation for the 21st century. *Journal of Gerontological Nursing, 26*(7), 8–17.

Bickel, W. K., Miller, M. L., Yi, R., Kowal, B. P., Lindquist, D. M., & Pitcock, J. A. (2007). Behavioral and neuroeconomics of drug addiction: Competing neural systems and temporal discounting processes. *Drug and Alcohol Dependence, 90S*, S85–S91.

Boustani, M., Zimmerman, S., Williams, C. S., Bruger-Galdini, A. L., Watson, L., Reed, P. S., et al. (2005). Characteristics associated with behavioral symptoms related to dementia in long-term care residents. *The Gerontologist, 45*(Special Issue No. 1), 56–61.

Buckwalter, K. C., Davis, L. L., Wakefield, B. J., Kienzle, M. G., & Murray, M. A. (2002). Telehealth for elders and their caregivers in rural communities. *Family & Community Health, 25*(3), 31–40.

Callahan, C. M., Kroenke, K., Counsell, S. R., Hendrie, H. C., Perkins, A. J., Katon, W., et al. (2005). Treatment of depression improves physical functioning in older adults. *Journal of the American Geriatric Society, 53*(3), 367–373.

Cohen, G. D. (2005). *The mature mind: The positive power of the aging brain.* New York: Basic Books.

Cotroneo, M., Kurlowicz, L. H., Outlaw, F. H., Burgess, A. W., & Evans, L. K. (2001). Psychiatric-mental health nursing at the interface: Revisioning education for the specialty. *Issues in Mental Health Nursing, 22*(5), 549–569.

Garibaldi, B., Conde-Martel, A., & O'Toole, T. P. (2005). Self-reported comorbidities, perceived needs, and sources for usual care for older and younger homeless adults. *Journal of General Internal Medicine, 20*(8), 726–730.

Gold, K., Kilbourne, A., & Valenstein, M. (2008). Primary care of patients with serious mental illness: Your chance to make a difference. *Journal of Family Practice, 57*(8), 1–14.

Hanrahan, N., & Sullivan-Marx, E. (2005). Practice patterns and potential solutions to the shortage of providers of older adult mental health services. *Policy Politics & Nursing Practice, 6*(3), 236–245.

Holden, D., & Dew, E. (2008). Telemedicine in a rural gero-psychiatric inpatient unit: Comparison of perception/satisfaction to onsite psychiatric care. *Telemedicine and e-Health, 14*(4), 381–384.

Hunkeler, E., Katon, W., Tang, L., Williams, J. W., Kroenke, K., Lin, E. H. B., et al. (2006). Long term outcomes from the IMPACT randomized trial for depressed elderly patients in primary care. *British Medical Journal, 332*(7536), 259–263.

Janken, J. K., & Dufault, M. A. (2002, January 24). Improving the quality of pain assessment through research utilization. *The Online Journal of Knowledge Synthesis for Nursing, 2C,* Article OJ0011. Retrieved May 22, 2004, from http://www.stti.iupui.edu/library/ojksn/case_study/cc_doc2c.html

Kaas, M., & Beattie, E. (2006). Geropsychiatric nursing practice in the United States: Present trends and future directions. *American Psychiatric Nurses Association, 12*(3), 142–155.

Kirchhoff, K. T. (2004). State of the science of translational research: From demonstration projects to intervention testing. *Worldviews on Evidence-Based Nursing, 1*(S1), S6–S12.

Kolanowski, A., & Piven, M. (2006). Geropsychiatric nursing: The state of the science. *American Psychiatric Nurses Association, 12*(2), 75–99.

Kurlowicz, L. H., Puentes, W. J., Evans, L. K., Spool, M. M., & Ratcliffe, S. J. (2007). Graduate education in geropsychiatric nursing: Findings from a national survey. *Nursing Outlook, 55*, 303–310.

Lindeman, C. (1975). Priorities in clinical nursing research. *Nursing Outlook, 23*(11), 693–698.

Loeb, S. J. (2009). Elders behind bars: Why we should care and what we should do. *Journal of Gerontological Nursing, 35*(7), 5–6.

Loeb, S. J., & AbuDagga, A. (2006). Health-related research on older inmates: An integrative literature review. *Research in Nursing & Health, 29*(6), 556–565.

Maas, M. (2004). Long-term care for older adults: Advocating for a new health-care paradigm. *Journal of Gerontological Nursing, 30*(10), 3–4.

Maas, M. L., & Buckwalter, K. C. (1996). Epilogue—gazing through the crystal ball: Gerontological nursing issues and challenges for the 21st century. In E.A. Swanson & T. Tripp-Reimer (Eds.), *Advances in gerontological nursing: Issues for the 21st century* (pp. 237–249). New York: Springer.

Maas, M. L., & Buckwalter, K. C. (2006). Providing quality of care in assisted living facilities: Recommendations for enhanced staffing and staff training. *Journal of Gerontological Nursing, 32*(11), 14–22.

Mahoney, D. (2005). The future of technology in mental health nursing—A nurse geropsychtechnologist? In K. D. Melillo & S. C. Houde (Eds.), *Geropsychiatric and mental health nursing* (pp. 387–393). Sudbury, MA: Jones and Bartlett.

McBride, A. B. (2000). Nursing and gerontology. *Journal of Gerontological Nursing, 26*(7), 18–27.

Morris, D. L. (2001). Geriatric mental health: An overview. *Journal of the American Psychiatric Nurses Association, 7*(6), S2–S7.

Morris, D. L., & Mentes, J. (2006). Geropsychiatric nursing education: Challenge and opportunity. *Journal of the American Psychiatric Nurses Association, 12*(2), 105–115.

Nadler-Moodie, M., & Gold, J. (2005). A geropsychiatric unit without walls. *Issues in Mental Health Nursing, 26*, 101–114.

National Center for Research Resources. (2009). *Clinical and Translational Science Awards.* Retrieved March 31, 2009, from http://www.ncrr. nih.gov/clinical_research_resources/clinical_ and_translational_science_awards

Pajarillo, E. J., Sers, A. J., Ryan, R. M., Headley, B., & Nalven, C. (1997). Consultation-liaison psychiatric nursing in long term care. *Journal of Psychosocial Nursing and Mental Health Services, 35*(8), 24–30.

Peek, C. J., & Heinrich, R. L. (2000). Integrating behavioral health and primary care. In M. E. Maruish (Ed.), *Handbook of psychological assessment in primary care* (pp. 43–91). Mahwah, NJ: Lawrence Erlbaum.

Puentes, W. J., Buckwalter, K., & Evans, L. K. (2006). Geropsychiatric nursing: Planning for the future. *Journal of the American Psychiatric Nurses Association, 12*(3), 165–169.

Puentes, W. J., & Evans, L. K. (2006). A dialogue with senior thought leaders in geropsychiatric nursing: Summary and synthesis. *Journal of the American Psychiatric Nurses Association, 12*(3), 161–164.

Reichman, W. E., Coyne, A. C., Borson, S., Negron, A. E., Rovner, B. W., Pelchat, R. J., et al. (1998). Psychiatric consultation in the nursing home: A survey of six states. *American Journal of Geriatric Psychiatry, 6*(4), 320–327.

Rosenblatt, A., Samus, Q. M., Steele, C. D., Baker, A. S., Harper, M. G., Brandt, J., et al. (2004). The Maryland assisted living study: Prevalence, recognition, and treatment of dementia and other psychiatric disorders in the assisted living population of central Maryland. *Journal of the American Geriatrics Society, 52*(10), 1618–1625.

Sackett, D. L., Straus, S. E., Richardson, W. S., Rosenberg, W., & Haynes, R. B. (2000). *Evidence-based medicine: How to practice and teach EBM.* London: Churchill Livingstone.

Smith, M., Buckwalter, K. C., & Maxson, E. (2002). Psychiatric and geriatric nurses together at the table: Evaluation of a combined conference. *Journal of the American Psychiatric Nurses Association, 8*(1), 3–8.

Smith, M., Mitchell, S., & Buckwalter, K. C. (1995). Nurses helping nurses: Development of internal specialists in long-term care. *Journal of Gerontological Nursing, 21*(3), 25–33. Reprinted in *Journal of Psychosocial Nursing, 33*(4), 38–42.

Smith, M., Mitchell, S., Buckwalter, K. C., & Garand, L. (1994). Geropsychiatric nursing consultation: A valuable resource in rural long-term care. *Archives of Psychiatric Nursing, 8*(4), 272–279.

Smith, M., Specht, J., & Buckwalter K. C. (2005). Geropsychiatric inpatient care: What is state of the art? *Issues in Mental Health Nursing, 26*(1), 11–22.

Stanley, J. (2009). Reaching consensus on a regulatory model: What does this mean for APRNs? *The Journal for Nurse Practitioners, 5*(2), 99–104.

Stevenson, C., & Naylor, M. D. (2005). Cognitively impaired older adults: From hospital to home. *American Journal of Nursing, 105*(2), 52–62.

Unutzer, J., Katon, W., Callahan, C. M., Williams, J. W., Hunkeler, E., Harpole, L., et al. (2002). Collaborative care management of late-life depression in the primary care setting: A randomized controlled trial. *JAMA, 288*(22), 2836–2845.

Vickery, K. (2003). The complex path to managing mental illness. *Provider, 29*(5), 18–22.

Wakefield, B. J., Buckwalter, K. C., & Gerdner, L. A. (1998). Biopsychosocial care of the elderly mentally ill. In M. A. Boyd & M. A. Nilhart (Eds.), *Psychiatric mental health nursing* (pp. 912–939). Philadelphia: Lippincott.

Zimmerman, S., Sloane, P. D., Eckert, J. K., Gruber-Baldini, A. L., Morgan, L. A., Hebel, J. R., et al. (2005). How good is assisted living: Findings and implications from an outcomes study. *The Journals of Gerontology, Social Sciences, 60*(4), S195–S204.

Appendices

Recommended Geropsychiatric Competency Enhancements for Entry Level Professional Nurses

Recommended Geropsychiatric Competency Enhancements for Entry Level Professional Nurses

Nurses care for older adults in health and illness across the full range of health care settings. Especially in late life, physical illness often precipitates and/or is accompanied by psychiatric symptoms. These recommended competency enhancement statements draw attention to the special needs of older adults with mental health concerns. They are not intended to 'stand-alone,' but rather to enhance existing or to-be-developed competencies for the entry level professional nurse.[1] The enhancements are organized within the existing *Older Adults: Recommended Baccalaureate Competencies and Cultural Guidelines for Geriatric Nursing Care*[2] developed in 2004 by AACN/HGNI. The geropsychiatric competency enhancements were drafted in Fall 2008 by the Geropsychiatric Nursing Collaborative (GPNC), a project supported by the John A. Hartford Foundation and housed at the American Academy of Nursing. They were reviewed by representatives of key professional organizations, revised, and then endorsed by the GPNC Core Competency Workgroup and National Advisory Panel and disseminated in early 2010 to all relevant professional organizations and schools of nursing for endorsement and utilization.

New competency enhancement statements and modifications to existing competencies are highlighted in yellow for ease in identification.

As revisions are made to existing competency documents, we recommend that the intent of these recommended enhancements be included and that the terms 'health,' 'illness,' 'frailty,' 'care' or 'disease' be broadly defined as both 'physical and mental.' Although physical and mental may be assumed, we believe that it is helpful to have both of these dimensions explicitly stated. Likewise, the term 'psychiatric disorder' should be used in combination with 'substance misuse disorder' to be more inclusive. It is further recommended that an expectation for the use of valid and reliable clinical assessment tools and evidence-based practices and processes be clearly stated and that gender, sexual orientation, and spirituality be made explicit when referring to cultural issues. Finally, the focus of these enhancements is on older adults; we recognize that the work of entry level nurses may have a lifespan perspective and, thus, some of these enhancements may also apply to other population groups.

---

[1] This competency enhancement document is one of seven developed and recommended by the Geropsychiatric Nursing Collaborative. The seven enhancement documents are aimed at the entry level nurse and the following groups of advanced practice nurses: gerontological NP and CNS, psychiatric NP and CNS, and other APRNs (NP and CNS) who care for older adults but are not prepared as gerontological experts, e.g., women's health, adult, family and acute care. A link to the entire set of enhancement documents can be found at http://www.aannet.org/GPNCresources. For more information, see www.aannet.org/GPNCgeropsych.

[2] AACN/HGNI (2004). Older Adults: Recommended Baccalaureate Competencies and Cultural Guidelines for Geriatric Nursing Care, available at www.aacn.nche.edu/Education/pdf/Gercomp.pdf

(continues)

APPENDIX A

Recommended Geropsychiatric Competency Enhancements for Entry Level Professional Nurses *(continued)*

Entry Level Gerontologic Nursing Competency Statements With Suggested Enhancements

1.	Recognize one's own and others' attitudes, values, and expectations about aging and their impact on physical and mental health care of older adults and their families.
NEW:	Identify opportunities for promoting mental and cognitive health of older adults and their families based on an assessment of strengths and resources.
2.	Adopt the concept of individualized care as the standard of practice with older adults.
3.	Communicate effectively, respectfully, and compassionately with older adults and their families, including those who are experiencing affective, behavioral and cognitive symptoms, recognizing and respecting generational and cultural differences.
4.	Recognize that sensation and perception in older adults are mediated by culture as well as functional, physical, cognitive, psychological, and social changes common in old age.
5.	Incorporate into daily practice valid and reliable tools to assess the functional, physical, cognitive, psychological, social, and spiritual status of older adults.
6.	Assess older adults' living environment with special awareness of the functional, physical, cognitive, psychological, social and social changes common in old age.
NEW:	Assess and implement evidence-based interventions to decrease disparities and enhance health promotion and therapeutic outcomes in individuals, families, communities and organizations across a range of health care settings.
7.	Analyze the effectiveness of individual, family and community resources in assisting older adults to achieve personal goals, maximize function, maintain independence and participate in decision-making regarding least restrictive living environments.
8.	Assess family knowledge of skills necessary to deliver mental and physical healthcare to older adults.
9.	Adapt technical skills to meet the functional, physical, cognitive, psychological, social, and endurance capacities of older adults.
10.	Promote adherence to a standard of individualized, restraint-free care in all healthcare settings.
11.	Prevent or reduce common risk factors that contribute to decline in mental and physical function, impaired quality of life, and excess disability in older adults.

Recommended Geropsychiatric Competency Enhancements for Entry Level Professional Nurses *(continued)*

12. Establish and follow standards of care to recognize, report and address physical and mental health outcomes of elder mistreatment.

13. Apply evidence-based standards to screen, immunize, and promote physically and mentally healthy activities in older adults.

NEW: Recognize normal, age-related physiological and cognitive changes as distinguished from pathology.

14. Recognize and manage geriatric syndromes and their psychiatric components common to older adults, considering relevant functional losses, cognitive impairment, and situational, developmental and transitional challenges.

15. Recognize the complex interaction of acute and chronic co-morbid physical and mental disorders and associated treatments common to older adults.

16. Use technology to enhance older adults' functioning (physical, social, cognitive and affective), independence, and safety.

17. Facilitate interdisciplinary and family communication as older adults transition across and between home, hospital, and nursing home, with a particular focus on the use of technology.

18. Assist older adults, families, and caregivers to understand and balance "everyday" autonomy and safety decisions, supporting the decisional capacity of older adults, including those with cognitive decline.

NEW: Support and advocate for older adults with cognitive, affective or behavioral symptoms in ethical, non-coercive decision-making with their families/caregivers related to everyday living, medical treatment, advance directives, and end of life care.

19. Apply ethical and legal principles to the complex issues that arise in care of older adults.

NEW: Appreciate issues related to decisional capacity, guardianship, financial management and durable and healthcare powers of attorney in the treatment of older adults.

20. Appreciate the influence of attitudes, roles, language, culture, race, religion, gender, and lifestyle on how families and assistive personnel provide long-term care to older adults.

21. Evaluate differing international models of geriatric physical and mental health care.

22. Analyze the impact of an aging society on its physical and mental health care systems.

(continues)

APPENDIX A

Recommended Geropsychiatric Competency Enhancements for Entry Level Professional Nurses *(continued)*

23. Evaluate the influence of legislative and payer systems on access, availability, and affordability of health care for older adults.

NEW: Ensure safe and effective transitions across levels of care between acute care and community-based long term care settings (e.g., Home, Assisted Living, Hospice, Nursing Homes) for older adults and their families.

24. Contrast the opportunities and constraints of supportive living arrangements on the mental health, function and independence of older adults and on their families.

25. Recognize the benefits of interdisciplinary team participation in physical and mental health care of older adults.

26. Evaluate the utility of complementary and integrative health care practices on health promotion and symptom management for older adults.

27. Involve, educate and, when appropriate, supervise family, friends and assistive personnel in implementing evidence-based practices for older adults, including those with cognitive, affective and/or behavioral symptoms, while sustaining the mental health and wellbeing of those providing the care.

28. Facilitate older adults' active participation in all aspects of their own health care.

29. Ensure quality and safety of care commensurate with older adults' vulnerability and frequency and intensity of care needs.

30. Promote quality end-of-life care for older adults, including those with cognitive impairment, which encompasses psychosocial care as well as pain and symptom management, as essential, desirable, and integral components of nursing practice.

Recommended Geropsychiatric Enhancements
for Gerontological Clinical Nurse Specialists

These recommended competency enhancement statements are not intended to 'stand-alone,' but rather to enhance existing or to-be-developed competencies for Gerontological Clinical Nurse Specialists.[1] The statements are organized within existing domains of the *Organizing Framework and CNS Core Competencies*[2] developed by NACNS in 2008. The geropsychiatric competency enhancements were drafted in Fall 2008 by the Geropsychiatric Nursing Collaborative (GPNC), a project supported by the John A. Hartford Foundation and housed at the American Academy of Nursing. They were reviewed by representatives of key professional organizations, revised, and then endorsed by the GPNC Core Competency Workgroup and National Advisory Panel and disseminated in early 2010 to all relevant professional organizations and schools of nursing for endorsement and utilization.

As revisions are made to existing competency documents,[3] we recommend that the intent of these recommended enhancements be included and that the terms 'health,' 'illness,' 'frailty,' 'care' or 'disease' be broadly defined as both 'physical and mental.' Although physical and mental may be assumed, we believe that it is helpful to have both of these dimensions explicitly stated. Likewise, the term 'psychiatric disorder' should be used in combination with 'substance misuse disorder' to be more inclusive. It is further recommended that an expectation for the use of valid and reliable clinical assessment tools and evidence-based practices and processes be clearly stated and that gender, sexual orientation, and spirituality be made explicit when referring to cultural issues. Finally, the focus of these enhancements is on older adults.

---

[1] This competency enhancement document is one of seven developed and recommended by the Geropsychiatric Nursing Collaborative. The seven enhancement documents are aimed at the entry level nurse and the following groups of advanced practice nurses: gerontological NP and CNS, psychiatric NP and CNS, and other APRNs (NP and CNS) who care for older adults but are not prepared as gerontological experts, e.g., women's health, adult, family and acute care. The entire set of enhancement documents can be accessed at www.aannet.org/GPNCresources. For more information, see www.aannet.org/GPNCgeropsych.

[2] NACNS (2008). Organizing Framework and CNS Core Competencies available at www.nacns.org/LinkClick.aspx?fileticket=22R8AaNmrUI%3d&tabid=94. Updated competencies specific to each of the three types of clinical nurse specialists (gerontological, psychiatric mental health, and other) were unavailable at the time of this work; thus, these geropsychiatric nursing enhancements were informed by those developed for the nurse practitioner role.

[3] We recognize that work is in process by the American Association of Colleges of Nursing (AACN) and the Hartford Institute for Geriatric Nursing (HIGN) to combine competencies for the Adult and Gerontological Clinical Nurse Specialist roles in accordance with the new Consensus Model. The GPNC enhancements were used to inform the work of the AACN and HIGN expert panels, however, the final AACN and HIGN documents are still in refinement at this time.

(continues)

APPENDIX B

Recommended Geropsychiatric Enhancements for Gerontological Clinical Nurse Specialists (*continued*)

A. Direct Care Competency	
NEW:	Conducts a comprehensive assessment that includes the differentiation of normal age changes from acute and chronic medical and psychiatric/substance misuse disease processes, with attention to commonly occurring atypical presentations and co-occurring health problems including cognitive impairment.
NEW:	Includes mental health alterations in the diagnosis of health status.
NEW:	Includes evaluation for elder mistreatment in overall assessment.
NEW:	Identifies and assesses factors that affect mental health including stressors that may be more common among older adults such as caregiving, multiple chronic illnesses, pain, relocation, trauma, cohort-specific stressors and losses such as financial (retirement), functional limitations (Instrumental Activities of Daily Living/Activities of Daily Living), changes in social network (death of family members and friends), and role (status changes).
NEW:	Uses valid and reliable clinical evaluation tools to evaluate common psychiatric/substance misuse disorders, such as depression, anxiety and delirium, as part of a complete health assessment and to monitor changes in status.
NEW:	Adapts assessment processes for persons with cognitive impairment and psychiatric/substance misuse disorders.
NEW:	Uses behavioral, environmental and pharmacological management strategies to ameliorate behavioral symptoms in individuals who have psychiatric/substance misuse disorders, including cognitive impairments.
NEW:	Remains sensitive to verbal cues and non-verbal behaviors in the communication patterns of older adults and their significant others with cognitive, neurological and speech and hearing impairments.
NEW:	Uses culturally appropriate, respectful communication that is adapted to patient's education, cognitive functioning, personal experience, psychiatric/substance misuse disorder, and mental health history.
NEW:	Monitors and evaluates the patient's response to and concomitant use of alcohol and recreational drugs, psychotropic and other medications including over-the-counter and herbal medication/product use, based on a thorough understanding of the principles of pharmacotherapeutics in older adults.
NEW:	Plans and implements care that promotes optimal function and minimizes development of complications, such as those from polypharmacy.
NEW:	Provides evidence-based brief intervention/crisis management and makes appropriate referrals to mental health care professionals and community agencies to address needs of individuals and families.

Recommended Geropsychiatric Enhancements for Gerontological Clinical Nurse Specialists *(continued)*

B. Consultation Competency

NEW: Serves as a clinical expert, clinical leader, and/or clinical consultant to other nurses in the care of older adults experiencing mental health issues.

C. Systems Leadership Competency

NEW: Coordinates transitions across levels of care between acute care and community-based long term care settings (e.g., Home, Assisted Living, Hospice, Nursing Homes) for older adults and their families.

NEW: Enhances interdisciplinary team function by contributing information about the assessment and care of older adults with psychiatric/substance misuse disorders and cognitive impairment.

NEW: Considers such factors as ability to pay for treatments related to fixed income (retired), entitlements (Medicaid and Medicare), and available resources when providing treatment to clients who may have financial limitations.

NEW: Leads quality improvement initiatives designed to improve the care of older adults with mental illness and cognitive impairment.

D. Collaboration Competency

No geropsychiatric enhancements recommended.

E. Coaching Competency

NEW: Analyzes the impact of aging and age-and disease-related changes in sensory/perceptual function, cognition, confidence with technology, and health literacy and numeracy on the ability and readiness to learn and tailors interventions accordingly.

NEW: Educates individuals, families, peers and groups to promote the knowledge and understanding of effective mental health promotion strategies, management of psychiatric/substance misuse disorders, and the interaction between physical and mental health/illness.

NEW: Assists older adults/caregivers/and their families to negotiate health care delivery systems, including mental health services.

F. Research Competency

NEW: Participates in geropsychiatric nursing research through the identification of older adults' problems, collection of data, and presentation and dissemination of findings.

(continues)

APPENDIX B

Recommended Geropsychiatric Enhancements for Gerontological Clinical Nurse Specialists *(continued)*

G. Ethical Decision-Making, Moral Agency and Advocacy
NEW: Applies knowledge of issues related to decisional capacity (including the balance between autonomy and safety), guardianship, financial management and durable and healthcare powers of attorney to the treatment of older adults.
NEW: Serves as leader, change agent and advocate within professional organizations for the behavioral and mental health needs of older adults.
NEW: Demonstrates awareness of personal and societal biases, especially ageism and stigma related to mental illness/substance misuse and dementia, and how these influence all aspects of the care of the older adult, including mental health promotion, screening, assessment, and treatment.
NEW: Assesses and incorporates into the treatment plan the patient's perceptions/interpretations of his or her physical and/or mental health/illness and care preferences as influenced by culture, sexual orientation, gender, ethnicity, and spirituality.
NEW: Engages in lifelong learning to assure currency in research and best clinical practices in geropsychiatric nursing.
NEW: Prevents or works to reduce common risk and environmental factors that contribute to psychiatric & behavioral symptoms.
NEW: Protects safety of elders and others in the community through legal reporting mechanisms when elder mistreatment, or destructive behaviors targeted at self or others, such as driving with cognitive impairment, are identified.
NEW: Demonstrates sensitivity to spirituality and culture when caring for older adults and their families who are at the end of life.
NEW: Advocates for health policy at the local, state, regional, and national level to reduce the impact of stigma on services for prevention and treatment of mental health problems and psychiatric/substance misuse disorders.
NEW: Uses knowledge to decrease barriers and gaps in systems that provide mental health services with particular attention to health disparities among the disadvantaged and older adults with differing culture, ethnicity, gender, sexual orientation, and spirituality.

APPENDIX C

Recommended Geropsychiatric Competency Enhancements for Gerontological Nurse Practitioners

Recommended Geropsychiatric Competency Enhancements for Gerontological Nurse Practitioners

These recommended competency enhancement statements draw attention to the special needs of older adults with mental health concerns. They are not intended to 'stand-alone,' but rather to enhance existing or to-be-developed competencies for Gerontological Nurse Practitioners.[1] The statements are organized within the existing *Nurse Practitioner Primary Care Competencies in Specialty Areas: Adult, Family, Gerontological, Pediatric, and Women's Health* developed by HRSA in 2002 and *National Organization of Nurse Practitioner Faculties Domains and Core Competencies of Nurse Practitioner Practice*[2] revised by NONPF in 2006. The geropsychiatric competency enhancements were drafted in Fall 2008 by the Geropsychiatric Nursing Collaborative (GPNC), a project supported by the John A. Hartford Foundation and housed at the American Academy of Nursing. They were reviewed by representatives of key professional organizations, revised, and then endorsed by the GPNC Core Competency Workgroup and National Advisory Panel and disseminated in Winter 2010 to all relevant professional organizations and schools of nursing for endorsement and utilization.

New competency enhancement statements and modifications to existing competencies are highlighted in yellow for ease in identification.

As revisions are made to existing competency documents,[3] we recommend that the intent of these recommended enhancements be included and that the terms 'health,' 'illness,' 'frailty,' 'care' or 'disease' be broadly defined as both 'physical and mental.' Although physical and mental may be assumed, we believe that it is helpful to have both of these dimensions explicitly stated. Likewise, the term 'psychiatric disorder' should be used in combination with 'substance misuse disorder' to be more inclusive. It is further recommended that an expectation for the use of valid and reliable clinical assessment tools and evidence-based practices and processes be clearly stated and that gender, sexual orientation, and spirituality be made explicit when referring to cultural issues.

[1] This competency enhancement document is one of seven developed and recommended by the Geropsychiatric Nursing Collaborative. The seven enhancement documents are aimed at the entry level nurse and the following groups of advanced practice nurses: gerontological NP and CNS, psychiatric NP and CNS, and other APRNs (NP and CNS) who care for older adults but are not prepared as gerontological experts, e.g. women's health, adult, family and acute care. A link to the entire set of enhancement documents can be found at www.aannet.org/GPNCresources. For more information, see www.aannet.org/GPNCgeropsych.

[2] HRSA (2002). Nurse practitioner primary care competencies in specialty areas: Adult, Family, Gerontological, Pediatric, and Women's Health, pp. 26–29 available at www.eric.ed.gov/ERICDocs/data/ericdocs2sql/content_storage_01/0000019b/80/1a/9d/20.pdf and NONPF (2006). National Organization of Nurse Practitioner Faculties Domains and Core Competencies of Nurse Practitioner Practice available at www.nonpf.com/associations/10789/files/DomainsandCoreComps2006.pdf.

[3] We recognize that work is in process by the American Association of Colleges of Nursing (AACN) and the Hartford Institute for Geriatric Nursing (HIGN) to combine competencies for the Adult and Gerontological Nurse Practitioner Specialties in accordance with the new Consensus Model. The GPNC enhancements were used to inform the work of the AACN and HIGN expert panels, however, the final AACN and HIGN documents are still in refinement at this time.

(continues)

APPENDIX C

Recommended Geropsychiatric Competency Enhancements for Gerontological Nurse Practitioners *(continued)*

Domain I: Health Promotion, Protection, Disease Prevention, & Treatment
I.A Assessment of Health Status
1. Analyzes the relationship between normal physiology and specific system alterations produced by aging and disease processes.
NEW: Adapts assessment processes for persons with cognitive impairment and psychiatric/substance misuse disorders.
NEW: Conducts a comprehensive assessment that includes the differentiation of normal age changes from acute and chronic medical and psychiatric/substance misuse disease processes, with attention to commonly occurring atypical presentations and co-occurring health problems including cognitive impairment.
NEW: Identifies and assesses factors that affect mental health including stressors that may be more common among older adults such as caregiving, multiple chronic illnesses, pain, relocation, trauma, cohort-specific stressors, and losses such as financial (retirement), functional (Instrumental Activities of Daily Living/Activities of Daily Living), social network (death of family members and friends), and role (status changes).
2. Assesses the developmental status regarding maintenance of self-identity through later and final stages of life.
3. Assesses the dynamic interaction between acute illness and known chronic health problems in older adults.
4. Assesses elders and caregivers for abuse and/or neglect.
5. Assesses for addictive behavior.
6. Assesses health/illness by conducting a complete health history in light of physiologic and psychosocial changes of aging.
NEW: Uses valid and reliable clinical evaluation tools to conduct a comprehensive mental health assessment across a range of psychiatric/substance misuse disorders that includes assessment of strengths and potential for improvement.
7. Performs a comprehensive physical exam considering physiologic changes of aging.
8. Performs a comprehensive functional assessment, including mental status, social support, and nutrition.
9. Assesses special risks of institutionalized older adults for common patterns of illness and communicable disease.
10. Assesses sexual function and sexual well-being in older adults.
11. Assesses roles, tasks, and stressors of informal system/family caregivers for older adults, especially the frail.

Recommended Geropsychiatric Competency Enhancements for Gerontological Nurse Practitioners *(continued)*

I.B	Diagnosis of Health Status
1.	Recognizes the commonly occurring conditions associated with aging, including differential diagnosis of delirium, dementia, and/or depression.
NEW:	Includes mental health alterations in the diagnosis of health status.
2.	Implements screening using appropriate, age-specific instruments and guidelines and interprets results in light of expected changes associated with aging.
3.	Applies knowledge of atypical presentations of disease seen with aging to the formulation of differential diagnoses.
NEW:	Differentiates psychiatric presentations of medical conditions, including psychiatric symptoms, from psychiatric/substance misuse disorders and arranges appropriate evaluation and follow-up.
4.	Plans diagnostic strategies and orders, performs, and interprets results of laboratory tests, clinical procedures, and other tests used in diagnosis and management of older adults with specific organ system alterations.

I.C	Plan of Care and Implementation of Treatment
1.	Treats acute and chronic illness and geriatric syndromes frequently manifested in older adults such as incontinence, falls, constipation, loss of functional abilities, dehydration, dementia, depression, delirium, and malnutrition.
NEW:	Uses behavioral, environmental, and pharmacological management strategies to ameliorate behavioral symptoms in individuals who have psychiatric/substance misuse disorders including cognitive impairments.
NEW:	Provides brief intervention/crisis management and makes appropriate referrals to mental health care professionals and community agencies to address needs of individuals and families.
2.	Adapts interventions to meet the complex needs of older adults and frail elders arising from normal changes of aging, multiple system problems, psychosocial, and financial issues.
NEW:	Remains sensitive to verbal cues and non-verbal behaviors in the communication patterns of older adults and their significant others with cognitive, neurological and speech and hearing impairments.
3.	Plans therapeutic interventions to restore or maintain optimal level of functioning and when appropriate plans for palliative care.
NEW:	Plans and implements care that promotes optimal function and minimizes development of complications, such as those from polypharmacy.

(continues)

APPENDIX C

Recommended Geropsychiatric Competency Enhancements for Gerontological Nurse Practitioners *(continued)*

4.	Prescribes medications with knowledge of pharmacodynamics and pharmacokinetic processes in older adults with high potential for adverse drug outcomes and polypharmacy.
NEW:	Monitors and evaluates the patient's response to and concomitant use of alcohol and recreational drugs, psychotropic and other medications including over-the-counter and herbal medication/product use, based on a thorough understanding of the principles of pharmacotherapeutics in older adults.
5.	Works with an interdisciplinary health care team to plan and deliver skilled gerontological care to older adults.
6.	Assists older adults or designated care agent in formulating advance directives, ethical decisions, and end-of-life care decisions.
NEW:	Applies knowledge of issues related to decisional capacity (including the balance between autonomy and safety), guardianship, financial management and durable and healthcare powers of attorney to the treatment of older adults.
7.	Prescribes and monitors ancillary therapies for older adults in various settings (e.g., physical therapy and nutritional therapy).
8.	Formulates and implements a plan of care related to sexual health and functioning in older men and women.
9.	Coordinates care within a context of potentially limited endurance, financial constraints, cultural considerations, family or caregiver needs, and ethical principles.
10.	Performs primary care procedures, including, but not limited to, wound debridement, pap tests, and microscopy.
11.	Applies research that is older adult-centered and contributes to positive change in the health of or health care delivered to older adults.
12.	Prevents or works to reduce common risk and environmental factors that contribute to: • decline in physical functioning, • impaired quality of life, • social isolation • excess disability in older adults • **NEW:** psychiatric & behavioral symptoms
II. Nurse Practitioner – Patient Relationship	
1.	Facilitates informed and appropriate transition of older adults from one level of care to another.
2.	Analyzes the impact of transitions in autonomy, relationships, and residence on the health/illness of older adults.

Recommended Geropsychiatric Competency Enhancements for Gerontological Nurse Practitioners *(continued)*

3. Assesses the impact of congregate/institutional living upon health/wellness of the residents and family.

4. Assists older adults and their families dealing with grief and bereavement.

5. Assists older adults, family members, and caregivers in maintaining the older adult's sense of autonomy.

NEW: Protects safety of elders and others in the community through legal reporting mechanisms when elder mistreatment or destructive behaviors targeted at self or others, such as driving with cognitive impairment, are identified.

NEW: Demonstrates awareness of personal and societal biases, especially ageism and stigma related to mental illness/substance misuse and dementia, and how these influence all aspects of the care of the older adult, including mental health promotion, screening, assessment, and treatment.

NEW: Uses culturally appropriate, respectful communication that is adapted to the patient's education, cognitive functioning, personal experience, psychiatric/substance misuse disorder, and mental health history.

III. The Teaching-Coaching Function

1. Adapts teaching-learning approaches to physiological changes associated with aging.

2. Analyzes the impact of aging and age-and disease-related changes in sensory/perceptual function, cognition, confidence with technology, and health literacy and numeracy on the ability and readiness to learn and tailors approaches accordingly.

3. Includes caregivers in teaching-learning activities when appropriate.

4. Creates an educational approach/learning environment for older adults, families, and caregivers with focus on optimal functioning.

NEW: Educates individuals, families, peers and groups to promote the knowledge and understanding of effective mental health promotion strategies, management of psychiatric/substance misuse disorders, and the interaction between physical and mental health/ illness.

5. Recognizes and utilizes the contributions of family and caregivers when eliciting information.

6. Elicits information skillfully about the patient's interpretation of health conditions given potential sensory and cognitive limitations of older adults, particularly the frail.

7. Demonstrates knowledge and skill in addressing sensitive topics with older adults such as sexuality, finances, mental health, substance abuse, and terminal illness.

(continues)

APPENDIX C

Recommended Geropsychiatric Competency Enhancements for Gerontological Nurse Practitioners *(continued)*

IV. Professional Role	
1.	Analyzes and applies theories of aging relevant to older adult roles, physical and psychological function and development.
2.	Advocates within nursing settings to create/enhance positive, health promoting environments and maintains a climate of dignity and privacy.
3.	Directs care and collaborates with non-professional caregivers and professional staff.
NEW:	Enhances interdisciplinary team function by contributing information about the assessment and care of older adults with psychiatric/substance misuse disorders and cognitive impairment.
NEW:	Serves as a clinical expert, clinical leader, and/or clinical consultant to other nurses in the care of older adults experiencing mental health issues.
NEW:	Demonstrates knowledge of the similarities and differences in roles of various health professionals providing mental health services, e.g., psychotherapist, psychologist, psychiatric social worker, psychiatrist, and advanced practice psychiatric nurse.
4.	Recognizes the importance of participation in community and professional organizations that influence the health of older adults and supports the role of the gerontological nurse practitioner.
NEW:	Serves as leader, change agent and advocate within professional organizations for the behavioral and mental health needs of older adults.
5.	Interprets the gerontological nurse practitioner role in primary and specialty health care to other health care providers and the public.
6.	Serves as a resource in the design and development of older adult community-based services.
NEW:	Engages in lifelong learning to assure currency in research and best clinical practices in geropsychiatric nursing.
NEW:	Participates in geropsychiatric nursing research through the identification of older adults' problems, collection of data, and presentation and dissemination of findings.
NEW:	Considers such factors as ability to pay for treatments related to fixed income (retired), entitlements (Medicaid and Medicare), and available resources when providing treatment to clients who may have financial limitations.

APPENDIX C

Recommended Geropsychiatric Competency Enhancements for Gerontological Nurse Practitioners *(continued)*

V. Managing and Negotiating Health Care Delivery Systems

1. Assists older adults/caregivers/and their families to negotiate health care delivery systems, including mental health services.

2. Uses up-to-date knowledge of regulatory processes and payer systems, i.e., Medicare/Medicaid, Centers for Medicare & Medicaid Services guidelines, managed care, and private sources, to deliver advanced practice service to the elderly.

VI. Monitoring and Ensuring the Quality of Health Care Practice

1. Assesses the impact of ageism and sexism on health care policies and systems.

2. Advocates for access to quality, cost-effective health care for older adults.

NEW: Leads quality improvement initiatives designed to improve the care of older adults with mental illness and cognitive impairment.

NEW: Advocates for health policy at the local, state, regional, and national level to reduce the impact of stigma on services for prevention and treatment of mental health problems and psychiatric/substance misuse disorders.

VII. Cultural & Spiritual Competence

NEW: Assesses and incorporates into the treatment plan the patient's perceptions/interpretations of his or her physical and/or mental health/illness and care preferences as influenced by culture, sexual orientation, gender, ethnicity, and spirituality.

NEW: Demonstrates sensitivity to spirituality and culture when caring for older adults and their families who are at the end of life.

APPENDIX D

Recommended Geropsychiatric Enhancements for Clinical Nurse Specialists Who Provide Care to Older Adults But Are Not Geriatric Specialists

Recommended Geropsychiatric Enhancements for Clinical Nurse Specialists Who Provide Care to Older Adults but are not Geriatric Specialists

These recommended competency enhancement statements are not intended to 'stand-alone,' but rather to enhance existing or to-be-developed- competencies for Clinical Nurse Specialists who provides care to older adults but are not geriatric specialists.[1] The statements are organized within existing domains of the *Organizing Framework and CNS Core Competencies*[2] developed by NACNS in 2008. The geropsychiatric competency enhancements were drafted in Fall 2008 by the Geropsychiatric Nursing Collaborative (GPNC), a project supported by the John A. Hartford Foundation and housed at the American Academy of Nursing. They were reviewed by representatives of key professional organizations, revised, and then endorsed by the GPNC Core Competency Workgroup and National Advisory Panel and disseminated in Winter 2010 to all relevant professional organizations and schools of nursing for endorsement and utilization.

As revisions are made to existing competency documents,[3] we recommend that the intent of these recommended enhancements be included and that the term: 'health,' 'illness,' 'frailty,' 'care' or 'disease' be broadly defined as both 'physical and mental.' Although physical and mental may be assumed, we believe that it i: helpful to have both of these dimensions explicitly stated. Likewise, the term 'psychiatric disorder' should be used in combination with 'substance misuse disorder' to be more inclusive. It is further recommended that an expectation for the use of valid and reliable clinical assessment tools and evidence-based practices and processes be clearly stated and that gender, sexual orientation, and spirituality be made explicit when referring to cultural issues. Finally, the focu: of these enhancements is on older adults; we recognize that the work of some advanced practice nurses may have a lifespan perspective, and, thus, many of these enhancements may also apply to other population groups.

---

[1] This set of competency enhancements is one of seven developed and recommended by the Geropsychiatric Nursing Collaborative. The others are aimed at the following groups of advanced practice nurses: geriatric NP and CNS, psychiatric NP and CNS, and other APRN [both NP and CNS] who care for older adults but are not prepared as geriatric experts, e.g., women's health, adult, family and acute care. A link to the entire set of enhancement documents can be found at www.aannet.org/GPNCresources. For more information, see www.aannet.org/GPNCgeropsych.

[2] NACNS (2008). Organizing Framework and CNS Core Competencies available at www.nacns.org/LinkClick.aspx?fileticket=22R8AaNmrUI%3d&tabid=94. Updated competencies specific to each of the three types of clinical nurse specialists (gerontological, psychiatric mental health, and other) were unavailable at the time of this work; thus, these geropsychiatric nursing enhancements were informed by those developed for the nurse practitioner role.

[3] We recognize that work is in process by the American Association of Colleges of Nursing (AACN) and the Hartford Institute for Geriatric Nursing (HIGN) to combine competencies for the Adult and Gerontological Clinical Nurse Specialist roles in accordance with the new Consensus Model. The GPNC enhancements were used to inform the work of the AACN and HIGN expert panels, however, the final AACN and HIGN documents are still in refinement at this time.

APPENDIX D

Recommended Geropsychiatric Enhancements for Clinical Nurse Specialists Who Provide Care to Older Adults But Are Not Geriatric Specialists *(continued)*

A. Direct Care Competency
NEW: Conducts a comprehensive assessment that includes the differentiation of normal age changes from acute and chronic medical and psychiatric/substance misuse disease processes, with attention to commonly occurring atypical presentations and co-occurring health problems including cognitive impairment.
NEW: Includes mental health alterations in the diagnosis of health status.
NEW: Includes evaluation for elder mistreatment in overall assessment.
NEW: Identifies and assesses factors that affect mental health including stressors that may be more common among older adults such as caregiving, multiple chronic illnesses, pain, relocation, trauma, cohort-specific stressors and losses such as financial (retirement), functional limitations (Instrumental Activities of Daily Living / Activities of Daily Living), changes in social network (death of family members and friends), and role (status changes).
NEW: Uses valid and reliable clinical evaluation tools to evaluate common psychiatric/substance misuse disorders, such as depression, anxiety and delirium, as part of a complete health assessment and to monitor changes in status.
NEW: Adapts assessment processes for persons with cognitive impairment and psychiatric/substance misuse disorders.
NEW: Uses behavioral, environmental and pharmacological management strategies to ameliorate behavioral symptoms in individuals who have psychiatric/substance misuse disorders, including cognitive impairments.
NEW: Remains sensitive to verbal cues and non-verbal behaviors in the communication patterns of older adults and their significant others with cognitive, neurological and speech and hearing impairments.
NEW: Uses culturally appropriate, respectful communication that is adapted to patient's education, cognitive functioning, personal experience, psychiatric/substance misuse disorder, and mental health history.
NEW: Monitors and evaluates the patient's response to and concomitant use of alcohol and recreational drugs, psychotropic and other medications including over-the-counter and herbal medication/product use, based on a thorough understanding of the principles of pharmacotherapeutics in older adults.
NEW: Plans and implements care that promotes optimal function and minimizes development of complications, such as those from polypharmacy.
NEW: Provides evidence-based brief intervention/crisis management and make appropriate referrals to mental health care professionals and community agencies with resources to address needs of individuals and families.

(continues)

APPENDIX D

Recommended Geropsychiatric Enhancements for Clinical Nurse Specialists Who Provide Care to Older Adults But Are Not Geriatric Specialists *(continued)*

B. Consultation Competency

No geropsychiatric enhancements recommended.

C. Systems Leadership Competency

NEW: Coordinates transitions across levels of care between acute care and community-based long term care settings (e.g., Home, Assisted Living, Hospice, Nursing Homes) for older adults and their families.

NEW: Works within an interdisciplinary team to promote the mental health and well-being of older clients and their families.

NEW: Considers such factors as ability to pay for treatments related to fixed income (retired), entitlements (Medicaid and Medicare), and available resources when providing treatment to clients who may have financial limitations.

NEW: Participates in quality improvement initiatives designed to improve the care of older adults with mental illness and cognitive impairment.

D. Collaboration Competency

NEW: Demonstrates knowledge of the similarities and differences in roles of various health professionals providing mental health services, e.g., psychotherapist, psychologist, psychiatric social worker, psychiatrist, and advanced practice psychiatric nurses.

E. Coaching Competency

NEW: Analyzes the impact of aging and age-and disease-related changes in sensory /perceptual function, cognition, confidence with technology, and health literacy and numeracy on the ability and readiness to learn and tailors interventions accordingly.

NEW: Educates individuals, families and groups to promote the knowledge and understanding of effective mental health promotion, management of psychiatric/substance misuse disorders, and the interaction between physical and mental health/illness.

NEW: Assists older adults/caregivers/and their families to negotiate health care delivery systems, including mental health services.

F. Research Competency

No geropsychiatric enhancements recommended.

APPENDIX D

Recommended Geropsychiatric Enhancements for Clinical Nurse Specialists Who Provide Care to Older Adults But Are Not Geriatric Specialists *(continued)*

G. Ethical Decision-Making, Moral Agency and Advocacy
NEW: Applies knowledge of issues related to decisional capacity (including the balance between autonomy and safety), guardianship, financial management and durable and healthcare powers of attorney to the treatment of older adults.
NEW: Advocates for the behavioral and mental health needs of older adults.
NEW: Demonstrates awareness of personal and societal biases, especially ageism and stigma related to mental illness/substance misuse and dementia, and how these influence all aspects of the care of the older adult, including mental health promotion, screening, assessment, and treatment.
NEW: Assesses and incorporates into the treatment plan the patient's perceptions/interpretations of his or her physical and/or mental health/illness and care preferences as influenced by culture, sexual orientation, gender, ethnicity, and spirituality.
NEW: Engages in lifelong learning that includes geropsychiatric nursing.
NEW: Prevents or works to reduce common risk and environmental factors that contribute to psychiatric & behavioral symptoms.
NEW: Protects safety of elders and others in the community through legal reporting mechanisms when elder mistreatment, or destructive behaviors targeted at self or others, such as driving with cognitive impairment, are identified.
NEW: Demonstrates sensitivity to spirituality and culture when caring for older adults and their families who are at the end of life.
NEW: Advocates for health policy at the local, state, regional, and national level to reduce the impact of stigma on services for prevention and treatment of mental health problems and psychiatric/substance misuse disorders.
NEW: Uses knowledge to decrease barriers and gaps in systems that provide mental health services with particular attention to health disparities among the disadvantaged and older adults with differing culture, ethnicity, gender, sexual orientation, and spirituality.

APPENDIX E

Recommended Geropsychiatric Competency Enhancements for Nurse Practitioners Who Provide Care to Older Adults But Are Not Geriatric Specialists

Recommended Geropsychiatric Competency Enhancements for Nurse Practitioners Who Provide Care to Older Adults but are not Geriatric Specialists

These recommended competency enhancement statements are not intended to 'stand-alone,' but rather to enhance existing or to-be-developed competencies for Nurse Practitioners who provide care to older adults but are not geriatric specialists. The enhancements are organized within the existing *Older Nurse Practitioner and Clinical Nurse Specialist Competencies for Older Adult Care* developed in 2004 by AACN/HGNI and placed within the seven NONPF domains.[2] The geropsychiatric competency enhancements were drafted in Fall 2008 by the Geropsychiatric Nursing Collaborative (GPNC), a project supported by the John A. Hartford Foundation and housed at the American Academy of Nursing. They were reviewed by representatives of key professional organizations, revised, and then endorsed by the GPNC Core Competency Workgroup and National Advisory Panel and disseminated in Winter 2010 to all relevant professional organizations and schools of nursing for endorsement and utilization.

New competency enhancement statements and modifications to existing competencies are highlighted in yellow for ease in identification.

As revisions are made to existing competency documents,[3] we recommend that the intent of these recommended enhancements be included and that the terms 'health,' 'illness,' 'frailty,' 'care' or 'disease' be broadly defined as both 'physical and mental.' Although physical and mental may be assumed, we believe that it is helpful to have both of these dimensions explicitly stated. Likewise, the term 'psychiatric disorder' should be used in combination with 'substance misuse disorder' to be more inclusive. It is further recommended that an expectation for the use of valid and reliable clinical assessment tools and evidence-based practices and processes be clearly stated and that gender, sexual orientation, and spirituality be made explicit when referring to cultural issues. Finally, the focus of these enhancements is on older adults; we recognize that the work of some advanced practice nurses may have a lifespan perspective, and, thus, some of these enhancements may also apply to other population groups.

---

[1] This competency enhancement document is one of seven developed and recommended by the Geropsychiatric Nursing Collaborative. The seven enhancement documents are aimed at the entry level nurse and the following groups of advanced practice nurses: gerontological NP and CNS, psychiatric NP and CNS, and other APRNs (NP and CNS) who care for older adults but are not prepared as gerontological experts, e.g., women's health, adult, family and acute care. A link to the entire set of enhancement documents can be found at http://www.aannet.org/GPNCresources. For more information, see www.aannet.org/GPNCgeropsych.

[2] AACN/HGNI (2004). Nurse Practitioner and Clinical Nurse Specialist Competencies for Older Adult Care, available at www.aacn.nche.edu/Education/pdf/APNCompetencies.pdf and NONPF (2006). National Organization of Nurse Practitioner Faculties Domains and Core Competencies of Nurse Practitioner Practice available at www.nonpf.com/associations/10789/files/DomainsandCoreComps2006.pdf.

[3] We recognize that work is in process by the American Association of Colleges of Nursing (AACN) and the Hartford Institute for Geriatric Nursing (HIGN) to combine competencies for the Adult and Gerontological Nurse Practitioner Specialties in accordance with the new Consensus Model. The GPNC enhancements were used to inform the work of the AACN and HIGN expert panels, however, the final AACN and HIGN documents are still in refinement at this time.

Recommended Geropsychiatric Competency Enhancements for Nurse Practitioners Who Provide Care to Older Adults But Are Not Geriatric Specialists *(continued)*

Domain 1 : Health Promotion, Protection, Disease Prevention, & Treatment
I.A Assessment of Health Status
1. Differentiate normal aging from illness and disease processes.
2. Use standardized assessment instruments appropriate to older adults if available, or a standardized assessment process to assess social support and health status, such as: function; cognition; mobility; pain; skin integrity; quality of life; nutrition; neglect and abuse.
NEW: Adapt assessment processes for persons with cognitive impairment and psychiatric/substance misuse disorders.
NEW: Conduct a comprehensive assessment that includes the differentiation of normal age changes from acute and chronic medical and psychiatric/substance misuse disease processes, with attention to commonly occurring atypical presentations and co-occurring health problems including cognitive impairment.
3. Assess for syndromes, constellations of symptoms that may be manifestations of other health problems, common to older adults, e.g., incontinence, falling, delirium, dementia, and depression.
NEW: Use valid and reliable clinical evaluation tools to conduct a comprehensive mental health assessment across a range of psychiatric/substance misuse disorders that includes assessment of strengths and potential for improvement.
NEW: Include evaluation for elder mistreatment in overall assessment.
4. Assess health status and identify risk factors in older adults.
NEW: Identify and assess factors that affect mental health including stressors that may be more common among older adults such as caregiving, multiple chronic illnesses, pain, relocation, trauma, cohort-specific stressors, and losses such as financial (retirement), functional (Instrumental Activities of Daily Living/Activities of Daily Living), social network (death of family members and friends), and role (status changes).
5. Assess the ability of the individual and family to manage developmental (life stage) transitions, resilience, and coping strategies.
6. Assess older adult's, family's, and caregiver's ability to execute plans of care.
7. Conduct a pharmacological assessment of the older adult, including polypharmacy, drug interactions, over-the-counter and herbal product use, and ability to obtain, purchase, and safely and correctly self-administer medications.

(continues)

APPENDIX E

Recommended Geropsychiatric Competency Enhancements for Nurse Practitioners Who Provide Care to Older Adults But Are Not Geriatric Specialists *(continued)*

8.	Assess for pain in the older adult, including the cognitively impaired, and develop a plan of care to manage.
I.B Diagnosis of Health Status	
9.	Identify both typical and atypical manifestations of chronic and acute illnesses and diseases common to older adults.
NEW:	Include mental health alterations in the diagnosis of health status.
NEW:	Differentiate psychiatric presentations of medical conditions, including psychiatric symptoms at the end of life, from psychiatric/substance misuse disorders and arrange appropriate evaluation and follow-up.
10.	Recognize the presence of co-morbidities and iatrogenesis in the frail older adult.
11.	Identify signs and symptoms indicative of change in mental status, e.g., agitation, anxiety, depression, substance use, delirium, and dementia.
12.	Interpret results of appropriate laboratory and diagnostic tests, differentiating values for older adults.
I.C Plan of Care and Implementation of Treatment	
13.	Promote and recommend immunizations and appropriate health screening.
14.	Prevent or work to reduce common risk and environmental factors that contribute to: • decline in physical functioning • impaired quality of life • social isolation • excess disability in older adults • **NEW:** psychiatric & behavioral symptoms
15.	Assist the patient to compensate for age-related functional changes according to chronological age groups.
NEW:	Remain sensitive to verbal cues and non-verbal behaviors in the communication patterns of older adults and their significant others with cognitive, neurological and speech and hearing impairments.
NEW:	Apply knowledge of issues related to decisional capacity (including the balance between autonomy and safety), guardianship, financial management and durable and healthcare powers of attorney to the treatment of older adults.

Recommended Geropsychiatric Competency Enhancements for Nurse Practitioners Who Provide Care to Older Adults But Are Not Geriatric Specialists *(continued)*

16. Refer and/or manage common signs, symptoms, and syndromes (with consideration of setting, environment, population, co-morbidities and multiple contributing factors), with specific attention to:

    - immobility, risk of falls, gait disturbance
    - incontinence
    - cognitive impairment (depression, delirium, dementia)
    - nutritional compromise
    - substance use/abuse
    - abuse or neglect (verbal, physical and sexual)
    - suicide or homicide ideations

NEW: Provide brief intervention/crisis management and make appropriate referrals to mental health care professionals and community agencies with resources to address needs of individuals and families.

NEW: Monitor and evaluate the patient's response to and concomitant use of alcohol and recreational drugs, psychotropic and other medications including over-the-counter and herbal medication/product use, based on a thorough understanding of the principles of pharmacotherapeutics in older adults.

NEW: Use behavioral, environmental, and pharmacological management strategies to ameliorate behavioral symptoms in individuals who have psychiatric/substance misuse disorders including cognitive impairments.

17. Maintain or maximize muscle function and mobility, continence, mood, memory and orientation, nutrition, and hydration.

NEW: Plan and implement care that promotes optimal function and minimizes development of complications, such as those from polypharmacy.

18. Use an ethical framework to address individual and family concerns about care-giving, management of pain, and end-of-life issues.

NEW: Coordinate transitions across levels of care between acute care and community-based long term care settings (e.g., Home, Assisted Living, Hospice, Nursing Homes) for older adults and their families.

19. Strive for restraint-free care, minimizing the use of physical and chemical restraints, and develop the most independent and protective setting possible.

(continues)

APPENDIX E

Recommended Geropsychiatric Competency Enhancements for Nurse Practitioners Who Provide Care to Older Adults But Are Not Geriatric Specialists *(continued)*

II. The Nurse Practitioner – Patient Relationship	
20.	Account for cognitive, sensory, and perceptual problems with special attention to temperature sensation, hearing and vision when caring for older adults.
NEW:	Use culturally appropriate, respectful communication that is adapted to patient's education, cognitive functioning, personal experience, psychiatric/substance misuse disorder, and mental health history.
NEW:	Demonstrate awareness of personal and societal biases, especially ageism and stigma related to mental illness/substance misuse and dementia, and how these influence all aspects of the care of the older adult, including mental health promotion, screening, assessment, and treatment.
21.	Recognize the heightened need for coordination of care with other health care providers and community resources with special attention to the frail older adult and those with markedly advanced age.
NEW:	Protect safety of elders and others in the community through legal reporting mechanisms when elder mistreatment or destructive behaviors targeted at self or others, such as driving with cognitive impairment, are identified.
22.	Develop caring relationships with patients, families, and other caregivers to address sensitive issues, such as driving, independent living, potential for abuse, end-of-life issues, advanced directives, and finances.
23.	Review treatment options and facilitate decision-making with the patient, family, and other caregivers or the patient's health care proxy.
III. The Teaching – Coaching Function	
24.	Consider age-related changes when executing teaching-coaching with regards to sensory and perceptual limitations, cognitive limitations, and memory changes.
25.	Utilize adult learning principles in patient, family, and caregiver education, such as timing of teaching, longer time to learn and respond, and need for individualized instruction, integration of information, and use of multiple strategies of communication.
NEW:	Analyze the impact of aging and age- and disease-related changes in sensory /perceptual function, cognition, confidence with technology, and health literacy and numeracy on the ability and readiness to learn and tailor interventions accordingly.
26.	Educate older adults, family, and caregivers about normal vs. abnormal events, physiological changes with aging, and myths of aging.
27.	Educate older adults, families, and caregivers about the need for preventive health care and end-of-life choices.

Recommended Geropsychiatric Competency Enhancements for Nurse Practitioners Who Provide Care to Older Adults But Are Not Geriatric Specialists *(continued)*

NEW: Educate individuals, families, peers, and groups to promote the knowledge and understanding of effective mental health promotion, management of psychiatric/substance misuse disorders, and the interaction between physical and mental health/illness.

28. Disseminate knowledge of skills required to care for older adults to other health care workers and caregivers through peer education, staff development, and preceptor experiences.

IV. Professional Role

29. Advocate within the health care system and policy arenas for the health needs of older adults, especially the frail and markedly advanced older adult.

NEW: Consider such factors as ability to pay for treatments related to fixed income (retired), entitlements (Medicaid and Medicare), and available resources when providing treatment to clients who may have financial limitations.

30. Articulate and promote to other health care providers and the public, the role within the healthcare team, of either the NP or CNS, and its significance in improving outcomes of care for older adults.

NEW: Work within an interdisciplinary team to promote the mental health and well-being of older clients and their families.

NEW: Demonstrate knowledge of the similarities and differences in roles of various health professionals providing mental health services, e.g., psychotherapist, psychologist, psychiatric social worker, psychiatrist, and advanced practice psychiatric nurse.

31. Create and enhance positive, health promoting environments that maintain a climate of dignity and privacy for older adults.

NEW: Engage in lifelong learning that includes geropsychiatric nursing.

NEW: Incorporate findings from research into mental health promotion and the assessment, treatment, and evaluation of mental health problems and psychiatric disorders affecting older adults and their families.

V. Managing and Negotiating Health Care Delivery Systems

32. Understand payment and reimbursement systems and financial resources across the continuum of care.

33. Promote continuity of care and manage transitions across the continuum of care.

NEW: Assist older adults/caregivers/and their families to negotiate health care delivery systems, including mental health services.

34. Communicate to other members of the interdisciplinary care team special needs of the older adult to improve outcomes of care.

(continues)

APPENDIX E

Recommended Geropsychiatric Competency Enhancements for Nurse Practitioners Who Provide Care to Older Adults But Are Not Geriatric Specialists *(continued)*

35.	Collaborate with the interdisciplinary geriatric and geropsychiatric care team to improve outcomes of care.
36.	Participate in the design and implementation of evidence-based protocols and processes of care to reduce adverse events common to older adults, such as infections, falls, polypharmacy.
VI. Monitoring and Ensuring the Quality of Health Practice	
37.	Address the impact of ageism, sexism, and cultural biases on health care policies and systems.
NEW:	Advocate for health policy at the local, state, regional, and national level to reduce the impact of stigma on services for prevention and treatment of mental health problems and psychiatric/substance misuse disorders.
NEW:	Use knowledge to decrease barriers and gaps in systems that provide mental health services with particular attention to health disparities among minority, disadvantaged and older adults with differing culture, ethnicity, gender, sexual orientation and spirituality.
38.	Use public and private databases to incorporate evidence-based practices into the care of older adults.
39.	Apply evidence-based practice using quality improvement methodologies in providing quality care to older adults.
40.	Use available technology to enhance safety and monitor the health status and outcomes of older adults.
41.	Facilitate access to hospice and palliative care to maximize a peaceful, pain-free, and compassionate death for patients with any end-stage disease, including dementia.
VII. Cultural & Spiritual Competence	
42.	Assess intergenerational differences in family members' beliefs that influence care, e.g., end-of-life care.
43.	Recognize the potential for cultural and ethnic differences between patients and multiple caregivers to impact outcomes of care.
44.	Assess patients' and caregivers' cultural and spiritual priorities as part of a holistic assessment.
NEW:	Assess and incorporate into the treatment plan the patient's perceptions/interpretations of his or her physical and/or mental health/illness and care preferences as influenced by culture, sexual orientation, gender, ethnicity, and spirituality.
NEW:	Demonstrate sensitivity to spirituality and culture when caring for older adults and their families who are at the end of life.

Recommended Geropsychiatric Competency Enhancements for Nurse Practitioners Who Provide Care to Older Adults But Are Not Geriatric Specialists *(continued)*

45.	Adapt age-specific assessment methods or tools to a culturally diverse population.
46.	Educate professional and lay caregivers to provide culturally competent care to older adults.
47.	Incorporate culturally and spiritually appropriate resources into the planning and delivery of health care.

Recommended Geropsychiatric Competency Enhancements for Psychiatric Mental Health Clinical Nurse Specialists

Recommended Geropsychiatric Competency Enhancements for Psychiatric Mental Health Clinical Nurse Specialists

These recommended competency enhancement statements draw attention to the special needs of older adults with mental health concerns. They are not intended to 'stand-alone,' but rather to enhance existing or to-be-developed competencies for psychiatric mental health clinical nurse specialists.[1] The statements are organized within the existing domains of the *Organizing Framework and CNS Core Competencies*[2] developed by NACNS in 2008. The geropsychiatric competency enhancements were drafted in Fall 2008 by the Geropsychiatric Nursing Collaborative (GPNC), a project supported by the John A. Hartford Foundation and housed at the American Academy of Nursing. They were reviewed by representatives of key professional organizations, revised, and then endorsed by the GPNC Core Competency Workgroup and National Advisory Panel and disseminated in Winter 2010 to all relevant professional organizations and schools of nursing for endorsement and utilization.

As revisions are made to existing competency documents, we recommend that the intent of these recommended enhancements be included and that the terms 'health,' 'illness,' 'frailty,' 'care' or 'disease' be broadly defined as both 'physical and mental.' Although physical and mental may be assumed, we believe that it is helpful to have both of these dimensions explicitly stated. Likewise, the term 'psychiatric disorder' should be used in combination with 'substance misuse disorder' to be more inclusive. It is further recommended that an expectation for the use of valid and reliable clinical assessment tools and evidence-based practices and processes be clearly stated and that gender, sexual orientation, and spirituality be made explicit when referring to cultural issues. Finally, the focus of these enhancements is on older adults; we recognize that the work of advanced practice psychiatric nurses may have a lifespan perspective and, thus, some of these enhancements may also apply to other population groups.

---

[1] This competency enhancement document is one of seven developed and recommended by the Geropsychiatric Nursing Collaborative. The seven enhancement documents are aimed at the entry level nurse and the following groups of advanced practice nurses: gerontological NP and CNS, psychiatric NP and CNS, and other APRNs (NP and CNS) who care for older adults but are not prepared as gerontological experts, e.g., women's health, adult, family and acute care. The entire set of enhancement documents can be accessed at www.aannet.org/GPNCresources. For more information, see www.aannet.org/GPNCgeropsych.

[2] NACNS (2008). Organizing Framework and CNS Core Competencies available at www.nacns.org/LinkClick.aspx?fileticket=22R8AaNmrUI%3d&tabid=94. Updated competencies specific to each of the three types of clinical nurse specialists (gerontological, psychiatric mental health, and other) were unavailable at the time of this work; thus, these geropsychiatric nursing enhancements were informed by those developed for the nurse practitioner role.

(continues)

APPENDIX F

Recommended Geropsychiatric Competency Enhancements for Psychiatric Mental Health Clinical Nurse Specialists (*continued*)

A. Direct Care Competency

NEW: Conducts a comprehensive assessment that includes the differentiation of normal age changes from acute and chronic medical and psychiatric/substance misuse disease processes, with attention to commonly occurring atypical presentations and co-occurring health problems including cognitive impairment.

NEW: Includes mental health alterations in the diagnosis of health status.

NEW: Evaluates for elder mistreatment in an assessment of violence and trauma.

NEW: Identifies and assesses factors that affect mental health including stressors that may be more common among older adults such as caregiver stress, multiple chronic illnesses, pain, relocation, trauma, cohort-specific stressors and losses such as financial (retirement), functional limitations (Instrumental Activities of Daily Living / Activities of Daily Living), changes in social network (death of family members and friends), and role (status changes).

NEW: Uses valid and reliable clinical evaluation tools to evaluate common psychiatric/substance misuse disorders, such as depression, anxiety and delirium, as part of a complete health assessment and to monitor changes in status.

NEW: Adapts assessment processes for persons with cognitive impairment and psychiatric/substance misuse disorders.

NEW: Uses behavioral, environmental and pharmacological management strategies to ameliorate behavioral symptoms in individuals who have psychiatric/substance misuse disorders, including cognitive impairments.

NEW: Remains sensitive to verbal cues and non-verbal behaviors in the communication patterns of older adults and their significant others with cognitive, neurological and speech and hearing impairments.

NEW: Uses culturally appropriate, respectful communication that is adapted to patient's education, cognitive functioning, personal experience, psychiatric/substance misuse disorder, and mental health history.

NEW: Monitors and evaluates the patient's response to and concomitant use of alcohol and recreational drugs, psychotropic and other medications including over-the-counter and herbal medication/product use, based on a thorough understanding of the principles of pharmacotherapeutics in older adults.

NEW: Plans and implements care that promotes optimal function and minimizes development of complications, such as those from polypharmacy.

NEW: Provides evidence-based brief intervention/crisis management and make appropriate referrals to other health care professionals and community agencies with resources to address needs of individuals and families.

APPENDIX F

Recommended Geropsychiatric Competency Enhancements for Psychiatric Mental Health Clinical Nurse Specialists *(continued)*

B. Consultation Competency

NEW: Serves as a clinical expert, clinical leader, and/or clinical consultant to other nurses in the care of older adults experiencing mental health issues.

C. Systems Leadership Competency

NEW: Considers such factors Coordinates transitions across levels of care between acute care, community-based, and institutional long term care settings (e.g., Home, Assisted Living, Hospice, Nursing Homes) for older adults and their families.

NEW: Works within an interdisciplinary team to promote the mental health and well-being of older clients and their families.

NEW: Considers such factors as ability to pay for treatments related to fixed income (retired), entitlements (Medicaid and Medicare), and available resources when providing treatment to clients who may have financial limitations.

NEW: Leads quality improvement initiatives designed to improve the care of older adults with mental illness and cognitive impairment.

D. Collaboration Competency

No geropsychiatric enhancements recommended.

E. Coaching Competency

NEW: Analyzes the impact of aging and age-and disease-related changes in sensory /perceptual function, cognition, confidence with technology, and health literacy and numeracy on the ability and readiness to learn and tailors interventions accordingly.

NEW: Educates individuals, families and groups to promote the knowledge and understanding of effective mental health promotion, management of psychiatric/substance misuse disorders, and the interaction between physical and mental health/illness.

NEW: Assists older adults/caregivers/and their families to negotiate health care delivery systems, including mental health services.

F. Research Competency

NEW: Participates in geropsychiatric nursing research through the identification of older adults' problems, collection of data, and presentation and dissemination of findings.

G. Ethical Decision-Making, Moral Agency and Advocacy

NEW: Applies knowledge of issues related to decisional capacity (including the balance between autonomy and safety), guardianship, financial management and durable and healthcare powers of attorney to the treatment of older adults.

NEW: Serves as leader, change agent and advocate within professional organizations for the behavioral and mental health needs of older adults.

Recommended Geropsychiatric Competency Enhancements for Psychiatric Mental Health Clinical Nurse Specialists *(continued)*

NEW: Recognizes one's own personal and societal ageist biases, especially stigma related to mental illness and dementia, and acknowledges the benefits of mental health promotion and psychiatric treatment for older adults.

NEW: Assesses and incorporates into the treatment plan the patient's perceptions/interpretations of his or her physical and/or mental health/illness and care preferences as influenced by culture, sexual orientation, gender, ethnicity, and spirituality.

NEW: Engages in lifelong learning to assure currency in research and best clinical practices in geropsychiatric nursing.

NEW: Prevents or works to reduce common risk and environmental factors that contribute to psychiatric and behavioral symptoms.

NEW: Protects safety of elders and others in the community through legal reporting mechanisms when elder mistreatment, or destructive behaviors targeted at self or others, such as driving with cognitive impairment, are identified.

NEW: Demonstrates sensitivity to spirituality and culture when caring for older adults and their families who are at the end of life.

NEW: Advocates for health policy at the local, state, regional, and national level to reduce the impact of stigma on services for prevention and treatment of mental health problems and psychiatric/substance misuse disorders.

NEW: Uses knowledge to decrease barriers and gaps in systems that provide mental health services with particular attention to health disparities among the disadvantaged and older adults with differing culture, ethnicity, gender, sexual orientation, and spirituality.

Recommended Geropsychiatric Competency Enhancements for Psychiatric Nurse Practitioners

Recommended Geropsychiatric Competency Enhancements for Psychiatric Nurse Practitioners

These recommended competency enhancement statements draw attention to the special needs of older adults with mental health concerns. They are not intended to 'stand-alone,' but rather to enhance existing or to-be-developed competencies for psychiatric nurse practitioners.[1] The statements are organized within the existing *Psychiatric-Mental Health Nurse Practitioner Competencies*[2] developed by NONPF in 2003. The geropsychiatric competency enhancements were drafted in Fall 2008 by the Geropsychiatric Nursing Collaborative (GPNC), a project supported by the John A. Hartford Foundation and housed at the American Academy of Nursing. They were reviewed by representatives of key professional organizations, revised, and then endorsed by the GPNC Core Competency Workgroup and National Advisory Panel and disseminated in Winter 2010 to all relevant professional organizations and schools of nursing for endorsement and utilization.

New competency enhancement statements and modifications to existing competencies are highlighted in yellow for ease in identification.

As revisions are made to existing competency documents, we recommend that the intent of these recommended enhancements be included and that the terms 'health,' 'illness,' 'frailty,' 'care' or 'disease' be broadly defined as both 'physical and mental.' Although physical and mental may be assumed, we believe that it is helpful to have both of these dimensions explicitly stated. Likewise, the term 'psychiatric disorder' should be used in combination with 'substance misuse disorder' to be more inclusive. It is further recommended that an expectation for the use of valid and reliable clinical assessment tools and evidence-based practices and processes be clearly stated and that gender, sexual orientation, and spirituality be made explicit when referring to cultural issues. Finally, the focus of these enhancements is on older adults; we recognize that the work of advanced practice psychiatric nurses may have a lifespan perspective and, thus, some of these enhancements may also apply to other population groups.

---

[1] This competency enhancement document is one of seven developed and recommended by the Geropsychiatric Nursing Collaborative. The seven enhancement documents are aimed at the entry level nurse and the following groups of advanced practice nurses: gerontological NP and CNS, psychiatric NP and CNS, and other APRNs (NP and CNS) who care for older adults but are not prepared as gerontological experts, e.g., women's health, adult, family and acute care. A link to the entire set of enhancement documents can be found at www.aannet.org/GPNCresources. For more information, see www.aannet.org/GPNCgeropsych.

[2] NONPF (2003). Psychiatric-Mental Health Nurse Practitioner Competencies, available at www.aacn.nche.edu/Accreditation/psychiatricmentalhealthnursepractitionercopetencies/FINAL03.pdf

APPENDIX G

Recommended Geropsychiatric Competency Enhancements for Psychiatric Nurse Practitioners *(continued)*

Domain 1: Health Promotion, Protection, Disease Prevention, & Treatment

I.A Assessment of Health Status

1. Obtains and accurately documents a relevant health history, with an emphasis on mental health history, for patients relevant to specialty and age.

   a. Performs a comprehensive physical and mental health assessment.

NEW: Adapts assessment processes for persons with cognitive impairment and psychiatric /substance misuse disorders.

   b. Performs a comprehensive psychiatric evaluation, that includes evaluation of mental status, current and past history of violence, suicidal or self-harm behavior, substance use, level of functioning, health behaviors, trauma, sexual behaviors, and social and developmental history.

NEW: Conducts a comprehensive assessment that includes the differentiation of normal age changes from acute and chronic medical and psychiatric/substance misuse disease processes, with attention to commonly occurring atypical presentations and co-occurring health problems including cognitive impairment.

2. Analyzes the relationship between normal physiology and specific system alterations associated with mental health problems, psychiatric disorders, and treatment.

3. Identifies and analyzes factors that affect mental health such as:

   a. genetics
   b. family
   c. environment
   d. psychodynamics
   e. culture & ethnicity
   f. spiritual beliefs and practices
   g. physiological processes
   h. coping skills
   i. cognition
   j. developmental stage
   k. socioeconomic status
   l. gender
NEW: m. substance misuse
NEW: n. stigma
NEW: o. sexual orientation
NEW: p. trauma, including elder mistreatment
NEW: q. caregiver stress

(continues)

APPENDIX G

Recommended Geropsychiatric Competency Enhancements for Psychiatric Nurse Practitioners *(continued)*

NEW:	r. multiple chronic illnesses
NEW:	s. pain
NEW:	t. relocation
NEW:	u. cohort-specific stressors, e.g., holocaust survivors
4.	Collects data from multiple sources using assessment techniques that are appropriate to the patient's language, culture, and developmental stage, including, but not limited to, screening evaluations, psychiatric rating scales, genograms, and other standardized instruments.
5.	Conducts a comprehensive multigenerational family assessment.
6.	Assesses the impact of acute and/or chronic physical illness, psychiatric disorders, and stressors on the family system.
7.	Performs a comprehensive assessment of mental health needs of a community.
8.	Performs and accurately documents appropriate systems and symptom-focused physical examinations, with emphasis on the mental status exam and neurological exam.
9.	Involves patients, significant others, and interdisciplinary team members in data collection and analysis.
10.	Synthesizes, prioritizes, and documents relevant data in a retrievable form.
11.	Demonstrates effective clinical interviewing skills that facilitate development of a therapeutic relationship.
12.	Assesses the interface among the individual, family, community, and social systems and their relationship to mental health functioning.
I.B Diagnosis of Health Status	
1.	Orders and interprets findings of relevant diagnostic and laboratory tests.
2.	Identifies both typical and atypical presentations of psychiatric disorders and related health problems.
3.	Differentiates psychiatric presentations of medical conditions from psychiatric disorders and arranges appropriate evaluation and follow-up.
4.	Develops a differential diagnosis derived from the collection and synthesis of assessment data.
5.	Diagnoses psychiatric disorders.

Recommended Geropsychiatric Competency Enhancements for Psychiatric Nurse Practitioners *(continued)*

6. Differentiates between exacerbation and reoccurrence of a chronic psychiatric disorder and signs and symptoms of a new mental health problem or a new medical or psychiatric disorder.

7. Diagnoses commonly occurring complications of mental health problems and psychiatric disorders, including physical health problems.

8. Evaluates the health impact of multiple life stressors and situational crises within the context of the family cycle.

9. Applies standardized taxonomy systems to the diagnosis of mental health problems and psychiatric disorders.

10. Evaluates potential abuse, neglect, and risk of danger to self and others, such as suicide, homicide, and other self-injurious behaviors, and assists patients and families in securing the least restrictive environment for ensuring safety.

I.C Plan of Care and Implementation of Treatment

1. Develops a treatment plan for mental health problems and psychiatric disorders based on biopsychosocial theories, evidence-based standards of care, and practice guidelines.

NEW: Plans and implements care that promotes optimal function and minimizes development of complications, such as those from polypharmacy.

2. Conducts individual, group, and/or family psychotherapy.

NEW: Provides brief intervention/crisis management and makes appropriate referrals to other health care professionals and community agencies with resources to address needs of individuals and families.

NEW: Remains sensitive to verbal cues and non-verbal behaviors in the communication patterns of older adults and their significant others with cognitive, neurological and speech and hearing impairments.

3. Treats acute and chronic psychiatric disorders and mental health problems.

4. Plans care to minimize the development of complications and promote function and quality of life using treatment modalities such as, but not limited to, psychotherapy and psychopharmacology.

5. Prescribes psychotropic and related medications based on clinical indicators of a patient's status, including results of diagnostic and lab tests as appropriate, to treat symptoms of psychiatric disorders and improve functional health status.

NEW: Monitors and evaluates the patient's response to and concomitant use of alcohol and recreational drugs, psychotropic and other medications including over-the-counter and herbal medication/product use, based on a thorough understanding of the principles of pharmacotherapeutics in older adults.

(continues)

APPENDIX G

Recommended Geropsychiatric Competency Enhancements for Psychiatric Nurse Practitioners *(continued)*

6. Educates and assists the patient in evaluating the appropriate use of complementary and alternative therapies.

7. Evaluates the impact of the course of psychiatric disorders and mental health problems on quality of life and functional status.

8. Manages psychiatric emergencies by determining the level of risk and initiating and coordinating effective emergency care.

9. Recognizes and accurately interprets the patient's implicit communication by listening to verbal cues and observing non-verbal behaviors.

10. Participates in community and population-focused programs that promote mental health and prevent or reduce risk of psychiatric disorders, including factors that contribute to decline in physical functioning, impaired quality of life, social isolation, excess disability in older adults, and psychiatric and behavioral symptoms.

11. Advocates for the patient's and family's rights regarding involuntary treatment and other medicolegal issues.

12. Coordinates the transition of patients and families among mental health care settings, general health care settings including acute care and community-based long term care settings (e.g., Home, Assisted Living, Hospice, Nursing Homes), and community agencies to provide continuity of care and support for the patient, family, and other health care providers.

13. Identifies, measures, and monitors clinical and related behavioral outcomes to determine the effectiveness and appropriateness of the plan of care.

14. Makes appropriate referrals to other health care professionals and community resources for individuals and families.

15. Applies ethical and legal principles to the treatment of patients with mental health problems and psychiatric disorders.

NEW: Applies knowledge of issues related to decisional capacity (including the balance between autonomy and safety), guardianship, financial management and durable and healthcare powers of attorney to the treatment of older adults.

16. Provides anticipatory guidance to individuals and families to promote mental health and to prevent or reduce the risk of psychiatric disorders.

17. Orders age appropriate tests and other procedures that provide data that contribute to the treatment plan.

18. Prescribes pharmacologic agents for patients with mental health problems and psychiatric disorders based on individual characteristics, such as culture, ethnicity, gender, religious beliefs, age, and physical health problems.

19. Ensures patient safety through the appropriate prescription and management of pharmacologic and non-pharmacologic interventions.

APPENDIX G

Recommended Geropsychiatric Competency Enhancements for Psychiatric Nurse Practitioners *(continued)*

Domain II. Nurse Practitioner–Patient Relationship

1. Manages the phases of the nurse practitioner-patient relationship.

   a. Utilizes interventions to promote mutual trust in therapeutic relationships.

   b. Maintains a therapeutic relationship over time with individuals, groups, and families to influence negotiated outcomes.

   c. Concludes therapeutically the nurse-patient relationship and transitions the patient to other levels of care, when appropriate.

NEW: Establishes and maintains a therapeutic relationship with older adults emphasizing culturally-appropriate empathy/reassurance, self-disclosure and comfort measures, including touch.

2. Applies therapeutic communication strategies based on theories and research evidence to reduce emotional distress, facilitate cognitive and behavioral change, and foster personal growth.

NEW: Uses culturally appropriate, respectful communication that is adapted to patient's education, cognitive functioning, personal experience, psychiatric/substance misuse disorder, and mental health history.

3. Monitors own emotional reaction and behavioral responses to others and uses this self-awareness to enhance the therapeutic relationship.

NEW: Demonstrates awareness of personal and societal biases, especially ageism and stigma related to mental illness/substance abuse and dementia, and how these influence all aspects of the care of the older adult, including mental health promotion, screening, assessment and treatment.

4. Uses the therapeutic relationship to promote positive clinical outcomes.

5. Identifies and maintains professional boundaries to preserve the integrity of the therapeutic process.

6. Analyzes the impact of duty to report and other advocacy actions on the therapeutic relationship.

NEW: Protects safety of elders and others in the community through legal reporting mechanisms when elder mistreatment or destructive behaviors targeted at self or others, such as driving with cognitive impairment, are identified.

Domain III. The Teaching-Coaching Function

1. Teaches patients and significant others about intended effects and potential adverse effects of treatment options.

NEW: Educates individuals, families, peers, and groups to promote the knowledge and understanding of effective mental health promotion strategies, management of psychiatric/substance misuse disorders, and the interaction between physical and mental health/illness.

(continues)

APPENDIX G

Recommended Geropsychiatric Competency Enhancements for Psychiatric Nurse Practitioners *(continued)*

2. Provides psychoeducation to individuals, families, and groups to promote knowledge, understanding, and effective management of mental health problems and psychiatric disorders.

3. Demonstrates sensitivity in addressing topics such as, but not limited to, sexuality, substance abuse, violence, and risk-taking behaviors.

4. Analyzes the impact of psychiatric signs and symptoms on the ability and readiness to learn and tailors approaches accordingly.

NEW: Analyzes the impact of aging and age-and disease-related changes in sensory/perceptual function, cognition, confidence with technology, and health literacy and numeracy on the ability and readiness to learn and tailors interventions accordingly.

5. Considers readiness to improve self-care and healthy behavior when teaching patients with mental health problems and psychiatric disorders.

Domain IV. Professional Role

1. Collaborates as a member of the interdisciplinary mental health and other health care team(s).

2. Provides consultation to health care providers and others to enhance quality and cost-effective services for patients and to effect change in organizational systems.

NEW: Considers such factors as ability to pay for treatments related to fixed income (retired), entitlements (Medicaid and Medicare), and available resources when providing treatment to clients who may have financial limitations.

3. Coordinates referral and ongoing access to primary and other health care services for patients.

4. Participates as leader, change agent and advocate in professional and community organizations that influence the health of patients (including older adults) with mental health problems and psychiatric disorders and supports the role of the psychiatric-mental health nurse practitioner.

5. Engages in and collaborates with others in the conduct of research to discover, examine, and test knowledge, theories, and evidence-based approaches to practice.

6. Advocates for the advanced practice psychiatric-mental health nurse's role to other health care providers; community, state, and federal agencies; and the public.

NEW: Serves as a clinical expert, clinical leader, and/or clinical consultant to other nurses in the care of older adults experiencing mental health issues.

7. Upholds ethical and legal standards related to the provision of mental health care.

APPENDIX G

Recommended Geropsychiatric Competency Enhancements for Psychiatric Nurse Practitioners *(continued)*

8.	Recognizes the importance of lifelong learning to be knowledgeable of relevant research and advances in clinical practice.
NEW:	Works within an interdisciplinary team to promote the mental health and well-being of older clients and their families.

Domain V. Managing and Negotiating Health Care Delivery System

1.	Utilizes ethical principles to create a system of advocacy for access and parity for mental health problems, psychiatric disorders, and addiction services.
2.	Influences health policy to reduce the impact of stigma on services for prevention and treatment of mental health problems and psychiatric disorders.
NEW:	Assists older adults/caregivers/and their families to negotiate health care delivery systems, including mental health services.

Domain VI. Monitoring and Ensuring the Quality of Health Care Practice

1.	Seeks consultation when appropriate to enhance one's own practice.
2.	Monitors relevant research to improve quality care.
NEW:	Leads quality improvement initiatives designed to improve the care of older adults with mental illness and cognitive impairment.
NEW:	Advocates for health policy at the local, state, regional, and national level to reduce the impact of stigma on services for prevention and treatment of mental health problems and psychiatric/substance misuse disorders.

Domain VII. Cultural and Spiritual Competence

1.	Recognizes the variability of the presentation of psychiatric signs and symptoms in different cultures.
2.	Acknowledges the influence of culture, ethnicity, and spirituality on the patient's perceptions of his or her psychiatric signs and symptoms.
NEW:	Assesses and incorporates into the treatment plan the patient's perceptions/interpretations of his or her physical and/or mental health/illness and care preferences as influenced by culture, sexual orientation, gender, ethnicity, and spirituality.
3.	Respects and integrates cultural, ethnic, and spiritual influences in designing a treatment plan for patients with mental health problems and psychiatric disorders.
NEW:	Demonstrates sensitivity to spirituality and culture when caring for older adults and their families who are at the end of life.
4.	Evaluates the impact of therapeutic interventions on the patient's cultural, ethnic, & spiritual identity and the impact of practices on outcomes of care.

Index

Pages numbers followed by b, f, and t denote boxes, figures, and tables, respectively.

A

Abilify (aripiprazole), 136t, 137t, 139, 213
absorption (drug), 124
abstract reasoning, 106
abuse
    elder. *See* elder mistreatment
    substance. *See* substance abuse
acamprosate (Campral), 246
access barrier model, 84
Action for Mental Health, 42
activities of daily living (ADLs)
    assessment, 105
    dementia and, 281
    limitations on, 6–7, 8f, 14
activity theory of aging, 20
activity-based therapies, 112, 165
    for dementia, 299–301
    for gambling, 406
acute confusion, 257
acute myopathy, 241
AD. *See* Alzheimer's disease
addiction, definition of, 228–229
ADLs. *See* activities of daily living
Administration on Aging (AoA), 13, 444–446
    caregiver resources, 354
    publications, 15–16b
adult children
    as caregivers, 339
    grief of, 344–345
adult day care, 291–292
advance care planning (advance directives), 427–429
    dementia and, 293–294
    psychiatric, 218–219

advanced practice nurses (APNs), 31–35, 220.
    See also geropsychiatric nurses
    clinical nurse specialist, 31, 165, 441
    cognitive–behavioral therapy and, 165
    mental health policy and, 441
    reimbursement for services, 454–457
    responsibilities, 388, 389
    role in end of life care, 424, 436
    self-employed, 455
A-FRAMES intervention model, 243
African Americans
    misdiagnoses, cultural differences and, 86–87
    response to caregiver role, 340–341
age stratification theory of aging, 20–21
age-related cognitive decline, 24–25
aging
    challenges of, 103
    demographics of, 3, 14–17, 439
    "successful", 18–19, 22, 103–104
    theories of, 17–21
"aging enterprise", 22
agitation
    antecedents, 315–317
    description of, 313–315
    drugs for, 322–324
    experimental interventions, 323b
    management of, 320–322
agnosia, 321
AIDS, caregiving roles and, 108
albumin, serum, 125
alcohol abuse, 229
    adverse health effects, 238–239
    assessment, 237–238

case studies, 235, 243
categories of, 236
prescription drugs and, 238
review of systems in, 239–242
treatment, 245–246
Alcoholics Anonymous, 242, 243, 245
alpha 1-acid glycoprotein levels, 125
alternative and complementary therapies, 112.
　　See also specific therapy
for anxiety, 190–191
for dementia, 298–299
Alzheimer's Association, 306
Alzheimer's disease (AD), 23–24, 104. *See also* dementia
case studies, 306–307
pharmacotherapy, 297–298
stress and, 40
wandering in, 324–326, 327b
ambivalence, intergenerational, 341
American Association on Intellectual and
　　Developmental Disabilities, 35
American Nurses Association (ANA)
publications, 12–13, 35–36
on role of nurse in end of life decisions, 430b
Standards of Clinical Nursing Practice, 35
American Nurses Credentialing Center (ANCC), 31
American Psychiatric Association, 123b
American Psychiatric Nurses Association (APNA), 32–34
American Recovery and Reinvestment Act of 2009, 447
amphetamines, 229
ANA. *See* American Nurses Association
ANCC (American Nurses Credentialing Center), 31
anemia, 241
anger, caregiver, 359–360
ANH (artificial nutrition and hydration), 428
anhedonia, 165
anima/animus, 19
Antabuse (disulfarim), 246
antianxiety drugs, 111, 139–141, 193–194.
　　See also specific drug
anticipatory grief, 434
anticonvulsants, 324. *See also specific drug*
antidepressants. *See also specific drug*
for anxiety, 193–195
categories of, 111, 128–129, 130t
for disruptive behaviors, 323
dosing and duration, 162t
mode of action, 130t
for sleep disorders, 383t, 386
suicide risk and, 134
withdrawal syndromes, 130–131, 134
antihistamines. *See also specific drug*
for sleep disorders, 383t, 386–387
antioxidants, 18

antipsychotics, 135–139. *See also specific drug*
adherence, promoting, 213–214
for agitation in dementia, 322–323
obesity and, 138
risks of, 212–213
second-generation, 135, 136t, 137t
typical and atypical, 164, 213
Antonovsky, Aaron, 39–40
anxiety
assessment and screening, 183–185
case studies, 196
causative agents and conditions, 181b, 182b
comorbid conditions, 162, 177–183
continuum of, 175
dementia and, 179, 180b
drugs to treat, 111, 139–141, 191–195
prevention, 191
rates among older adults, 176–177
research, 175–176
resources, community and family, 195
symptoms in older adults, 178b
treatment, 185–195
anxiolytics, 111, 139–141, 193–194. *See also specific drug*
AoA. *See* Administration on Aging
APNA (American Psychiatric Nurses Association),
　　32–34
APNs. *See* advanced practice nurses
apraxia, 321
Aricept (donepezil), 297
aripiprazole (Abilify), 136t, 137t, 139, 213
arrhythmias, 240
*The Art of Aging: A Doctor's Prescription
　　for Well-Being*, 39
art therapy, 113, 296–297
arthritis, 104
artificial nutrition and hydration (ANH), 428
Asian Americans
cultural competency and, 89–91
mind-body relationship, 86
assertive community programs, 218
assertiveness training, 107–108
assessment and screening. *See also specific test or tool*
anxiety, 183–185
cognitive impairment, 57
comprehensive mental health, 53–54, 105–107
delirium, 261–265
dementia, 277–283
depression, 151–156
psychosis, 209–212
therapeutic environment for, 281–283
assisted living, 467
for dementia, 292
ataque de nerviosis, 78–79

attention
    assessment, 282
    defined, 22
autonomy, 321
Awareness–Assessment–Negotiation Model, 78
azapirones, 193–195

B

Bandura, Albert, 39
barbiturates, 230, 385–386. *See also specific drug*
barriers to care, 14, 84f, 149, 426, 443
basic needs, meeting, 320–321
Bazelon Center for Mental Health Law, 219t
Beck Depression Inventory, 86, 87, 107
"Beers Criteria", 126
Behavior Care intervention, 356
behavioral observation, 211–212
Behavioral Pathologic Rating Scale for
    Alzheimer's Disease, 277
Behavioral Risk Factor Surveillance System, 6
Benadryl (diphenhydramine), 386
benzodiazepines, 111, 139–140. *See also specific drug*
    for anxiety, 193
    distribution of, 124
    in medical detoxification, 245–246
    for sleep disorders, 382–384
    user profile, 230
bereavement, 40, 433. *See also* grief
bibliotherapy, 191
biological theories of aging, 18–19
bipolar disorder, 205–206
blindness, sleep disorders and, 368
bone density, alcohol abuse and, 241
botanical therapies. *See* dietary supplements
buprenorphine, 246
bupropion (Wellbutrin), 132t, 133
    for gambling, 405
    side effects, 163
buspirone (Buspar), 140
    for anxiety, 193–195

C

caffeine, 231
CAGE questionnaire, 232
CALM Tools for Living, 187
caloric restriction, 18
CAM (Confusion Assessment Method), 262–263
Campral (acamprosate), 246
cancer, 104
    alcohol abuse and, 242
    sleep disorders and, 372
cannabis, 229
Caplan, Gerald, 41

carbamazepine (Tegretol), 405
cardiopulmonary resuscitation (CPR), success
    rate of, 427–428
cardiovascular disease, 104, 240
care managers, for depression, 168
caregiver. *See also* family
    anger, 359–360
    assessment, 351–354
    burden, 168, 218, 339–340
    case studies, 360
    coping strategies, 342
    grief, 344–351
    health effects, 342–344
    interventions, 303–305
    roles, 108
    support, 340–341, 354–360
    well-being, 336–338
Caregiver Well-Being Scale, 336–338, 351
case management, 217
case studies
    alcohol abuse, 235, 243
    Alzheimer's disease, 306–307
    anxiety, 196
    caregivers, 360
    Comprehensive Mental Health Assessment tool, 61–68b
    cultural competence, 89–91
    delirium, 255–256
    dementia, 286
    depression, 169
    elder mistreatment, 419
    end of life, 435
    gambling, pathological, 407
    mental health promotion, 115–116
    nursing paradigm, 46–47
    schizophrenia, 222
    sleep disorders, 390–391
    substance abuse, 244
CASI (Cognitive Abilities Screening Instrument), 279
casinos, 396, 407
CC (collaborative care) models, 188–189
Celexa (citalopram), 405
cellular aging theory, 18
Center for Health Workforce Studies, 31
Center for Mental Health Services, 454
CERAD (Consortium to Establish a Registry for
    Alzheimer's Disease), 278
CERAD assessment tools, 278
certified nursing assistants (CNAs), 305
CES-D, 87
Charles Bonnet syndrome, 208
CHCs (community health centers), 446
chloral hydrate, 385
cholinergic deficiency, 258

chronic grief, 434
chronic homelessness, 11
chronic illness
    anxiety and, 179–180
    impact of, 104, 109
chronic worry, versus adaptive worry, 184
chronicity of mental illness, 8–9
chronobiology, 368
circadian rhythms
    agitation and, 316
    sleep regulation and, 368–369
cirrhosis, 239–240
citalopram (Celexa), 405
Clinical Institute Withdrawal Assessment Scale, 245
clinical nurse specialist (CNS), 31, 165, 441
Closing the Gap: A National Blueprint to Improve the Health of Persons with Mental Retardation, 10
clozapine (Clozaril), 136t, 137t, 138, 213
clubhouses, 218
CMHA. *See* Comprehensive Mental Health Assessment tool
CNAs (certified nursing assistants), 305
CNS (clinical nurse specialist), 31, 165, 441
cocaine, 229–230
cognition
    assessment, 57, 105–106
    changes in aging, 22–25
    developmental model, 295
    impairment, 179, 315
Cognitive Abilities Screening Instrument (CASI), 279
cognitive–behavioral therapy, 112
    for anxiety, 186–188
    collaborative care models, 187
    for depression, 164, 165–166
    in home care, 187–188
    for insomnia, 375–378, 391
    in primary care, 186–187
    for schizophrenia, 216
    for substance abuse, 243
Cohen-Mansfield Agitation Inventory, 277, 325
collaborative care (CC) models, 188–189
community health centers (CHCs), 446
community management skills, 216
community mental health movement, 41–42
Community Mental Health Services Block Grants, 446
community residences, 292
community resources, 195
community services, 114, 217–218, 445–446
community-based interventions, for early-stage dementia, 295
competence
    cultural, 87–91
    personal, 21
complementary therapies. *See* alternative and complementary therapies

complicated grief, 434
comprehension, assessment of, 106
Comprehensive Mental Health Assessment (CMHA) tool, 53–54
    case studies, 61–68b
    history and overview, 57–59
    McHugh and, 61
    objectives, 59
computer–telephone integrated system (CTIS), 356
confusion, acute, 257
Confusion Assessment Method (CAM), 262–263
Consensus Statement on the Upcoming Crisis in Geriatric Mental Health, 31
Consortium to Establish a Registry for Alzheimer's Disease (CERAD), 278
consultation, mental health, 113
continuity theory of aging, 20
coping strategies, caregiver, 342
Cornell Scale for Depression in Dementia, 151, 155f, 277
counseling
    for gambling, 405–406
    mental health, 110
CPR (cardiopulmonary resuscitation), success rate of, 427–428
CRASH, 88
creatinine, serum, 125
Criminalization of Individuals with Severe Psychiatric Disorders, 12
crisis, maturational versus situational, 109–110
crisis intervention, 110–111, 215
crisis theory, 41
critical gerontology theory, 22
cross-linking theory, 18
Crowe, Marie, 55
crystallized intelligence, 23
CTIS (computer–telephone integrated system), 356
cultural competence, 87–91
    case studies, 89–91
Cultural Influences on Mental Health Model, 88
culture
    affect and, 107
    beliefs about mental illness and, 77–78
    caregiver role and, 340–341
    defined, 76
    formulation of, 80t
    help-seeking behavior and, 83
    influence of, 43
    normative behavior and, 86
culture-bound syndrome, 79
Cymbalta (duloxetine), 132t, 133
cytochrome P-450 isoenzymes, 125, 126, 380

D

dance and movement therapy, 113
day care, adult, 291–292
day treatment programs, 217–218

death. *See* end of life care
death vigils, 433
dehydration, terminal, 428
delayed grief, 434
delirium, 206–207
   assessment and evaluation, 261–265
   case studies, 255–256
   clinical features, 264t
   dementia and, 260, 263
   diagnostic criteria, 257
   documentation, 267–269
   drugs for, 266
   ethics and, 269
   incidence rates, 256
   pathophysiology, 258
   progression of, 260
   resources, 269–270
   reversible causes of, 263–265
   risk factors, 258, 259t, 266
   safety and recovery, 265–267
   subtypes, 259–260
   terminology, 257
   underdiagnosis, 260–261
Delirium Abatement Program, 267
DELIRIUM diagnostic tool, 263–265
Delirium Observation Screening, 262
Delirium Rating Scale, 262
Delirium Symptom Interview, 262
delusions, 203, 205
   paranoid, 206
dementia, 23–24, 25, 104. *See also* Alzheimer's disease
   antipsychotics and, 135
   anxiety and, 179, 180b
   assessment, 273, 277–283
   behavioral and psychological symptoms, 276–277
   care environments, 291–294
   case studies, 286
   causes, 275
   clinical features, 264t
   delirium and, 260, 263
   depression and, 151
   diagnosis, 283–285
   Down's syndrome and, 9
   interventions, 294–306
   in literature and films, 303b
   neurobiology of, 275–276
   nursing role in, 287
   pain and, 319
   problem behaviors in, drugs to treat, 324t
   psychosis in, 207
   resources, 306
   wandering in, 324–326, 327b
Dementia Mood Picture Test, 318
Dementia Screening Questionnaire for Caregivers, 278
demographics of aging, 3, 14–17, 439

denial
   family, 283, 286
   patient, 285
deoxyribonucleic acid (DNA), 18
Depakote (valproate), 405
Department of Veterans Affairs (DVA), 452–453
dependency, physical, 228
depression
   assessment and screening, 151–156
   care managers, 168
   caregiver, 342–343
   case studies, 169
   clinical features, 264t
   comorbid conditions, 162, 177–179, 440
   consequences of, 147–148
   drugs to treat, 161–164
   etiology, 150–151
   illness as etiologic factor in, 149–150, 158b
   major. *See* major depression
   minor, 156, 163–164
   nursing interventions, 166, 167b
   risk factors, 150
   stigma and shame, 149
   suicide and, 148
   symptoms of, 149, 159b
   treatment, 160–161
desipramine, 129
desvenlafaxine (Pristiq), 132–133
Desyrel. *See* trazodone
determinism, 37
detoxification, medical, 242
development in aging, 21–22
diagnosis. *See also specific disorder*
   communicating, 284–285
   nursing, 54, 68b
Diagnostic and Statistical Manual of Mental Disorders (DSM IV), 24–25, 53
   critique of, 55, 56–57
   delirium and, 258
   diagnosis example, 68b
   history of, 54
   multiaxis systems, 56
dietary supplements, 112–113. *See also specific supplement*
   drug interactions with, 122, 127
   for sleep disorders, 380–382
diphenhydramine (Benadryl), 386
Discomfort Scale for Patients with Dementia of the Alzheimer's Type, 318
disease management skills training, 216
disenfranchised grief, 434
disengagement theory of aging, 20
distribution (drug), 124–125
disulfarim (Antabuse), 246
divorce, 102
DNA (deoxyribonucleic acid), 18

documentation, 267–269
doll therapy, 300
Domains and Core Competencies of Nurse Practitioner Practice, 34
donepezil (Aricept), 297
dopamine D2 receptor, 136
dopaminergic drugs, 404
Down's syndrome, 9
drug(s). *See also* pharmacotherapy; *specific drug*
    absorption, 124
    of abuse, 229–231. *See also* substance abuse
    to avoid in older adults, 126
    depression induced by, 159b
    distribution, 124–125
    economic considerations, 127
    at end of life, 428–429
    excretion, 125–128
    interactions, 122, 126, 137t
    for medical detoxification, 245–246
    metabolism, 125
    pharmacodynamic changes, age-related, 125–128, 191
    pharmacokinetic changes, age-related, 123–125, 241
    prescribing process, 128f
    prescription, abuse of, 230
    in psychiatric stabilization, 41
    side effects, monitoring, 298
    sleep decreased by, 388b
    toxicity, agitation and, 316–317
Drug Interactions (website), 123
DSM IV. *See Diagnostic and Statistical Manual of Mental Disorders*
duloxetine (Cymbalta), 132t, 133
DVA (Department of Veterans Affairs), 452–453
dysphoria, 108
dysthymia, 156

E
eating difficulties, 326–328
EBP. *See* evidence-based practice
EDGE (Electronic Dementia Guide for Excellence), 306
education
    geropsychiatric nurses, 33–35, 471–472
    patient, 114, 190, 389, 406
EEGs (electroencephalograms), 374
Effexor (venlafaxine), 131–132, 163
ego, 37
ego integrity, 19–20
elder mistreatment (EM)
    assessment and screening, 414–418
    case studies, 419
    incidence and prevalence, 412
    institutional, 413–414
    legal concerns, 418
    perpetrators, characteristics of, 413

prevention, 418–419
    referral, 418
    reporting, 414
    risk factors, 412
    theories, 413
    types, 411–412, 412t
electroconvulsive therapy, 166
electroencephalograms (EEGs), 374
electromyograms (EMGs), 374–375
Electronic Dementia Guide for Excellence (EDGE), 306
electro-oculograms (EOGs), 374–375
EM. *See* elder mistreatment
"emergence of the person" in dementia, 276–277
EMGs (electromyograms), 374–375
emotional functioning, 106–107
    assessment, 282
encephalopathy, Wernicke's, 240–241
end of life care. *See also* advance care planning; grief
    assessment, 431–432
    case studies, 435
    dying process, 432–433
    future of, 436
    hospice and palliative care, 424–426
    quality care, barriers to, 426
    role of nurse in, 430b
endocrine theory, 18
Enhanced Care intervention, 356
environment
    agitation in response to, 317
    dementia care, 291–294
    modification, 301–302, 321–322
    therapeutic, 281–283
Environmental Skill-Building Program, 356
EOGs (electro-oculograms), 374–375
Epidemiological Catchment Area survey, 13
EPS (extrapyramidal symptoms), 135–136
Epworth Sleepiness Scale, 391
Erikson, Erik, 19, 37–38, 39
error theories of aging, 18
Eskalith (lithium carbonate), 405
Essentials of Psychiatric Mental Health Nursing in the BSN Curriculum, 33, 34
ethics, 218–220
    delirium and, 269
    dementia and, 284–285
ethnic elders, 73–76, 81–82. *See also* culture; minority populations
    barriers to mental health care, 83–84
    disparities in quality of care, 84–87
ethnicity
    defined, 76–77
    impact of, 103
euthanasia, active, 430b

evidence-based practice (EBP), 469–470
  depression models, 168–169
  National Registry of Evidence-Based Programs and Practice, 168
  nursing protocols, 470–471
Evidence-Based Practice Implementation Resource Kits, 454
exaggerated grief, 434
excretion (drug), 125–128
Exelon (rivastigmine), 297
exercise, insomnia and, 378
Expert Consensus Guidelines for Using Antipsychotic Agents in Older Patients, 164
extrapyramidal symptoms (EPS), 135–136

F

Faces Pain Rating Scale, 318
family. *See also* caregiver
  education, 216–217
  influence of, 82
  nurse's relationship with, 305
  role in diagnosis of dementia, 283–285
  support from, 107, 114, 195, 218
Family Involvement in Care (FIC), 305
fatigue, versus sleepiness, 368
FDA warnings, 134, 135
federally funded programs, 443–454.
        See also Medicaid; Medicare
feminism
  influence on geropsychiatric nurses, 43–44
  theories of aging, 22
FIC (Family Involvement in Care), 305
financial issues. *See also* poverty
  abuse/exploitation, 412t
  drug therapy, 127
  income statistics for older adults, 16b
  wellbeing, 104
fluvoxamine (Luvox), 405
forensic nursing, 37
Forensic Nursing: Scope and Standards of Practice, 35–36
Frankl, Viktor, 39
free radical theory, 18
freebasing, 230
Freud, Sigmund, 37–39
functional status, assessment of, 6–7

G

GABA receptors, 382
GAD (generalized anxiety disorder). *See* anxiety
GADSS (Generalized Anxiety Disorder Severity Scale), 185
galantamine (Reminyl), 297
Gamblers Anonymous (GA), 404–405
gambling, pathological
  among older adults, 396–397
  assessment and diagnosis, 397–404

case studies, 407
follow-up, 406
Internet, 406–407
pharmacotherapy, 405
prevalence, 395–396
GAPNA (Gerontological Advanced Practice Nurses Association), 32, 33
gastrointestinal disorders, alcohol abuse and, 239–240
gay men. *See* homosexuals
gender, impact of, 102. *See also* men; women
General Practitioner Assessment of Cognition, 57
generalized anxiety disorder (GAD). *See* anxiety
Generalized Anxiety Disorder Severity Scale (GADSS), 185
generativity, 19
Geodon (ziprasidone), 136t, 137t, 139, 213
Geriatric Anxiety Inventory, 184–185
Geriatric Depression Scale, 107, 211
Geriatric Depression Screening tool, 151, 154f
Geriatric Michigan Alcoholism Screening Test (MAST-G), 232–233
Geriatric Nursing Education Consortium, 472
Gerontological Advanced Practice Nurses Association (GAPNA), 32, 33
gerontological nurses. *See also* geropsychiatric nurses
  education and training, 31–32
  information system, 38f
  standards of practice, 36t
Gerontological Society of America, 123b
geropsychiatric nurses
  education and training, 33–35, 471–472
  expanded roles for, 468–469
  future of, 465–472
  influences, 42–44
  mental health policy, role in, 441–443
  new settings for, 468
  reimbursement issues, 454–457
  research, needed, 469–470
  standards of practice, 35–37
  theoretical foundations, 37–44
The Geropsychiatric Nurses Collaborative (GPNC), 34
Getting Started: A To Do List for Graduate Nurse Practitioners in Massachusetts, 455
ghost sickness, 79
ginkgo biloba, 112
ginseng, 113
Glossary of Culture-Bound Syndromes, 79
Golden Living project, 467
GPNC (The Geropsychiatric Nurses Collaborative), 34
grief, 40–41, 433–435
  caregiver, 344–351
group activities, 295–296
group therapy, 216

H

hallucinations, 203, 205
  Charles Bonnet syndrome, 208
  delirium, 206
haloperidol (Haldol), 405
harm reduction, 243
Hartford Institute for Geriatric Nursing, 270
Hayflick, Leonard, 18
health, definition of, 147
healthcare costs, 439–450
healthcare proxies. *See* advance care planning
healthcare reform, 457–460
Healthy IDEAS: Identifying Depression, Empowering
    Activities for Seniors, 168
Healthy People 2010, 122, 148
help-seeking behavior, 83
hematological conditions, 241
hepatic function, 125, 239
hepatitis, 239–240
herbal supplements. *See* dietary supplements
hierarchy of human needs, 19, 39
Hispanic Americans, 78–79
history, patient, 183–184
  elder mistreatment screening, 414–416
  psychosis, 209–211
HIV/AIDS, caregiving roles and, 108
home environment, modifying, 301–302, 321–322
home health care, 292
homelessness, 10–12
  chronic, 11
  federal programs, 451–452
  public cost, 11
homeostatic process, 368–369
homicide, schizophrenia and, 215
homosexuals, 13
  disenfranchised grief, 434
hormones, depression and, 150
hospice care, 424–425
  for dementia, 293–294
Hospital Anxiety and Depression Scale, 185
Hospital Elder Life program, 266
housing, 217
HUD section 232, 446–447
human development, stages of, 19
hypersexuality, 328–329
hyponatremia, 130

I

IADLs. *See* instrumental activities of daily living
iatrogenesis, 41
ICD (International Classification of Diseases), 53, 55–56
id, 37
IDDs. *See* intellectual and developmental disabilities
idioms of distress, 78

illness, chronic
  anxiety and, 179–180
  impact of, 104, 109
illusions, 206
immune function, alcohol abuse and, 241–242
immunological theory, 18
Impressions of Medication, Alcohol, and Drug Use
    in Seniors, 233–235
Improving Mood: Promoting Access to Collaborative
    Treatment (IMPACT), 168, 188
impulse control disorders, 404
incarceration, as risk factor, 12–13
"incident to" provisions, 455
income. *See also* financial issues; poverty
  statistics for older adults, 16b
  Supplemental Security, 452
indemnity insurance companies, 456
individual-focused intervention, 215–216
individualism, 19
"informal caregiving", 335
inpatient units, geropsychiatric, 467–468
insomnia, 373–374. *See also* sleep disorders
institutional factors, mental health promotion and, 4
instrumental activities of daily living (IADLs)
  assessment, 105
  in dementia, 281
  limitations on, 6–7, 8f, 14
intellectual and developmental disabilities (IDDs)
  nursing specialization, 36t
  risks and recommendations, 9–10
  terminology, 35
*Intellectual and Developmental Disabilities Nursing:
    Scope and Standards of Practice*, 10
intelligence
  changes in, 23
  defined, 22
intergenerational ambivalence, 341
International Association of Forensic Nurses, 35–37
International Classification of Diseases (ICD),
    53, 55–56
International Society for Education and Research
    in Psychiatric–Mental Health Nursing
    (SERPN), 34
Internet gambling, 406–407
Internet resources, 123, 355b
interpersonal processes, 4
Interpersonal Relations in Nursing, 44
interpersonal therapy, 164
interventions, nursing. *See also specific intervention*
  anxiety, 185–191
  delirium, 265–267
  dementia, 294–306
  depression, 166
  gambling, pathological, 404–406

mental health promotion, 110–114
    sleep disorders, 375–382
    substance abuse, 247–249
intrapersonal factors, mental health promotion and, 4

J

John A. Hartford Institute for Geriatric Nursing, 306
judgment, assessment of, 106
Jung, Carl, 19

K

kava, 112–113
kidney function, 125
    alcohol abuse and, 241
Kleinmann, Arthur, 43
koro, 79
Korsakoff's syndrome, 241

L

language, assessment of, 282
learning
    assessment, 282
    defined, 22
legal concerns, 218–219, 418
legislation, 442, 444, 447
lesbians. *See* homosexuals
Lewy body dementia, 207
Lie/Bet questionnaire, 404
life expectancy, 16, 423–424
light, circadian rhythms and, 368
light therapy, 378–380
Lindemann, Erich, 40
lithium carbonate (Eskalith), 405
liver function, 125, 239
living arrangements, 13
living wills. *See* advance care planning
loneliness, 108–109
long-term care facilities, 292–293
Luvox (fluvoxamine), 405

M

major depression, 156
    psychosis in, 205
    unipolar, drugs for, 161t
managed care organizations, 456
Man's Search for Meaning, 39
MAOIs (monoamine oxidase inhibitors), 130, 164
marginalized groups, examples of, 4
marijuana, 229
marital status, 13
Marwit–Meuser Caregiver Grief Inventory
    (MM-CGI), 345–351
masked grief, 434
Maslow, Abraham, 19, 39

massage therapy
    for agitation in dementia, 323b
    for sleep disorders, 380
MAST-G (Geriatric Michigan Alcoholism Screening Test),
    232–233
McHugh, Paul, 55, 60–61
MCI (mild cognitive impairment), 23, 24b
Medicaid, 447–449
    reimbursement, 456
    reliance on, as stressor, 104
Medicare, 449–451
    Hospice Benefit, 425
    reimbursement, 149, 455–456
    reliance on, as stressor, 104
medication. *See* drug(s); pharmacotherapy; *specific drug*
melatonin, 369
    receptor agonists, 383t, 387
Memorial Delirium Assessment Scale, 262
memory
    assessment, 106, 282
    changes, 23–24
    defined, 22
    types, 23
Memory and Behavior Problems Checklist, 1990R, 325
Memory Impairment Screen, 57
men
    as caregivers, 335–336, 339, 343, 357–358
    gay. *See* homosexuals
    homeless, 11
    suicide among, 13
mental disorders. *See also specific disorder*
    categorizing and treatment planning, 61
    chronicity of, 8–9
    contributing factors, 108–110
    defined, 5
    disability and, 5–6
    epidemiology, 121
    in ethnic elders, 75
    explanatory models of, 77–78
    serious and persistent, 7–9
    underdiagnosis, 440
    underreporting, 14
mental health
    defined, 3, 101
    integration, 458–459
    stressors impacting, 102–105
Mental Health: A Report of the Surgeon General, 3, 4–5,
    13, 177
Mental Health America, 219t
Mental Health Atlas, 148–149
mental health care
    access to, 83–84
    federally funded programs, 443–454
    integration with primary care, 468

quality of, 84–87
sociostructural context of, 83
underutilization, 5, 340
mental health parity, 441–442
Mental Health Parity Act (MHPA), 442
Mental Health Problems of Prison and Jail Inmates, 37
mental health promotion, 472. *See also* public policy
case studies, 115–116
clinical research, 114–115
global initiatives, 148–150
levels of, 101–102
models, 3–4
resources, 114
themes, 4–5
therapeutic interventions, 110–114
Mental Illness and Homelessness, 11
mental retardation. *See* intellectual and developmental disabilities
metabolic theory of aging, 18
metabolism (drug), 125
methadone, 246–247
MHPA (Mental Health Parity Act), 442
"middle adulthood", 39
middle age, stages of, 19
mild cognitive impairment (MCI), 23, 24b
mind-body relationship
Asian Americans and, 86
community mental health and, 42
removed from DSM, 54
Surgeon General's report (1999), 147
Mini-Cog, 57, 211
Mini-Mental State Examination (MMSE), 53, 57, 68b, 279
for delirium, 261
for psychosis, 211
sample items, 58
wandering risk assessment, 325
minor depression, 156
drugs to treat, 163–164
minority populations, 13. *See also* ethnic elders
definition of, 77
projected growth of, 17
statistics, 15b, 16b
mirtazapine (Remeron), 132t, 133, 163
MM-CGI (Marwit–Meuser Caregiver Grief Inventory), 345–351
MMSE. *See* Mini-Mental State Examination
mobility impairment, 6–7
Modified Caregiver Strain Index, 351, 352–353f
monoamine oxidase inhibitors (MAOIs), 130, 164
"mood congruent/incongruent", 205
mood stabilizers, 324
mortality rates, historical, 423–424
musculoskeletal conditions, 104, 241
music therapy, 113, 302–303, 322, 323b
myopathy, acute, 241

N
NAEH (National Alliance to End Homelessness), 11
nafazodone (Serzone), 131
naltrexone (Narcan), 247, 405
NAMI (National Alliance on Mental Illness), 218, 219t
Narcotics Anonymous, 242, 243
Nardil (phenelzine), 130
National Adult Day Services Association, 292
National Alliance on Mental Illness (NAMI), 218, 219t
National Alliance to End Homelessness (NAEH), 11
National Council on Problem Gambling (NCPG), 406
National Institute on Aging, 24, 123b
National Institute on Drug Abuse (NIDA) treatment principles, 242
National Law Center on Homelessness and Poverty, 11
National Opinion Research Center (NORC) screen, 395–396, 402–403f
National Registry of Evidence-Based Programs and Practice (NREPP), 168
National Sleep Foundation, 367
National Social Life, Health, and Aging Project, 412
National Survey on Drug Use and Health, 227–228
Native Americans, 79
NCPG (National Council on Problem Gambling), 406
NEECHAM Confusion Scale, 262
need-driven dementia-compromised behavior model, 294–295
nefazodone, 164
negative automatic thoughts record, 165–166
neglect, 412t
neurodevelopmental sequencing model, 295
neuroimaging, 150
neuroleptics, 111
neurological disorders, 240–241
Neuropsychiatric Inventory, 277
NHC (Nursing Home Collaborative), 466–467
nicotine, 231
nicotine replacement therapies, 247
NIDA (National Institute on Drug Abuse) treatment principles, 242
non-rapid eye movement (NREM) sleep, 370
nonselective serotonin reuptake inhibitors (non-SSRIs), 131–134
NORC (National Opinion Research Center) screen, 395–396, 402–403f
normative behavior, 86
nortriptyline, 129
NREPP (National Registry of Evidence-Based Programs and Practice), 168
Nuland, Sherwin, 39
Numerical Rating Scale, 318
nurses
advanced practice. *See* advanced practice nurses
dementia care training, 304–305
geropsychiatric. *See* geropsychiatric nurses

role in assessment and intervention, 149, 166, 167b, 220
    standards of practice, 36t
Nursing: Concepts of Practice, 44
nursing diagnosis, 54, 68b
Nursing Home Collaborative (NHC), 466–467
nursing homes
    abuse in. *See* elder mistreatment
    impact on caregivers, 304
    nursing initiatives, 466–467
    placement in, 13
    as stressor, 104–105
nursing interventions. *See* interventions, nursing
nursing paradigm, 45f, 46–47
nursing protocols, 470–471
    Psychogeriatric Nursing Assessment, 277–278
    suicide, 160
nursing theories, 44
Nursing's Social Policy Statement, 12–13

O

obesity, antipsychotics and, 138
OBRA (Omnibus Budget Reconciliation Act), 127–128
obstructive sleep apnea syndrome (OSAS), 371–372
olanzapine (Zyprexa), 136t, 137t, 138
    for gambling, 405
    for psychosis, 213
*Older Adults: Recommended Baccalaureate Competencies
    and Curricular Guidelines for Geriatric Nursing
    Care*, 32
Older Americans Act, 444
Older Americans Resources and Services, 279
"oldest-old" persons, 14
omega-3 fatty oils, 113
Omnibus Appropriations Act of 2009, 444
Omnibus Budget Reconciliation Act (OBRA), 127–128
On Death and Dying, 424
One in 100: Behind Bars in America 2008, 12
opioids, 230–231
    dependence on, 246–247
Orem, Dorothea E., 44
organizational factors, mental health promotion and, 4
OSAS (obstructive sleep apnea syndrome), 371–372
Outline for Cultural Formulation (CF), 79–80

P

pain
    assessment, 317–319
    end of life, 432
    management, barriers to, 319–320
Pain Assessment in Advanced Dementia Scale, 318
Pain Intensity Scale, 318
palliative care, 425–426
pancreatitis, alcohol abuse and, 239
paranoid delusions, 206
Parkinson's Disease, 104

Parnate (tranylcypromine), 130
partial hospitalization programs, 217–218
Passion Flower, 113
Pathways study, 283–284
Patient Health Questionnaires (PHQs), 151, 152–153f
patient history. *See* history, patient
Patient Self-Determination Act of 1990, 427, 430b
Peck, Robert, 19–20
peer groups, 20
Peplau, Hildegarde E., 44
periodic limb movement disorder (PLMD), 373
personality
    theories, 37–39
    types, 20
person–environment fit theory, 21
"personifications", 38
pets, therapeutic use of, 113
pharmacodynamic changes, age-related, 125–128, 191
pharmacokinetic changes, age-related, 123–125
    alcohol abuse and, 241
pharmacotherapy, 111. *See also* drug(s); *specific drug*
    for Alzheimer's disease, 297–298
    for anxiety, 191–195
    challenges and considerations, 122–128
    for depression, 161–164
    for gambling, 405
    for psychosis, 212–214
    recommendations, 191
    for sleep disorders, 382–388
phase-advanced sleep pattern, 369–370, 379
phase-delayed sleep pattern, 370, 378, 379–380
phenelzine (Nardil), 130
phenomenological theory, 22
PHQs (Patient Health Questionnaires), 151, 152–153f
physical abuse, 412t
physical dependency, 228
physical examination, 183
    elder mistreatment screening, 416
    end of life, 431
physical functioning, assessment of, 105
physical health, as risk factor, 13–14
physical neglect, 412t
Physician's Desk Reference for Herbal Medicines, 122, 380
piperazines, 164
Pittsburgh Sleep Quality Index, 391
Planned Lifetime Assistance Network, 218
plants, therapeutic use of, 113
PLMD (periodic limb movement disorder), 373
PLST. *See* progressively lowered stress threshold
political economy of aging theory, 21
polyneuropathy, 240
polypharmacy
    defined, 127
    psychosis and, 207–208
polysomnograms (PSGs), 375

portable automated multisensory intervention devices, 300
posttraumatic stress disorder, 55
poverty. *See also* income
    as risk factor, 13
    statistics, 17
Practice Parameters for the Medical Therapy of Obstructive Sleep Apnea, 372
Practice Parameters for the Use of Light Therapy in the Treatment of Sleep Disorders, 379, 380
President's New Freedom Commission on Mental Health, 3, 147
    goals, 148, 457–458
Preskorn, Sheldon, 126
Prevention of Suicide in the Primary Care Older Adults Collaborative Trial (PROSPECT), 168
preventive care, 214–215, 472
primary care
    cognitive–behavioral therapy in, 186–187
    mental health integration with, 468
primary groups, mental health promotion and, 4
Principles of Drug Abuse Treatment, 242
Principles of Preventive Psychiatry, 41
prisons, 12–13
Pristiq (desvenlafaxine), 132–133
problem-solving treatment (PST), 191
Profile of Older Americans, 15–16b
prognostication, 429
programmed theories of aging, 18
Programs of All-Inclusive Care for the Elderly, 447–448
Progress Report on Alzheimer's Disease 2001-2002, 24
progressively lowered stress threshold (PLST), 40
    for caregivers, 304
    dementia and, 294
Projects for Assistance in Transition from Homelessness, 451–452
Protection and Advocacy for Individuals with Mental Illness, 452
PSGs (polysomnograms), 375
PST (problem-solving treatment), 191
psychiatric stabilization, 41
psychiatric–mental health nurses, standards of practice for, 36t
psychiatry
    geriatric, resources for, 123
    interactive perspectives of, 61
psychoanalytic and personality theories, 37–39
psychodynamic nursing theory, 44
psychodynamic therapy, 112
Psychogeriatric Nursing Assessment Protocol, 277–278
psychological abuse, 412t
psychological assessment, end of life, 431
psychological dependency, 228
psychological neglect, 412t

psychological theories of aging, 19–20
psychosis. *See also specific disorder*
    assessment and screening, 209–212
    crisis intervention, 215
    diseases associated with, 203–205, 207
    epidemiology, 208–209
    ethical and legal issues, 218–220
    nursing role, 220
    onset, 206t, 209
    polypharmacy and, 207–208
    risk factors, 209
    substance abuse and, 207–208
    symptoms, 203, 204t
    treatment, 212–218
    types, 203, 209
psychosocial changes, anxiety and, 180–183
psychosocial development, theory of, 39
psychosocial therapies, 111–112, 113, 164, 215–218
psychotropic drugs. *See also specific drug*
    prevalence of use among older adults, 126–127
    role of, 111, 122
public policy (mental health), 4
    agenda for older adults, 457–460
    considerations, 459–460
    geropsychiatric nurses, role of, 441–443

Q

questions, phrasing of, 184
quetiapine (Seroquel), 136t, 137t, 139, 213

R

race, definition of, 76
racism, impact of, 103
ramelteon (Rozerem), 386–387
rapid eye movement (REM) sleep, 370
"rate of living" theory (metabolic theory of aging), 18
Rating Anxiety in Dementia Scale, 185
REACH II intervention, 356–357
recall, definition of, 23
receptor response, altered, 125
referral, 113
reimbursement for APN services, 454–457
relaxation training (RT), 189, 378
Remeron (mirtazapine), 132t, 133, 163
reminiscence therapy, 112, 296
Reminyl (galantamine), 297
renal function, 125
    alcohol abuse and, 241
research
    anxiety, 175–176
    geropsychiatric nursing, 469–470
    mental health promotion, 114–115
    substance abuse, 231
"resistance resources", 39–40

resources
    anxiety, 195
    caregiver, 354
    clinician, 359
    community, 195
    delirium, 269–270
    dementia, 306
    geriatric psychiatry, 123
    Internet, 123, 355b
    mental health promotion, 114
    schizophrenia, 219t
Resources for Enhancing Alzheimer's Caregiver Health
    (REACH), 356–357
respite programs, caregiver, 358–359
restless leg syndrome (RLS), 372
restraints, 266
review of systems, 239–242
Revised Algase Wandering Scale, 325
risperidone (Risperdal), 136t, 137t, 138, 213
rivastigmine (Exelon), 297
RLS (restless leg syndrome), 372
Rosen, Gerald, 55
Rozerem (ramelteon), 386–387
RT (relaxation training), 189, 378

S

S-adenosylmethionine (SAM-e), 113
SAMHSA (Substance Abuse and Mental
    Health Services Administration),
    227–228, 454
SCDNT (self-care deficit nursing theory), 44
schizophrenia
    case studies, 222
    characteristics, 206t
    epidemiology, 208–209
    in ethnic minorities, 86, 103
    homicide and, 215
    nursing role, 220
    psychosocial therapies, 215–218
    resources, 219t
    symptoms, 205
Schizophrenia Patient Outcomes Research Team
    recommendations, 215
SCN (suprachiasmatic nucleus), 368
*Scope and Standards for the Nurse Who Specializes
    in Developmental Disabilities and/or Mental
    Retardation*, 35
*Scope and Standards of Advanced Practice Registered
    Nursing*, 441
*Scope and Standards of Gerontological Nursing
    Practice*, 441
*Scope and Standards of Psychiatric-Mental Health
    Nursing Practice*, 35
second-generation antipsychotics, 135, 136t, 137t

sedative hypnotics, 230. *See also specific drug*
    considerations for prescribing in elderly, 384–385
    discontinuing, 387–388
selective serotonin reuptake inhibitors (SSRIs), 130–131.
    See also specific drug
    for anxiety, 193
    common, 131t
    for depression, 161–162
    side effects, 163
self-actualization, 19
self-care, caregiver, 354
self-care deficit nursing theory (SCDNT), 44
Selye, Hans, 39
senior centers, 453–454
"sense of coherence", 39–40
sensory impairment, agitation and, 315
Seroquel (quetiapine), 136t, 137t, 139, 213
serotonin syndrome, 130
serotonin-norepinephrine reuptake inhibitors
    (SNRIs), 133–134
SERPN (International Society for Education
    and Research in Psychiatric–Mental
    Health Nursing), 34
service contracts, 69–70t
service delivery models, nursing home, 466
Serzone (nafazodone), 131
SET (structural ecosystem), 356
sexual abuse, 412t
sexual disturbances, 328, 328–329
sexuality, 19
shame (stigmatization), 81, 149, 219–220
Short Geriatric Depression Scale, 325
Short Portable Mental Status Questionnaire, 106, 279
SHORT-CARE instrument, 11
Simple Descriptor Scale, 318
"simple pleasures" therapy, 299–300
simulated presence therapy, 300–301
sleep
    institutional schedules for, 388–389
    physiology of, 368–370
    quality of life and, 367
"sleep architecture", 370
sleep cycles, 370, 371b
sleep diaries, 374, 375, 391
sleep disorders
    assessment, 374–375
    in caregivers, 351–353
    case studies, 390–391
    common, 371–374
    in dementia, 326
    education and counseling for, 389
    follow-up, 389
    nursing interventions, 375–382
    pharmacotherapy, 382–388

referral and consultation, 389
REM disorder, 370
sleep hygiene, 376, 377b
Sleep in America poll, 367
sleep patterns, 369–370
sleep restriction, 376–377
sleepiness, fatigue versus, 368
smoking cessation, 231
    drugs to support, 247
    Medicare coverage, 451
SNRIs (serotonin-norepinephrine reuptake inhibitors),
    133–134
social constructionist theory, 22
social ecology model of health promotion, 3–4
"social equilibrium", 21
social exchange theory, 20
social isolation, 108–109, 339
social learning theory, 39
Social Managed Care Plans, 450–451
social roles, 21, 109
Social Services Block Grant (SSBG) program, 452
social skills training, 107–108, 216
social support, 107, 340–341
sociological theories of aging, 20–21
sociology, influence of, 42–44
somatization, 79
South Oaks Gambling Screen (SOGS), 396, 397, 398–401f
spirituality, 39
    end of life assessment, 431
spouses
    as caregivers, 339
    grief of, 344–345
SSI (Supplemental Security Income), 452
SSRIs. *See* selective serotonin reuptake inhibitors
St. John's wort, 112, 162
The State of Aging and Health in America, 6, 14
state programs, 444–445
stigmatization, social, 81, 149, 219–220
stimulants, 229–230
stimulus control, 376
    for gambling, 406
storytelling, 282, 283, 296
stress response, 39–40
stroke, alcohol abuse and, 241
structural ecosystem (SET), 356
Study to Understand Prognoses and Preferences for Out-
    comes and Risks of Treatments (SUPPORT), 426
subculture theory of aging, 20
substance abuse. *See also* alcohol abuse
    case studies, 244
    comorbid conditions, 229
    defined, 228
    federal initiatives, 454
    homeless persons and, 11

Medicare coverage, 451
nursing interventions, 247–249
prevalence among older adults, 227–228
psychosis and, 207–208
research, 231
screening, 231–235
treatment, 242–247
Substance Abuse and Mental Health Services
    Administration (SAMHSA), 227–228, 454
subsyndromal delirium, 258
subsyndromal depression, 440
"successful aging", 18–19, 22, 103–104
suicide
    assisted, 430b
    depression and, 148
    nursing protocol for, 160
    risk factors, 13, 157
    statistics for older adults, 121
Sullivan, Harry Stack, 37–38
"sundown syndrome", 316
superego, 37
supernatural beliefs, 78
Supplemental Security Income (SSI), 452
support groups
    caregiver, 304
    gambling, 405
supportive therapy, 189–190
suprachiasmatic nucleus (SCN), 368
Surgeon General's reports, 3–5, 13, 147, 149, 166, 177

T
tardive dyskinesia (TD), 135
TCAs (tricyclic antidepressants), 128–129, 163–164
technology
    geropsychiatric nurses and, 469
    to monitor wandering, 326, 327b
Tegretol (carbamazepine), 405
telomeres, 18
Ten-Point Clock Test, 279–281
"terminal drop", 23
therapeutic touch, 299
thiamine deficiency, 240–241
third party payers, 454–457
Three P Model of Insomnia, 375
Time Slips, 296
topiramate (Topamax), 405
transgenerational violence, 413
tranylcypromine (Parnate), 130
trazodone (Desyrel), 132t, 133–134
    for disruptive behaviors, 323
    side effects, 164
    for sleep disorders, 386
treatment. *See* interventions, nursing; *specific therapy*
tricyclic antidepressants (TCAs), 128–129, 163–164

trust
  ethnic elders, 81–82
  between nurse and patient, 212
Try This: Best Practices in Nursing Care of Older Adults, 470
Two Process Model of Sleep Regulation, 368, 369f

U
uncomplicated grief, 434
underutilization of care, 5, 340
unipolar major depression, 161t
United States Conference of Mayors, 11
United States Department of Housing and Urban
    Development, 11

V
valerian, 113
validation therapy, 112
valproate (Depakote), 405
vascular dementia (VaD), 275, 276
venlafaxine (Effexor), 131–132, 163
Verbal Descriptor Scale, 318
veterans, support for, 452–453
"victim blaming", 12
video respite, 300
violence, transgenerational, 413
visual acuity, 109
    in assessment, 282
vulnerable populations, 7–13

W
wandering, 324–326
    interventions for, 327b
wear and tear theory, 18

weight changes, 328
Wellbutrin. *See* bupropion
Wellstone-Domenici Parity Act, 442
Wernicke's encephalopathy,
    240–241
WHO. *See* World Health Organization
withdrawal
    alcohol, 238–239, 245
    antidepressant, 130–131, 134
women, 13
    alcohol abuse and, 236–237
    as caregivers, 335–336, 339,
        343, 354
    depression and, 6
    gay. *See* homosexuals
    homeless, 11
    insomnia and, 367, 373
    longevity and living arrangements, 102
    psychosis more prevalent in, 209
    social roles, 43–44
    statistics, 15b
World Health Organization (WHO)
    health definition, 147
    mental health policies, 4
    publications, 148–149
World Health Report of 2006, 149
World Population Ageing 2007, 14
worry, chronic versus adaptive, 184

Z
ziprasidone (Geodon), 136t, 137t, 139, 213
Zyprexa. *See* olanzapine